**Clinical Surgery in General:**
RCS Course Manual

*For Churchill Livingstone*

*Publisher:* Lucy Gardner
*Indexer:* John Sampson
*Production Controller:* Mark Sanderson
*Sales Promotion Executive:* Caroline Boyd

# Clinical Surgery in General:
## RCS Course Manual

Edited by

### R. M. Kirk MS FRCS
Honorary Consulting Surgeon, Royal Free Hospital, London

### Averil O. Mansfield ChM FRCS
Consultant Surgeon, St Mary's Hospital and Medical School, London, UK

### John Cochrane MS FRCS
Penrose May Tutor, Royal College of Surgeons of England, London;
Consultant Surgeon, Whittington Hospital, London, UK

CHURCHILL LIVINGSTONE
EDINBURGH LONDON MADRID MELBOURNE NEW YORK AND TOKYO 1993

CHURCHILL LIVINGSTONE
Medical Division of Longman Group UK Limited

Distributed in the United States of America by Churchill
Livingstone Inc., 650 Avenue of the Americas, New York,
N.Y. 10011, and by associated companies, branches and
representatives throughout the world.

First published 1993

ISBN 0-443-04574-7

**British Library Cataloguing in Publication Data**
A catalogue record for this book is available from the British
Library.

**Library of Congress Cataloging in Publication Data**
Clinical surgery in general/edited by R.M. Kirk, Averil O.
  Mansfield, John Cochrane.
      p. cm.
    Includes index.
    ISBN 0-443-04574-7
    1. Surgery. I. Kirk, R. M. (Raymond Maurice) II.
Mansfield, Averil O. III. Cochrane, John, FRCS.
    [DNLM: 1. Surgery, Operative. 2. Surgery. WO 100
C64125 1993]
RD31.C645 1993
617- -dc20
DNLM/DLC
for Library of Congress                          93-6785
                                                    CIP

The
publisher's
policy is to use
paper manufactured
from sustainable forests

Produced by Longman Singapore Publishers (Pte) Ltd.
Printed in Singapore

# Contents

# Contributors

**Wynne Aveling** MA MB BChir FRCA
Consultant Anaesthetist, University College and
Middlesex School of Medicine, London, UK

**John Bancewicz** BSc (Hons) ChM FRCS
Reader in Surgery, University of Manchester,
Manchester; Consultant Surgeon, Hope
Hospital, Salford, Manchester, UK

**Tom Bates** FRCS
Consultant Surgeon, The William Harvey
Hospital, Ashford, UK

**T. G. Brennan** MB BSc FRCS FRCSI
Consultant Surgeon, St James's University
Hospital, Leeds; Honorary Senior Lecturer,
University of Leeds, UK

**B. Brozović** MD PhD FRCPath
Consultant Haematologist, North London Blood
Transfusion Centre, London, UK

**Laura J. Buist** MD FRCS
Surgical Registrar, Liver Unit, Queen Elizabeth
Hospital, Birmingham, UK

**Clive A. C. Charlton** MB BS FRCS
Member of the Court of Examiners of the Royal
College of Surgeons; Consultant Urologist, Royal
United Hospital, Bath, UK

**John Cochrane** MS FRCS
Penrose May Tutor, Royal College of Surgeons
of England, London; Consultant Surgeon,
Whittington Hospital, London, UK

**Timothy Cooke** MB ChB
St Mungo Professor of Surgery, University of
Glasgow, Glasgow; Honorary Consultant
Surgeon, Glasgow Royal Infirmary, Glasgow,
UK

**Carmel A. E. Coulter** FRCP FRCR
Consultant in Clinical Oncology, St Mary's and
the Middlesex Hospital, London, UK

**Richard A. Cowie** MB ChB FRCSE (SN)
Consultant Neurosurgeon, Hope Hospital,
Salford and Royal Manchester Children's
Hospital, Manchester, UK

**David L. Crosby** MB FRCS
Consultant Surgeon, University Hospital of
Wales, Cardiff, Wales, UK

**M. K. H. Crumplin** MB FRCS
Consultant Surgeon, Maelor Hospital, Wrexham,
Wales, UK

**Alfred Cuschieri** MD ChM FRCSEd FRCS (Eng)
Professor and Head of Department of Surgery,
Ninewells Hospital and Medical School,
University of Dundee, Dundee, Scotland, UK

**D. M. Davies** FRCS
Consultant Plastic Surgeon, Charing Cross
Hospital, London, UK

**Len Doyal** BA MSc
Senior Lecturer in Medical Ethics, St
Bartholomew's and The London Hospital
Medical Colleges, London, UK

**Peter A. Driscoll** BSc FRCS (Ed)
Senior Lecturer in Accident and Emergency
Medicine, University Department of Accident
and Emergency Medicine, Hope Hospital,
Salford, Manchester, UK

**Hugh Dudley** CBE ChM FRCS (E) FRACS FRCS
Emeritus Professor, University of London, UK

**Brian W. Ellis** MB FRCS
Consultant Surgeon, Ashford Hospital, Ashford,

Middlesex; Chairman Hounslow and
Spellthorne H. A., District Audit Advisory
Committee, UK

**A. M. Emmerson** MB FRCPath FRCP (G)
Professor and Head of Microbiology, University
Hospital, Queen's Medical Centre, Nottingham,
UK

**Jane Fothergill** MB ChB MRCP FRCS (Ed)
Consultant in Accident and Emergency
Medicine, St Mary's Hospital, London, UK

**Charles S. B. Galasko** MSc ChM FRCS (Eng)
FRCS (Ed)
Professor of Orthopaedic Surgery, University of
Manchester; Clinical Director, Department of
Orthopaedic Surgery, Salford Hospital, Salford,
Manchester, UK

**J. B. Garland** MD FRCS (Eng) FRCS (Ed)
Consultant Urologist, Salford Royal Hospital,
North Manchester General Hospital and Royal
Manchester Children's Hospital, Manchester, UK

**Nicholas J. Goddard** MB FRCS DipChirMain (Paris)
Consultant Orthopaedic Surgeon, Royal Free
Hospital, London, UK

**P. J. Guillou** BSc MD FRCS
Professor of Surgery, St James's University
Hospital, Leeds; Formerly Professor of Surgery,
Imperial College of Science, Technology and
Medicine; Director, Academic Surgical Unit, St
Mary's Hospital, London, UK

**I. R. Haywood** FRCS
Brigadier L/RAMC; Consultant Surgeon,
Defence Medical Services; Formerly Joint
Professor of Military Surgery, RCS England and
RAM College, Queen Elizabeth Military
Hospital, Woolwich, UK

**Nigel D. Heaton** FRCS
Senior Registrar in Surgery, King's College
Hospital, Denmark Hill, London, UK

**Edward R. Howard** MS FRCS
Senior Lecturer (Hon) and Consultant Surgeon,
Kings College Hospital, London, UK

**R. A. Huddart** BA MB BS MRCP
Registrar, Department of Radiotherapy, Royal
Marsden Hospital, Sutton, Surrey, UK

**Miles Irving** MD ChM FRCS
Professor of Surgery, Manchester University,
Manchester; Honorary Consultant Surgeon,
Hope Hospital, Salford, Manchester, UK

**Jennifer Jones** BSc FRCP FFARCS
Consultant Anaesthetist in Charge of Intensive
Care Unit, St Mary's Hospital, London, UK

**R. A. C. Jones** MB FRCS
Consultant Neurosurgeon, Hope Hospital and
Royal Manchester Children's Hospital, Salford,
Manchester, UK

**R. M. Jones** MD FRCA
Professor and Head of Academic Department of
Anaesthetics, Imperial College and St Mary's
Hospital Medical School, London

**Martin Jourdan** BSc PhD MS FRCS
Consultant Surgeon and Reader in Surgery,
Guy's Hospital, London, UK

**Leela Kapila** FRCS
Consultant Paediatric Surgeon, University
Hospital, Nottingham, UK

**Greg Keogh** FRACS
Senior Registrar, Royal Infirmary, Glasgow, UK

**R. M. Kirk** MS FRCS
Honorary Consulting Surgeon, Royal Free
Hospital, London; Formerly Member of Council,
Royal College of Surgeons, England; Examiner
for FRCS Glasgow; Formerly Member of Court
of Examiners, Royal College of Surgeons,
England; Examiner for Primary FRCS England

**Roop Kishen** MBBS DA MD FFARCS
Consultant in Intensive Care Medicine and
Anaesthesia, Hope Hospital, Salford,
Manchester; Honorary Lecturer in Anaesthesia,
University of Manchester, Manchester, UK

**Anna C. Kurowska** MB BS BSc BA MRCP
Consultant in Palliative Medicine, Whittington
Hospital, London; Deputy Medical Director,
Edenhall Marie Curie Centre, London, UK

**David John Leaper** MD ChM FRCS FRCS (Ed)
Consultant and Senior Lecturer, University
Department of Surgery, Southmead Hospital,
Bristol, UK

**Roderick A. Little** PhD MRCPath
Professor of Surgical Science, Head of MRC
Trauma Group; Director, North Western Injury
Research Centre, University of Manchester,
Manchester, UK

**Richard Lloyd** FDSRCS FRCS
Consultant Maxillofacial Surgeon, Hope
Hospital, University of Manchester Medical
School, Manchester, UK

**Paul McMaster** MA MD ChM FRCS FICS
Consultant Surgeon, Liver Unit, Queen
Elizabeth Hospital, Birmingham, UK

**Kevin Mackway-Jones** MA MRCP FRCS
Senior Registrar in Accident and Emergency
Medicine, University Department of Accident
and Emergency Medicine, University of
Manchester, Hope Hospital, Salford,
Manchester, UK

**Averil O. Mansfield** ChM FRCS
Consultant Surgeon, St Mary's Hospital and
Medical School, London, UK

**Roger Marcuson** MChir FRCS FRCS (Ed)
Consultant Vascular Surgeon, Hope Hospital,
Salford, Manchester, UK

**David Marsh** MD FRCS
Senior Lecturer and Honorary Consultant in
Orthopaedic Surgery, Clinical Sciences Building,
Hope Hospital, Salford, Manchester, UK

**R. S. Maurice-Williams** FRCS FRCP
Consultant Neurosurgeon, The Royal Free
Hospital, London, UK

**John F. Moorhead** MB FRCP
Consultant, Nephrology and Transplantation,
The Royal Free Hospital, London, UK

**Muntzer Mughal** FRCS ChM
Consultant Surgeon, The Royal Preston Hospital
and Chorley District Hospital, UK

**Jonathan Noble** MB ChM FRCSE FRCS
Consultant Orthopaedic Surgeon and Honorary
Lecturer in Orthopaedic Surgery, University of
Manchester Medical School, Hope Hospital,
Salford, Manchester, UK

**Susan M. O'Reilly** MB BCh MRCP (I)
Lecturer and Honorary Senior Registrar, Cancer
Research Campaign Laboratories, Department of
Medical Oncology, Charing Cross Hospital,
London, UK

**Jason Payne-James** MB FRCS (Ed & Eng)
Forensic Medical Examiner, London; Honorary
Senior Research Fellow, Department of
Gastroenterology and Nutrition, Central
Middlesex Hospital, London

**A. L. G. Peel** MA MChir FRCS
Consultant Surgeon, Department of Surgery,
North Tees Hospital, Stockton-on-Tees, UK

**Michael Pietroni** MB BS FRCS
Consultant Surgeon, Whipps Cross Hospital,
London, Regional Adviser in Surgery; Associate
Dean, British Postgraduate Medical Federation,
London, UK

**Michael W. Platt** MB BS FRCAnaes
Senior Lecturer, St Mary's Hospital Medical
School (Imperial College of Science, Technology
and Medicine in the University of London);
Honorary Consultant Anaesthetist, St Mary's
Hospital, London, UK

**Mohamed Y. A. Rady** MB BChir MA (Cantab) MD
(Cantab) MRCP (UK) FRCS (Ed) FRCS (Eng)
Lecturer in Accident and Emergency Medicine,
University of Manchester, UK; Currently,
Resuscitation Research Fellow, Henry Ford
Hospital, Detroit, USA

**Raymond Ross** MB ChB FRCSEd FRACS
Consultant Orthopaedic Surgeon, Hope
Hospital, Salford, Manchester; Honorary
Assistant Lecturer, University of Manchester,
Manchester, UK

**Gordon J. S. Rustin** MD MSc FRCP
Senior Lecturer in Medical Oncology, Charing
Cross Hospital, London; Consultant, Mount
Vernon Hospital, Northwood, Middlesex, UK

**Michael Schachter** BSc MB MRCP
British Heart Foundation Senior Research
Fellow, Department of Clinical Pharmacology, St
Mary's Hospital Medical School, London, UK

**J. E. Scoble** MB MRCP
Consultant Physician, Kings College Hospital,
London, UK

**William S. Shand** MD FRCS FRCSEd
Consultant Surgeon, St Bartholomew's and
Homerton Hospitals, London; Honorary
Consultant General Surgeon, St Mark's
Hospital for Diseases of the Rectum and Colon,
London, UK

**Jean Simpson** BSc MSc
Audit Co-ordinator, Houslow and Spelthorne
Health Authority, Middlesex, UK

**J. A. R. Smith** PhD FRCS (Eng) FRCS (Ed)
Consultant General Surgeon, Northern General
Hospital NHS Trust, Sheffield; Honorary
Lecturer in Surgery, University of Sheffield,
Sheffield, UK

**J. J. T. Tate** MS FRCS
Senior Registrar in General Surgery, Royal Free
Hospital, London, UK

**Adrian Tookman** MRCP
Consultant in Palliative Medicine, Royal Free
Hospital, London; Medical Director, Edenhall
Marie Curie Centre, London, UK

**Robin Touquet** RD FRCS DCH
Consultant in Accident and Emergency
Medicine, St Mary's Hospital and St Charles'
Hospital, London, UK

**Tom Treasure** MD MS FRCS
Consultant Thoracic and Cardiac Surgeon, St
George's Hospital, London, UK

**Christopher Wastell** MS FRCS
Professor of Surgery, Chelsea and Westminster
Hospital, London, UK

**Stewart Watson** FRCS MRCP
Consultant in Plastic and Hand Surgery, Plastic
Surgery and Burns Unit, Withington Hospital,
Manchester, UK

**Malcolm H. Wheeler** MD FRCS
Consultant Surgeon, University of Wales and
Royal Infirmary, Cardiff, Wales, UK

**David J. Whitby** MB BS FRCS
Senior Lecturer, Department of Plastic and
Reconstructive Surgery, Honorary Clinical
Research Fellow, Department of Cell and
Structural Biology, University of Manchester,
Manchester, UK

# Preface

Radical changes have taken place in the FRCS examination. It is taken early in surgical training and in the past was the sole formal test of surgical knowledge. The introduction of Intercollegiate Specialist Assessment Board examinations of surgeons towards the end of training in their selected specialty, has allowed the curriculum for the FRCS examination to be re-assessed. In the past the accent was on knowledge of general surgery but it is now on surgery in general.

As a result, candidates are expected to be able to utilize their acquired knowledge of basic science to solve clinical problems. There is less emphasis on particular diseases and individual operations, more weight is placed on general principles. The College Course for the Clinical Surgery in General (CSiG) part of the FRCS has, pari-passu, undergone a radical change. This text reflects the changes that have taken place and many of the contributors are teachers on the Course, or examiners.

There are many excellent textbooks of clinical surgery and we have not tried to compete with them. However, surgeons in training are expected to acquire and practise clinical skills, so we advise them to read widely, in textbooks, reviews and original articles, in addition to acquiring experience while looking after patients.

1993

R.M.K.
A.O.M.
J.C.

# Acknowledgements

The royalties are intended to go to the Royal College of Surgeons of England for the Audiovisual Unit. We are grateful to our many contributors for foregoing financial rewards. In particular, Professor Miles Irving undertook to recruit colleagues who have contributed the section on Trauma, and Professor Ron Jones has not only contributed chapters but has drawn in colleagues and cooperated in covering a range of topics.

Mrs Angela Christie has drawn, with great skill, many of the illustrations.

Miss Oonagh Collins, Step Course Administration at the Royal College of Surgeons, has been a valuable link between the Editors and Publisher.

We have had enthusiastic support and co-operation from the staff of Churchill Livingstone particularly Peter Richardson, Lucy Gardner, Miranda Bromage and Janice Urquhart. Thanks also goes to Graham Wild and John Sampson.

# Introduction

*R. M. Kirk   A. O. Mansfield   J. Cochrane*

The purpose of this manual is to help you to apply the knowledge of the basic sciences to clinical practice. Of course, even if you are able to do this you will still not have a complete grasp of surgery. The reason is that much practice is still based not on science but on empiricism — that is, as a result of the accumulated experience of your predecessors who have observed the effects of their actions, and compared different methods. You will, during your own practice, add to and modify the pool of knowledge. The methods of determining the effectiveness of, for example, various treatments, have been refined by the careful application of statistical methods and the neutralization of bias.

It is not our intention to produce a definitive textbook of surgery. We wish to introduce you to some of the areas of knowledge with which you must be familiar, in whatever branch of surgery you intend to practice. At the end of most chapters, and at the end of the book, are lists of references for further reading.

Expand your knowledge from clinical textbooks which offer generally accepted knowledge and practices, but remember that they cannot be completely up to date because of delays in preparing, publishing and distributing them. Critically read surgical journals. Original articles offer you not only more up-to-date knowledge but also the opportunity to judge if the authors have planned and carried out investigations logically, measured the results accurately, and drawn valid conclusions from them. Authoritative reviews provide a digest of current thinking but do not rely too heavily upon them, because it is valuable for you to read the literature and make up your own mind, rather than act on received wisdom.

The best time to read up a subject is when you are about to see, or have just seen, a relevant clinical problem. Your knowledge of the patient provides a 'peg' on which to hang the new information you acquire, so that you avoid the need to learn a list of facts. Notes read in a clinical vacuum, and taken at lectures, that you may never read again, do not remain in your memory. Listen carefully to your seniors, ask questions when a suitable opportunity occurs, and watch the development of events, noting the outcome of the action taken. At frequent intervals review and organize your knowledge. It is valueless unless it is accessible and usable. The prospect of examinations serves a valuable purpose quite apart from the assessment by the examiners: it drives you to identify gaps in your knowledge, complete it, and organize it.

In addition to acquiring knowledge on which you can draw, you must develop attitudes which enable you to use it effectively. You are not training to become a mere technical wizard, who, placed before a patient, can carry out an operation with panache. Of course you wish to become a surgeon for personal satisfaction, enjoyment of the skilful use of techniques and so on. However, the successful practice of surgery is succinctly expressed in the American aphorism, 'Choose well, cut well, get well'. It must be the correct operation, on the correct patient, who is brought to surgery in the best possible condition and will be carefully monitored thereafter. 'Choose well' is, therefore, as important as 'Cut well'.

Our satisfaction as surgeons also depends upon our confidence that we are serving our patients sympathetically as well as effectively. We are immensely privileged that we are trusted by people who often have no previous knowledge of us, to make good decisions on their behalf and carry out the necessary actions with skill and care. We require a wide range of qualities to fulfil all these functions. There have been many attempts to list the unique characteristics that together make a good surgeon. Apart from technical competence, we need stamina, good inter-personal and communications skills, 'common sense', decisiveness, ability to withstand stress, leadership, the humility to admit error, self-motivation and, perhaps above all, integrity. This last, elusive quality is important. None of us has all the required attributes in full measure: we need to recognize the deficiencies and determine to compensate for them to the best of our ability.

# 1. Clinical history and examination

*R. M. Kirk*

## Should you read this chapter?

Maybe you think you are already too experienced to need instruction. If you think that, then you are definitely lacking self-knowledge. Of all the skills you require in surgery and in medicine generally, taking a history, examining the patient and interpreting your findings are paramount. They form the base from which you work. If you take the wrong diagnostic path all the rest of your activities are misdirected.

A high proportion of examination candidates cannot carry out the basic procedures of diagnosis. Some have never been taught properly, some have picked up bad habits, some are simply not thorough and logical in their approach. Examiners are unforgiving of failure in the clinical assessments, however knowledgeable the candidates may be about rare diseases and the latest surgical procedures.

Unfortunately many candidates are unsure of what is expected of them, both when taking a history and examining the patient. They are also unsure about the best way of presenting their findings and conclusions.

The next time you sit before a new patient, try to analyse the sequence of your questions, your motivation in asking them in that manner, and your interpretation of the answers. Similarly, when you have completed the physical examination, ask yourself if there is anything you missed out and why you forgot it.

The mechanism of diagnosis is complex. You do not carry a ranked list of causes for each presenting feature in your head. From your accumulated experience, reading, and listening to others, you develop associations in your mind. The over-

weight multiparous lady with postprandial upper abdominal symptoms forms a pattern which triggers the possibility of gallstones — or reflux oesophagitis. In a similar fashion, the discovery of a particular physical sign may trigger the need to look elsewhere. For example, when you discover an enlarged lymph node in the neck, you should automatically remember to examine the drainage area of the gland — and the remainder of the reticuloendothelial system.

## History

There are two parts to taking the history — determining the cause of the complaint that has brought the patient to you, and determining the general state and feelings of the patient. Do not differentiate between taking a history from a surgical patient and taking one from a medical patient. When making decisions about management it is important to have as much relevant information as possible. If you embark on surgical treatment after concentrating on a localized lesion you will be unprepared if complications develop.

### Prime complaint

Do not passively listen and record the patient's words. The danger of this is that it leaves the direction of the discussion to the patient: it is vital that you control and lead the interview. This entails asking a question, letting the patient answer it, then cutting in at the correct moment to ask for clarification, ask a supplementary question, or change tack. Too early an interruption causes resentment but if the opportunity is

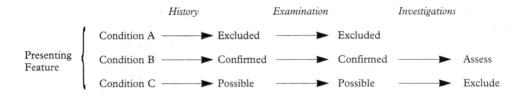

**Fig. 1.1**  The presenting feature may suggest a number of diagnoses. Each step is intended to exclude or confirm each diagnosis. You hope to end with only one diagnosis, with the others confidently excluded.

missed the patient is likely to go off at a tangent and resist being brought back to your line of thought.

The object of questions about the presenting symptom is to determine the anatomical site of the lesion causing it. Does function of the suspect system affect the symptom, does the symptom affect the function of the system? The same line of questioning must be applied to all suspect systems. The intention is that one system may be confidently implicated and the others are exonerated (Fig. 1.1).

Supplementary questions are intended to reveal a pattern – a group of features that form a syndrome. As a likely diagnosis enters your mind you will ask about other features that are usually associated with it. Pattern recognition is an important aid to diagnosis. Indeed, experienced clinicians do not take a history in isolation but observe the person who is giving it and often make a provisional diagnosis within a few seconds (Fig. 1.2). Treat such a diagnosis merely as a working hypothesis, useful for the present, to be tested and abandoned at once if it is refuted.

| Young child | Appendicitis |
| Young woman | Gynaecological |
| Young man | Hernia, appendicitis |
| Middle-aged woman | Gynaecological, diverticulosis coli |
| Middle-aged man | Diverticulosis coli |
| Elderly woman | Gynaecological, cancer colon |
| Elderly man | Cancer colon |

**Fig. 1.2**  The presenting patient prejudices the clinician. If you are seeing a patient with lower abdominal pain, the diagnoses that you first consider are influenced by the type of patient.

As the origin of the presenting symptom is localized, its severity, duration, mode of onset and general effects must be determined.

### General assessment

Now carefully assess each body system by means of questions about its function now and in the past. There are sets of fairly standard questions that may reveal malfunctions. If the patient answers 'Yes' to the question 'Are you short of breath when climbing stairs?' the possibilities of cardiorespiratory disease and anaemia immediately spring to mind.

Ask what the patient thinks about the cause of the symptoms. The answers provide guidance in deciding how to explain the problem and give reassurance.

## Examination

### Where is the local lesion?

If there is a localized lesion, first determine exactly where it is. This entails reviewing the structures in the area and carrying out tests to find out whether they lie over or under the lesion and whether it is attached to them. Examples are upward movement of a structure attached to the trachea when the patient swallows, and intra-abdominal tenderness to palpation that is allayed when the patient is asked to perform a manoeuvre that tenses the overlying abdominal muscles. If you know where the lesion is and know the structures you can usually deduce the likely diagnosis in this patient. Do not distress the patient by clumsy, painful palpation; except in some emergencies it is never necessary and is counter-productive because the patient guards against your examination, preventing you from gaining vital information.

*What are the characteristics of a lump?*

You should already know the site. Now determine the size, shape, surface, consistency and special characteristics. For example, is it tender, hot, pulsatile, reducible, bilateral, fluctuant, coloured, translucent? Is there a cough impulse, overlying inflammation, oedema or vascularity? What is the effect of movement or function of the part?

Remarkably, we all miss diagnoses not because they are obscure but because we do not assiduously follow the routines which we learned at the beginning of clinical training.

*General examination*

Develop the skill to carry out rapidly a complete examination of the patient. In this way you familiarize yourself with the range of normality and can rapidly and confidently detect abnormalities.

Thoughtless, repeated observation, palpation and other examinations are a waste of time and may be distressing for the patient. Try to examine everything once, concentrating on the findings. A common fault is to 'go through the motions' of, for example, palpating lymph nodes to impress the patient, or an examiner, rather than to obtain crucial information.

However, a single examination may be misleading. Physical signs often change rapidly in acute conditions, so when in doubt repeat the examination after an interval.

## Diagnosis

You now hope to have a reasonably confident diagnosis, have eliminated other causes for the presenting features, and have made an assessment of the physical and mental state of the patient.

Suitable investigations can now be ordered, to corroborate the working diagnosis, to exclude others more certainly, and to assess the severity or anatomical site of an identified condition.

A firm diagnosis may not always be possible but sufficient information may be gained to plan a course of action. In a patient with an 'acute' abdomen the information often allows you to make a clinical decision to perform exploratory laparotomy, further investigation, medical treatment, to ask a specialist in another field, or to observe the patient for a limited period and reassess the clinical features.

If you are still in doubt after taking a history and examining the patient, do not necessarily rush to order investigations in the hope that 'something will turn up'. Of course, intelligently selected investigations may be invaluable in confusing cases. All too often they are instruments for vacillation. It is often more profitable and less time consuming to go back to the beginning and retake the history, repeat the examination, or ask a colleague to do so with an open mind.

On many occasions the given history may differ markedly from the first, perhaps because you have misinterpreted what the patient has said, or allowed the patient to take charge and been led astray.

Some questions and signs have a high discriminatory value, others do not. A clinical feature or test may give a falsely positive prediction of the dignosis. Two or three points that suggest one diagnosis may be of less value than one that has a high discriminatory capacity. For example, the diagnosis of acute, uncomplicated appendicitis is often mistakenly made because the pain is in the right iliac fossa, the patient has gastrointestinal symptoms and is tender in the iliac fossa. However, if there is also tenderness in the left iliac fossa, this must either be complicated, i.e. perforated appendicitis, or another diagnosis must be considered.

When in doubt between the likely, i.e. the most common, diagnosis and a less frequent but important diagnosis, do not lightly pass over the important one. It is dangerous to miss a rarer but serious condition.

## Record

All the effort you have put into elucidating the problem may be lost if you do not make a careful record that can be read and understood by others

— and by yourself. Although various devices for recording are available, they sometimes fail. Even if you have dictated into a recording machine, write the details as well.

Having recorded the findings in the history and the examination, state your conclusions, your policy and what emerged from your discussion with the patient. If you intend to arrange investigations, state what you have in mind. If you arrange treatment, state what monitoring procedures should be carried out.

## Think

Have you missed anything? Have you rushed to the wrong conclusion? Is there a vital question that you could ask, or a physical sign to test your provisional diagnosis?

Remember your obligations to the patient, not just to make a correct diagnosis but also to give reassurance that you have excluded a serious alternative condition. For example, the confident discovery that minimal haemorrhoids, which may not even warrant any treatment, are the cause of rectal bleeding does not absolve you from carrying out sigmoidoscopy and any other tests to exclude large bowel cancer.

## Discuss

In the past, informing the patient, discussing and explaining possible actions and their consequences were often casually performed. This is no longer tolerable. Listen to the patient and if necessary change your policy of management. Do not forget to inform relatives in appropriate circumstances.

## Emergency

You cannot obsessively stick to a routine in some situations. A patient may have airway obstruction, calamitous bleeding, be in excruciating pain, be mentally disarranged, violent or unconscious. In each case you must quickly and accurately determine the cause of the emergency state, correct it and deal with lesser conditions as the opportunities occur. It is particularly important to record everything, otherwise some vital consideration may be missed when routines are broken. When the emergency condition is under control, meticulously carry out a thorough assessment.

When a number of emergencies present at the same time you must apply triage (from the French, *trier* = to pick out). In principle this recognizes that loss of life is more important than loss of a limb.

# 2. Investigations

*M. C. Pietroni*

There are two elements to the investigation of a surgical problem. The first is the formulation of the correct question that requires an answer and the second is the selection of the most appropriate test to answer the question posed. Investigations are commonly employed:

1. to establish a diagnosis
2. to choose between alternative plans of action
3. to establish preoperative fitness for surgery
4. for medicolegal reasons.

By the time a history has been taken and the patient has been examined a hypothesis is already emerging.

What do you need to know? Define it. Do not request all the 'thyroid function tests' you know just because the patient has a goitre.

A man of 52 with a lump in the groin that appears on coughing and disappears on lying down probably has a hernia. Do not embark on a series of investigations to exclude, for example, a lymphoma of the nodes in the groin. If the man has a missing testicle, however, or symptoms of prostatic obstruction, or is hypertensive then investigate him to answer the questions:

1. Where is the missing testicle?
2. Does he need an operation on his prostate?
3. Is he fit for day-case surgery?

Now choose the most appropriate investigation. Select the most convenient, safest and cheapest method that is likely to give a firm answer. Do not embark on a series of sequential investigations which waste time and money. Choose the right one first.

In order to be able to do this you need to have a clear idea of what investigations can do for you.

Never hesitate to ask advice from the specialists. Seek the radiologist's, the haematologist's and the microbiologist's help if you wish to find the swiftest way to answer your question.

## HAEMATOLOGY

Most laboratories now use analysers that give all the common haematological indices when only a haemoglobin (Hb) estimation is required. Be careful to interpret these values in the light of the patient's general condition. For example, dehydrated patients have a high Hb and packed cell volume (PCV) because of haemoconcentration. Patients who are heavy smokers or who have chronic obstructive airways disease also have raised Hb levels. Smoking and carbon monoxide in patients with vascular disease also raise the Hb. These high levels in vascular patients lead to increased blood viscosity which in turn contributes to symptoms. Remember that patients with rheumatoid arthritis often have a low Hb. Allow for this if such a patient has a haematemesis.

The Hb level by itself is insufficient to establish the transfusion requirements in acute blood loss. In the first few hours after blood loss it cannot answer the question 'How much blood has been lost?' The body's physiological responses to shock produce a reduction in the capacity of the circulation. It is only after many hours that haemodilution produces a representative cellular/plasma ratio, when the PCV is a better guide.

The level of the white blood count (WBC) is a valuable indicator but not an accurate diagnostic tool. When raised it gives useful corroborative evidence of infection. When normal it does not exclude infection. By itself it cannot answer the question 'Has this patient got appendicitis?'

In the presence of overwhelming sepsis a low or normal level indicates an inability of the patient's immune system to react to infection. Levels of 15–18 000 WBC cm$^{-3}$ generally indicate intermediate degrees of infection, while levels over 20 000 WBC cm$^{-3}$ suggest life-threatening sepsis. Trends are more useful than absolute levels. A falling white count in a clinically improving patient suggests response to treatment.

It is possible to label granulocytes with radioactive phosphorus. The cells aggregate in septic foci and can be localized using a gamma camera if the site of infection cannot be detected clinically computed tomography (CT) scanning has generally superseded this test.

Always seek the haematologist's help when analysing bleeding disorders and coagulopathies. In the presence of massive blood loss and whenever six or more units of blood have been transfused, check the prothrombin time (PT), kaolin cephalin clotting time (KCCT) and platelet counts to identify any prolonged bleeding tendency. The result may indicate the need to infuse fresh frozen plasma or platelets. In cases of suspected disseminated intravascular coagulopathy (DIC) the haematologist's help is essential. Measure fibrinogen degradation products and fibrinogen titres and measure the thrombin time. These results will assist in assessing the need for platelets, cryoprecipitate and fresh frozen plasma.

Patients with deep venous thrombosis (DVT) or pulmonary embolism (PE) require anticoagulation. Use the activated partial thromboplastin time (APTT), for heparin therapy and the PT for patients on warfarin. The laboratory results will usually be expressed as international normalized ratios (INR), to aid therapeutic adjustments. Measure heparin levels in the circulating blood or factor 10 levels in cases of massive thrombosis, where heparin consumption can be unpredictable. Once the patient has been stabilized the frequency of testing can be gradually reduced to once weekly and eventually to once monthly.

Perform a sickle cell test on all patients from the Middle East, the Indian subcontinent and on those of African and Mediterranean extraction. Hypoxia and dehydration are especially danger-

ous in these patients as a sickle cell crisis may be so induced.

When ordering blood for cross-matching do not overestimate the need. Order blood grouping with saving of the serum for operations of medium severity such as cholecystectomy and thyroidectomy. The transfusion of blood postoperatively is rarely required here.

Discuss cases of suspected lymphoma with the haematologist. It may be that if the peripheral blood picture shows involvement (as in chronic lymphatic leukaemia) there will be no need for lymph node biopsy. This will avoid a general anaesthetic and a bone marrow sample can be taken under local anaesthetic instead. If you do need a lymph node biopsy (see below) then do not forget that the haematologist can help as well as the histopathologist. Immunocytochemistry can give valuable prognostic information and can distinguish between T-cell and B-cell lymphomas. Formalin fixation destroys this information. Collect the dry lymph node in liquid nitrogen or if this is not available cut the node sharply in half and do an imprint on a slide, which is then airdried.

## HISTOPATHOLOGY

A biopsy is a sample of tissue. Ensure that it is a representative sample. The pathologist can comment only on the tissue presented by the surgeon. The more information you give the more useful and detailed is the pathologist's report. Cytology refers to the examination of cells and is inherently not as reliable as histology, which looks at architectural detail too.

Cytological examination of the spun-down deposit of fluids can often diagnose cancer. This is the simplest way to diagnose malignancy in pleural effusions and in ascites. Urine cytology is also useful, especially as a monitoring test in patients with known urothelial tumours. Avoid painful, expensive procedures when simple ones will do. Sputum cytology when positive may avoid the need for bronchoscopy and biopsy.

Fine-needle aspiration (FNA) cytology is a valuable diagnostic tool in lesions of the breast and thyroid. Radiologically guided aspirates can also be obtained from organs within the abdominal cavity.

Take FNA of palpable breast lesions when you wish to establish the diagnosis preoperatively or when you think you can avoid surgery. The finding of malignant cells establishes the diagnosis but a negative result does not exclude malignancy. Positive and negative results are operator dependent so interpret them with care. FNA is particularly useful with impalpable breast lesions. These are usually shown on mammography as clusters of microcalcification. Ensure your FNA sample is taken with radiological guidance. Speak to your histopathologist about his attitude to a positive FNA result. If you wish to proceed to definitive breast surgery he may prefer histological proof of cancer first. Centres with great expertise will accept a cytological result alone.

The cytologist can say that a thyroid lesion is a cancer but the distinction between a follicular adenoma and a follicular carcinoma is not easily made by this method. Invasion of the capsule is the key factor and fine-needle aspirates and even needle biopsies do not supply this tissue.

The best biopsy is the whole lesion. You only need a biopsy if you have different management options in mind. Most skin lesions are best removed in toto. If you must sample the lesion take a representative portion. In the rectum and colon orientate your specimen on a piece of filter paper before immersing it in formalin. This preserves the normal architectural relationships of the layers. Avoid taking biopsies of polyps. Take the whole lesion. If this is not possible ensure you sample the base, not the tip of the lesion. You need to know about invasion. At gastroscopy do not biopsy the centre of the ulcer; this just yields necrotic tissue. Take several samples at the periphery. At oesophagoscopy you may want to establish a diagnosis of oesophagitis but you also need to know the nature of the mucosa proximally. Take labelled biopsies at intervals of 2 cm.

Try not to take biopsies of lymph nodes. Wherever possible take at least one whole node and do not crush or alter its anatomy. When this is not possible take a wedge, preserving if possible the capsule. The pathologist is not just giving a report on cellular detail but also on altered anatomy. Remember to send a sample to the microbiologist if you suspect tuberculosis. Immunocytochemistry will be required with lymphomas. Either send an unfixed sample in liquid nitrogen or carry out an imprint as mentioned before.

The smaller the sample the greater is the degree of expertise required of the pathologist. This can be a problem with deep-seated organs (abdominal masses, liver and pancreas) where only a needle biopsy is available. Sample carefully. A false negative may be due to a sampling error.

Remember that the pathologist is able not only to make the diagnosis but also to give you useful information about prognosis. You want to know about clearance margins, depth of invasion, cellular differentiation, numbers of nodes and presence or absence of metastases. Make it easy for him by giving as much information as possible. Label and orientate your specimen and identify specific portions you want examined when sending very large specimens.

## MICROBIOLOGY

A pus swab contains a representative sample of organisms from an infected source only briefly. Some organisms die because they are anaerobic (e.g. *Streptococcus faecalis*) because they are delicate (e.g. *Neisseria*), or because the other organisms in the sample proliferate faster and overwhelm them. Lose no time therefore between taking the swab and transferring it to an appropriate medium for culture. If pus is available then collect a quantity and send that, rather than a swab, to the microbiologist. Pus swabs (in Stewart's transport medium) should be stored at 4°C when taken at night time. Do ensure they are sent to the laboratory the next day.

Taking swabs for culture without careful thought may cause you to miss the diagnosis. Make sure you ask the correct question in order to select the best method of answering it. For example, the detection of amoebic dysentery is not accomplished by taking a swab for culture but by examining a fresh specimen immediately under the microscope. If you can see blood-stained mucus through the sigmoidoscope then take a sample of that rather than sending a stool specimen. When investigating diarrhoea send three fresh stool specimens taken on three separate days.

Tell the microbiologist whether the urine specimen you send is a midstream specimen or a catheter specimen. Always interpret the culture report in the light of the microscopy report. More than 15 pus cells per microlitre of urine is generally taken as a significant result. Remember that tuberculosis may present as a sterile acid pyuria. Occasionally pus cells are seen in great numbers in the absence of any growth on culture. This usually implies a recent operation (e.g. a transurethral resection of the prostate) or the presence of an antibiotic. Do let the microbiologist know about antibiotic therapy.

This is especially important when taking blood cultures. Whenever possible take blood before starting antibiotic therapy. If this is not possible then let the microbiologist know. He will add β-lactamase to the culture medium in order to neutralize the effect of penicillin or cephalosporin.

When investigating urethral discharges remember that non-specific urethritis and chlamydial infections are difficult to diagnose. Special transport media are required. The gonococcus is a delicate organism and fresh samples swiftly examined are vital to establishing a bacteriological diagnosis.

Always seek the help of the microbiologist whenever you deal with super-added infection, especially in transplant patients and in the immunocompromised (as in HIV infections or in patients on chemotherapy). *Pneumocystis carinii* is the commonest opportunistic infection here. The picture can, however, become quite complicated, partly because several infective agents can become involved (bacterial, viral, fungal) and partly because the picture may change from day to day.

It is a wise precaution to test all jaundiced patients or those with a history of jaundice for the hepatitis antigen. A positive result for hepatitis B alerts medical, nursing and laboratory staff of the risks of needle-stick injury. Testing for HIV seropositivity is a controversial subject. It is well known that the incidence is highest in homosexuals, their partners and offspring and in drug addicts. Confining HIV testing to this group may

well miss many others who may be carriers. At present there is no consensus on who should be tested, when the test should be done or how often it should be repeated. There are complicated and unresolved questions over the rules of consent. Naturally the implications of a positive result are enormous. It seems wise therefore to obtain informed consent and to perform the test whenever the clinical need seems appropriate. You will need to counsel patients carefully both before doing the test and afterwards if the result is positive.

## BIOCHEMISTRY

Modern laboratories use the autoanalyser. All the common biochemical indices are measured even if only one has been requested. The results are expressed as concentrations per unit volume of blood. Blood loss, dehydration, infusion and transfusion will therefore affect the result. This is especially important when dextrose or lipids are being infused. Avoid a tourniquet if you want calcium levels. Potassium leaches out of cells so avoid delay in delivering the sample for analysis.

Remember you are sampling plasma. You are only indirectly discovering what is going on inside cells. Potassium levels, for instance, reflect poorly the intracellular potassium. The plasma amylase is only transiently raised in the plasma during pancreatitis. Hormone, enzyme and drug levels are affected by the levels of the plasma proteins, so allow for this when interpreting results.

You need information about electrolyte balance in patients with dehydration and intestinal obstruction. Sodium, potassium and bicarbonate levels will assist you in judging fluid and acid–base balance. The rate at which laboratory values change will dictate how often these tests should be performed. There is no need to repeat these tests on a daily basis if the changes are not clinically significant. The body's homeostatic mechanisms are usually very good but if the physiology of the lungs or kidneys is impaired then you will need information more often.

Be careful with dehydrated patients who have diabetes as well as intestinal obstruction. Use glucose and potassium levels as well as the electrolytes in gauging transfusion requirements. Keep an eye on the levels of urea and creatinine. Any element of renal failure in addition will make therapeutic judgements difficult.

In surgery the investigation of the jaundiced patient is now a radiological rather than a biochemical exercise. However, the balance between the levels of bilirubin, alkaline phosphatase and the transaminases will give valuable additional information. Obstruction is always characterized by high bilirubin and alkaline phosphatase levels. The latter often lag behind the bilirubin when the obstruction has been relieved. Hepatocellular damage is usually reflected more in the transaminases, which are then disproportionately raised.

Use hormone assays intelligently when investigating thyroid disease. There is scarcely ever a need for all the thyroid function tests to be performed. What do you want to know? Hypothyroidism is reflected in a low total thyroxine ($T_4$) and high levels of thyroid-stimulating hormone (TSH), while hyperthyroidism will produce high levels of total $T_4$ and triiodothyronine ($T_3$). Measuring the levels of free $T_3$ and $T_4$ is not necessarily helpful or reliable and the levels may mislead in patients with protein abnormalities, the pregnant and the elderly. If your patient is on maintenance therapy judge his control clinically. Do not be swayed by the biochemical levels. Thyrotoxic patients controlled with propranolol will still have abnormal biochemical levels even though they are well controlled clinically.

## RADIOLOGY

Once again phrase the question you want answered and then choose the right investigation. Too many indiscriminate radiological examinations are carried out. Discuss difficult cases with the radiologist. Remember that X-rays are shadows. An X-ray report is an expression of an opinion on the interpretation of shadows on a particular occasion. It is not infallible. Plain films are used for the demonstration of differences between penetration characteristics of different tissues in a particular locality. They are of course unsurpassed in the demonstration of fractures and tumours of bone. However, secondary deposits in an osteoporotic spine may be difficult to outline. Choose a bone scan.

X-ray the skull and the cervical spine in recent severe head and neck trauma. The presence or absence of a skull fracture does not often alter the management of the patient but it is most important not to miss cervical spine fractures. You will need to immobilize the head and neck as a matter of urgency if such a fracture exists.

The chest X-ray is excellent for outlining lung tumours since they are outlined by relatively normal air-containing lung. It is easy to miss masses near and behind the mediastinum, however, and the straight line of a left lower lobe collapse can be missed behind the left heart border if the X-ray penetration is not exactly right. In the presence of past surgery or radiotherapy to the lung the chest X-ray does not easily discriminate between past events and a new tumour. Choose CT or magnetic resonance imaging (MRI) (see later).

Plain X-rays of the breast (mammograms) use high-resolution X-ray films and rays with special penetration characteristics. The dosage is low and mammograms may be repeated on several occasions for screening purposes. Be reluctant to use them under the age of 45 since the younger breast is denser than the postmenopausal breast. The fine spiculate calcification of breast cancer is difficult to recognize against the dense stroma in the younger age groups.

Use plain X-rays in the renal tract when looking for renal calculi but remember that uric acid stones are not opaque. Be careful how you interpret calcified lesions and learn to distinguish the difference between phleboliths and calculi.

Plain X-rays are invaluable in outlining hollow organs in the abdomen because of the contrast between air-containing bowel and surrounding tissues. Because of this they are helpful in intestinal obstruction. The position but not the nature of the obstruction can usually be inferred. Small bowel can usually be distinguished from large bowel by the disposition of the loops and the presence of the ladder pattern of the valvulae conniventes.

Differences in penetration characteristics can be enhanced by using tomography, and an extension of this process is CT scanning. CT scanning gives superb cross-sectional views of any region of the body. Pictures can be enhanced either by adding contrast media to hollow organs or by simultaneous arteriography.

CT scanning has revolutionized the investigation of disease. It is now the investigation of choice for outlining problems within the chest and abdomen whenever the questions posed are:

- How extensive is this lesion?
- Has it spread into adjacent structures?
- Is it resectable?

In appropriate cases a CT-guided needle biopsy will also give a histological diagnosis.

MRI is the latest advance in this field. External magnets cause realignment of the protons of hydrogen nuclei. They then resonate and emit signals which can be picked up. This therefore allows a three-dimensional image to be constructed and pictures may be taken from any angle. MRI is particularly useful in the central nervous system as lipids have a high content of hydrogen atoms. The distinction between vessels, tumour, inflammatory lesions and surgical scars is more easily demonstrated using MRI than CT scanning.

Ultrasound examinationof the abdomen is of course quicker and cheaper and may give the answer just as reliably as CT or MRI in many cases, but you are more likely to move from ultrasound to CT or MRI than vice versa when the first investigation has failed. An exception is with carcinoma of the pancreas. Weight loss has caused the fat to disappear and the outlines may appear blurred or indistinct on CT, whereas the ultrasound scan may readily outline a pancreatic mass.

Ultrasound is particularly useful in the biliary and urogenital systems. The contrasts between fluid-filled organs, normal tissue and stones leads to variations in echogenicity. Portable systems now make this a valuable diagnostic tool in the out-patient department. Be careful in your interpretation of negative results. Small uncalcified stones may be missed. If there is any clinical doubt about the common bile duct use endoscopic cholangiography rather than ultrasound. Ultrasound is of primary importance in establishing whether a lesion is solid or cystic. For this reason it is particularly useful in the breast, in the thyroid and with testicular lesions. It may also answer this question in the chest, abdomen or pelvis. It is especially useful in the pelvis because the urine-filled bladder provides a better contrasting background than does air-filled bowel. Intra-cavity ultrasound is a more recent advance. Tumour extent can be gauged in the oesophagus, vagina and rectum. Rectal endosonography can, in addition, help in outlining complex sphincter defects.

The investigation or disease in hollow organs is traditionally accomplished by using contrast media. The organ is then outlined. Double-contrast studies with air enable fine mucosal details to be identified in the gastrointestinal tract. Use this examination when you wish to outline polyps of the small bowel or mucosal abnormalities in small bowel malabsorption states, in Crohn's disease and in ulcerative colitis. Cancers of the stomach, colon and rectum can also be useful outlined this way. Endoscopy, however, is usually a quicker and more certain way of establishing the diagnosis, especially since there is simultaneous access to biopsy. A negative endoscopy is more reliable than a negative barium study. Use barium studies when you wish to outline gross disease, or for the small bowel where the organ is not generally accessible to endoscopy. Local factors in your hospital will determine whether upper gastrointestinal endoscopy and colonoscopy are easily obtained. If they are then use this facility in preference to barium studies. Of course, barium studies can be used in addition, especially by surgeons who do not do their own endoscopies.

Barium studies are better than endoscopy for the assessment of functional disease of a hollow organ. Better still for motility disorders use oesophageal or rectal manometry. Barium and especially cine-barium studies of swallowing and defaecation give good pictures of the functioning organ. Manometry will quantify the problem.

The bladder is of course normally investigated by cystoscopy but contrast radiology has a place, especially in the demonstration of reflux (especially so in children). The bladder is filled with contrast and pictures are taken during micturition (micturating cystogram).

Radio-imaging is a method of outlining a problem within an organ by using radio-isotopes. The radio-isotope chosen is one that has a particular affinity for the organ under investigation. The resulting pictures are called radioactive scans. They do not have the anatomical clarity of other methods, but they highlight changes in physiology in the organ. Used in the investigation of thyroid disease you can demonstrate increased, reduced or absent function in a palpable lump. You might be able to show other impalpable lesions or a retrosternal thyroid enlargement. Subtraction scans may demonstrate a parathyroid adenoma by taking two types of scan (one demonstrating vascularized organs and the other the thyroid) and subtracting one from the other. Use liver scans or pancreatic scans to help you in distinguishing between tumours and benign lesions already shown in the liver, spleen and pancreas on CT scanning. Gallium scanning helps in the distinction between hepatomas and secondary deposits in the liver.

Use bone scans when looking for lesions in the spine which may be too small to show with conventional radiography. It is the increased vascularity of the lesion (inflammatory or malignant) which reveals its presence. You will still need to seek confirmation of its nature by other means (e.g. biopsy).

Radioactive scans in the genitourinary tract are used in showing dynamic as opposed to anatomical differences. Conventional iodine-based contrast radiology gives poor pictures in the presence of obstruction. Use DTPA (diethylene tetramine pentaacetic acid) to show the pelvis and ureter, or DMSA (dimercaptosuccinic acid) to show the cortex or when you suspect the presence of differences in function between the two kidneys (e.g. renal artery stenosis or after long-standing obstruction on one side has been relieved).

## THE VASCULAR SYSTEM

Learn to use Doppler ultrasound scans on all your vascular patients. Do it yourself and get used to the problems of siting the probe accurately and using the correct angulation. Do not press too hard. You will occlude the vessel. Accustom yourself to the sharp-peaked biphasic waveform of normal vessels. Obstructed vessels show a low-frequency long-duration waveform with very little delay before the next waveform. The *portable* Doppler ultrasound is an invaluable tool in the out-patient department, the ward and the operating theatre and you should learn to diagnose problems by ear. Sophisticated machinery in the vascular laboratory gives you a paper readout with an analysis of waveform characteristics. Use this together with vascular imaging to establish the site of the lesion, its severity, and whether it can be relieved or not. Use Doppler ultrasound in conjunction with a proximally placed sphygmomanometer cuff to find the occluding pressure. The two lower limb pressures can be compared with each other and with the pressure in the arm (pressure index = ankle pressure/arm pressure). This gives you an idea of the severity of the problem. You can use this as a simple non-invasive monitoring tool in the out-patient department.

The standard imaging technique for the vascular system is the retrograde (Seldinger) transfemoral arteriogram. The catheter is passed up the aorta and films are taken of the arterial tree. The procedure although invasive is safe and produces reliable pictures. There is a risk of initiating intimal dissection or dislodgement of a thrombus in the presence of severe aortic disease or in the presence of aneurysms. Some surgeons feel that the presence of an aortic aneurysm is a contraindication to the retrograde transfemoral route. Always look carefully at the aortic bifurcation. If there is any doubt about disease at this level the radiologist should take lateral views. In the presence of a proximal lesion the distal arterial tree is sometimes difficult to demonstrate. Beware of attributing this to distal occlusion when the cause is really one of underfilling. Look carefully at the region of the origin of the profunda artery and the popliteal trifurcation. The vessels in the leg are often overlain by bony outlines and a good peroneal artery can easily be missed behind the fibular shadow. Look carefully for patency of the dorsal pedal arch.

If the femoral artery is impalpable or occluded then choose a translumbar or axillary (or brachial) route. In many centres a more popular alternative would be digital subtraction angiography (DSA). Indeed this has supplanted femoral arteriography in many centres. The translumbar route gives excellent pictures but there are dangers of haematoma, haemorrhage and intimal dissection. It should be avoided in the presence of aneurysmal disease. If the puncture site is above the renal arteries there are risks associated with too much contrast entering the renal circulation too suddenly.

The axillary or brachial route requires more expertise and should be performed only by radiologists doing this on a regular basis. Once again there is a problem with local vessel damage and with haematoma. Occasional damage to the brachial plexus has been reported.

DSA should now be available to most vascular centres. The dye is injected via a peripheral vein.

Large quantities are required and this occasionally gives rise to problems of hypotension. The pictures obtained are often almost as good as with conventional arteriograms but dilutional problems result in inferior pictures of the distal vascular tree.

Duplex scanning is the most recent development in this field. A combination of ultrasound scanning and measurements of the velocity of the flowing blood allows a computer-generated image of the vessel to be displayed. It is not invasive and is therefore repeatable. It is a useful screening test especially in the surveillance of infrageniculate anastomoses.

# 3. Decision making

*R. M. Kirk*

Surgical practice varies remarkably. A patient with a particular condition may be treated expectantly by one surgeon and operated upon by another. In theory, once the diagnosis of a common condition is made, it should be possible to determine the best action from previous trials. However, many important surgical and other decisions cannot be made with mathematical precision. We each interpret selectively the available information, depending upon our characters, philosophy and previous experience. We often cannot logically justify why we made a particular decision, any more than we can give the real reasons why we studied medicine, chose a surgical career, or chose a particular life partner.

Attempts to apply reason may be thwarted because the problem is too complex, with too many imponderables. Too often the aspects that can be tested objectively are unimportant while the crucial aspects are not amenable to objective testing in our present state of knowledge. This should not deter us from attempting to deduce the implications of different courses of action. Some surgeons appear to get better results than others; perhaps they have exceptional inborn technical skills, but often they make a higher percentage of decisions that prove to be correct. Those of us who are less 'lucky' need to study how they make their decisions, and copy them. The great golfer Gary Player is reputed to have said 'The more I practise and the harder I try, the luckier I get'.

## Incomplete information

Decision making is facilitated if all the required information is available. However, in surgical practice we never have a complete knowledge of the physical and psychological state of the patient and of the extent and severity of the condition. Moreover, it is often necessary to take some action even before all the available information reaches us.

## Discriminating features

A frequent cause of failure, especially among inexperienced clinicians, is indiscriminate over-collection of information, resulting in confusion. Long lists can be composed of the presenting features of recognized conditions but if all the features are given equal 'weight' the possible interpretations are multiplied. Identify the cardinal features (Latin *cardinis* = a hinge, i.e. on which the diagnosis hinges), and base decisions on them.

## Distracting pressures

It is rare to have but a single patient on whom to concentrate. Other patients and other activities need attention. Rank these demands in order of priority, remembering that this order is not static. In battles and major disasters the calls may be overwhelming. Select those whose lives can be saved by quick action, setting aside for the moment those requiring too much time and those whose lives are not endangered. This often agonizing series of decisions is called 'triage' (Old French *trier* = to pick, select).

## Insight

The solution to a puzzle often appears apparently spontaneously as the result of a shift in the way that the problem is viewed. For this reason, when time permits, put aside the subject when an impasse is reached and reconsider it later.

## Provisional decisions

All decisions must be provisional. They rest on incomplete knowledge and on the interpretation of events at the time they are made. The situation may alter rapidly from progression of the presenting condition and from the effects of your response. The initial plan may be called the *strategy*. By monitoring and responding to the situation you alter the *tactics*. Too often, initially good management fails because it is not reviewed and revised in the light of subsequent changes. Be willing to accept that your actions are incorrect early, and change tactics. Most people find the admission of error to be painful and a few will not, for this reason, accept that they have made a mistake. Such people should not take up a surgical career.

## Anticipation

Actively look for predictable features that will affect your decisions. After selecting a course of action, do not totally reject the ones you have passed over. Consider the ill-effects your action may produce if you have misjudged the condition, and be ready to change it if necessary. Your management may, of itself, produce predictable effects that should be anticipated, recognized, and corrected if necessary.

## Preparation

Standard reactions are appropriate in certain conditions. Examples are external haemorrhage, respiratory obstruction and cardiac arrest. Of course standard management will not save everyone and indeed may rarely be inappropriate. Nevertheless, such routines are likely to save the greatest number of lives. Whenever you can identify a routine reaction that is safe and acceptable, learn it and practise using it. Regrettably, many medical practitioners prove to be inexpert when tested in procedures such as administering cardiac resuscitation.

## Personal and acquired experience

In the distant past clinicians based their decisions on their own experience, supplemented by advice from those colleagues with whom they came into contact. Their reaction to a condition was determined by what they had seen or heard previously. With the availability of written treatises they were given access to wider experience. We are fortunate in being able to survey the accumulated experience of our colleagues throughout the world. However, it remains our own responsibility to view what we read critically. The validity of a report must be judged on the clarity and logic of the investigation and the soundness of the interpretation. It is not always necessary to be statistically competent to detect flaws in the construction of an experiment or the conclusions drawn from the findings.

## Personal audit

Whether or not others review your results, make sure that you look back on your successes and failures. A successful outcome does not necessarily signify that you have acted wisely, nor does failure necessarily denote that your actions were at fault. Sometimes you conclude that the patient has recovered in spite of errors in your management. At other times your may console yourself that your decisions were correct but the problems were overwhelming or there were factors which you could not be aware of. Identify, admit and learn from your mistakes. Some people, claiming to be experienced, have merely repeated the same mistakes over a long period. Remember the statement of the novelist, Thomas Hardy, 'Experience is as to intensity, not as to duration.'

## Essentials for good decisions

1. Identify the discriminating features which override less reliable, perhaps contradictory features.

2. Do not be obsessed with your personal, perhaps limited, experience, which may not be typical.

3. Critically read the surgical literature to determine the best action to take in standard circumstances. Keep up to date since evidence

gathered at one time is not necessarily of permanent value as fresh assessments are made.

4. If you make a decision to act, do not continue doggedly with it. The decision is only for the time that it was made.

5. Constantly monitor the condition of the patient to note the effect of the action and be ready to change course if necessary.

6. Whenever you have a difficult decision to make, ask yourself, 'If my selected course of management fails, can I justify it to the patient, to my peers, and most importantly to myself?'

7. Do not be too proud to ask advice. Outlining the problem to a colleague often clarifies your own thoughts.

8. Learn from your mistakes — and your successes.

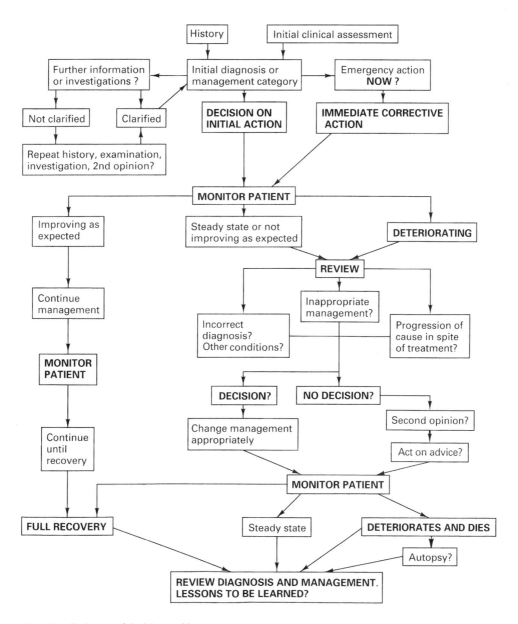

**Fig. 3.1** Pathways of decision making

# 4. Influence of coexisting medical disease

*R. M. Jones*

About half of adult patients presenting for surgery will have a coexisting disease unrelated to the pathological process necessitating surgery. This proportion is increased in the elderly and patients presenting for emergency surgery. The morbidity and mortality associated with surgery and anaesthesia are increased in patients with coexisting disease and the more significant the coexisting disease the greater the risk (Buck et al 1987). The medical diagnoses most commonly associated with an increase in surgical morbidity and mortality are:

1. ischaemic heart disease
2. congestive cardiac failure
3. hypertension
4. chronic respiratory disease
5. diabetes mellitus
6. cardiac arrhythmias
7. anaemia.

It can be seen that pre-existing cardiac-related problems account for the most significant increase in operative risk. The aims of management of patients presenting for surgery with pre-existing medical disease(s) are threefold:

1. to diagnose the presence of pre-existing medical disease and make an accurate assessment of the degree of the problem
2. to ensure that the patient's medical condition is optimized before surgery
3. to consider the potential for drug interactions arising from the use of anaesthetic and other drugs administered in the operative and perioperative period with those that the patient is taking long term.

All patients presenting for surgery should have a full clinical history and examination performed, including details of concurrent drug therapy, previous medical history and history of allergy. Depending on the nature of the coexisting medical disease and that of the planned surgery, additional specialized investigations may subsequently be needed. Young (<45 years), fit patients undergoing minor elective surgery do not need routine blood haematology or chemistry, a chest X-ray or an electrocardiogram (ECG).

## CARDIOVASCULAR DISEASE

### Coronary artery disease

Coronary atherosclerosis is the commonest type of cardiovascular disease; it is probably the single most common underlying factor in the production of operative morbidity and mortality (Aitkenhead el al 1989). The preoperative evaluation must include an assessment of diseases associated with the development of coronary atherosclerosis, e.g. systemic arterial hypertension, diabetes mellitus and smoking. The degree of activity that precipitates symptoms of myocardial ischaemia must be assessed and the presence or absence of congestive heart failure should be noted (does the patient also become breathless on exertion?). Patients with a degree of heart failure in addition to ischaemia have often had a previous myocardial infarction and may be taking digoxin. Concurrent drug therapy should be noted and almost without exception this should be continued until the time of surgery (see section on concurrent drug therapy). The drugs most frequently encountered are:

1. nitrates (e.g. glyceryl trinitate)
2. β-adrenergic antagonists
3. calcium antagonists
4. angiotensin enzyme converting inhibitors
5. digoxin.

It is important to remember that the preoperative ECG is normal in 20–50% of patients with proven ischaemia. Smokers should be encouraged to stop smoking at least 12 hours before surgery in order to decrease the percentage of carboxyhaemoglobin present in the blood and minimize the cardio-vascular side-effects of nicotine. It is also important to differentiate chest pain of gastrointestinal origin (e.g. hiatus hernia) from ischaemic cardiac pain. This may necessitate a specialist opinion and subsequent investigations such as a thallium scan.

The basis of management depends on the fact that myocardial ischaemia will occur whenever the balance between myocardial oxygen supply and demand is disturbed, so that demand exceeds supply. The major determinants of myocardial oxygen supply are:

1. the coronary perfusion pressure (the aortic diastolic pressure minus the left ventricular end-diastolic pressure)
2. diastolic time.

The major determinants of myocardial oxygen demand are:

1. increasing heart rate
2. increasing inotropic state
3. afterload — the impedance to left ventricular ejection (the systemic arterial pressure is an approximate determinant of afterload)
4. preload — the left ventricular end-diastolic pressure.

In the perioperative period factors that decrease supply and/or increase demand must be avoided. It can be seen that an increase in heart rate and an increase in preload will be especially deleterious as they will increase myocardial oxygen demand and decrease myocardial oxygen supply. During the perioperative period a decrease in systemic arterial pressure to a significant degree (a decrease in diastolic pressure greater than 20% of the patient's normal resting diastolic pressure is a useful guide) must not be allowed to occur because this decreases coronary perfusion pressure, which is very poorly tolerated in patients with multiple sites of coronary artery narrowing. Good pain management postoperatively is essential, as the presence of pain will lead to hypertension and tachycardia.

## HYPERTENSION

Moderate or marked, long-standing, untreated hypertension increases perioperative morbidity and mortality, and is a significant risk factor for the production of coronary atherosclerosis. Patients with sustained systemic arterial hypertension (systolic >160 mmHg, diastolic >110 mmHg) should be satisfactorily stabilized on antihypertensive therapy before elective surgery of any type or duration. Patients with long-standing moderate to marked hypertension should be assumed to have coronary atherosclerosis, even in the absence of overt signs and/or symptoms of ischaemic heart disease, and managed appropriately. Antihypertensive therapy is associated with its own unique considerations for anaesthetic and surgical management, the specific issues depending upon the medication the patient is taking (see section on concurrent drug therapy).

## HEART FAILURE

This implies an inadequacy of heart muscle secondary to intrinsic disease or overloading. The latter may be due to an increase in volume (an increase in intravascular volume or valve incompetence) or pressure (systemic arterial hypertension or aortic stenosis). It is usual for one ventricle to fail before the other, but disorders that damage or overload the left ventricle are more common (e.g. ischaemic heart disease, systemic arterial hypertension), and hence symptoms attributable to pulmonary congestion are usually the presenting ones. Left ventricular failure is the most common cause of right ventricular failure and if this supervenes dyspnea may actually decrease as right ventricular output decreases, leading to a reduction in pulmonary congestion. Conventionally, congestive heart failure refers to the combination of left and right ventricular failure with evidence of (and symptoms relating to) systemic and pulmonary venous hypertension.

Physiologically, heart failure may be thought of as the failure of the heart to match its output in order to meet the body's metabolic needs. Treatment is aimed at normalizing this imbalance. Thus, cardiac output can be improved or metabolic needs decreased. Traditionally, digitalis glycosides have been thought of as mediating their beneficial effects by improving cardiac output. Vasodilators can also be used to decrease peripheral demand.

In the preparation of the patient before surgery, digitilization remains the basis of treatment for the patient in heart failure (although its value in failure that is predominantly right-sided is open to question). Digitilization is particularly indicated in patients with atrial fibrillation or flutter, and when congestive heart failure is marked or of recent onset. Diuretics still have a role, but with the increase in use of vasodilators this is a diminishing one.

The operative mortality and morbidity of patients with well-compensated heart failure is small; however, surgery in the presence of decompensated heart failure is associated with a particularly high mortality and if the operation cannot be delayed peri- and intraoperative haemodynamic monitoring should be comprehensive. For major surgery this would indicate the use of a balloon-tipped pulmonary artery catheter; measurement of cardiac output and pulmonary capillary wedge pressure (a determinant of left ventricular preload) will allow the construction of ventricular function curves to guide in the selection of appropriate cardiovascular therapy. Postoperative admission to a high-dependency unit or an intensive care facility (with the ability to measure and adjust preload, afterload and cardiac output) is indicated.

## CONGENITAL HEART DISEASE

Eisenmenger's syndrome is the commonest form of symptomatic congenital heart disease seen in adult patients. This consists of pulmonary hypertension with a reversed or bidirectional shunt usually through a large atrial or ventricular septal defect. Patients have a very high pulmonary vascular resistance and this renders the underlying defect inoperable (short of heart–lung transplantation), although they may live for many years and patients up to the age of 50 or 60 years may be encountered who present for incidental noncardiac surgery. Systemic arterial hypotension in the perioperative period will increase right to left shunting and worsen hypoxia. Other problems include air embolus during surgery, and postoperative thromboembolism and infective endo-

carditis. Because of the danger of life-threatening haemoptysis, patients are usually not taking prophylactic anticoagulants. However, preoperative subcutaneous heparin is usually safe and early ambulation should be encouraged to minimize the risks of thromboembolism. All patients should receive prophylactic antibiotics. During the siting of intravenous lines it is important to avoid getting air in the tubing.

## ACQUIRED VALVULAR HEART DISEASE

### Mitral stenosis

This is nearly always of rheumatic origin, but symptoms do not appear until the valve area is reduced to less than 2.5 cm$^2$, i.e. half the normal valve area. This may take 20 years following the episode of rheumatic fever. As valve area decreases below 2cm$^2$, an increase in left atrial pressure is required at rest to maintain cardiac output. A valve area below 1cm$^2$ is severe mitral stenosis and is associated with a left atrial pressure in excess of 20 mmHg, and even at rest cardiac output may be barely adequate; there is pulmonary hypertension. Eventually right ventricular failure supervenes and atrial fibrillation is common. Patients with mild to moderate mitral stenosis and sinus rhythm tolerate surgery well. All patients should receive antibiotic prophylaxis. Fluid balance should be carefully monitored, as over-transfusion may precipitate pulmonary oedema whereas under-transfusion will compromise left ventricular filling. Similarly, changes in heart rate are poorly tolerated, and during surgery the anaesthetist will use a technique which minimizes changes in cardiac parameters. If major surgery is to be undertaken, with the possibility of large blood loss, consideration should be given to monitoring pulmonary capillary wedge pressure by means of a balloon-tipped flow-directed catheter. Unless the patient is taking oral anticoagulants a local anaesthetic technique may be used for surgery, although a high spinal or epidural block may be associated with adverse cardiovascular effects (systemic arterial hypotension) and should be employed with caution.

Patients who are dyspneic at rest and have a fixed and reduced cardiac output, present a significant risk during surgery. Digoxin should be continued up until the time of operation and plasma electrolytes checked, as hypokalaemia will increase the incidence of rhythm disturbances. These patients may have to be ventilated electively postoperatively.

## Aortic stenosis

Valvular aortic stenosis is commonest in elderly males, although it may occur at any time of life. The aetiology is diverse and includes congenital, rheumatic, senile and mixed forms. It must be remembered that it is most common in patients in whom the incidence of ischaemic heart disease is also high. As in mitral stenosis, moderate degrees of stenosis of the aortic valve do not appreciably increase the risks of surgery. However, severe aortic stenosis is associated with an increased peri-operative morbidity and mortality. Systemic arterial hypotension must be avoided at all times, because it will compromise coronary perfusion. Thus, peripheral vasodilatation, hypovolaemia and myocardial depression are all poorly tolerated. A change in cardiac rhythm is also poorly tolerated, as the atrial component to ventricular filling is essential to maintain normal cardiac output.

For major procedures it is advisable to monitor left ventricular filling pressure as higher than normal filling pressures are needed to maintain cardiac output.

## CARDIOMYOPATHIES

Using echocardiography, three principal forms of cardiomyopathy are described:

1. Congestive or dilated cardiomyopathy: this may be associated with toxic, metabolic, neurological and inflammatory diseases. There is decrease in contractile force of the left or right ventricle, resulting in heart failure.

2. Hypertrophic or obstructive cardiomyopathy: this is an autosomal dominantly inherited condition, in which there is hypertrophy and fibrosis which mainly affects the interventricular septum, but may involve the whole of the left ventricle.

3. Restrictive cardiomyopathy: this is a rare form of cardiomyopathy and the main feature is the loss of ventricular distensibility due to endocardial or myocardial disease. Restrictive cardio-myopathy in many ways resembles constrictive pericarditis, and the endocardial disease may produce thromboembolic problems.

Table 4.1 summarizes the treatment and management of these patients.

## DISTURBANCES OF CARDIAC RHYTHM

### Atrial fibrillation

This is the most commonly encountered disturbance of cardiac rhythm and it is important to define the disease process causing the fibrillation. These are:

1. ischaemic heart disease
2. rheumatic heart disease, especially mitral stenosis
3. pulmonary embolism
4. bronchial carcinoma
5. thyrotoxicosis
6. thoracotomy.

If there appears to be no underlying cause, the rhythm disturbance is usually termed 'lone' atrial fibrillation. The atrial discharge rate is usually between 400 and 600 impulses per minute, but the atrioventricular (AV) node cannot conduct all these impulses, so that some fail to reach the ventricle or only partially penetrate the node, and this results in a block or delay to succeeding impulses. Ventricular response is therefore irregular, but seldom more than 200 impulses per minute; the use of drugs or the presence of disease of the AV node often causes the response rate to be lower than this. The medical management of patients with atrial fibrillation must include the management of the underlying cause of the rhythm disturbance. It is important to ensure that the fibrillation is well controlled, i.e. that the response rate of the ventricle is not too rapid. Digitalis alkaloids remain the primary method of slowing AV nodal conduction, but if these fail to control the response rate, verapamil or β-adrenergic antagonists are usually effective. If surgery is urgent the latter may be given by slow intravenous injection (e.g. using propranolol, administering 1 mg aliquots every 2–3 minutes — to a maximum of 10 mg — with the aim of decreasing the ventricular response rate to less than 100 beats

**Table 4.1**  Cardiomyopathies: diagnosis and treatment

|  | Congestive (dilated) | Hypertrophic (obstructive) | Restrictive |
|---|---|---|---|
| Presenting signs/symptoms | Heart failure | Syncope | Heart failure |
|  | Rhythm disturbance | Dyspnea | Eosinophilia |
|  | Systemic emboli | Angina<br>Rhythm disturbance<br>Systolic murmur appearing during long-standing hypertension |  |
| Treatment | Diuretics<br>Vasodilators<br>Antiarrhythmics<br>Anticoagulants | Antiarrhythmics<br>β-adrenergic antagonists<br>Anticoagulants | Steroids<br>Cytotoxic agents |

per minute). Intravenously administered verapamil should not be used in conjunction with β-adrenergic antagonists as this may precipitate complete heart block. Occasionally cardioversion will restore sinus rhythm, although this is unusual if the atrial fibrillation has been long standing.

## Atrial flutter

The causes of this disturbance of cardiac rhythm are similar to those of atrial fibrillation, and the perioperative considerations are principally those of the underlying disease process. Atrial flutter is less commonly seen than atrial fibrillation. Although control of ventricular rate is more difficult in flutter, unlike fibrillation cardioversion is often successful. In patients with a very rapid ventricular rate, verapamil administered intravenously will often reduce the rate and may be used in an emergency; occasionally it will restore sinus rhythm.

## HEART BLOCK

There are two basic types of heart block:

1. atrioventricular heart block
2. intraventricular conduction defects.

## Atrioventricular heart block

This may be incomplete (first or second-degree AV block), or complete (third-degree AV block). In first-degree heart block the PR interval of the ECG exceeds 0.21 seconds but there are no dropped beats and the QRS complex is normal.

It does not always imply significant underlying heart disease, but is seen in patients on digitalis therapy. It is important not to expose the patient to any drug in the perioperative period which will further decrease AV nodal conduction (e.g. halothane anaesthesia, β-adrenergic antagonists or verapamil).

There are two types of second-degree heart block: Mobitz types one and two. Mobitz type one block is also known as the Wenckebach phenomenon and this is usually associated with ischaemia of the AV node or the effects of digitalis. There is a progressive increase in the length of the PR interval until the impulse fails to excite the ventricle and a beat is dropped. As a generalization, patients with this type of heart block do not require a pacemaker prior to surgery, and should it be necessary the administration of atropine will often establish normal AV conduction. Mobitz type two block is less common than type one and is a more serious form of conduction defect and may be a forerunner to complete AV block. The atrial rate is normal and the ventricular rate depends on the number of dropped beats, but it is commonly 35–50 beats per minute. The net result is that of an irregular pulse. The ECG indicates that there are more P waves than QRS complexes but the PR interval, if present, is normal. It is probably acceptable to undertake minor surgery in patients with Mobitz type two block without the need for the insertion of a prophylactic pacemaker. However, in these circumstances drugs such as atropine and isoprenaline should be immediately at hand, and the means for temporary pacing should be available. Prophylactic pacemaker insertion is indicated for major surgery, especially if this is likely to result in significant blood loss and associated haemodynamic instability.

Third-degree heart block is also termed complete heart block. It may result from conduction defects located within the AV node, bundle of His, or the bundle branch and Purkinje fibres. An escape pacemaker emerges at a site distal to the block (e.g. if the impulses are blocked within the AV node, the bundle of His usually emerges as the subsidiary pacemaker). In general, the more distal the site of the escape pacemaker, the more likely is the patient to suffer symptoms such as dyspnea, syncope or congestive heart failure and to need permanent ventricular pacemaker therapy. Pacemaker therapy is always indicated before surgery, although in emergency situations (such as complete heart block appearing intraoperatively) various drugs may be tried to increase the heart rate. Atropine may be of value if the escape pacemaker is junctional. Isoprenaline may be of value if the escape pacemaker is more distal.

### Intraventricular conduction defects

Left bundle branch block is always associated with heart disease. The QRS complex is wide (>0.12 seconds). A hemiblock occurs if only one of the two major subdivisions (anterior and posterior) of the left bundle is blocked. The QRS complex is not prolonged in left hemiblocks. Left anterior or posterior hemiblock may occur with right bundle branch block and it is generally considered that left anterior plus right bundle branch block is not an indication for temporary pacemaker therapy before surgery, but that left posterior plus right bundle branch block is an indication for a pacemaker. The latter patients are at risk of developing complete heart block. Right bundle branch block is not invariably associated with underlying heart disease. The principal significance lies in its association with a left posterior hemiblock, as there is then a risk of complete heart block; in these patients a temporary pacemaker is indicated before surgery and anaesthesia.

## PACEMAKERS

The patient with a pacemaker can safely undergo surgery and anaesthesia, but it is important to review the medical condition that gave rise to the need for pacemaker therapy. The usual indications for a pacemaker are:

1. congenital or acquired complete heart block
2. sick sinus syndrome
3. bradycardia, associated with syncope and/or hypotension.

Acquired complete heart block is probably the commonest indication, the underlying cause for this usually being ischaemic heart disease. The patient should be specifically asked about the return of symptoms such as syncope, which may indicate that the pacemaker is failing to capture the ventricle (or atria if an atrial pacemaker is present). The heart rate should be within a couple of beats per minute of the pacemaker's original setting. It is important to determine the type of pacemaker that has been implanted and the time that it was put in.

All patients with pacemakers are normally regularly reviewed in a pacemaker clinic. Whenever a pacemaker is in situ, atropine, adrenaline and isoprenaline should be available for use in the event of pacemaker failure. During surgery, diathermy is usually safe but some precautions are needed (Simon 1977):

1. The indifferent electrode of the diathermy should be placed on the same side as the operating site and as far away from the pacemaker as possible.

2. The use of diathermy should be limited to short bursts of 1–2 seconds at intervals not greater than every 10 seconds.

3. The anaesthetist should check the patient's pulse when the diathermy is used for inhibition of pacemaker function (Aitkenhead et al 1989, Simon 1977).

## RESPIRATORY DISEASES

### Asthma

Patients with asthma have bronchospasm, mucus plugging of airways and air trapping. These result in a mismatch of ventilation and perfusion and total effective ventilation may be severely impaired. A number of exogenous and endogenous stimuli may produce reversible airway obstruction. The most active chemical mediators are histamine and the leukotrienes. Expiration is prolonged, functional residual capacity and residual volumes are increased and vital capacity is decreased. Bronchospasm may be aggravated by anxiety, by instrumentation of the upper airway, by foreign material or irritants in the upper airway, by pain, and by drugs. The latter include morphine, papaveretum, unselective β-adrenergic antagonists, and various anaesthetic drugs including tubocurarine and anticholinesterases. In taking the clinical history, special attention should be paid to factors which precipitate an attack and the patient's normal drug therapy should be reviewed. If at all possible, the timing of surgery should be arranged to coincide with a period of remission of symptoms. The patient's normal bronchodilator therapy should be continued up until the time of surgery, and consideration should be given to the provision of preoperative chest physiotherapy. It is important to allay preoperative anxiety and suitable premedication should be prescribed. Diazepam, pethidine, promethazine and atropine are considered free from bronchospastic activity. If the patient is taking steroid therapy, additional doses may be needed in the perioperative period (see the section on concurrent drug therapy). In the postoperative period, careful attention should be paid to pain management, together with the use of nebulized or intravenous bronchodilators if this is necessary. Local anaesthetic techniques are often suitable in the severe asthmatic undergoing suitable surgery and appropriate techniques can be used to provide postoperative analgesia (e.g. epidural blocks). In the perioperative period, the following are indications for the use of intermittent positive pressure ventilation in asthmatics:

1. distress and exhaustion
2. systemic arterial hypotension or significant disturbance of cardiac rhythm
3. an arterial oxygen tension of less than 6.7 kPa or an arterial carbon dioxide tension of greater than 6.7 kPa, associated with an increasing metabolic acidosis in the face of maximum medical therapy.

### Chronic bronchitis and emphysema

A patient with chronic bronchitis will have had a cough with sputum production on most days for three months of the year for at least two years. The patient with emphysema will have destruction of alveoli distal to the terminal bronchioles and loss of pulmonary elastic tissue. Patients with chronic bronchitis are often smokers (see section on smoking), and have irritable airways leading to coughing and some degree of reversible airways obstruction in response to minimal stimulation. Patients with emphysema experience airway closure with air trapping and therefore inefficient gaseous exchange. Chronic bronchitis and emphysema commonly coexist in the same patient. Many of the considerations in the perioperative period that apply to the asthmatic patient also apply to patients with chronic bronchitis and emphysema; there are, however, some additional points to note. These diseases are usually slowly progressive and may eventually result in a respiratory reserve that is so low that the patient is immobile and dyspneic at rest, and even speaking and eating may be difficult. It is important that elective surgery should take place during the months in which symptoms are least noticeable; this is usually during the summer. Every effort should be made to persuade smokers to quit their habit. If the patient requires major surgery, and if the disease is severe, elective tracheostomy and postoperative ventilation may be called for. These will facilitate the clearing of secretions, and thus gaseous exchange, during the postoperative period when diaphragmatic splinting and pain or respiratory depression may cause acute respiratory insufficiency.

### Smoking

Cigarette smoking has wide-ranging effects on the cardiorespiratory, immune systems and on haemostasis (Jones 1985). It is a common cause of perioperative morbidity, and smokers have about six times the incidence of postoperative respiratory complications compared with non-smokers. Smokers may have arterial carbon monoxide concentrations in excess of 5%; the resultant carboxyhaemoglobin decreases the amount of haemoglobin available for combination with oxygen, and inhibits the ability of haemoglobin to give up oxygen (i.e. the oxygen dissociation curve is shifted to the left). Carbon monoxide also has a negative inotropic effect. Nicotine increases heart rate and systemic arterial blood pressure. Thus, carbon monoxide decreases oxygen supply, while nicotine increases oxygen demand and this is of particular significance in patients with is-chaemic heart disease. In these patients, it is especially important that patients stop smoking for 12–24 hours before surgery; this will result in a significant improvement in cardiovascular function (the elimination half-lives of carbon mono-xide and nicotine are a few hours).

However, the respiratory effects of smoking, especially mucus hypersecretion, impairment of tracheobronchial clearance, and small airway narrowing take at least six weeks before there is any improvement in function after smoking ces-sation. Similarly, the effects of smoking on immune function (smokers are more susceptible to post-operative infections) require at least six weeks before improvement occurs. Many smokers will complain that they find it difficult to clear their mucus if they stop smoking, and will use this as an excuse not to stop smoking before surgery; there may be some substance to this claim but it does not outweigh the benefits of stopping. It is important that the risks of smoking are empha-sized to smokers, and they should be encouraged to stop smoking for as long as possible before elective surgery.

## ENDOCRINE DYSFUNCTION

### Thyroid gland

Excluding diabetes, disorders involving the thyroid gland account for about 80% of endocrine disease. There are two practical issues for the surgeon and anaesthetist. First, there are problems related to the local effects of a mass in the neck. These include airway problems and the potential for difficult tracheal intubation. Second, there are problems associated with the generalized effects of an excess or deficiency of hormone. Patients with hyperthyrodism must be made euthyroid and properly prepared before surgery. Propylthiouracil (average daily dose 300 mg) inhibits hormone synthesis and blocks the peripheral conversion of thyroxine to triiodothyronine. As a generaliza-tion, the larger the gland the longer it takes to achieve the euthyroid state. The vascularity of the gland can be considerably decreased by seven days' treatment with potassium iodide solution. Pro-pranolol is an alternative treatment to thiouracil, and 60–120 mg daily for two weeks may be the only treatment required, and is now routinely used at many centres.

The management of the properly prepared patient should cause few problems. An emergency operation in a poorly or non-prepared patient is associated with significant risk and should be avoided if at all possible. Cardiovascular compli-cations are potentially life threatening and intra-venous propranolol should be considered before induction of anaesthesia (using 0.5–1.0 mg in-crements every 5 minutes to decrease the resting heart rate by 10 beats per minute). Disturbances of cardiac rhythm, hypoxia and hyperthermia may all occur. If appropriate, a local anaesthetic technique may be the method of choice. Hypo-thyroidism is not uncommon, especially in elderly patients. Cardiac output is low and blood loss is poorly tolerated. However, blood transfusion must be given with caution in order to avoid over-loading the circulation. It has been said that in hypothyroidism the respiratory centre is less re-sponsive to hypoxia and hypercarbia, so that it may be necessary to ventilate patients electively in the postoperative period. These patients are especially sensitive to opioid analgesics and these should be used with caution in the perioperative period. The patient's temperature should be monitored and measures taken to prevent hypo-thermia; hypothermia will aggravate the circu-latory and respiratory depression.

### Pituitary gland

In hypopituitarism, the varying involvement of the several hormones which the anterior pituitary produces leads to a variety of clinical presenta-tions; amenorrhoea in females and impotence in males are common presenting features. If hypo-pituitarism is unrecognized, there is a greatly in-creased perioperative risk of hypoglycaemia, hypothermia, water intoxication and respiratory failure. If the diagnosis is known, planned substi-tution therapy is indicated before surgery. Oral hydrocortisone, 15 mg twice daily, is administered. This is increased during the operative period;

thyroxine is also given and the dose slowly increased to about 0.15 mg daily, and the plasma thyroxine level is measured.

Acromegaly is caused by excessive production of pituitary growth hormone. This results in overgrowth of bone, leading to an enlarged jaw and kyphoscoliosis, as well as connective tissue and viscera. There is cardiomegaly, early atherosclerosis and systemic arterial hypertension, and diabetes mellitus is common. Management should include consideration of all associated conditions and the anaesthetist will carefully assess the patient, as tracheal intubation may be difficult.

Deficiency of antidiuretic hormone results in diabetes insipidus. A water deprivation test is used to differentiate diabetes insipidus from compulsive water drinking, and measurements are made of urine and plasma osmolarity. When the plasma osmolarity reaches about 295 mosmol l$^{-1}$ normal patients will concentrate their urine but patients with diabetes insipidus cannot do so. If the syndrome is differentiated from compulsive water drinking, the operative management of these patients is usually uncomplicated. The patient should receive a bolus of 100 milliunits of vasopressin intravenously before surgery and during the operation 100 milliunits h$^{-1}$ are administered by continuous infusion. Isotonic solutions, such as 0.9% sodium chloride, may then be administered with minimal risk of water depletion or hypernatraemia. Plasma osmolarity should be monitored perioperatively (the normal range is 284–285 mosmol/ l$^{-1}$).

## Adrenal gland

Adrenocorticol insufficiency is known as Addison's disease. It may present in acute and chronic forms and may be due to disease of the gland itself or to disorders of the anterior pituitary or hypothalamus. A patient with adrenocortical insufficiency undergoing surgery presents a major problem. The cardiovascular status of the patient and the blood glucose and electrolytes must be measured. The patient is prepared by infusing isotonic sodium chloride and glucose solutions, in order to correct hypernatraemia and hypoglycaemia. The day before surgery, an intramuscular injection of 40 mg methylprednisolone

is administered. Before induction of anaesthesia a further 100 mg hydrocortisone is administered, and for major surgery an infusion of hydrocortisone should be given during the operation. Hydrocortisone has approximately equal glucocorticoid and mineralocorticoid effects. Postoperatively, the dose of hydrocortisone is decreased from 100 mg twice daily to a replacement dose of about 50 mg daily.

Adrenocorticol hyperfunction is commonly iatrogenic. Whatever the aetiology, these patients will have glucose intolerance manifest as hyperglycaemia or frank diabetes mellitus, systemic arterial hypertension (possibly associated with heart failure) and electrolyte disturbances, especially hypocalaemia and hypernatraemia. Protein breakdown leads to muscle weakness and osteoporosis. Muscle weakness will be aggravated by obesity, and respiratory function should be carefully assessed before surgery, as well as postoperatively. Osteoporosis may lead to vertebral compression fractures and patients should be positioned during surgery with great care. Prolonged immobilization after surgery will lead to further demineralization of bone and hypercalcaemia may lead to the formation of renal calculi. Vitamin D therapy may therefore be needed in the postoperative period.

Aldosteronism may be primary (an adrenocortical adenoma — Conn's syndrome) or secondary, in which the condition is associated with an increase in plasma renin secretion (e.g. the nephrotic syndrome and cardiac failure). Patients will have hypokalaemia and hypernatraemia, which may be associated with systemic arterial hypertension. If the diagnosis is made before surgery, the administration of spironolactone (up to 300 mg daily) will reverse hypertension and hypokalaemia.

## Phaeochromocytoma

These catecholamine-secreting tumours may produce sustained or intermittent arterial hypertension. During surgery, arterial hypertension and disturbances of cardiac rhythm are common, due to the release of adrenaline and noradrenaline into the circulation. Prolonged secretion of these produces not only arterial hypertension but also a contracted blood volume; α- and β-adrenergic

**Table 4.2**  Severity of diabetes

| | Type of surgery | |
| --- | --- | --- |
| | Minor | Intermediate/major |
| Controlled by diet | No specific precautions | Measure blood glucose 4-hourly: if >12 mmol l$^{-1}$ start dextrose–insulin infusion. Avoid i.v. dextrose |
| Controlled by oral agents | Omit medication on morning of operation and start when eating normally postoperatively | Omit medication and monitor blood glucose 1–2-hourly; if >12 mmol l$^{-1}$ start dextrose–insulin infusion |
| Controlled by insulin | Unless very minor procedure (omit insulin when nil by mouth) give dextrose–insulin infusion during surgery and until eating normally postoperatively | |

blockade will help to reverse both these effects. It is important that preoperative α-adrenergic blockade is not complete, for the following reasons:

1. It may cause preoperative postural syncope.

2. It may cause difficulties in controlling the profound hypotension that sometimes occurs after tumour removal.

3. A rise in systemic blood pressure on tumour palpation is a useful sign in searching for small tumours or metastases.

Phenoxybenzamine is the agent usually used to induce partial α-adrenergic blockade. Careful preoperative preparation using α- and β-adrenergic blockade, as well as the introduction of anaesthetic techniques that promote cardiovascular stability, have greatly decreased the mortality of patients undergoing surgery for removal of a phaeochromocytoma, from 30–45% in the early 1950s to less than 5% recently.

## PANCREAS

### Diabetes mellitus

Even minor surgery is associated with an increase in basal metabolic rate and protein breakdown with nitrogen loss and some degree of glucose intolerance. Thus, surgery in a patient with preexisting glucose intolerance, whether this is known or not, will further exacerbate metabolic derangement. Diabetes is also a potent risk factor in the development of coronary artery disease and patients may have diabetic neuropathy which may cause

autonomic nervous system dysfunction, leading to a lability in arterial blood pressure. Before surgery, the cardiovascular status of the patient should be carefully reviewed and blood pressure taken both supine and erect to test for the possibility of autonomic neuropathy; the preoperative control of blood glucose is assessed and should be adequate. In the perioperative period it is important to monitor the patient by estimating blood glucose concentrations, rather than urinary glucose measurements, which are too insensitive for appropriate surgical patient management. It is important to treat ketoacidosis before surgery, including urgent surgery, if at all possible. Sepsis markedly increases insulin requirements. Patients undergoing cardiac bypass surgery may also have increased insulin requirements.

Table 4.2 summarizes the regimes suitable for minor and more major surgery in diabetics that are either controlled by diet alone, by oral hypoglycaemic agents, or with insulin. Chlorpropamide is a sulphonylurea with a very long duration of action and hypoglycaemia is a particular concern in patients taking this agent; it should be stopped 48 hours before planned surgery and the blood sugar measured regularly after the patient becomes nil by mouth.

Patients taking long-acting insulin preparations should be converted to Actrapid insulin, 8-hourly, using the same total insulin dose, and surgery should be scheduled for the early morning if possible. A number of regimes for the infusion of dextrose-insulin have been described but the common aim is to maintain the blood glucose between 6 and 12 mmol l⁻¹. One method is to add 10 mmol of KCl and 6–12 units Actrapid insulin (precise dose depending upon the blood sugar measured 1 hour before surgery) to 500 ml of 5% dextrose and to give 100 ml h⁻¹ starting half an hour before surgery. The blood sugar is measured at least 2-hourly during surgery and the amount of insulin adjusted to maintain the blood sugar between 6 and 12 mmol l⁻¹. Following surgery blood sugar and plasma potassium are measured at least 4-hourly.

Postoperatively, as soon as the patient starts eating, those who are normally treated with oral hypoglycaemics may need subcutaneous insulin for a few days before oral therapy is recommenced. Patients normally treated with insulin can be converted to 8-hourly Actrapid insulin to a total equal to the normal preoperative dose. After three days the original regime can usually be restarted (i.e. using long-acting insulins). In the perioperative period lactate-containing fluids (e.g. Hartmann's solution) should be avoided in diabetics. If oral feeding has not started within 72 hours of surgery, consideration should be given to the institution of parenteral nutrition.

## OBESITY

Life expectancy is decreased by obesity, and operative morbidity and mortality increase with increasing weight. In moderate obesity, the patient presenting for surgery should be instructed to decrease weight and given appropriate dietary advice. They should also be carefully examined for the presence of conditions with which obesity is commonly associated; these include diabetes mellitus and systemic arterial hypertension. Patients who are double or more their ideal weight are usually termed morbidly obese. These patients present a number of problems to both surgeon and anaesthetist. Their preoperative cardio-respiratory status should be carefully assessed and as these patients are at an increased risk of inhalation of gastric contents all of them should receive appropriate antacid therapy before surgery. Obesity is one of a number of conditions that will lead to an increase in postoperative deep vein thrombosis and associated thromboembolic phe-

nomena; they should receive appropriate preoperative prophylaxis for this. Transport and positioning of morbidly obese patients may cause difficulties and occasionally two standard operating tables used side by side may be needed. Intravenous access may be difficult and non-invasive methods of monitoring arterial blood pressure may be inaccurate. Therefore, an intra-arterial line is indicated for all but the most minor procedures. This will also enable arterial blood gases to be monitored in the intra- and postoperative period. Patients may need continued ventilatory support after surgery.

## BLOOD DISORDERS

Primary blood disorders produce a wide range of clinical manifestations, which may affect any organ in the body. Conversely, there are nearly always some changes in the blood accompanying general medical and surgical disorders. Thus, haematological investigations form an important part of the assessment and subsequent monitoring of most disease processes.

### Anaemia

This is defined clinically as a reduction in haemoglobin level below the normal range for the individual's age and sex. It becomes clinically apparent when the oxygen demand of the tissues cannot be met without the use of compensatory mechanisms. Although the level of haemoglobin at which elective surgery should be postponed will vary according to the precise medical status of the patient and the type of surgery planned, as a generalization a level of 10 gdl⁻¹ is commonly accepted as one below which preoperative anaemia should be treated before surgery. It is important to realize that a blood transfusion to raise the haematocrit should be carried out at least 48 hours before the preoperative procedure, as this period of time will allow full recovery of the stored erythrocytes' oxygen-carrying capability. In order to minimize the risk of transmitting the human immunodeficiency virus (HIV), transfusion should be undertaken only if the urgency of surgery necessitates this. Tissue oxygenation appears to be maximal at around a haemoglobin concentration of 11 gdl$^{-1}$ (tissue oxygenation depends upon cardiac output, peripheral vascular resistance, blood viscosity and blood oxygen-carrying capacity). Patients with ischaemic heart disease are likely to suffer more from the consequences of decreased oxygen-carrying capacity from untreated anaemia, and it is especially important to treat preoperative anaemia in these patients.

## Haemoglobinopathies

These are characterized by the presence of abnormal haemoglobins in the blood. Haemoglobin S is an abnormality in the amino acid sequence of the haemoglobin. When a deoxygenated haemoglobin molecule becomes distorted, this may lead to capillary occlusion and tissue hypoxia. The disease is inherited and it may be in the heterozygous or homozygous form. The former (HbAS) does not usually cause problems during surgery as the molecular distortion, known as sickling, only occurs at very low oxygen saturations. However, in the homozygous state (HbSS), there is a real risk of sickling during surgery and this may cause tissue infarction. Screening tests are available for the presence of haemoglobin S and electrophoresis is used to determine the exact nature of the abnormality. During surgery it is important to avoid low oxygen tensions and thus an elevated inspired oxygen concentration is used, and the patient is kept warm and well hydrated in order to maintain cardiac output and avoid circulatory stasis. If very major surgery is planned, where there is the possibility of perioperative hypoxia, for example pulmonary surgery, an exchange transfusion should be considered in an attempt to raise the levels of haemoglobin A to 40%–50%. Patients with haemoglobin C and haemoglobin SC should be managed in a similar way to those with haemoglobin SS.

## Haemophilia

Before surgery in patients with haemophilia A or B the concentration of the coagulation factors should be increased to a level that will minimize bleeding, and this concentration should be maintained until healing has occurred. It is important to seek specialist advice in determining the dosage of factors required. Cryoprecipitate and fresh frozen plasma or factor IX fraction are used to manage bleeding episodes, but the patients should be tested for antibodies to the products. If these are present, only life-saving operations should be contemplated. If cryoprecipitate or freeze-dried factor IX concentrate are administered, complications include viral hepatitis and allergy, and adrenaline and hydrocortisone should always be immediately at hand during their administration.

## RENAL DISEASE

### Chronic renal failure

This is said to be present when chronic renal impairment, from whatever cause, results in abnormalities of plasma biochemistry. Usually, this happens when the glomerular filtration rate (GFR) has fallen to less than 30ml min$^{-1}$. Management before surgery depends on the severity of the renal failure. Patients in late and terminal degrees of chronic renal failure (GFR <10 ml min$^{-1}$) may already have commenced on dialysis. If not, dialysis should be performed before surgery if at all possible. Dialysis does not reverse all the adverse effects of chronic renal failure; for example, systemic arterial hypertension and pericarditis may still be present. In addition, patients who are dialysed very soon before surgery may have cardiovascular lability during anaesthesia and surgery because they may have a relatively contracted blood volume. These patients are also vulnerable to infection, anaemia, blood coagulation defects, electrolyte disturbances and psychological problems. It is important to define the degree of renal failure present before surgery, and review the dialysis regime. Blood biochemistry, coagulation and haemoglobin must be checked. There should be a careful assessment of cardiorespiratory function and the patient's normal medication reviewed. The latter may well include antihypertensive drugs (see section on concurrent drug therapy). A careful search should be made for the presence of occult infection and all patients should have a preoperative chest X-ray. The susceptibility to infection is compounded in transplant patients by the administration of immuno-suppressive drugs, and prophylactic antibiotics may be necessary preoperatively and postoperatively. Chest physiotherapy may also be needed. Procedures such as arterial or central venous cannulation must be carried out under strict aseptic conditions. Before, during and after surgery, fluid and electrolyte balance must be very carefully monitored.

### The nephrotic syndrome

The clinical association of heavy proteinuria, hypoalbuminaemia and generalized oedema is usually referred to as the nephrotic syndrome. The hypoalbuminaemia is the result of urinary albumin loss and the syndrome becomes apparent if more than 5 g of protein are lost per day, and the plasma albumin concentration falls to less than 30 g l⁻¹. It is important to define the underlying cause of the nephrotic syndrome. Before surgery, the plasma protein and electrolyte levels must be estimated and corrected as indicated. An albumin infusion (up to 50 g) will restore circulating blood volume and may in itself initiate a diuresis. An alteration in plasma proteins will cause changes in drug effect due to an alteration in drug binding. The anaesthetist may use more conservative doses of some of his drugs. Central venous cannulation is advisable for all but the most minor surgery.

## HEPATOCELLULAR DISEASE

The patient with pre-existing liver disease is at an increased risk during surgery, especially if the pressure gradient across the liver is greater than 12 mmHg, suggesting a significant degree of portal hypertension. Perioperative mortality is probably in excess of 50% in the presence of marked ascites, raised bilirubin, reduced albumin ($<25$ g l⁻¹) and prolonged prothrombin time. In contrast to obstructive jaundice, if hepatocellular disease is responsible for decreased prothrombin synthesis, parenteral administration of vitamin K will not correct the situation. In patients with hepatocellular disease, the safety of hospital personnel must be borne in mind and all patients should be screened routinely for hepatitis B.

Infection control precautions should be instituted if this is positive. In the presence of excess bleeding, especially if clotting factors are known to be reduced preoperatively, fresh blood and plasma should be transfused. Blood should be given slowly in the presence of moderate to severe liver disease, because citrate clearance will be reduced. The presence of jaundice from whatever cause brings with it some specific problems in the operative period.

### Obstructive jaundice

The haemoglobin of red cells is the major source of bilirubin. Jaundice due to biliary tract obstruction which decreases the gastrointestinal uptake of vitamin K will often cause a prolonged prothrombin time. This usually responds to intramuscular vitamin K, 10 mg daily for two days preoperatively. There is an increased incidence of postoperative renal failure in patients with preoperative jaundice. The precise cause is unclear; it may be due to endotoxin produced from the patient's own bowel flora, or to obstruction of renal tubules by pigment. It is especially important to maintain good hydration and urine output intraoperatively as well as postoperatively. It is therefore essential to monitor closely urine output, and if this falls below (30 ml h⁻¹) mannitol should be used. Mannitol is an osmotic diuretic and 250 ml of 10% solution should be infused over 30 minutes. During surgery, close monitoring of cardiac status should be undertaken; jaundice itself tends to cause a bradycardia although other rhythm disturbances may occur. As in all situations, if the prothrombin time is prolonged, regional anaesthetic techniques are contraindicated.

## NEUROLOGICAL DISEASE

### Multiple sclerosis

The aetiology of this disease of temperate climates has become clearer in recent years. It appears that in genetically susceptible individuals activated T-cells and macrophages responding to environmental triggers interact with type 1 astrocytes, causing a disruption of the blood–brain barrier and a leak of immune mediators into the nervous system. This causes demyelination. Patients may present for incidental surgery or surgery associated with alleviation of the complications, e.g. implantation of extradural stimulating electrodes. In order to decrease perioperative morbidity, careful preoperative examination is needed. Patients may have a labile autonomic nervous system associated with postural hypotension. Muscle atrophy may lead to significant kyphoscoliosis and this may result in a restrictive form of pulmonary disease. Urinary tract infections commonly occur, but the patients must be carefully examined to identify other infective foci. An elevation in temperature is the one definite factor known to precipitate an exacerbation of the disease, so that all but the most urgent surgery should be postponed until the patient is free from infection. Epilepsy is not uncommon in patients with multiple sclerosis.

## Epilepsy

This term refers to a variety of types of recurrent seizure produced by paroxysmal neuronal discharge from various parts of the brain. Seizures may have a cerebral cause (e.g. tumour) or be due to a systemic disorder (e.g. uraemia, hypercalcaemia). The symptomatology is variable and seizures may cause total loss of consciousness or only a minimal alteration in awareness. The disease occurs in all age groups, with an incidence of about 1%. About 75% of patients have no recognizable underlying cause. If there is an underlying cause, the surgical management should take this into account. Otherwise management is usually uncomplicated; it is important that the patient's usual anticonvulsant medication be continued until the time of surgery and restarted as soon as possible postoperatively, if necessary using drug parenteral administration (see section on concurrent drug therapy). Anticonvulsant drugs such as phenytoin lead to induction of liver microsomal enzymes, and thus the patient's response to a variety of drugs that may be given during the perioperative period may be altered.

## Myasthenia gravis

This is an autoimmune disease of the neuromuscular junction, involving the postjunctional acetyle-

choline receptors. Specific autoantibodies have been identified and microscopic changes in the membrane demonstrated. The disease is characterized by muscle weakness of fluctuating severity, most commonly effecting the ocular muscles. Facial and pharyngeal muscle weakness also occurs, leading to dysarthria and dysphagia. It can occur at any age in life, but is most frequently seen in the fourth decade. There is an association with thymic enlargement and thymomas, both benign and malignant. About two-thirds of patients without a thymic tumour will improve after thymectomy, although the outlook is less good for patients with tumour, whether this is excised or not. Inhibitors of the enzyme cholinesterase (e.g. edrophonium, neostigmine, pyridostigmine) are used in the treatment of myasthenia gravis, as are drugs which suppress the immunological response and eliminate circulating antibodies. The latter has now become the first line of treatment and 90% of patients will benefit from the use of azathioprine or steroids.

Patients may present for thymectomy or incidental surgery, and the surgical management depends upon the nature of the operation and severity of the disease. As usual, the patient's normal medication must be continued up until the time of surgery. If the disease is severe, or major thoracic or upper abdominal surgery is planned, elective postoperative ventilation is advisable and occasionally a tracheostomy will be required, but this should only be needed if ventilation is prolonged and excess secretions are a problem. Respiratory failure in myasthenic patients may be secondary to either a myasthenic or a cholinergic crisis. Assisted ventilation should be instituted and anticholinesterase drug therapy stopped, and then cautiously reintroduced after testing with small doses of intravenous endrophonium (2–5 mg). Elective postoperative ventilation may also be advisable for lesser forms of surgery, including thymectomy, if the patient's preoperative vital capacity is less than 2 litres or there is a history of intercurrent respiratory problems. Following surgery, the requirements for anticholinesterase and other drug therapy may be changed and it is important to titrate drug dosage against clinical response. It should remembered that over-treatment can cause weakness just as can undertreatment. Postoperatively, the adequacy of ventilation can best be assessed by repeated blood gas measurement and therefore, before surgery, there are advantages to the placement of an intra-arterial line. This will also facilitate accurate cardiovascular monitoring during surgery.

## ALCOHOLISM AND DRUG ABUSE

Addiction is characterized by psychological dependence, change in tolerance and a specific withdrawal syndrome. Drugs including alcohol are used in susceptible individuals in order to obtain oblivion or excitement. Aetiological factors include psychiatric illness, personality disorders and social pressures. It should be remembered that many addicts abuse more than one drug. In general, it is advisable to maintain normal doses of the addict's usual drug in the immediate pre- and postoperative periods. The perioperative period is not the best time to attempt to wean a patient from his addition and it may only serve to precipitate an acute withdrawal reaction. Addicts may not admit to their addiction and the first sign that there is a problem may be the appearance of a withdrawal syndrome.

Specific organ damage may result from drug addiction. Alcohol gives rise to liver damage and can progress to cirrhosis, and thus change in protein synthesis, altered glycogen storage and susceptibility to hypoglycaemia. In addition, alcoholics are prone to bleeding, especially from the gastrointestinal tract, and there may be hypomagnesaemia. They may also have cardiomyopathy, and careful assessment of cardiovascular status is necessary in the alcoholic patient. Solvent or glue sniffers may have hepatic or renal damage and bone marrow suppression. Addicts to opioids will often have used contaminated needles and syringes and there is a high incidence of hepatitis and liver damage and also of infection with the HIV virus (see section on AIDS later). If sudden hypotension occurs in the operative or postoperative period in a narcotic addict, if other obvious causes are excluded, this may respond to the administration of intravenous morphine.

## PSYCHIATRIC DISEASE

Anxiety and concern are a normal reaction of patients to forthcoming surgery and anaesthesia. A significant proportion of the population will suffer from an affective disorder at some time in their lives. A depressive illness is the commonest affective disorder and treatment may involve psychotherapy, antidepressant drug therapy or, if the disorder is severe, electroconvulsive therapy. It is important that the patient's preoperative drug therapy is continued although both tricyclic antidepressants and monoaminoxidase inhibitors significantly interact with the drugs used during anaesthesia (see section on concurrent drug therapy). Before surgery both a psychiatrist and an anaesthetist should be consulted and many anaesthetists would prefer that the drugs be continued up until the time of surgery, and their anaesthetic technique modified to take account of the potential for drug interactions. It should not be forgotten that severe affective disorders are accompanied by a very significant mortality rate in terms of suicide, and supportive drug therapy should not automatically be withdrawn before planned surgery unless there is a very good reason to do so. The postoperative course in patients with a depressive illness may be more prolonged and these patients should be treated with appropriate forbearance.

## ACQUIRED IMMUNE DEFICIENCY SYNDROME (AIDS)

This is thought to be caused by infection with a retrovirus, the human immunodeficiency virus (HIV). Infection is most common in homosexual men and in users of drugs that are injected by needles which can be infected. However, it may also be seen in patients who have received infected blood products (e.g. haemophiliacs). The disease is not very infectious and is transmitted primarily in blood, and there is little evidence to support transmission via saliva or airborne transmission. It is thought that the risk of infection in medical and allied professions is low, unless accidental inoculation has occurred. This issue of routine preoperative screening is controversial, (see Chapter 9).

## SURGERY IN THE ELDERLY

Although patients over the age of 65 comprise

**Table 4.3**

| | |
|---|---|
| Oral contraceptives | Maintain for minor or peripheral procedures and institute prophylaxis against deep vein thrombosis, before surgery. Stop one complete monthly cycle before abdominal (esp. pelvic) surgery |
| Anticoagulants | Stop oral agents several days before surgery and substitute heparin if continued anticoagulant is necessary. The action of heparin can be rapidly reversed with protamine |
| Agents used in diabetes | See section on diabetic management |
| Levodopa | Omit dose before surgery |
| Monoamine oxidase inhibitors | Significant potential for drug interactions causing severe physiological disturbance. Discuss with psychiatrist and anaesthetist and treat each case on its merits. |
| Steroids | Supplement with hydrocortisone 100 mg i.v. 30 min before surgery, repeated 3-hourly during surgery, reducing slowly postoperatively to the patient's preoperative dose. Treat similarly if taking large dose regularly, any time during 3 months before surgery |

only 22% of the surgical caseload, they are reported to account for 79% of perioperative deaths. The mortality of surgery in elderly patients is significantly higher in those suffering from serious coexisting medical conditions. In a study of 100 000 surgical operations, the relative risk of dying within seven days, comparing patients over 80 with those under 60, was 3, but the risk factor comparing patients having symptomatic medical disease with those having none was over 10 (Cohen et al 1988). Not only do elderly patients have an increased likelihood of coexisting disease, but physiological function in general decreases with age. As a generalization, many physiological functions decrease by about 1% per annum after the age of 30 (e.g. cardiac output, glomerular filtration rate, renal blood flow). Respiratory function also declines with age (maximum breathing capacity decreases from about 100 l/min at 20 to 30 l/min at 80). The elderly are also more sensitive to the majority of drugs that might be used in the perioperative period, (e.g. diazepam has a half-life measured in hours that is approximately equal to subject age in years). As in all other situations where a patient presents for surgery with a significant coexisting disease, the morbidity and mortality associated with surgery can be reduced to a minimum after careful preoperative evaluation and optimizing the patient's condition.

## CONCURRENT DRUG THERAPY

It is a general rule that any patients stabilized on long-term drug therapy should continue to take the normal medication until the time of surgery, and that this should be recommenced as soon as possible following surgery. If the patient is unable to take drugs by mouth, then appropriate parenteral administration is required. This is especially important for patients taking drugs such as antiepileptics, antiarrhythmics or antihypertensives. A thorough knowledge of the pharmacokinetic and pharmacodynamic profile of the individual drugs is needed, in order that the appropriate doses and interval between doses is arrived at for parenteral administration. A number of drugs (e.g. propranolol) undergo extensive first-pass liver metabolism after oral administration and drugs such as this need much lower doses administered parenterally than they do orally. Admission to hospital for surgery gives the opportunity to review the appropriateness of long-term drug therapy and dosage, and this may be especially important in elderly patients as they are more likely to suffer from toxic symptoms. The nature of some operations may mean that the need for continued drug therapy has to be reviewed postoperatively, or the dosage of the drugs may need to be altered. An example of this would be a myasthenic patient undergoing thymectomy. Although the majority of patients stabilized on long-term therapy should continue their normal drugs up until the time of surgery, there are a number of drugs whose administration or dosage will need to be modified before surgery (see Table 4.3 for the more important examples of these).

## REFERENCES

Aitkenhead A R, Barnett D B 1989 Heart disease. In: Vickers M D, Jones R M (eds) Medicine for anaesthetists. Blackwell, London, p 4

Buck N, Devlin H B, Lunn J N 1987 The report of a confidential enquiry into perioperative deaths. Nuffield Provincial Hospitals Trust, London

Cohen M M, Duncan P G, Tate R B 1988 Does anesthesia contribute to operative mortality? Journal of the American Medical Association 260: 2859–2863

Jones R M 1985 Smoking before surgery: the case for stopping. British Medical Journal 290: 1763–1764

Simon A 1977 Perioperative management of the pacemaker patient. Anesthesiology 46: 127–131

# 5. Trauma

*Guest Editor: Miles Irving*

PART 5.1
## ORGANIZATION OF ACCIDENT AND EMERGENCY DEPARTMENT AND MAJOR DISASTER PLANS

*D. W. Yates*

## Organization of accident and emergency

A broad spectrum of surgical problems are seen in the accident and emergency (A&E) department, ranging from paronychia, to Colles' fracture and major head injury. Staff may be able to offer complete care to some patients and for others they may initiate management which will be either continued within the hospital or shared with doctors in the community. It is essential that those working in A&E departments acknowledge these differing systems of care and, if appropriate, integrate their assessment and treatment with those who may be involved subsequently.

The A&E department should be organized so that the needs of presenting patients can be determined rapidly and appropriate management initiated as quickly as possible.

## Walking wounded

All patients who present as 'walking wounded' should be assessed within a few minutes of arrival by a senior nurse who can determine the priority of the case and give an estimate of the waiting time. Initial care by the nurse, including the ordering of X-rays, is under consideration in some A&E departments.

Sometimes patients present with problems which may be better dealt with elsewhere. It is unwise to manage this problem of 'inappropriate attenders' at an administrative level, by drawing up criteria which can be applied by the reception staff. All presenting patients should be assessed by a doctor or by a suitably trained senior nurse. A decision can then be taken about the most appropriate method of treatment.

Waiting may be inevitable and advantage should be taken of this to disseminate information about accident prevention and health promotion. Entertainment and drinks should also be available. A note adjacent to any drink dispenser should advise the patient not to drink if treatment may include general anaesthesia.

Layout of the minor treatment area should encourage the doctors to walk to the patients rather than vice versa. Treatment cubicles should be multi-purpose, each with a trolley, chair and foot-rest. Couches are less adaptable and are best avoided. Small wounds can be cleaned, dressed and sutured in these cubicles. Provision of rooms for special procedures should be resisted, with the exception of dentistry, ophthalmology and otolaryngology. A dental chair for the former and a darkened room with appropriate equipment for the latter are valuable. A slit lamp should be available in the A&E department or in an adjacent out-patient facility.

Information can be displayed in the minor treatment area about the services in the local community. These should be used as far as possible to complete the care of patients with minor wounds and infections. For example, sutures can usually be removed by nurses at health centres, and tetanus prophylaxis, initiated in the A&E department, can be completed by the general practitioner.

The management of patients with minor injuries is best standardized by the use of protocols, agreed with the appropriate specialists and frequently reassessed with regard to adherence and validity. Good examples are the care of mild head injury, the use of X-rays to assess ankle injury and prescription of analgesics and antibiotics.

## Stretcher cases

Patients with more severe injuries must be treated in a separate part of the department. An experienced nurse must be available at all times to make a rapid assessment of arriving patients and allocate them to the correct part of the department. Some will be directed immediately into the resuscitation area, others into adjacent cubicles. Ideally the latter should be on an open plan, with monitoring facilities. The nurses' station and doctors' working area must be nearby, preferably within sight of all these patients.

The Resuscitation Room should be spacious and able to accommodate at least two patients. It can be considered as a short-term intensive care area. Most equipment should be wall mounted or suspended, to leave the floor clear. Built-in X-ray equipment is a great advantage. Equipment at each trolley position should be identical so that staff can work in a familiar, consistent environment. Oxygen and suction must be immediately available. A 500 ml bag of crystalloid solution is connected to a giving set, prepared ready for use and discarded if not used within 12 hours, to avoid the risk of infection. An automatic blood pressure machine saves nursing time and a pulse oximeter is now considered an essential part of a resuscitation bay. A defibrillator and other components of an advanced cardiac life support system must be available also. Central venous pressure is less often determined nowadays in the initial management of the multiply injured patient, but the equipment must be at hand. Pressure devices to hasten rapid transfusion and warming plates to heat up transfused blood are also necessary.

Packs of sterile equipment should be procedure orientated. Those most commonly required will be for venous cut-down, urinary catheterization, chest drain insertion, pericardiocentesis and peritoneal lavage. A thoracotomy set should also be available. It is reasonable to keep the more expensive pelvic external fixator pack in the main operating theatre on immediate standby. These latter two sets are required rarely in the A&E department, but can be life saving. A polaroid camera, used to record the initial appearance of a compound limb injury, allows appropriate dressings to be applied and left undisturbed until definitive operation. Frequency of wound inspection correlates with the frequency of infection. Close liaison between the resuscitation area and the hospital pathology laboratory is essential. If arterial blood gas analysis cannot be carried out rapidly, consider purchasing an analyser for the resuscitation room.

Maintain a close working relationship with the intensive care unit and the theatres for efficient and rapid management of a seriously ill or injured patient. Equipment used in these two areas should be compatible. The resuscitation trolley must be fitted with portable oxygen and suction. A portable ventilator must be available in the A&E department to accompany the patient on what can be a hazardous journey to another part of the hospital. Compact monitors facilitate the continuous monitoring of ECG, blood pressure and other variables during inter- and intra-hospital transfer.

Observation beds adjacent to the A&E department are a valuable resource for the management of patients with mild head injury and minor medical problems. They may also be used for the recovery of patients who have had general anaesthetics in the A&E department — although this is now an increasingly unusual occurrence.

Most procedures which require a general anaesthetic for routine management will be carried out in the main operating theatre. However, a theatre is a necessary part of any A&E department. It should be used for the assessment and initial management of more extensive limb wounds and for the performance of joint reductions and fracture manipulations under local or regional anaesthetic block. The theatre should be adjacent to the resuscitation room, so that critically injured patients can undergo immediate surgery. This will rarely be required but can be life saving.

## Teaching and research

There is a welcome trend to appoint more senior medical staff to A&E departments, but there continues to be a fairly rapid turnover of junior doctors. The combination of inexperience and the wide spectrum of conditions which can present to the department demands a major commitment to teaching. This must be carried out formally at regular departmental meetings and informally 'on the shop floor'. The development of treatment protocols as outlined above greatly simplifies this process. A programme of continuing clinical audit is essential and the conduct of research in the department encourages a healthy introspection. In all these aspects of the A&E department's work it is essential that the staff liaise with their colleagues in the surgical teams within the hospital, with the paramedics in the ambulance service and with the general practitioners in the community.

## MAJOR INCIDENTS

Major incidents pose special problems to the hospital service. A sudden influx of patients overloads the normal system of assessment in the receiving area of the A&E department. The poor quality of information serves to confuse the situation. Most major incidents can be expected to produce a large number of a particular type of injury (e.g. burns, crush injuries, skin lacerations by glass) rather than the usual mixture seen in everyday clinical practice. This may lead to rapid overloading of some aspects of the hospital inpatient system.

For these reasons it is necessary to adopt a different system of initial assessment and management. Much more attention must be given to identifying the correct priorities. More senior staff will be required at the reception point in the A&E department to carry out this task. Assume that the normal lines of communication will be severely stretched. Back-up systems must be available. This is particularly important in relation to communication between the scene of the incident and the hospital and between the hospital and members of staff who are at home.

Staff within the hospital at the time of the emergency are either given specific tasks which they can carry out throughout the incident, or asked to 'act up' for more senior colleagues who are called in from home. Their tasks should be clearly listed on 'action cards' held both in their own department and in the A&E department.

A team of 'key personnel', the A&E consultant, senior hospital nurse and the senior administrator should coordinate the response from a communications centre in the A&E department. A senior clinician should be appointed as the chief triage officer to sort patients in the reception area. Ideally one doctor and at least one nurse should be delegated to look after each patient in the major treatment area. Senior surgeons assess priorities for operative intervention and the intensive care staff and anaesthetists should be closely involved in the initial resuscitation of the critically injured. Those patients relegated to the minor treatment areas must be carefully assessed and treated by a separate group of doctors. As a general principle patients are admitted through one receiving area and transferred from the theatre to one postoperative area. This greatly simplifies initial assessment and postoperative care. The help of radiologists in assessing those requiring X-rays is invaluable and can best be provided by asking one radiologist to work in the A&E department both to assess patients' radiological needs and also to help in the interpretation of films.

The provision of a medical and nursing team to work at the scene of a major incident can seriously deplete the hospital's resources. In metropolitan areas an ideal solution is the provision of out-of-hospital care by staff from an adjacent district. Staff should only be sent out from a host district if the hospital can make up the resulting staff shortfall from within its own resources. Plans for a major incident cannot be expected to be comprehensive and cover all possible contingencies. The most effective response will be achieved if staff have a clear idea of their potential sphere of responsibility, can expect to work in a familiar environment and can clearly identify lines of command and communication. An occasional rehearsal of the call-out system reminds staff of these objectives and helps to keep the dust off the major incident plan. Finally, a major incident causes a lot of stress amongst staff and appropriate action must be taken to recognize and treat this.

**Table 5.1**   Models of A&E care

| | |
|---|---|
| 1. Immediate<br>e.g. hypovolaemic<br>shock | Initial assessment and<br>resuscitation. Stabilization prior<br>to transfer |
| 2. Planned<br>e.g. shoulder<br>dislocation | Treatment protocols, agreed with<br>in-patient team. Subsequent care<br>as in-patient or out-patient |
| 3. Shared<br>e.g. minor burn | Initial care in A&E. Follow-up<br>shared with community |
| 4. Comprehensive<br>e.g. mallet finger | Initial treatment and any<br>necessary follow-up in A&E<br>department |

## PART 5.2
## FIRST AID, TRANSPORT AND TRIAGE
*K. Mackway-Jones*

It must be remembered that the trauma victim presenting in the resuscitation room was injured some time before arrival. In the intervening period a whole series of people, both professional and non-professional, have either had a hand in treatment or have made decisions about care. Since the so-called 'golden hour' begins at the time of injury, these treatments and decisions can have a profound effect on outcome.

## FIRST AID

### General points

First aid may either be carried out by suitably trained bystanders, or by professional ambulance personnel who have been called to the scene. Whatever the training or status of the provider the principles remain the same.

On arriving at the scene of an accident it is tempting to begin treatment straight away. Remember however, that treatment is not the priority. Help must be summoned, and the safety of both the first aid provider and the victim considered. Only when these factors have been dealt with should an evaluation of the injuries be made and treatment commenced (Fig. 5.2.1).

**S** hout for help

**A** pproach with care

**F** ree from danger

**E** valuate

**Fig. 5.2.1**   The SAFE approach.

### Evaluation and treatment

Evaluation and treatment must be carried out in a sensible and methodical manner. The main concerns are for the patency of the airway, the protection of the cervical spine, the maintenance of adequate breathing, and the maintenance of an adequate circulation (Fig. 5.2.2).

**A** irway and cervical spine

**B** reathing

**C** irculation

**Fig. 5.2.2**   The ABC of evaluation and treatment.

It is important to carry out the evaluation in this order, and to treat any problems as they are discovered; there is little point in assessing breathing if the airway is not patent, nor in restoring circulation if breathing (and therefore oxygenation) is inadequate.

### Airway and cervical spine control

The first assessment of airway patency should be made by asking the victims whether they are all right. The ability to answer this question immediately assures the first aider that the airway is patent. If the casualty is unable to answer then the airway should be investigated. Foreign material (such as vomit, false teeth and extrinsic debris) should be removed from the mouth using the finger-hook technique shown in (Fig 5.2.3.)

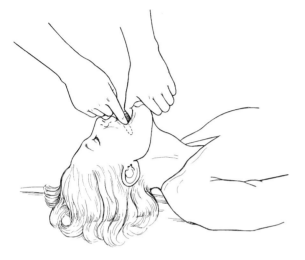

**Fig. 5.2.3**    Finger hook.

If this does not work then eliminate the possibility that the tongue is obstructing the airway. The mandible should be moved anteriorly using the jaw thrust manoeuvre shown in (Fig 5.2.4.)

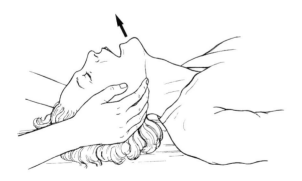

**Fig. 5.2.4**    Jaw thrust.

Take care at all times to protect the cervical spine. This is best achieved by having a helper maintain in-line cervical stabilization until equip-ment such as rigid cervical collars and spine boards are available. Avoid techniques for clearing the airway which involve neck movement (such as 'head tilt/chin lift') following trauma, as they may exacerbate cervical spine injuries.

## Breathing

Once the airway has been cleared assess the presence and adequacy of breathing. Feel for exhaled breath and observe chest movements. If the casualty is not breathing at all then start artificial respiration. If no equipment is available use mouth-to-mouth or mouth-to-nose methods. The mouth-to-mask technique shown in Figure 5.2.5 is more efficient and is less unpleasant for the rescuer. Many first aiders now carry these devices and if one is available, use it.

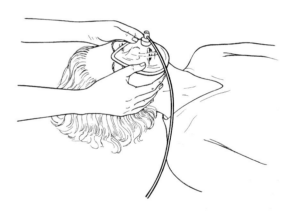

**Fig. 5.2.5**    Mouth-to-mask rescue breathing.

Adequacy of breathing is more difficult to assess. Observe the respiratory rate and the depth and pattern of respiration. If breathing is inadequate, seek treatable causes such as chest compression from extrinsic sources, and sucking wounds. Stabilize paradoxical segments. Once equipment has arrived at the scene more invasive procedures, such as needle thoracostomy for tension pneumothorax, may be performed if skilled persons are present. Administer oxygen at the highest possible concentration as soon as it is available.

## Circulation

Determine the presence or absence of circulation by palpation of a large central artery; in the adult feel the carotid or femoral arteries but in the young child the brachial artery is the site of choice. If the pulse is absent then commence closed chest cardiac massage as shown in Figure 5.2.6.

Look for sites of external bleeding and achieve haemostasis by applying direct pressure. Fractures should then be immobilized to limit further blood loss and reduce pain.

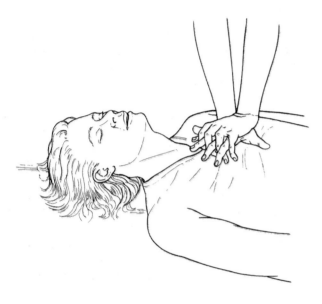

**Fig. 5.2.6**   Closed chest cardiac massage.

## TRANSPORT

Transfer from the scene of an accident to hospital will generally be by ambulance, although helicopters are increasingly available. If the transfer time is short then long procedures carried out prior to leaving the scene merely delay the time at which definitive care can be provided. Therefore in this situation limit the 'packaging' of the casualty for transfer to life-saving manoeuvres, such as securing the airway for transport, procedures necessary to stop further injury occurring, such as spinal immobilization, and standard quick procedures, such as the provision of high-flow oxygen. In rural areas, and in trapped patients where transfer times are longer, it is justifiable to undertake longer procedures at the scene to try and achieve more stability during transport.

Once 'packaged' the move to hospital should be as fast as possible without causing further harm to the casualty, or endangering the lives of the crew or public.

## TRIAGE

### General points

Triage, meaning to sift or to sort, was first used by Napoleon's Surgeon Marshall, Baron Larrey, to improve battlefield care. His aim was to provide optimum care to the maximum number of casualties by ensuring that they were treated in order of need, rather than in the order in which they arrived at the dressing station. This idea is now a cornerstone of military medicine and has wide application in civilian practice.

### Triage application

Employ triage principles whenever the number of casualties exceeds the capacity to provide optimum care. Thus appropriate situations for the use of triage range from the road accident with two casualties and only one helper, to major disasters where there may be thousands of victims. Whatever the situation modern triage is dynamic rather than static; continual reassessment allows priorities to be changed according to the changing state of the patient, and depending on the stage of care. The different stages at which triage decisions should be made are summarized in Figure 5.2.7.

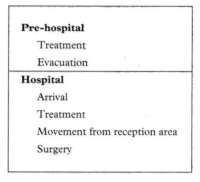

**Fig. 5.2.7**   Stages of care requiring triage decisions.

| Category | Priority | Name | Colour |
|----------|----------|------|--------|
| 1 | First | Immediate | Red |
| 2 | Second | Urgent | Yellow |
| 3 | Third | Delayed | Green |
| 4 | Fourth | Expectant | Blue |
| 5 | | Dead | White |

**Fig. 5.2.8** The five-category system.

## Triage categories

The categories into which casualties are sorted are generally referred to as priorities. The five-category system shown in Figure 5.2.8 is widely used.

The first priority group consists of patients who require immediate life-saving treatment, for example airway clearing or thoracostomy for tension pneumothorax. The second group comprises those patients requiring urgent treatment (generally surgery) whose lives are not in immediate danger. The aim is to deliver definitive care to these patients within 6 hours. The third group is made up of patients who can withstand a delay to definitive care of more then 6 hours.

The fourth group includes patients whose injuries are so severe as to be non-survivable, and those patients whose injuries are such that the time taken to treat them would seriously compromise the treatment of other casualties. Circumstances will dictate whether such a group has to be defined. Casualties in this category are treated expectantly until all first priority patients have been treated. Their evacuation and treatment, should they survive long enough, therefore begins after group one cases and before group two.

The final category consists of the dead.

## Triage methods

The most experienced person present should carry out triage. Three broad approaches to making triage decisions are possible. These are discussed below.

### Anatomical

This method requires that the nature of the injuries suffered by the casualty are discovered, and that the urgency of the injuries is then assessed. While this is the definitive method for triage, and can be used once the casualty has reached hospital, it has many disadvantages in the pre-hospital setting. First, it is time consuming, requiring a full secondary survey. Second, it requires complete exposure of the patient, something that is frequently neither possible nor desirable out of hospital. Finally, in order to make a correct triage decision a wide medical knowledge is required; thus this method can only be used by senior staff experienced in trauma care.

### Physiological

In this method the consequence rather than the nature of the injury is assessed. Established physiological measures of injury, such as the trauma score or the simpler revised trauma score are used, and the priority assigned on a predetermined scale. This method has the advantage that it is quick and reproducible, and can be applied by any suitably trained member of the emergency service. Furthermore any deterioration in the casualty's condition is quickly spotted. Certain of the measured variables, in particular systolic blood pressure, may be difficult to assess out of hospital. Clinical approximations, for instance the widely used rule that an absence of a radial pulse indicates a blood pressure of less than 90 systolic, are accurate enough to be used in these situations.

### Mixed

This method is essentially a combination of the anatomical and physiological methods discussed above. Initial triage decisions ('first-look triage') are made on the basis of a primary survey of the airway, breathing and circulation. Priority cases are identified at this stage. Later a physiological score is obtained. If enough time is available and conditions are satisfactory a secondary survey can be undertaken. This approach has the advantage that it is quick and allows more to be done if time allows.

## Triage documentation

Once triage decisions have been made using the categories and methods described above, it is

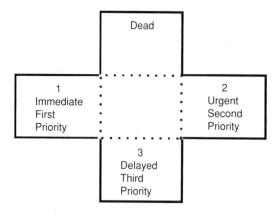

**Fig. 5.2.9**   Single card and cruciform triage labels.

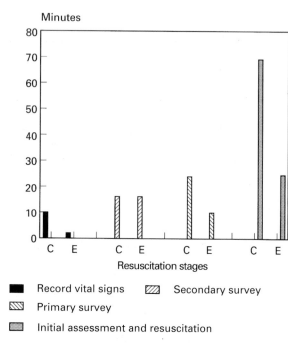

■ Record vital signs   ▨ Secondary survey

▧ Primary survey

▦ Initial assessment and resuscitation

**Fig. 5.3.1**   Differences in resuscitation times in unit C.

important that the casualties are clearly marked by priority. This is usually achieved by using triage labels. Labels should be visible, clearly marked by priority (both by colour and text), easily attached, and allow for easy changes in priority as the casualty's condition changes. Space should be available for notes on diagnosis and treatment.

Two types of label are in widespread use: the single card system (such as the Thames label) and the cruciform system (such as the Cambridge label). These types are depicted in Figure 5.2.9. The cruciform label is suitable for use during dynamic triage, and can be used from point of injury to point of definitive care. The single label appears simpler to use, but is much more limited in application.

---

## PART 5.3
## INITIAL TREATMENT , RESUSCITATION AND PRIMARY ASSESSMENT
### *P. Driscoll*

---

A fully integrated team of trained doctors and nurses needs to be present to deal with trauma victims when they arrive at the hospital. The team needs to work in an efficient and organized manner so that the trauma patient receives a rapid primary evaluation with resuscitation of the vital functions, followed by a more detailed secondary survey leading to definitive care.

The most efficient team organization is achieved by having each team member carrying out individual tasks simultaneously. This process is known as 'horizontal organization'. The least efficient technique, in which each task is carried out sequentially, is known as 'vertical organization'. If tasks are to be performed simultaneously, precise allocation of tasks to each team member is essential, or else there is chaos. Each procedure is divided into manageable units and allocated to individual team members by a designated team leader. These tasks must be divided evenly among the team to prevent overloading of any particular member.

When these organizational changes were introduced into a particular trauma unit significant reductions in resuscitation times were achieved (Fig. 5.3.1) (Driscoll & Vincent 1992). In particular the time to complete the life-saving procedures of primary survey and resuscitation (see above) fell by over 50% to 11.6 minutes. This is known to correlate with the physiological changes in the patient in the resuscitation room

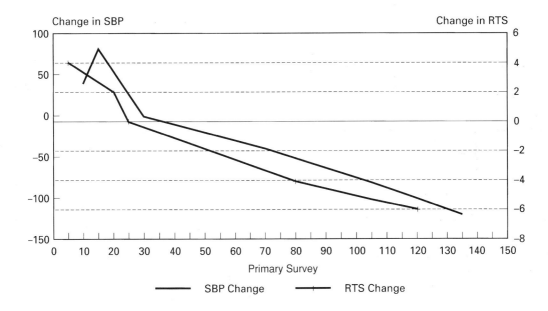

**Fig. 5.3.2** Variation in SBP and RTS with change in TLSP.

(Fig 5.3.2). There is also a direct relationship between this time period and the long-term survival of the patient.

## PREPARATION

In most situations the hospital will be warned about the imminent arrival of the trauma patient. During this time equipment should be checked, a team leader designated and tasks allocated (Table 5.3.1) (Driscoll & Skinner 1991). Protective clothing should be worn with gloves, glasses and aprons being compulsory for all team members, because blood and body fluids should be considered potentially HIV and hepatitis positive. All team members should have been immunized against tetanus and hepatitis B.

## PRIMARY SURVEY AND RESUSCITATION

The objectives of this phase in the resuscitation are to identify and correct any immediately life-threatening conditions (ATLS course manual 1988). (Table 5.3.2) describes a list of priorities. It is important to realize that assessment and resuscitation are carried out simultaneously by the trauma team and not sequentially as implied by this list. Problems should be anticipated and prepared for rather than reacted to. If there is any deterioration in the patient at any stage of the resuscitation then reassess the patient in the A to D order (Table 5.3.2).

When the patient arrives the team members should already be in position in the resuscitation room. The trauma victim is then transferred from

**Table 5.3.1** Trauma team tasks

| | |
|---|---|
| Team leader | Carries out the primary and secondary survey. Coordinates the trauma team |
| Anaesthetist | Airway and neck control, ventilation and fluid balance |
| A doctor | All other procedures |
| Two nurses | Help the doctors, record vital signs, attach monitors and remove the patient's clothes |

**Table 5.3.2** Priorities for the trauma team during the primary survey and resuscitation

| | |
|---|---|
| A | Airway and cervical spine control |
| B | Breathing |
| C | Circulation and haemorrhage control |
| D | Dysfunction of the central nervous system |
| E | Exposure |

the stretcher to the trolley by one of a variety of methods depending on the nature of the suspected injuries. The chosen method needs to be coordinated by the team leader so there is no rotation of the spinal column or exacerbation of pre-existing injuries. Lines and leads need to be freed beforehand so that they do not become disconnected or snagged.

## Airway and cervical spine

Secure a patent airway while maintaining in-line neck stabilization. It is safer to assume there is a cervical spine fracture in any multiply injured patient, especially if there is evidence of trauma above the clavicle. This injury can only be ruled out by clinical judgement, combined with a full cervical radiological series which is carried out during the secondary and definitive phases of the resuscitation. In the meantime stabilize the neck with a rigid collar, sand bags and tape. While these are being put in place, hold the head secure between the palms of the hands.

Simultaneously, while clasping the head, ask the patient his name. A logical response with a normal voice indicates the airway is patent and that sufficient oxygenated blood is perfusing the brain. A non-verbal response could mean the airway is partially obstructed. No response could mean a complete obstruction or an unconscious patient.

In either of the latter two circumstances open the mouth and clear any debris with either Magill forceps or a rigid sucker. Pliable suckers should never be used in this situation as they block easily and they can be pushed through a fractured base of skull into the cranial vault.

The tendency to vomit is high in trauma patients because many have eaten a meal immediately prior to the trauma. Since it is impractical to manage these patients on their side, constant supervision in the supine position is required. If vomiting starts, make no attempt to turn the patient's head to one side unless the cervical spine has been cleared. If the patient is secured to a back board then the whole board can be turned. When a backboard is not used suck the vomit away as it appears in the mouth. Once the mouth is clear, pull the jaw (and hence the tongue) forward, using either the jaw thrust or chin-lift technique.

If the airway is clear and secure and the patient has a gag reflex then give 100% oxygen via a tight-fitting mask — preferably a Hudson type — which will maximize the inspired oxygen concentration. This will achieve a fraction of inspired oxygen ($FiO_2$) of over 0.8. If the airway is unstable and there is no gag reflex, then insert an oropharyngeal airway and oxygenate the patient with 100% oxygen via a bag-valve mask device with a reservoir bag attachment. A two-person technique is preferable to ensure a tight seal between the mask and face. This can produce an $FiO_2$ of over 0.9. If the patient is semi-conscious then a nasopharyngeal airway may be better tolerated. An oropharyngeal airway can precipitate vomiting, cervical movement and a rise in intracranial pressure.

At this stage, the decision to intubate is dependent on the stability of the airway and the patient's respiratory effort. If there is a reduced gag reflex and inadequate ventilation then the patient should be intubated. This is the only safe way to protect the airway because mask ventilation can distend the stomach and induce vomiting. Endotracheal intubation must follow a period of pre-oxygenation by the ventilatory circuits previously described.

In certain situations, such as major facial injury or swelling, it may prove impossible to intubate the patient. In these cases, perform a surgical cricothyroidotomy if the patient is over 12 years old. A needle cricothyroidotomy is safer for patients under 12 years of age.

## Breathing

Strip the thorax of all clothing and inspect it for marks, holes and movement. The respiratory rate has to be counted because it is a sensitive measurement of thoracic problems as well as being an invaluable indicator of haemorrhagic shock (Table 5.3.3). An early sign of respiratory compromise is shallow ventilation with a rate over 20/min.

Check the neck for swellings, distended veins and abnormal tracheal position. Listen to both sides of the chest, anteriorly as well as in the axil-

**Table 5.3.3**    Classification of hypovolaemic shock according to blood loss (Baskett 1991)

|  | 1 | 2 | 3 | 4 |
|---|---|---|---|---|
| Blood loss | | | | |
| Litres | 0.75 | 0.8–1.5 | 1.5–2.0 | >2.0 |
| % | <15 | 15–30 | 30–40 | >40 |
| Blood pressure | | | | |
| Systolic | Normal | Normal | Reduced | Very low |
| Diastolic | Normal | Raised | Reduced | Very low |
| Pulse | <100 | 100–120 | 120 (weak) | >120 (very weak) |
| Capillary refill | Normal | >2 s | >2 s | Undetectable |
| Respiratory rate | Normal | Normal | >20/min | >20/min |
| Urinary flow rate (ml h$^{-1}$) | >30 | 20–30 | 10–20 | <10 |
| Skin colour | Normal | Pale | Pale | Pale/cold |
| Mental state | Alert | Anxious/aggressive | Drowsy/aggressive | Drowsy/unconscious |

**Table 5.3.4**    Immediately life-threatening thoracic conditions

1.  Tension pneumothorax
2.  Cardiac tamponade
3.  Open chest wound
4.  Massive haemothorax
5.  Flail chest

la, to determine if there is equal air entry and also over the epigastrium, to ensure the stomach is not being ventilated. If there is no air entry to both sides then there is either complete obstruction of the upper airway or an incomplete seal between face and mask. If there is a difference between air entry on both sides then there is a local thoracic problem, such as a foreign body in the bronchus, or a haemo- or pneumothorax.

Five immediately life-threatening thoracic conditions need to be excluded (Table 5.3.4). Their signs and symptoms will be discussed in detail in Chapter 5.10.

If a tension pneumothorax is suspected, drain it immediately. Initially insert a 14g cannula into the pleural cavity, in the second intercostal space, in the mid-clavicular line. This gains enough time for a definitive chest drain to be inserted in the fifth intercostal space in the mid-axillary line.

An opening in the chest wall greater than two-thirds the size of the trachea allows air to preferentially enter the pleural space by this portal during inspiration. Cover the defect and insert a chest drain in order to prevent a tension pneumothorax from developing.

If a pericardial tamponade is suspected and the patient is in extremis then treat it initially with a needle pericardiocentesis. This may gain enough time for the definitive thoracotomy which will be required.

**Circulation**

A rapid assessment of the grade of shock is necessary. Important information can be gained quickly by observing the skin, pulses and conscious level (Table 5.3.3). A rapid, thready pulse may indicate early hypovolaemia but there are other causes for it. An irregular pulse after trauma is usually an indicator of cardiac impairment. If the carotid pulse can be felt then there is at least 50% of the blood volume still present. Unconsciousness results from a drop of 50% in the blood volume.

Compress all overt haemorrhage points with a pressure dressing instead of wasting valuable time trying to isolate and clamp bleeding vessels. Use tourniquets only when the limb is considered unsalvageable.

Insert two large-bore (14g or 16g) cannulas peripherally, because the rate of fluid administration is determined by the cannula's diameter and inversely by its length. Central veins are potentially more dangerous to cannulate. The ideal place is the antecubical fossa but this may not be possible if there is vascular damage to the upper limb.

Once the first cannula is in position, draw off 20 ml of blood before connecting it to two 0.5-litre bags of colloid. These have to be infused quickly if there is any evidence of hypovolaemia. Send the blood for urea/electrolytes, full blood count and blood grouping. If there is any difficulty aspirating blood do not jeopardize the cannula. Instead connect it to an intravenous giving set and commence infusion. Blood can then be taken from the femoral artery or vein. An arterial sample also needs to be taken for blood gas analysis.

Assess adequate resuscitation quantitatively by monitoring the same parameters used to define shock (Table 5.3.3). Therefore measure the blood pressure, pulse pressure, heart and respiratory rates. After the secondary survey, monitor the Glasgow Coma Score (GCS), urinary output and arterial blood gases. Every trauma patient needs to be connected to an ECG monitor. Dysrythmias may indicate cardiac contusion (see Chapter 5.10) or hypothermia. Suspect hypoxia or hypovolaemia in trauma patients with bradycardia, aberrant conduction or premature beats. Electromechanical dissociation could indicate a tension pneumothorax, massive hypovolaemia or cardiac tamponade.

If the patient has a low blood pressure then approximately 30% of the blood volume has been lost already. These patients require typed blood, which should only take 10–15 minutes to prepare. Typed blood is also needed when there is only a limited response following infusion of 2 litres of colloid. Reserve uncrossed matched blood for patients with grade 4 shock. The time taken to cross-match blood fully can only be afforded in the first two grades of shock (Table 5.3.3). Warm all intravenous fluids before infusion to prevent iatrogenic hypothermia.

**Table 5.3.5**    Conscious level assessment in the primary survey

| | |
|---|---|
| A | Alert |
| V | Responds to verbal stimuli |
| P | Responds to painful stimuli |
| U | Unresponsive |

## Dysfunction

The brain and spinal cord can then be assessed rapidly by determining the conscious level, pupillary response and by asking the patient to wiggle the toes and squeeze the doctor's hands. In the primary survey make only a quick assessment of the conscious level. A useful mnemonic for this is AVPU (Table 5.3.5). This will be augmented with the GCS during the secondary survey. A decrease in the conscious level may indicate a fall in the cerebral oxygenation or perfusion. If such a change is detected, reassess the A, B and Cs before considering an intracranial cause. Similarly, movement of the hand and toes are gross tests of the spinal cord. Augment these with a detailed examination in the secondary survey.

## Exposure

At the end of the primary survey remove the patient's remaining clothing. Take care that the spine is not accidently moved during this procedure. If there are sufficient personnel present take the opportunity to log-roll the patient. Remove any debris and palpate the whole vertebral column for tenderness and deformity. Auscultate the lung fields before log-rolling the patient back into the supine position. Take care to prevent the patient becoming cold by using covers between examinations and by keeping the resuscitation room warm.

## MECHANISM, HISTORY AND REASSESSMENT

Interview the ambulance personnel in order to determine the exact time and mechanism of injury, the initial pre-hospital state and what treatment had been instituted and to what effect.

The body's elastic tissue rebounds to its original position following trauma and so the true extent can be missed when the patient is seen initially in the resuscitation room. Therefore, if the patient has been a victim of a road traffic accident, enquire about the direction and magnitude of the forces by obtaining a description of the vehicle's deformation. This information is invaluable in increasing the team's awareness to particular patterns of injury.

The patient's relevant history should be taken by one member of the team but it can be delayed until the end of the secondary survey. A useful mnemonic for this is listed in Table 5.3.6.

**Table 5.3.6**    Relevant history

| | |
|---|---|
| A | Allergies |
| M | Medicines |
| P | Past medical history |
| L | Last meal |
| E | Event mechanism |

The team leader should then assess the full situation. The airway, breathing and circulation need to have been stabilized before moving on to the detailed head-to-toe assessment in the secondary survey. Check that the blood has been sent to the laboratory, that the vital signs are being recorded and that all the immediately life-threatening conditions have been excluded or treated.

REFERENCES

ATLS course manual 1988 American College of Surgeons, Chicago
Baskett P 1991 Management of hypovolaemic shock. In: Skinner D, Driscoll P, Earlam R (eds) ABC of major trauma. BMJ Publications, London
Driscoll P 1990 The influence of trauma team organization on patient resuscitation time. Journal of Emergency Medicine 8:387
Driscoll P, Skinner D 1991 Initial assessment and management — 1: Primary survey. In: Skinner D, Driscoll P, Earlam R (eds) ABC of major trauma. BMJ Publications, London

PART 5.4
## SECONDARY ASSESSMENT AND THE PLANNING OF TREATMENT
*M. Mughal*

Secondary assessment is the complete and systematic examination of the patient, ensuring that no injury is missed. It must not be started until the primary survey has been completed, any immediately life-threatening injuries identified and resuscitation begun. Any investigations required are planned at this stage. Ideally one doctor keeps a constant check on the airway, breathing and circulation while another carries out the secondary assessment. This begins with the examination of the head, working in an orderly sequence to the neck, chest, abdomen, extremities, the back and the neurological system.

Inspect the head for lacerations and bruising and palpate it for fractures. Examine the eyes for injury and visual acuity, the nose and ears for foreign bodies, bleeding and cerebrospinal fluid leak, and the mouth for dental and soft tissue injuries. The neck is examined after removal of the cervical collar if applied, while an assistant holds the head firmly. Gently palpate the cervical spine for tenderness and a step, indicating dislocation. Examine the trachea for deviation, and the jugular veins for an indication of the central venous pressure. This is an appropriate time to obtain a lateral X-ray of the cervical spine, if indicated, while one person holds the head steady and another pulls down on the arms to get the shoulders out of the way of the X-ray beam, so that all seven cervical vertebrae, including the C7–T1 junction, will be seen.

Examine the chest for bruising, penetrating wounds, deformity, asymmetry of expansion, paradoxical movement, tenderness over the ribs and sternum. Percuss and auscultate both front and back after carefully log-rolling the patient. A tension pneumothorax will have been detected and treated during the primary survey, but a small simple pneumothorax, haemothorax or flail segment may be detected only at this stage. Cover open wounds with clean occlusive dressings. If the signs are those of a simple pneumothorax without respiratory distress, obtain a chest X-ray to confirm clinical findings, which are not infallible, before inserting a chest drain. Chest drainage is not without morbidity and the only exception to waiving a chest X-ray in these circumstances is when there is an urgent need to intubate and ventilate the patient. Auscultate the precordium for heart sounds, which are muffled in cardiac tamponade, the other signs of which are distended neck veins and hypotension (Beck's triad). Suspect myocardial contusion in blunt frontal chest injury with sternal tenderness. Commence ECG monitoring, which may reveal arrythmias and myocardial ischaemia. Examine the abdomen next, not forgetting the back. Inspection for wounds and bruising is a valuable indicator of underlying visceral injury but palpation for tenderness is often unreliable. It is useless if the patient is unconscious or has sustained a high spinal cord transection; even if it is elicited in a responsive patient, it may be only a reflection of abdominal wall injury. Palpate the pelvis for fractures, the external genitalia for bruising and blood at the external urethral meatus, and the perineum for bruising and tenderness indicating the possibility of urethral disruption. Always perform a rectal examination, noting anal tone, loss of which may indicate a serious spinal cord injury, the position of the prostate gland, which may be high in complete disruption of the membranous urethra, and noting the presence of blood or bony spicules. Similarly carry out a vaginal examination.

Examine the limbs for soft tissue, bony and neurovascular injury. Correct any deformities and splint the limb as soon as possible to avoid further neurovascular damage. Record the state of the peripheral circulation before and after such a manoeuvre. Splinting of fractured limbs decreases pain, reduces the incidence of fat embolism and facilitates transfer. Examine the spine after log-rolling the patient. Inspect for bruising, palpate for tenderness and deformity, and test for motor and sensory deficit. Assess the neurological status using the Glasgow Coma Scale.

Carefully record the examination findings and any investigations planned. Take blood for a blood count, serum electrolytes and any other specific tests, and for grouping and cross-matching if indicated. Order essential plain X-rays in most cases of serious injury, particularly if blunt, of the cervical spine, chest and pelvis. Other imaging techniques, such as computed tomography (CT) scans, angiograms, intravenous urograms and urethrograms may be required. Plan them according to need and priority, ensuring that the patient is not shunted back and forth to the X-ray department. A nurse and doctor must accompany the patient during such investigations, to supervise positioning and ensure uninterrupted resuscitation. A diagnostic peritoneal lavage may also be indicated at this stage but must only be carried out after consultation with the general surgeons.

While waiting for the results of investigations, obtain as much information as possible about the circumstances relating to the injury and the patient's medical history. This may be gained from the patient, any friends and relatives, witnesses and ambulance personnel. Specifically ask and record information about allergies, medication, tetanus immunization status and last meal. Administer analgesia when necessary, preferably intravenous morphine, titrating the dose against response. In cases of penetrating injury, give a single dose of a broad-spectrum antibiotic and take necessary antitetanus measures. Since many injuries have medicolegal implications, carefully save and label any significant debris, clothing or implements extracted from wounds, as forensic evidence.

Plan treatment according to the injuries identified and facilities available. List all the injuries in order of priority and, if the facilities required to treat them are available locally, call the appropriate specialists. Each can then carry out a detailed assessment of the injury in his field and a final treatment plan can be drawn up. Arrange theatre time, anaesthetists, blood, special instruments, assistance and intensive care facilities. With foresight and careful planning the patient with multiple injuries can have many injuries treated at one session and definitively, thus avoiding morbidity and minimizing disability.

PART 5.5
# WOUND MANAGEMENT
*D. J. Whitby*

Although wound healing has long been of interest to investigators, the results of most studies, until recently, have had little effect on the practical management of wounds. Consequently many surgeons' knowledge of wound healing has been very limited and their approach to wound management has been empirical. Our knowledge of wound healing is expanding rapidly as new techniques in cell and molecular biology allow study of the underlying mechanisms which control this process. These studies suggest that, for the first time, it may be possible to control normal wound healing, so that the quality of wound healing is improved, with less scar formation, and the rate of wound healing is increased. Biotechnology companies have identified wound care and wound manipulation as one of the likely growth areas in health care in the coming decades and are investing large capital sums to develop products to improve wound healing. Because of these developments, surgeons are likely to have an increasing variety of options available when they are treating wounds, and a basic knowledge of wound healing will be essential so that sensible wound management decisions can be made.

## WOUND HEALING

Soft tissue injuries heal by a complex series of cellular events leading to connective tissue formation and repair by scar formation. The process is continuous, but it is convenient to consider it in three phases.

### Phase 1: inflammation

Tissue injury, with disruption of vessels, activates platelets and initiates the coagulation cascade, producing a clot in the wound and generating biologically active substances which cause vasodilation, increased capillary permeability and oedema. These substances are also chemoattractant to polymorphonucleocytes (PMNs) and monocytes, and act as potent growth factors for fibroblasts and endothelial cells.

PMNs are present in the wound within a few hours and their numbers increase during the first 24–48 hours. Macrophages, arising by local proliferation and from circulating blood monocytes, are present within 24 hours and both cell types act to remove cellular debris, foreign material and bacteria by phagocytosis. PMNs prevent infection and remove necrotic tissue but their role is not essential to tissue repair as clean wounds will heal in the absence of PMNs. Macrophages are critical to wound healing and reduction in their numbers will slow or stop wound healing. Part of this central role is due to the secretion by macrophages of growth factors which stimulate proliferation of fibroblasts, endothelial cells and smooth muscle cells and extracellular matrix deposition by fibroblasts. These processes start after three to four days and are characteristic of phase 2 of wound healing.

### Phase 2: cell proliferation and matrix formation

As tissue debris and clot are removed, fibroblasts migrate into the wound, endothelial migration and proliferation produce new capillaries, and matrix synthesis of collagen, proteoglycans and glycoproteins occurs. Production of this vascular 'granulation tissue' occurs in all adult wound healing — it is prominent in open wounds left to heal by secondary intention, but less obvious in incised, primarily repaired wounds. Epithelial migration and proliferation re-establishes epidermal continuity and the clot covering the surface of the wound is lost. As matrix production, and particularly collagen synthesis, continues the mechanical strength of the wound increases, with approximately 50% of the normal strength of skin regained by six weeks after injury.

### Phase 3: matrix remodelling

For practical purposes a wound is healed by the end of phase 2, but significant changes occur during phase 3, which is prolonged and in children may last two or more years. The scar becomes less vascular and less cellular, while collagen synthesis and degradation continue. Reorientation of collagen fibrils occurs and the tensile strength of the scar increases (although not to the level of undamaged tissue). However, the normal tissue structure is not restored and because of its inelastic nature the scar may cause long-term problems by restricting function and growth.

## Wound contracture

In wounds where tissue loss has occurred, which are left to heal by secondary intention, contraction of granulation tissue in the wound reduces the size of the tissue defect. There is some evidence that the cell responsible for this process is the myofibroblast — a fibroblast with contractile properties — although the exact role of this cell is unresolved. Although reducing the size of the tissue deficit is of benefit in wound healing, the distortion and scar formation produced by the process inhibit function in certain areas of the body (particularly on the face and around joints).

## WOUND MANAGEMENT

Wound closure aims to restore tissue integrity, while preserving function and minimizing deformity. The basic objective of wound management is to produce optimal conditions in the wound so that uncomplicated healing occurs. As well as direct treatment of the wound, the general condition of the patient will affect wound healing and due consideration needs to be given to the patient's overall care. Malnutrition, present prior to the injury or associated with extensive injuries, will impair wound healing . Anaemia and vascular disease, by impairing oxygen delivery to the wound, will also have an adverse effect. Certain diseases, by altering the balance between host resistance and bacterial invasion, make infection more likely. Uncontrolled diabetes, alcoholism, malignant disease, chemotherapy and immunosuppression all increase the risk of wound infection and subsequent impaired wound healing.

Deciding on the timing and method of wound closure depends on whether the wound is clean or contaminated, and whether or not there is tissue loss. The natural inclination of surgeons is to close a wound at the earliest opportunity. However, immediate closure of a wound is not always required, unless vital structures are exposed, and closure of a wound which is contaminated by bacteria and contains devitalized tissues runs the risk of wound infection, with wound breakdown and further tissue loss. In the worst instances aerobic and anaerobic infections may become life threatening. Infection, foreign bodies and devitalized tissue in the wound all prolong the inflammatory phase of healing and may delay connective tissue formation.

In most traumatic wounds the size and site of the wound does not determine the timing of closure, except in particular cases (see below). There are three alternatives methods of wound closure: primary closure, delayed primary closure and healing by secondary intention.

## Primary closure

Clean wounds are suitable for primary repair, either by direct suture if tissue loss is minimal or by reconstruction with skin grafts or flaps if tissue has been destroyed.

In the strictest sense only non-traumatic, surgical wounds can be considered free of bacterial contamination. However, many traumatic wounds are suitable for primary repair if adequate debridement (see below) and cleansing of the wound are carried out soon after the time of injury.

## Delayed primary closure

In wounds with significant contamination, soft tissue closure should be delayed until four to five days after the injury. Heavily contaminated wounds and those containing devitalized tissue require debridement soon after injury and the wound is then left open, covered with appropriate dressings. In the four to five days after injury the wound develops resistance to infection and may then safely be closed, either by direct suture or by skin graft or flap if there is tissue loss. The nature of the mechanism which produces this enhanced resistance to infection has not been clearly defined, but probably relates to the inflammatory response generated from the time of injury, with increased numbers of PMNs and macrophages present in the wound at the time of delayed closure.

If the wound involves the pleura or peritoneum then these cavities and the overlying muscle can be closed after debridement, with appropriate drainage, and the skin and subcutaneous tissue left open for delayed primary repair. Similarly, wounds exposing vessels, nerves, open joints and tendons may require appropriate primary coverage of these structures, with delayed repair of the overlying skin.

The aim of debridement should be to remove all devitalized tissue, all foreign bodies and all tissue which has been bacterially contaminated. Sharp excision of tissue, under local or general anaesthetic, is the most effective method. The limits of devitalized muscle and skin may be difficult to determine at the initial procedure. Tissue colour, texture, bleeding and, for muscle, contraction when squeezed briefly with forceps, will act as a guide to tissue viability. In the trunk and limbs it may be possible to excise back to obviously healthy tissue, without creating significant functional impairment or producing a wound which requires reconstructive procedures to close. However, if tissue viability is in doubt at the initial exploration or the debridement is less radical in order to preserve potentially viable, vital structures, a further exploration and debridement may be required 48 hours later, prior to delayed primary closure as a third stage.

## Healing by secondary intention

Wound with full-thickness loss of skin and soft tissue will heal slowly, without surgical attempts to appose damaged tissue, by secondary intention. The defect closes by a combination of wound contracture, epithelial migration and connective tissue formation, usually producing significant scar formation. In heavily contaminated wounds this is the safest way to allow wound healing but scar formation restricts its use in the face and hands to small areas of tissue loss. On the trunk and limbs, away from joints, it may be appropriate but the process is slow where there is a significant tissue loss, and modern methods of reconstruction will often allow delayed repair of the defect, improving function and shortening the patient's stay in hospital.

## Facial wounds

Facial and scalp wounds in particular are usually suitable for primary closure, even with significant contamination, as the highly vascular tissues are resistant to infection. For the same reason wound debridement in facial skin can be less extensive than in the limbs or trunk, in order to preserve this specialized tissue and minimize deformity. Injuries with significant tissue loss should be referred for assessment by a reconstructive surgeon soon after the patient's admission, so that an appropriate plan of treatment can be devised.

## Trunk and limb wounds

Modern reconstructive techniques, involving free and pedicled tissue transfers, allow much greater freedom in the management of complex wounds in these areas. Wounds which may have significant tissue loss, exposure of vital structures and heavy contamination used to be difficult to manage, and healing with delayed primary closure or by secondary intention often resulted in gross deformity and loss of function. Transfer of well-vascularized muscle and myocutaneous flaps can allow primary closure of these wounds and greatly improved function. This may involve an extensive surgical procedure early in the patient's treatment, but if the patient's general condition is satisfactory this type of reconstructive surgery will significantly reduce the number of surgical procedures required and reduce the hospital stay for the patient, as well as producing functionally better long-term results. One area in which this approach has been shown to be particularly effective is in the management of open fractures of the lower tibia, reducing the incidence of non-union and osteomyelitis.

The results of reconstructive surgery for these wounds is improved if the surgery is carried out soon after injury, preferably within 48 hours. In order for this to be possible the trauma surgeon needs to anticipate these potential problems and involve a plastic surgeon soon after the patient's admission, preferably at the time of initial assessment of the wound.

## High-velocity wounds

Wounds from handguns are caused by low-velocity bullets and are adequately managed by primary or delayed primary wound closure as outlined above. However, the type of wound produced by high-velocity (high-energy) rifle bullets or weapon fragments requires special consideration. As a high-velocity fragment passes through the body, energy is released and absorbed by the tissues, which are accelerated outwards, destroying a large volume of surrounding tissues and producing a cavity 30–40 times the diameter of the fragment. This cavity is short lived and the pressure within it is sub-atmospheric. As the cavity collapses air, clothing, dirt and bacteria are sucked into it, producing a grossly contaminated wound. The amount of soft tissue damage produced by these weapons relates to the energy absorbed by the tissues and this in turn depends on the nature of the damaged tissue. Elastic tissues, such as skin, and low-density tissue, such as lung, are relatively resistant to damage, while high-density tissue, such as muscle, liver and brain, sustain very extensive damage.

The external appearance of these wounds is deceptive as the entry and exit wounds may be small, because of the skin's elasticity, while the underlying wound is large. Skin excision can be limited to obviously damaged areas but extensive incisions through skin and deep fascia are required to expose the full extent of the wound. In the limbs adjacent tissue compartments may require fasciotomies to prevent the development of compartment syndromes. Careful wound debridement is then carried out, which often requires extensive excision of damaged muscle. Delayed primary closure of the wound is performed and immediate coverage of exposed vital structures may be required, as discussed above.

## Wound drainage

If the appropriate method of wound closure has been chosen, drainage of soft tissue wounds is usually not required. If good haemostasis is not possible in a wound closed primarily (which is unusual) then closed suction drainage may be required. Communication of the wound with the peritoneal or pleural cavities may require appropriate drainage of these areas. Wounds closed by delayed primary repair should not require drainage.

## Antibiotic prophylaxis

Adequate wound debridement and appropriate choice of wound closure are the main factors in preventing wound infection, but antibiotics may be required because of the nature of the wound or because of pre-existing conditions which make a patient more susceptible to infection. A decision to use antibiotics should be based on an assessment of the degree of contamination of the wound, the patient's general condition, the length of time between injury and wound debridement and the type of wound closure involved.

Soft tissue injuries which have been heavily contaminated (particularly if perforation of abdominal viscera has occurred), injuries exposing fractures or open joints and injuries which breach the dura usually require antibiotics. Coexisting diseases, which alter the body's defence mechanisms, as discussed above, will make infection more likely.

A short course of broad-spectrum intravenous antibiotics, started prior to surgical procedures, is usually most effective, as this produces tissue levels which eliminate bacteria from the wound as the tissues are manipulated during debridement and closure. Patients at risk of developing bacterial endocarditis, because of cardiac disease or vascular implants, also require antibiotic prophylaxis.

## Tetanus prophylaxis

Adequate wound debridement and antibiotic prophylaxis in potentially contaminated wounds are important. However, many wounds contaminated by soil are relatively minor and a wound is only identified in 60% of reported cases of tetanus. Active and passive immunization should

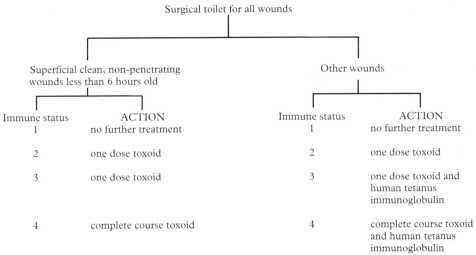

**Categories of immune status**
1  Previous complete course of toxoid or a booster dose within last 5 years
2  Previous complete course of toxoid or a booster dose between 5 and 10 years ago
3  Previous complete course of toxoid or a booster dose 10 years ago
4  No complete course of toxoid or immune status unknown

**Fig. 5.5.1** Tetanus prophylaxis. Reproduced by permission of Butterworth-Heinemann Ltd.

therefore be considered in all patients with contaminated wounds. A suitable system for non-immune patients is given in (Fig 5.5.1.)

**Wound dressings**

New materials and technologies are providing an ever-changing variety of wound dressings, each aimed at specific types of wounds. These dressings may have beneficial effects on wound healing but many of the manufacturers' claimed benefits have yet to be effectively proven. Choosing the most appropriate dressing for a particular wound requires assessment of the requirements of the wound and knowledge of the properties of the dressing.

Wound dressings may have a physiological role, to provide an optimal wound environment, a physical role to protect the wound and a psychological role to shield the wound from the patient. To optimize the microenvironment in a wound the ideal wound dressing would have several properties, including the following:

1. Allow gaseous exchange while maintaining high humidity in the wound. This maintains $PO_2$ and pH at appropriate levels, while epithelialization proceeds more rapidly in a moist environment.

2. Remove wound exudate containing cellular debris. Excess wound exudate makes bacterial infection more likely and the presence of foreign material prolongs the inflammatory phase of healing.

3. Maintain wound temperature close to body core temperature. This allows mitosis and phagocytosis to proceed at optimal levels.

4. Be impermeable to bacteria.

5. Be non-adherent, non-allergenic and free from toxic and particulate contaminants. Adherent dressings damage new epithelium when they are changed and by causing further tissue damage they prolong the inflammatory phase of wound healing. Toxic and particulate contaminants in the dressing will also prolong the inflammatory phase.

6. Conform to wound contour.

The present range of wound dressings combines these properties to varying degrees. Further developments in dressings will be made in these areas but a new generation of dressings will probably be biologically interactive with the wound. The incorporation of components of the extracellular matrix and growth factors into dressings may allow manipulation of the healing process in order to increase the rate and quality of normal wound healing and improve the treatment of chronic wounds.

---

## PART 5.6
# THE MANAGEMENT OF HEAD INJURIES
## R. A. C. Jones

---

'Care more for the individual patient than for the special features of the disease'
*Sir William Osler*

Head injury, as a disease entity or pathological process, proves difficult to define accurately, covering as it does a wide spectrum of injury to the scalp, skull, orbital and facial anatomy, and to the central nervous system. A practical definition, covering those areas with which the surgeon is concerned when faced with a 'head injury', is 'trauma which carries some risk of damage to the brain', since management is directed towards mitigating the effects of the injury on the brain, so preventing further damage, promoting as full a recovery as possible.

Epidemiologically, head injury is an important entity because of its prevalence amongst the young, especially males, in most societies, both developed and developing, providing the leading cause of death and disability below the age of 45 years. Thus, of deaths due to accident, head injury is the immediate cause in 70%; males account for 70% of accidents.

Head injury is unpredictable in its early course; one may not categorize, or give a grade of severity to, the majority of injuries, in the early post-traumatic phase, since a complication may dramatically alter the further course, and the outcome. The unpredictability of head injury makes any form of 'triage' unreliable, since the apparently trivial injury may cause death, from cerebral compression, or other secondary complication, while an apparently severe head injury at the outset may (especially in the young) attain a better level of recovery than initially predicted. Thus, each patient demands individual attention and careful assessment, with prompt intervention where indications arise. There is no process with which the surgeon deals which carries a greater number of potential pitfalls; perhaps no treatment more rewarding than the timely relief of a life-threatening complication. The ubiquity of head injury demands a knowledge on the part of all surgeons of its management.

## Definitions

*Minor head injury.* An injury giving rise to no, or brief, amnesia for events surrounding the blow or incident. The patient, having recovered from the immediate effects, should at no point during observation be worse than confused. The definition requires modification in certain specific injuries, producing localized damage, e.g. depressed skull fracture.

*Major head injury.* An injury giving rise to coma from the moment of injury, and persisting over the ensuing 6 hours or more, with or without any complicating secondary phenomena.

*Retrograde amnesia (RA).* The time interval between the subject's last recollection and the time of injury; an unreliable indicator of severity.

*Post-traumatic amnesia (PTA).* Widely accepted as a good guide to the severity of injury, as judged at the outset of treatment, in those with seemingly minor and moderate injuries. The interval can be assessed by observers, as the interval from impact (usually identifiable) to the point at which a fully alert state is achieved.

*Glasgow Coma Score (GCS).* Widely accepted method of evaluating a patient's neurological function at all stages after injury, avoiding ambiguity of former descriptions, e.g. 'semi-conscious', 'drowsy', allowing clear distinction between an alert state, with speech, and all stages of altered activity to unresponsiveness. Its strength lies in simplicity, multi-disciplinary application, and ease of recording. Its weakness in infants and small children is self-evident, commanding special vigilance in treating the very young.

*Secondary injury.* The primary injury sustained by the brain at the moment of impact seldom causes immediate death. A severe acceleration–deceleration injury may cause irrecoverable brain stem damage, death ensuing within several hours, but more commonly deterioration is caused by secondary phenomena. These include hypoxaemia and ischaemia, brain oedema or compressive intracranial haematoma, or a combination of these. Such secondary effects may be preventable or treatable.

*Multiple injuries.* In respect of head injury this implies major injury to at least one other system, involving the chest or abdomen, spine, or limbs. The importance lies in the effect on mortality rate, through difficulties of diagnosis in the comatose patient and in the effect on overall management.

*Closed head injury.* Injury to the head with or without skull fracture (linear, depressed, basal) with no clinical evidence of communication with the exterior. The majority of severe acceleration — deceleration injuries are of this type. There may be extensive scalp, facial or orbital bruising, but the absence of cerebrospinal fluid (CSF) fistula via the nose or ear, or the absence of laceration communicating with a vault fracture, implies no risk of contamination of the intracranial contents.

*Open head injury.* One in which there is evidence of communication with the exterior, heightening the risk of infection. Such communication may be via a breech in the scalp overlying a fracture, or via the skull base, made evident by frank CSF fistula (via nose or ear) or by radiological evidence of intracranial air (aerocoel).

*Depressed skull fracture.* This may be closed or open (compound). It is commoner in blunt injury to the head, less common in traffic accidents, and noted for the focal nature of the cerebral damage. Thus such patients may not show the deep levels of coma seen in more diffuse brain injury, and an alert state may be at variance with the apparently extensive nature of the injury at first assessment. Minor degrees of depression of the skull contour, i.e. no more than the thickness of the skull vault on a suitable X-ray projection, may require no active treatment, especially if the scalp is intact. More extensive depression requires intervention.

*Intracranial haematoma (ICH).* A major cause of deterioration after injury, especially in those patients whose initial (primary) injury seemed minor. Haematoma may form anywhere within the cranium, be arterial or venous in origin, lie extra- or subdurally or lie within the cerebral (or cerebellar) parenchyma. Acute extradural haematoma, from middle meningeal arterial bleeding, occurs characteristically after an apparently minor head injury with full recovery of consciousness before deterioration. It constitutes one of the most urgent of neurosurgical interventions. Acute subdural haematoma occurs, conversely, in those usually suffering a more severe primary injury, with altered consciousness from the outset, but such acute, usually venous, bleeding may allow, as in extradural haematoma, a lucid or relatively lucid interval during which the patient may talk.

## MANAGEMENT OF HEAD INJURY

### Initial assessment

The time of the incident and the mode of injury provide a useful guide in predicting the immediate course of the injury process. Local examination of the head and neck, and examination of other systems, will be modified by knowledge of the mode of the injury. All road accident injuries require full and careful examination, looking particularly for injury to other systems. Conversely, assault and many industrial injuries remain confined to the head, where depressed fracture is relatively commoner.

Neurological examination should record the level of awareness, or depth of coma, the pupillary signs, and lateralizing neurological signs in the limbs. Of particular importance is the presence or absence of speech, and the quality of such speech, as designated in the Glasgow Coma Scale.

**Table 5.6.1**    Guidelines for the management of patients with head injury

---

A. Criteria for skull X-ray after recent head injury

The presence of one or more of the following indicates the need for a skull x-ray in patients with a history of recent head injury:

1. Loss of consciousness or amnesia at any time
2. Neurological symptoms or signs
3. Cerebrospinal fluid or blood from the nose or ear
4. Suspected penetrating injury or scalp laceration, bruising or swelling
5. Alcohol intoxication
6. Difficulty in assessing the patient (e.g. the young, epilepsy)

---

B. Criteria for hospital admission after recent head injury

The presence of one or more of the following:

1. Confusion or any other depression of the level of consciousness at the time of examination
2. Skull fracture
3. Neurological signs or significant headache or persistent vomiting
4. Difficulty in assessing the patient (e.g. alcohol, the young, epilepsy)
5. Other medical conditions (e.g. haemophilia)
6. The patient's social conditions or lack of responsible adult/relative

Note:
a. Post-traumatic amnesia with full recovery is *not* an indication for admission
b. Patients sent home should be given written instructions about possible complications and appropriate action

---

C. Criteria for consultation with a neurosurgical unit

Presence of one or more of the following:

1. Deterioration
2. Depression of the level of consciousness *or* focal neurological signs *or* fits with or without skull fracture
3. Disorientation or other neurological disturbance persisting for more than 12 hours even if there is no skull fracture
4. Coma continuing after resuscitation
5. Suspected open injury of the vault or the base of the skull
6. Depressed fracture of the skull

**Table 5.6.2**    Guidelines for the management of patients with head injury

| | | |
|---|---|---|
| Well orientated | | Home with head injury sheet and to care of responsible relative |
| | | *or* if no responsible relative, ADMIT |
| Well orientated with:    Skull X-ray:<br>a. scalp laceration,    not positive<br>   bruising or swelling,<br>   or | | HOME with head injury sheet and to care of responsible relative |
| b. Clinical signs of closed fracture,<br>   or | | *or* if no responsible relative, ADMIT |
| c. Known loss of consciousness,<br>   or | | |
| d. Amnesia    positive | | ADMIT — OBSERVE |

| | | |
|---|---|---|
| 1. Disorientated<br>   or worse, or    Skull X-ray: | | ADMIT |
| 2. Alcohol/difficult to assess, or | | Consult neurosurgeons |
| 3. Stable focal signs | | |
| 4. Open skull fracture<br>   (CSF or blood from nose,<br>   ear or wound) | | |
| 5. Severe headache | | |
| 6. Persistent confusion for<br>   12 hours | | |

| | | |
|---|---|---|
| 1. Deteriorating<br>   consciousness | | Urgent referral to neurosurgeons |
| 2. Developing focal signs | | |
| 3. Dilating pupil, slowing<br>   pulse, rising blood<br>   pressure | | |

## Special points

'Confusion' may prove to be dysphasia, and therefore of localizing value, particularly in blunt injury to the dominant hemisphere, usually left.

Minor asymmetry of signs in the limbs, for instance reflex asymmetry, is of relatively little value in the overall assessment of the patient.

View the fundus if the degree of any orbital haematoma allows, but the absence of papilloedema is of little help. Never dilate the pupils artifically for fundoscopy.

The examination of children requires modification, and the degree of cooperation is of little value, since a small child may be uncooperative though alert. The presence of extensor plantar responses below the age of 18 months of age is a normal finding.

In states of altered awareness, certain signs may not be elicited, because of the absence of patient cooperation. Thus visual field defects, and sensory deficit in the limbs cannot be assessed without patient cooperation.

Take note of previous alcohol intake, and make due allowance, though always erring on the side of caution.

Subsequent management after first assessment may be dictated by the observance of guidelines provided for management, (Table 5.6.1, summarized in Table 5.6.2). but take an early opportunity to commence an observation chart, especially noting the presence or absence of speech.

Skull X-ray is of special value when either blunt or penetrating injury is suspected, particularly in assault, and when injury involves the orbit or face. All open injuries require skull X-ray.

X-ray the cervical spine on all closed acceleration–deceleration injuries. Portable films are to be discouraged, but pay due attention to the patient's clinical course while visiting the X-ray department, since deterioration can occur during this period, when observation may be less than satisfactory.

## INTERVENTION

After initial assessment of severity, resuscitation carries a high priority. The airway must always be secured, if necessary by tracheal intubation. The circulation must be assessed, with due consideration of the rarity (except in children) of hypotension due to intracranial events; falling blood pressure raises the likelihood of blood loss in another territory.

In the comatose patient, intracranial events have a relatively low priority against securing the airway and establishing the full extent of any associated injuries. Priority should be given to the security of the patient for transfer, between departments or hospitals. Plain and computed X-ray examination should not be undertaken hastily, until stability is achieved, except in those patients showing rapid deterioration after being accessible to speech.

### Operations

*Wound toilet.* This is desirable where there is extensive scalp or facial laceration, even when a subsequent operation is likely, this being preferable to allowing undue bleeding or spread of contamination. In the case of persisting coma, after resuscitation and X-ray examination, including CT scan, the further care lies in the ambit of the intensive care unit or neurosurgical high-dependency area. Subsequent treatment is undertaken in collaboration with experienced anaesthetists, with the placing of a device for the monitoring of intracranial pressure, and treatment by mannitol, ventilation continuing until it is deemed safe to allow the patient spontaneous respiration.

*Extradural heamatoma.* This is best relieved by craniotomy, after CT scan has identified the lesion, in a typical temporal location, or in a more unusual frontal or parietal site. Hence the value of CT scanning. Where deterioration is rapid, and facilities preclude such scanning, intervention must be based on clinical and radiological localization — scalp bruising, ipsilateral pupillary enlargement, lateralized vault fracture; craniotomy remains the preferred operation, after initial burr-hole relief of intracranial hypertension, in the line of the proposed craniotomy. Craniectomy affords less satisfactory access and an inferior cosmetic outcome.

*Acute subdural haematoma.* This demands generous craniotomy, since evacuation of the haematoma will often expose the need for cortical haemostasis or resection (e.g. frontal or temporal lobectomy). The benefits of such decompression may be considered to be enhanced in certain situations by the exclusion of the bone flap during withdrawal.

*Depressed skull fracture.* This seldom requires hasty intervention. Open depressed fracture of the vault requires judicious toilet, debridement, exploration and repair of any dural laceration, removal of any foreign material, and, frequently, primary cranioplasty using the (cleaned) bone fragments. Subsequent late cranioplasty is thus avoided in many cases, given modern antibiotic cover. Such an antibiotic regime, covering operation and the first postoperative week, would be cefuroxime 1.5 g i.v., t.d.s. or flucloxacillin 1 g i.v. and ampicillin 1 g q.d.s.; attitudes to antibiotic philosophy vary, and advice from a microbiologist is advised. Repair of basal CSF fistulae is an elective neurosurgical procedure, when persisting leakage is confirmed by investigation using CT scanning and CSF enhancement.

*Post-traumatic hydrocephalus.* This requires elective investigation and the placing of a suitable shunt; attitudes differ as to type and timing.

## PITFALLS IN MANAGEMENT

1. The alcohol factor — the frequency of the association between alcohol intake and head injury — demands vigilance, and the exclusion of alcohol as a reason for clinical deterioration.

2. Lack of information about the injury — especially in blunt injury about the head; orbital, and (occasionally) pharyngeal penetration.

3. The seemingly trivial childhood injury, with little or no external stigma, and no radiological evidence of fracture. Extradural haematoma may be mistaken for an intercurrent childhood ailment.

4. Non-accidental injury, usually in infants, where the stated mode of injury seems unlikely to have produced the injury noted, or where there is inconsistency in the account provided.

5. Injury to another system, especially bleeding in the chest or abdomen, producing unexpected hypotension.

6. Intercurrent medical condition, for instance spontaneous intracranial haemorrhage, occurring perhaps during a fracas, simulating major head injury.

7. A patient with an apparently minor head injury who having been discharged, returns to the accident department with headache, or unexpected behavioural disturbance, e.g. confusion, incontinence. Such patients require scanning.

8. Occipital fissure fracture should raise the possibility of posterior fossa haematoma; although rare, when they occur — especially in childhood — deterioration can be abrupt.

9. Early post-traumatic epilepsy, especially in children, may be confused with deterioration from secondary phenomena, especially compression by haematoma.

10. Injury to the vertex of the skull, with or without depressed fracture, may produce a venous injury to the sagittal sinus. An extradural haematoma at the vertex should be treated conservatively if the clinical state allows, and a depressed fracture at the vertex should be treated with great caution. Operative venous haemorrhage from the sagittal sinus may be catastrophic.

11. An apparent disproportionate weakness in the upper limbs, unassociated with other focal abnormality, may be due to brachial plexus injury, especially in motor-cycle accidents.

While those with major injuries, and especially those who require operative intervention, receive adequate follow-up as an out-patient and rehabilitation where required, those with minor and moderate head injury are commonly dismissed without arrangements for review, and left to make their own way back to their previous level of activity. Since injury to the head gives rise to much post-traumatic symptomatology, with psychological and social implications, those recovering from such injuries should be seen and counselled and appropriate steps taken to secure their return to their former level of activity.

### FURTHER READING

Report of the working party on head injuries. R.C.S. England June 1986

Teasdale G, Galbraith S 1980 Acute traumatic intracranial haematoma. In-progress in neurological surgery, Vol. 10. Karger, Basel.

Teasdale G, Jennett B, 1974 Assessment of coma and impaired consciousness: a practical scale. Lancet ii : 81–84

Jennett B, Teasdale G, 1980 Management of head injuries. Davies, Philadelphia

## PART 5.7
# SPINAL FRACTURES
## *R. A. Cowie*

### Instance and aetiology

Of the 10–15 per million of the population who suffer significant spinal cord injury in the UK each year, 55% occur in the cervical, 35% in the thoracic and 10% in the lumbar regions of the spine. Approximately 55% are due to road traffic accidents, where injuries to motor-cyclists are twice as common as car occupants. Accidents which occur at home, or at work, account for 22% of admissions, sporting activities 18% and assault 5%. Analysis of fatalities after road traffic accidents indicate that 20% have severe spinal cord injury, often in the upper cervical spine.

## Management at scene of accident

The spinal cord is at risk of further injury if the handling of the patient is less than optimal. The patient must be supervised while he is extracted from the scene of the accident, transferred to hospital and throughout the period of clinical and radiological evaluation until the spine has been stabilized.

Patients who are conscious may complain of neck or back pain and, on occasion, pain originating from nerve root compression. The victim may complain of sensory disturbance and weakness whose neurological level corresponds to the site of the spine injury.

With the unconscious patient, spinal injury should be suspected if the mechanism of injury indicates the neck has been at risk, or if there is evidence of an impact on the head. The head and neck should be kept in a neutral position, avoiding flexion, extension or rotation through gentle longitudinal traction. If cardiopulmonary resuscitation or intubation is required then an assistant should maintain gentle traction during laryngoscopy. Otherwise the unconscious patient can be rolled into the lateral position with the head supported to keep the neck in a neutral alignment. Avoid the three-quarter prone position as this induces rotation of the neck. Undertake rapid assessment of respiratory function, patency of the airway and associated abdominal or limb injuries. In patients who have sustained spinal cord trauma, narcotic analgesics can critically depress respiration, and orotracheal suction may stimulate a vagal reflex and aggravate bradycardia.

The patient is transferred after the application of a spinal board with an integral head and neck splint. Alternatively, a collar can be employed. During transfer, it is important to monitor the adequacy of ventilation and to keep the patient warm to avoid hypothermia.

## Management at receiving hospital

A full history should be obtained from the patient, witnesses of the accident and the ambulance crew. A thorough general examination is then necessary as spinal injuries are often associated with multiple trauma; 20% have severe head injuries, 15% chest injuries and a few abdominal injuries. The assessment of intra-abdominal trauma in those who have high spinal cord injury is difficult because of paralysis of the abdominal wall muscles and a secondary ileus, obscuring conventional signs. Peritoneal lavage should be considered.

Specific signs of spinal injury include evidence of local abrasion or bruising, a gibbus or widening of the interspinous gap. Priapism may be present when the spinal cord lesion is above the sacral neurological segments.

Careful neurological evaluation is necessary to assess the level and extent of the cord damage. Record light touch, pinprick and joint position sensitivity, taking care to include the perineum. Record motor power according to the Medical Research Council Scale, and also limb, abdominal wall, anal and bulbocavernous reflexes.

## Radiological evaluation

The patient should be supervised directly by a doctor who ensures that the whole of the spine is kept in the neutral position. Good-quality films are necessary and this may mean transfer of the patient to the X-ray department. A lateral view of the cervical spine generally reveals a fracture or dislocation. Scrutinize the alignment of the vertebral bodies and the normal lordotic curve which is formed by the posterior aspects of the vertebral bodies. A crush fracture and subluxation may be revealed. The width of the gap between the spinous processes may be increased if there is a torn intraspinous ligament. A prevertebral haematoma (soft tissue shadow greater than 5 mm) may indicate an underlying fracture. A unilateral locked-facet joint produces a degree of rotation of the spine above the level of injury. It is most important that the whole length of the cervical spine should be displayed; this may require downward traction of the arms by an assistant during the X-ray.

Examination of the craniocervical junction should include a transoral view to help diagnose a fracture of the atlas, the odontoid peg, or axis. On occasion, the spinal cord can suffer damage after hyperextension injury without fracture or subluxation, particularly in elderly patients who have degenerative spondylosis and a small spinal canal.

The thoracic and lumbar spine should be X-rayed with lateral and anteroposterior views. Pay attention to the presence of a paravertebral haematoma.

Computed tomography of the injury produces much useful additional information, including the display of the cervicothoracic region.

## Management of spinal injury

### Cervical spine

Patients with an unstable fracture dislocation will require reduction and stabilization via skull traction. Restoration of the dislocation relieves neurological compression and splints the spine.

### Thoracolumbar injuries

The majority of patients are managed without surgery, using pillows to make a contoured surface on which the patient lies. This allows restoration of the normal alignment of the spine. However, certain fractures may be dealt with by open reduction and fixation using a spinal rod system. There is little evidence that this offers any advantage to neurological recovery, though when the lesion is incomplete and there is evidence of compression of neural tissue by bone fragments, open decompression, reduction and fixation may be advantageous.

## Complications of cord injury

### Respiratory complications

Impairment of respiratory function is common after injury to the cervical spinal cord, through paralysis of the intercostal muscles, or the anterior horn cells of the phrenic nerve (C3, 4, 5).

Associated thoracic injuries, such as rib fractures or pulmonary trauma, may be present. Patients who are paralysed have difficulty expectorating mucus, so that partial collapse of the lung and ventilation–perfusion disorders are common. Hypoxia can lead to cardiac arrest. Patients at risk should have continuous monitoring of oxygen saturation, chest X-ray and bronchoscopy as needed.

### Cardiovascular complications

When the sympathetic outflow has been interrupted by spinal cord injury, the resting vagal tone produces bradycardia and hypotension. Excessive intravenous fluid administration will cause pulmonary oedema. Pharyngeal suction stimulates the vagus and aggravates bradycardia and liability to cardiac arrest. Atropine treatment may be required. These problems are aggravated when the vasomotor paralysis leads to hypothermia.

### Urinary tract

Insert a small-bore urinary catheter to avoid over-distension of the atonic bladder. Later a suprapubic catheter or intermittent self-catheterization may be used as alternatives. There is an increased risk of bladder calculi in paraplegic patients because of hypercalciuria secondary to paralysis and immobility. Urinary catheters should be changed regularly. It is most important to avoid urinary infection wherever possible, so that ascending infection and chronic damage can be prevented.

### Gastrointestinal complications

Paralytic ileus develops in the first few days after injury and oral fluids should be withheld. A nasogastric tube will be required to reduce gastric distension and pressure on the diaphragm. Acute peptic ulceration with haematemesis or perforation is occasionally encountered; shoulder pain may be the only clinical complaint.

### Thromboembolism

There is a high risk of deep venous thrombosis

and pulmonary embolism in the early phases of para- or tetraplegia. It is the commonest cause of death in those who survive the initial injury. Prophylaxis with subcutaneous heparin and anti-thromboembolism stockings should be considered.

*Skin pressure sores*

Ischaemic necrosis of the skin occurs as the result of unrelieved pressure, usually at bony prominences, such as heel, sacrum, ischial tuberosity and the greater trochanter. Patients should be turned every 2 hours manually or on a mechanical bed or Stryker frame. The sore may affect skin, fat, muscle or deep structures. Excision and plastic reconstruction may be required. Joint contractures should be prevented by physiotherapy and splintage.

## Transfer to spinal unit

The specialized facilities needed for the lifelong care of patients with spinal cord injury are concentrated at supra-regional spinal cord centres. Here the specialized nursing, physiotherapy, occupational therapy and social support services can be provided. The majority of patients are able to return to their homes and rejoin society.

## Prognosis for recovery

Approximately one-third of patients with high complete lesions die within 12 months of the injury. It is difficult to forecast recovery in partial lesions, though improvement may continue for several years. Principal causes of morbidity and mortality are renal failure, pressure sores and respiratory infections.

FURTHER READING

Bedbrook GM (ed) 1981 The care and management of spinal cord injuries. Springer-Verlag, New York
Bedbrook GM (ed) 1985 Lifetime care of the paraplegic patient. Churchill Livingstone, Edinburgh
Grundy D, Russell J, Swain A 1986 ABC of spinal cord injury. British Medical Journal Publications, London

## PART 5.8
# MAXILLOFACIAL INJURIES
*R. Lloyd*

## Signs and symptoms

*Fractures of the zygomatic complex*

These injuries frequently present with bruising and oedema around the eye — 'black eye'. Subconjunctival haemorrhage will be present with any fracture involving the orbital walls. Numbness over the distribution of the infraorbital nerve is usually present, and step deformities and flattening of the cheek prominence may be palpable.

Isolated orbital fractures may cause restriction of ocular movements and diplopia due to trapping of extraocular muscles.

*Fractures of the middle third of the facial skeleton*

These injuries commonly occur at three classical levels, described by the French surgeon, Le Fort (Fig. 5.8.1). At the lower level, the Le Fort I fracture line is transverse, from above the alveolar ridge to the pterygoid region. There may be only swelling of the upper lip and mobility of the maxilla when it is gripped between finger and thumb and gently moved forwards. The upper and lower teeth may not meet correctly on biting.

The Le Fort II fracture extends from the nasal bones into the medial orbital wall and crosses the infraorbital rim. The Le Fort III fracture is the most severe, and the central third of the face is detached from the cranial base. In these higher-level fractures bruising and swelling around the eyes will be present. Subconjunctival haemorrhage is often seen and nasal haemorrhage and cerebrospinal fluid rhinorrhoea may be profuse. The maxilla will be mobile, as above.

*Fractures of the mandible*

These can occur at several common sites (Fig. 5.8.2), notably though the neck of the condylar process, between the posterior alveolar margin and the angle, and anteriorly between the alveo-

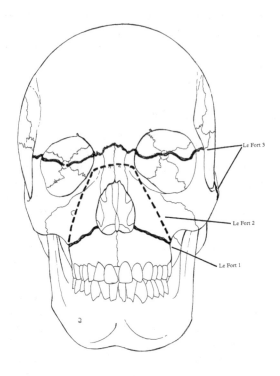

**Fig. 5.8.1**  Common sites of fracture of the midface.

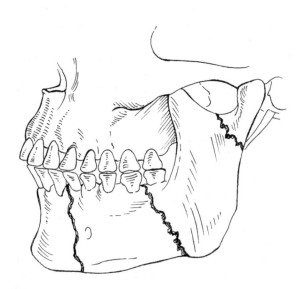

**Fig. 5.8.2**  Common sites of fracture of the mandible.

lar margin anterior to the premolar teeth to the lower border of the mandible. They may be unilateral or bilateral. Bruising and swelling over the fracture site will be present. Haemorrhage from the mouth or rarely the ear may occur. Crepitus and mobility can be demonstrated on palpation across the fracture site and a sublingual haematoma may be present. Numbness of the lower lip on the affected side and difficulty occluding the teeth are common findings.

### Radiology

Detailed radiography may not be possible in the initial stages of management of the multiply injured patient, and should be deferred until the patient is stabilized. If, however, a computed tomographic scan is being performed for suspected intracranial damage, views of the facial bones on the scan may be obtained.

For mid-face fractures of the maxilla and zygomatic region, occipitomental views are required, as well as a lateral skull radiograph. For the mandible, lateral obliques and a postero-anterior view are necessary, or if available an orthopantomogram.

---

PART 5.9
## UROLOGICAL INJURIES
*J. B. Garland*

---

Urological injury is rarely life threatening but frequently has long-term complications. It is rarely an isolated injury and is frequently associated with orthopaedic and abdominal trauma. Close cooperation with specialist colleagues in assessment, planned investigation and ultimately surgery is necessary.

### General principles of management

1. Clinical assessment of shock and establishment of baselines
2. Look for bruising over the kidney, and the perineum in urethral injuries, tissue swelling in scrotal injuries, bleeding at the

external meatus in urethral injuries. Feel for tenderness in the renal angle with capsular haematoma, and rigidity and guarding over a ruptured bladder

3. Radiological investigation in trauma
   a. Intravenous urography (IVU) is essential to establish function, non-function or partial function of kidneys, and anatomical integrity of the kidneys, ureters and bladder
   b. Urethrogram and cystogram for suspected urethral and bladder injury to identify the site of damage
   c. Ultrasonic scanning (U/S) is a useful ancillary investigation to confirm injury and identify collections of blood and urine in perirenal collections and full bladders

4. Principles of surgery
   a. To control haemorrhage, including nephrectomy for severely damaged kidney, and evacuate clot
   b. Provision of drainage to prevent the accumulation of urine and blood, which can lead to abscess formation and subsequent Gram-negative septicaemia
   c. Stenting (splinting) of anastomosis; positioning an indwelling stent (a special ureteric catheter) or a urethral catheter channels urine through an anastomosis and stops leakage and morbidity

5. Long-term follow-up of patients for late complications
   a. Hypertension and non-function in renal injuries
   b. Frequency and urgency in bladder injuries
   c. Impotence and stricture formation in urethral injuries.

## Kidney and ureter

The kidney is covered by perinephric fat and is enclosed in Gerota's fascia. Traumatic bleeding will be limited if this is intact. Capsular haematoma is also limited by the intact capsule. The kidney is retroperitoneal, and if bleeding occurs to any degree structures are difficult to identify and nephrectomy is often required to control bleeding. A preoperative IVU is therefore absolutely necessary.

Isolated kidney injuries are commonly sports injuries. Major trauma is likely to be associated with intra-abdominal rupture of viscus and bowel, haemopneumothorax, multiple fractures and brain injury, and renal injury is usually a minor consideration.

## Bladder and membranous urethra

These injuries are undoubtedly the commonest form of urological trauma and need to be considered together, as the mode of injury — crush injuries with partial or complete disruption of the pelvic ring — is the same, as is the initial management (cystogram if possible, and IVU) and treatment.

A typical patient will have had a catheter passed while being resuscitated. Clear urine indicates no injury. A small amount of blood-stained urine suggests an extraperitoneal extravasation from a ruptured bladder. No urine indicates intraperitoneal rupture of the bladder. Confirmation is by cystogram. If catheter drainage is established and signs are minimal there is little indication for exploration. If signs of intra-abdominal injury are present, exploration is necessary after an IVU to indicate the presence and function of one or two kidneys. If no catheter can be passed a urethrogram indicates the site of obstruction, such as a complete membranous urethral rupture or, surprisingly, contrast passing into the bladder.

Urological surgical treatment takes second place to orthopaedic and general surgical treatment, but opportunity should be taken to establish urethral catheter drainage under a general anaesthetic if not already carried out. If this is impossible, establish suprapubic drainage of the bladder and the prevesical space.

## Anterior urethra

This is common in the construction industry. Falling astride scaffolding, beams and ladders causes pain, swelling and ventral penile bruising over the site of injury. The patient is unable to pass urine with a true rupture and may be distressed. After a lesser injury a submucosal haematoma makes micturition painful and slow but possible. Ideally, a urethrogram would show continuity of the urethra or the site of injury and the degree of extravasation.

Attempt to pass a catheter into the bladder and leave it to drain for seven to ten days. If it will not pass, insert a suprapubic catheter. At a subsequent exploration the haematoma is evacuated, traumatized urethra is excised and oblique anastomosis performed to minimize stricture formation.

## Testis

Surprisingly for an organ that is subcutaneous, rupture of the testis is uncommon. The scrotal position, and cremasteric retraction of the testis with activity, protect the testis from all but a direct injury. The frictionless surface of the tunica vaginalis allows the testis to evade the direct effects of a blunt injury. The type of injury, a large scrotal haematoma and painful testicle are indicative of rupture.

Exploration is mandatory, with evacuation of clot and suture of the tunica albuginea. Testicular atrophy can occur after exploration but is inevitable without it.

## Penis

Fracture of the penis is a rare complication of excessive forcible bending of the erect organ. One or both corpora cavernosa ruptures, producing a large subcutaneous haematoma and detumescence.

Initial catheterization should be followed by anterior exploration, evacuation of the haematoma and suture of the laceration. Fibrosis of the corpora and poor distal erection are likely with conservative treatment but less so with exploration.

---

PART 5.10
# CHEST INJURIES
*J. Bancewicz*

---

## Penetrating injuries

The management of penetrating injuries to the chest clearly depends on what has been injured inside the chest. However, the nature of the injury is itself dependent to a large extent on the instrument that has been used.

### Knives

Fortunately most knife wounds do not produce serious injury. If the thorax has been entered there may be a pneumothorax or haemothorax and the only treatment that is required is a chest drain. Massive or continuing blood loss require thoracotomy. In many cases the bleeding will be from injured intercostal vessels, but clearly all intrathoracic structures are at risk. Wounds in the lower parasternal area or the epigastrium may penetrate the heart, causing cardiac tamponade. Remember that wounds in the lower chest may penetrate the diaphragm.

### Missiles

Missile injuries require more active treatment than most knife wounds. Low-velocity missiles, such as a bullet from a handgun, will probably remain in the chest, whereas high-velocity missiles often pass completely through, leaving a large exit wound and causing severe shock-wave damage which is often fatal. Most modern rifles are high-velocity weapons. Bomb fragments are often propelled at high velocity in the immediate vicinity of the explosion.

High-velocity weapons cause extensive tissue damage beyond what is visibly injured. Extensive debridement of injured tissue is required. Low-velocity missiles that enter the chest should be removed at thoracotomy, followed by conservative debridement. Low-velocity missiles may ricochet within the thorax and lodge in unexpected places far from the entry site. For this reason they may penetrate the diaphragm in the most unexpected circumstances.

### Injury to the oesophagus

The oesophagus is rarely injured by knives or missiles. It is a small target within the chest and if it is injured it is likely that there will be serious injury to the aorta or heart, with fatal consequences.

## Non-penetrating injuries

### Injury to the chest wall

Blunt injury to the chest is much more common than penetrating injury, causing pain and depression of respiration. Hypoxia is a particular hazard in combined head and chest injury.

### Rib fractures

Even 'minor' rib injuries suppress respiration and the ability to cough, threatening the elderly and those with pre-existing lung disease. Fracture of the first rib always indicates a serious injury and is a useful prognostic indicator.

Pain from fractured ribs may be controlled by oral or parenteral analgesics, infiltration with lignocaine, or intercostal nerve blocks.

### Flail chest

There is a mobile section of chest wall with double fractures of several ribs. Although paradoxical respiration, with to and fro movement of air between lungs (pendulluft) occurs, the volume of air that moves in this way is small. More important is the pain and instability of the chest wall that makes respiration and coughing difficult, often accompanied by serious lung contusion. Analgesia, careful fluid balance, physiotherapy and repeated blood gas analysis are important. Treat hypoxia by tracheal intubation and ventilation. Fixation of rib fractures is controversial.

### Fracture of sternum

Sternal fractures are painful, troublesome and often associated with myocardial injury. If displaced they are best dealt with by open reduction and fixation with wires or pins. Cardiac monitoring for dysrhythmia is essential.

### Pneumothorax

Pneumothorax is the commonest complication of chest injury. Treat small ones expectantly. Otherwise insert a chest drain, especially if positive pressure ventilation is required, or when transferring the patient to another hospital.

Tension pneumothorax presents as severe respiratory distress or cardiac arrest. Immediately insert a chest drain. In emergencies insert a widebore intravenous cannula.

Pneumothorax is usually due to minor lung lacerations that seal very quickly. A persistent fistula requires repair.

### Haemothorax

Haemothorax or haemopneumothorax always demands drainage, otherwise infection and empyema develop quickly. Blood in the chest usually defibrinates and remains fluid, but clotted haemothorax demands a limited thoracotomy to evacuate it. Massive or continuing bleeding requires thoracotomy for control.

### Chest drains

Prompt, skilful insertion of a chest drain can be life saving. However, unskilful insertion can be painful and dangerous. Do not insert using sharp trocar points. Make a small incision in the chest wall down to the pleura. Enter the thorax with a haemostat and enlarge the hole to finger size. Now safely introduce the drain.

### Pulmonary contusion

Pulmonary contusion is the commonest complication of injury to the chest wall. Initial X-rays may well be normal. Severe contusion produces hypoxia. Avoid fluid overload and use mechanical ventilation if hypoxia persists.

### Pulmonary laceration

A large laceration may produce marked air leakage or bleeding, requiring thoracotomy.

### Rupture of trachea or bronchus

Rupture of trachea or main stem bronchi may produce dramatic subcutaneous emphysema (the 'Michelin Man' syndrome) or massive intrapleural air leakage. Immediately pass a bronchoscope before passing an endotracheal tube. Tracheal intubation and ventilation increase the leakage from a ruptured bronchus. Thoracotomy and repair is the treatment of choice.

### Rupture of diaphragm

Rupture of the diaphragm is related to increased abdominal pressure rather than thoracic injury, associated with other intra-abdominal injuries. Perform laparotomy, rather than thoracotomy.

## Cardiac Injuries

### Myocardial contusion

Anterior chest injuries often cause myocardial contusion. Cardiac performance, dysrhythmias and ECG signs are similar to infarction. Monitor the patient continuously for a few days and take care with fluid balance.

### Injury to valve structures

Injury to the valves may occur with severe trauma. Rupture of chordae tendinae may cause incompetence of the mitral or tricuspid valves. This may occur several days after injury and the diagnosis may be missed for many months.

### Cardiac tamponade

Cardiac tamponade is most commonly seen after knife injuries since missile injuries, or rupture after blunt trauma, are often fatal. The venous pressure is often raised in a hypotensive patient. Pericardiocentesis may improve the patient for a short time to allow transfer to an operating theatre. However, thoracotomy may be required in the emergency room.

## Injury to thoracic aorta

Rupture of the thoracic aorta may occur in severe deceleration injuries. Most injuries are fatal, but it is possible to survive partial rupture, usually of the descending aorta between the left subclavian artery and the ligamentum arteriosum. Widening of the mediastinum on a chest X-ray may raise

suspicion of the injury. Confirmation of the diagnosis requires aortography and repair should be performed promptly after diagnosis. Cardiac bypass is used by some, but is not essential.

### FURTHER READING

Trinkle J K 1971 Flail chest and pulmonary contusion. In : Trinkle J K, Grover F L (eds) Management of thoracic trauma victims. Lippincott, Philadelphia, pp 39–45

## PART 5.11
# ABDOMINAL INJURIES
*M. Irving*

The injured abdomen, although a relative rarity compared with other injuries, remains a difficult diagnostic area and a source of major morbidity and mortality.

It is traditional to classify abdominal injury into blunt and penetrating and this still stands. On the other hand, advances in imaging and better monitoring of cardiorespiratory status following injury now mean that many traditional techniques for managing abdominal injury have been modified or superseded.

## Mechanisms of blunt injury

There are three principal damaging forces in blunt abdominal injury. The first is direct compression, where the applied force squeezes the viscus between the abdominal wall and the vertebral column, such as can occur with a seat belt injury. The second force is a shearing mechanism that is applied obliquely and affects viscera at points where they are anchored such as at the peritoneal attachments at the duodenojejunal flexure, the spleen and the ileocaecal junction and the vascular attachments of the liver. Finally, there are the bursting forces that occur in viscera at points away from the site of compression, for example at the apex of a loop of bowel . All these forces can combine to produce compression, bruising and ischaemic injury to the abdominal viscera and the abdominal walls, including the diaphragm and the structures in the retroperitoneum.

## Mechanisms of penetrating injury

These injuries are characteristically those seen as the result of war, terrorism and interpersonal violence. Penetrating injury is of two broad types. First, there is the knife injury, commonly resulting from stabbing. Second, there is the firearm injury. Stabbing will tend to produce well-defined injuries largely confined to the track of the offending weapon, with minimal or serious consequences depending upon what has been transgressed. On the other hand, firearms injuries will produce penetration associated with a degree of tissue destruction which varies with the type of shot used and the kinetic energy it dispenses in its passage through the body, according to whether it is high or low velocity.

## General principles of diagnosis

In dealing with any abdominal injury the two major questions to be asked are: is there abdominal visceral injury producing peritonitis and/or haemorrhage sufficient to require operation; and are there defects in the abdominal wall and viscera that need repair? These questions are important now that some bleeding and some disrupted viscera can be managed conservatively. Obviously, ruptured gut causing peritonitis will always require operation to close the defect. As always, the history is of importance when assessing the situation, and in particular an account of the mechanism of the accident is vital. Features particularly worthy of elicitation in the case of motor vehicle accidents are whether or not the victim was wearing a seat belt, the position of passengers within the vehicle, and whether there is a possibility of a distended stomach, uterus or bladder. Injury to the structures above and below the abdomen, i.e. the thorax and the pelvis or femurs, are indicative of a high risk of associated abdominal injury. Once a history has been taken, the patient should receive a thorough physical examination, as described previously, which will elicit clinical evidence of abdominal wall and visceral problems. Special investigations which will aid accurate diagnosis are diagnostic peritoneal lavage, ultrasound, conventional radiography, computerized axial tomography (CAT) scanning and laparoscopy. Increasing sophistication of imaging techniques means that the importance of some of them is changing. While there is no doubt that peritoneal lavage is an extremely sensitive way of detecting blood in the peritoneal cavity, ultrasound is also equally effective and has the additional advantage of demonstrating the organ which is damaged. It also allows an opportunity for assessment of whether or not conservative treatment may be instituted as in the case of a ruptured liver or spleen.

## General principles of treatment of abdominal injuries

Resuscitation and stabilization as described previously are the important first steps. Failure to achieve stabilization, associated with clear evidence of continuing intra-abdominal bleeding such as a distending abdomen, is a definite indication of the need for urgent operation. However, such a situation is unusual and the more likely scenario is that a period of stabilization can be achieved during which diagnostic measures can be undertaken and a treatment plan formulated. Certain injuries formerly routinely operated on can now successfully be treated by a conservative approach combined with strict observation. Thus, a stabbing injury that is associated only with local tenderness around the entry site and without evidence of continuing blood loss or spreading peritonitis can successfully be managed with observation only, unless the above-mentioned complications develop, at which time operation will be necessary. Similarly, as indicated below, ruptured solid viscera which cease to bleed can be managed without operation. On the other hand, continuing haemorrhage, spreading peritonitis, evisceration and defects in the abdominal wall all require immediate surgical repair.

## Abdominal wall injuries

Rupture of the muscles of the anterior abdominal wall can occur spontaneously, when the rectus abdominis tears during coughing or vigorous abdominal exercise. More frequently, the anterior abdominal wall muscles will tear during acute compression by a seat belt in a deceleration injury. Such defects should be suspected when there is circumferential imprinting of clothing marks on the anterior abdominal wall, itself a sign that there is probably associated severe intra-abdominal injury. Palpation of the contracting abdominal wall will usually reveal that the fingers can be inserted into the defect caused by the ruptured muscle.

Rupture of the diaphragm is also a common accompaniment of intra-abdominal compression. It can be difficult to diagnose as the radiological signs may be few if the gut that has been forced through the tear has reduced spontaneously into the abdomen. A high degree of suspicion must always be maintained in patients who have sustained abdominal compression injuries.

## Visceral injuries

The spleen is the most commonly damaged viscus within the abdominal cavity. Damage can vary from minor capsular tears, through lacerations to total fragmentation. It is now recognized that the spleen is an important immunological organ which should be preserved if the rare but lethal condition of overwhelming post-splenectomy infection is to be avoided. Because of this the days when all ruptured spleens were automatically removed have long since passed. There is no doubt that in children even badly damaged spleens will heal spontaneously, provided haemorrhage ceases, and it is now perfectly acceptable to treat an injured spleen in a child by resuscitation and observation as long as one can be assured that there is no accompanying visceral injury that requires operation. The same principle applies in the adult, although operation is more frequently required to control bleeding and repair parenchymal tears. Damaged spleens can be repaired by suture or partial splenectomy. Additionally, techniques have been described to repair even shattered spleens by enclosing them in an absorbable mesh, but this is probably unwise and severely damaged spleens should still be removed. The practice of wrapping splenic fragments in omentum in an attempt to preserve some of their immunological function is now largely discredited as being ineffective and prone to complications.

## Liver injuries

Injury to the liver can vary from simple laceration caused by blunt injury through to fragmentation, cavitation and devascularization. Penetrating injury can result in injuries varying from simple tracks caused by knife blades through to the cavitating lesions caused by a bullet traversing the liver substance, with its associated shock waves. The management of liver injuries has changed radically over recent years. It is now recognized that many, even quite severe injuries, can be treated conservatively, even without operation. Certainly stab wounds and simple lacerations, if they stop bleeding, do not need operation. The availability of accurate imaging using CAT scanning and ultrasound combined with direct visualization of the liver using laparoscopy enable the surgeon to see whether or not conservative management is feasible. Indications for operation include uncontrollable bleeding resulting in persistent hypovolaemic shock, and fragmentation resulting in widespread devitalization. Control of haemorrhage within the liver substance is achieved by suture ligation. Packing of the liver substance to control bleeding, once frowned upon, is now acceptable again. On the other hand, lobectomy to remove a severely damaged lobe is now rarely considered necessary, it being accepted that more conservative measures can be successful. The major problems encountered result from laceration of hepatic veins behind the liver. These difficult injuries are best managed by internal bypass and repair. Delayed haemorrhage can result in haemobilia, with blood draining into the gastrointestinal tract through the biliary tree. Such cases can be treated by interventional radiologists using embolization.

## Pancreas

Damage to the pancreas results either from blunt injury compressing the pancreas against the vertebral column, or from penetrating injury.

Pancreatic injury is often difficult to diagnose and thus is easily missed for several days. Immediate signs are a rise in amylase and the demonstration either on imaging or at operation of an upper abdominal retroperitoneal haematoma.

Treatment of pancreatic injuries involves resection of devitalized tissue, diversion of secretions from the remaining pancreatic tissue into the gastrointestinal tract and widespread drainage of the retroperitoneum.

### Intestine and mesentery

Small and large bowel can be divided either by blunt injury resulting in compression, shearing and laceration, or by penetrating injury. Devitalization of the bowel can result from laceration of the mesentery. Bowel is particularly prone to damage at the points where it transfers from intraperitoneal to retroperitoneal areas, i.e. the duodenojejunal flexure and the ileocaecal junction. Treatment involves resection of the devitalized bowel with end-to-end anastomosis. Primary repair of colonic wounds is acceptable, but where there is gross faecal contamination or extensive associated injury, resection of the damaged bowel with exteriorization of both ends remains the safest policy.

## PART 5.12
# VASCULAR TRAUMA
## *R. Marcuson*

Vascular injuries have occurred throughout history. Wars have always led to trauma. Spears and knives may be sharper and bullets have higher velocity, but other causes of vascular trauma now occur. The appalling incidence of road traffic accident-related trauma remains far too high. Doctors of all specialities may cause iatrogenic vessel damage and drug abusers damage their vessels. We still injure ourselves and each other either deliberately or accidentally, with disastrous consequences to life and limb. The surgeon's ability to repair damage has improved and there is much evidence in the literature to support this. To achieve these results, however, it is clear that early diagnosis and early repair are essential. Whatever the nature of the injury, vascular damage is always a possibility and must *actively* be excluded by appropriate history taking, examination and if necessary specialist investigation.

### AETIOPATHOLOGY

Arteries and veins may be damaged by sharp or blunt trauma. The result is haemorrhage or thrombosis and often a combination of both.

Incised or penetrating wounds occur from bullets or high-velocity projectiles, knife wounds, spears, arrows or by falling or being pushed onto sharp objects. A number of vascular injuries are caused by medical, surgical or radiological interventional procedures. Free bleeding is the rule. Arterial bleeding is pulsating and can be torrential, while venous bleeding tends to well up from the wound. Internal haemorrhage may lead to significant hypovolaemia without any other signs. Alternatively the haemorrhage may be contained within a cavity or fascial compartment with major consequences, for example mediastinal shift due to haemothorax, pericardial tamponade or tracheal compression due to cervical haematoma. Rarely artery and vein are involved in such a way as to produce an arteriovenous fistula leading either to high output cardiac failure or an arteriovenous aneurysm.

Closed injury may be of the deceleration type or direct blunt injury. Deceleration leads either to avulsion of smaller branches of large arteries, for example branches of the superior mesenteric artery near the duodenojejunal junction, or rupture of large vessels at the junction of their free course and a fixed part as at the distal aortic arch/descending thoracic aorta junction.

Blunt injury usually leads to an intimal tear which is a focus for intravascular thrombus formation. Transverse tears may also lead to flap formation. Progression either to distal embolism or total vessel thrombosis is a significant risk. Some 3–5% of carotid artery trauma is said to be due to blunt injury either from direct blows to the neck or from whiplash injury.

## PRINCIPLES OF MANAGEMENT

### History

There is always time to obtain at least a brief history. Valuable information is derived from a knowledge of the mechanism of the injury and the degree of violence involved, the weapon used and the time of the incident.

### Arrest of haemorrhage

External haemorrhage can frequently be controlled by local pressure. Larger vessels, for example the femoral artery in the groin, may rarely require the application of a (vascular) clamp in the accident and emergency department. Tourniquets should be used with care.

Internal haemorrhage may require urgent surgery. Within the thorax, for example, major haemorrhage from the great vessels can demand emergency fourth or fifth space thoracotomy, either from the left or right side, if necessary with a trans-sternal extension. Large De Bakey-type vascular clamps are applied. Great vessel injury may, however, become stable with mediastinal tamponade. Thus mediastinal widening greater than 8 cm on the postero-anterior chest X-ray is an indication for angiography to evaluate aortic integrity.

In abdominal trauma, laparotomy may be required as an emergency. The source of the haemorrhage is usually obvious in such cases. Aortic, renovascular and vena caval haemorrhage may be tamponaded by the retroperitoneum. Proximal and distal vascular control is advisable before exploring the haematoma.

Arrest of venous bleeding can be particularly difficult. After removal of a pack, local control may be obtained by judicious use of two 'swabs on sticks', angled retractors or balloon catheters.

### Correction of blood volume deficit

Major blood loss occurs rapidly in vascular trauma. Rapid volume replacement with appropriate fluids is essential and large-bore peripheral intravenous cannulae are frequently required. Massive blood transfusion may be required and can lead to coagulopathies which require correc-tion with platelets and appropriate clotting factors. Hypothermia may also occur. Adult respiratory distress syndrome (ARDS) may develop in the postoperative period.

### Management of the airway

This is a particular problem associated with neck injuries. Early surgical exploration, usually via a long incision anterior to the sternomastoid muscle, is mandatory for active external haemorrhage and an expanding cervical haematoma. A careful watch must be kept for the development at any stage of laryngeal oedema or tracheal compression.

### Diagnosis and treatment of ischaemia

In limb trauma, either penetrating or blunt, arterial thrombosis may occur. Note that at initial examination the peripheral pulses may be present, only to be lost when the thrombosis occurs — this is an evolving situation and repeated formal examination and pulse recording are necessary.

The assessment of the limb for ischaemia may be difficult. Hypovolaemia leads to a reduction in pulse volume and capillary perfusion which can give the impression of arterial occlusion. Restoration of the circulating volume may lead to reappearance of the pulses. Atherosclerotic occlusion may pre-date the injury. Pain may also cause vasoconstriction. The use of hand-held Doppler probes may also be confusing. Flow can be detected distal to an occlusion due to a collateral circulation and may give false reassurance to the inexperieced user.

The diagnosis of arterial spasm is suspect. This is particularly so where the radial pulse is lost in supracondylar fracture of the humerus, and arterial trauma should be presumed until proven to the contrary. Either the brachial artery has been compressed between the bone fragments or an intimal tear has occurred, leading to thrombosis. If the peripheral circulation does not return following reduction of the fracture, exploration is mandatory.

Basic neurological function, i.e. power and sensation, must also be recorded. Loss of function from the time of injury suggests nerve damage, while later loss may indicate arterial occlusion and ischaemic neurological dysfunction.

Arterial thrombosis will lead to the classical five 'P's, and restoration of flow as soon as possible is essential for optimum recovery. Delay for formal arteriography is probably best avoided — it is very easy to 'lose' another hour. If doubt exists as to the site or the presence of arterial occlusion an 'on-table one-shot' arteriogram is easily and rapidly performed.

At an early stage a decision must be taken with regard to primary amputation. Where the trauma has caused vascular, neurological and severe bone injury this may be the best way to achieve early rehabilitation. In patients with pre-existing vascular disease primary amputation should be particularly considered. An on-table arteriogram may be very helpful here.

In many vascular injuries there is soft tissue and bone injury. Modern fracture management can be very time consuming and it is important to remember that re-establishment of arterial flow takes precedence over all other repairs. It is the time from arterial occlusion which counts and not the time from the start of the surgical procedure. Thus after an appropriate exposure an internal shunt is placed in the artery (and vein if necessary) and held in place by sialastic vessel loops. It is now possible to define more accurately nerve and soft tissue damage. Rigid bone fixation is then carried out, after which the vessel and if necessary nerve repairs are performed.

## Repair of the vessel injury

### Arterial repair

Simple ligation may be the best option. For example, intercostal arteries (the commonest source of vascular injury in chest trauma) can be ligated with impunity. The radial *or* ulnar (but *not* both) can usually be ligated but Allen's test must be performed first. End arteries and all larger arteries cannot be ligated without significant sequelae and must be repaired or bypassed.

Simple transverse injuries can be repaired by direct suture. Interrupted sutures should be used on all arteries smaller than 10 mm in diameter.

Longitudinal clean wounds can be repaired by lateral suture provided no significant narrowing occurs. A vein patch is required for any vessel narrower than 10 mm in diameter. Ragged breaches of the wall or thrombotic occlusions due to intimal damage must be excised back to normal vessel and formally repaired. Vessels greater than 10 mm in diameter may be repaired with Dacron or PTFE prostheses — for very large vessels the risk of infection may have to be accepted and broad-spectrum antibiotic given as appropriate. The recently described rifampicin bonding to gelatin-coated Dacron prostheses may have a place in this situation. In the lower limb, smaller arteries should be repaired with segments of contralateral saphenous vein by interposition or bypass. Cephalic vein from the injured arm may be used in the upper limb. Interrupted sutures should be used for end-to-end anastamoses using three or four-point circumferential stay sutures to prevent distortion.

### Venous repair

Venous injury is present in about 50% of cases of arterial trauma. In general, ligation of smaller veins is well tolerated. The upper limb veins, up to the axillary vein, can usually be ligated without late sequelae. This is not true for the lower limb, where venous repair should be carried out for popliteal vein injury and for all more proximal veins.

Simple tears may be repaired by lateral suture but patching is necessary if any narrowing occurs. Larger veins require composite reconstruction using panels of vein or fashioning a wide-bore tube by spiralling saphenous vein and suturing it over a stent. Externally reinforced PTFE is an alternative but probably not as successful.

There is low pressure within the venous circuit — special care is necessary with suture placement, particularly at end-to-end anastomoses, where interrupted sutures should be used. Systemic anticoagulation to prevent thrombotic failure of venous repairs is indicated but should be used with caution because of potential haemorrhagic complications due to the extent of the trauma. Low-dose heparin prophylaxis should particularly be used in lower-limb cases.

## Management of the soft tissue injury

All dead tissue must be excised at the primary procedure. Quite large amounts of tissue may need to be removed along with all foreign material. The police may require fragments of bullets or embedded material for forensic examination.

In both upper and lower limb vascular injury, reperfusion is often associated with compartment syndromes. Prophylactic compartment decompression should be undertaken.

Soft tissue loss frequently accompanies vascular trauma. Primary cover of vascular anastomoses may not be easily achieved. Muscle rather than skin cover should be provided if at all possible by muscle rotation flaps, covered if necessary by split skin grafts. More extensive tissue loss may require free transfer of myocutaneous flaps using microvascular techniques. If this is not possible in the emergency situation, an antiseptic-soaked pack may be left in the wound but early definitive tissue cover is required.

FURTHER READING

Vascular trauma 1988 Surgical Clinics of North America 68: 4

PART 5.13
# PERIPHERAL NERVE INJURIES
*D. Marsh*

Division of peripheral nerves differs from injuries to other structures in one important respect: it involves transection of cells. The distal portion of the neurone must die, since it has no connection with the cell body, and restitution of a functioning unit can only be achieved by a process of *regeneration*, as opposed to repair. The aims of the surgeon are to optimize the conditions for this biological process to take place, by applying the principles of wound care and causing minimal additional tissue damage to the nerve, and to maximize the benefit from a given level of regenerative response by accurate coaptation of the cut ends and good rehabilitation.

## Structure and function of a peripheral nerve

The neurones making up a nerve trunk are grouped into fascicles. In the more proximal segments there is considerable crossing over and rearrangement between fascicles, but more distally (below the elbow, for example) the fascicular arrangement is constant and predictable, and corresponds to the eventual motor and cutaneous branches. Some nerves, such as the ulnar nerve, have small numbers of well-defined fascicles; others, such as the median nerve, have large numbers of smaller ones.

Understanding the connective tissue framework of the nerve is essential for thinking about nerve repair. The outermost layer is the *epineurium*, whose chief characteristic is its mechanical strength. It is usually in a state of longitudinal tension, which is why the ends of a cut nerve spring apart. Each fascicle is surrounded by *perineurium*; this functions as a blood–nerve barrier and determines the biochemical environment of the nerve tissue. The individual axons are invested in *endoneurium*, which forms conduits guiding each axon to the appropriate end organ.

The nerve is nourished by an internal longitudinal plexus of vessels, fed at intervals by perforators from the adventitia. This plexus becomes occluded if the nerve is subjected to undue tension, otherwise it can support the nerve trunk even when it has been lifted from its bed over quite a distance. The cell body and axonal parts of the neurone communicate with each other chemically by means of a highly efficient, two-way axoplasmic transport system. This carries transmitter substances centrifugally under normal conditions and structural proteins during regeneration after injury. It also carries, to the cell body, signalling molecules from the end organs or from axons which are damaged; these influence the nucleus in its control of the cell.

## Surgical pathology of nerve injury

Blunt trauma to a nerve may produce a temporary block in the conduction of impulses, but leave intact the axonal transport system. The axon distal to the injury does not die and complete functional recovery can be expected; this is *neuropraxia.* More severe trauma will interrupt axonal transport and cause Wallerian degeneration: the distal axon dies, the myelin sheath disintegrates and the Schwann cells turn into scavenging macrophages which remove the debris. The cell body embarks on a pre-programmed regenerative response usually known as chromatolysis, since it involves disappearance of the Nissl granules which are the rough endoplasmic reticulum of the normal cell. An entire new set of ribosomes appear, dedicated to the task of reconstruction, and by their efforts axon sprouts emerge from the axon proximal to the lesion and grow distally. Injury of this severity is *axonotmesi*s; it eventually produces a good functional result because the endoneurial tubes are intact and the regenerating axons are therefore guaranteed to reach the correct end organs.

Laceration or extreme traction produces *neurotmesis*, which also leads to Wallerian degeneration distally and chromatolysis proximally, followed by either cell death or axonal regeneration. In this case, the final functional result is bound to be much worse than in any injury which leaves the endoneurial tubes intact. The axon sprouts have to traverse a gap filled with organizing repair tissue; presumably the chances of any given axon regenerating down its original conduit are vanishingly small. Axons which do reach the distal stump have then to grow towards the periphery — this they traditionally do at a rate of 1 mm per day. Axons which fail to enter the distal stump may form a tender neuroma, symptoms from which may be exceedingly troublesome. Progress may be monitored clinically by the Tinel sign — 'electric' feelings in the territory of the nerve produced by light percussion over regenerating axon tips — whether in the distal portion of the nerve or in a neuroma.

Motor axons have the capacity to produce collateral sprouts once they enter muscle, leading to abnormally large motor units with relatively good return of strength. Sensory axons often fail to reinnervate the specialized receptors which form the basis for the sense of touch and this, together with the mismatching of axons with conduits, means that sensory recovery is invariably poor, except in the very young. In the hand this means a poor functional result.

**Diagnosis of nerve injury**

Most peripheral nerve injuries occur in the upper limb, at hand or wrist level, and they may lead to substantial disability and handicap. It is generally agreed (though not easy to prove scientifically) that delay of more than a few days leads to a worse result from repair. For this and other (e.g. medicolegal) reasons, it is important not to miss nerve injuries in the casualty department. Unfortunately it is very easy to do so: motor function may be thought to be inhibited by pain rather than paralysed, and patients often swear they can feel touch in an area supplied by a nerve which is subsequently found to be completely divided. The only safe policy is as follows:

- In penetrating wounds, test every nerve which could conceivably have been damaged.
- Formally test every relevant muscle, since partial lesions are common.
- For the same reason, test the entire relevant skin territory.
- Do not ask 'Can you feel this?'; set a discrimination task that can only be accomplished with intact sensibility, such as distinguishing sharp from blunt correctly on several applications.
- Test for absent sweating, especially in the fingers, by running a plastic pen over the skin: the pen skids easily over abnormally dry skin.
- Record findings in the notes.
- Have a very low threshold for formally exploring the wound.

**Treatment**

Suture of peripheral nerves needs to be done gently and with precision; it should not be done at 4 o'clock in the morning unless dictated by associated injuries. The wound will not deteriorate significantly in 12 hours or so, provided it is covered with something like a betadine soak and the injured part is continuously elevated. The most senior surgeon available should perform or supervise the procedure on the next available list.

Remember you are there to assist the biology, not to 'fix' the nerve. Even the most delicate instruments, used with the greatest magnification, are blunt and clumsy on the scale of axons. Handle the nerve very gently; do not let the wound dry out; use bipolar diathermy; perform the simplest procedure that brings the nerve ends together neatly. Direct, end-to-end suture is preferable, provided it can be achieved without excessive tension or flexion of adjacent joints. If not, then interposition graft consisting of strands of expendable cutaneous nerve, such as medial cutaneous nerve of forearm or sural nerve, is better. Nerve ends should be approximated somehow at the first procedure to prevent shortening and, since nerve is relatively resistant to infection, it is often best to repair a nerve primarily, even in a wound which is too contaminated to close. The strongest indication for delayed definitive repair is when it is impossible to assess primarily how much of the proximal and distal stumps is viable.

## Factors affecting outcome

The end result of peripheral nerve repair is dictated, above all else, by the age of the patient at the time of injury and suture. Young children can regain sensory function which is at least comparable to normal; older patients cannot. This may well be more a result of CNS plasticity, allowing better processing of abnormal afferent signals, than better regeneration peripherally. Compared to this, the difference we can make by early diagnosis, good surgery and excellent rehabilitation is small. Nonetheless, that is the only difference we *can* make, and we should go for it.

Positive symptoms, such as paraesthesiae, neuroma or causalgia, will often dictate a poor result more powerfully than negative symptoms of numbness or weakness.

In the end the patients determine the outcome by the extent to which they accept the permanent deficit and learn to work round it. Much depends on their job and whether, or at what stage, they can return to it. It is important to help the patient reassume responsibility in this way by giving good prognostic advice, the services of an experienced hand therapist and prompt expert treatment of neurogenic pain if it arises.

## Future prospects for treatment

Forty years ago the argument was all about the timing of nerve repair: primary versus secondary. Ten years ago it was all about surgical technique: whether to use a microscope, whether to suture individual fascicles. Now the question is whether the science of neurobiology will yield any useful adjunctive therapies to use alongside surgical repair. The army of people addressing this question is large because the lessons learned may eventually be of value for the huge numbers of people suffering central nervous lesions, as well as the small numbers suffering peripheral damage.

Several agents have been found to enhance peripheral nerve regeneration in experimental animals; very soon we shall start to see the results of clinical trials. Before accepting the conclusions of such work, be convinced that the measures of outcome reported are valid. Beware of sensory tests that look neat but are notoriously difficult to perform rigorously. If you see two-point discrimination values, for example, look to see if the paper gives any information about how they were obtained or by whom. Place most reliance on quantitative functional tests, such as picking up and object recognition. Above all, look at the design of the trial: was there a control group consisting of cases which were truly comparable, especially as regards their age?

---

PART 5.14.
# HAND INJURIES
*J. Noble*

---

With the hand we construct, condemn and caress. Its importance as an organ is represented by the size of its representation on the cerebral cortex.

## Assessment

Consider:
1. skin loss and viability
2. contamination
3. swelling
4. infection or potential infection

5. integrity of the flexor tendons
6. integrity of the extensor tendons
7. integrity of the nerves
8. integrity of the vessels
9. signs of fracture/dislocation at the wrist, carpometacarpal, metacarpal and phalangeal joints
10. signs of instability or ligamentous injury at the metacarpophalangeal and interphalangeal joints.

Avoid these pitfalls:

1. Do not staunch bleeding by shoving in haemostats, because you may damage nearby nerves.

2. Beware of degloving injuries, as occurs when a ring is avulsed. Degloved skin will not heal unless it is reapplied as a free or vascularized graft without tension.

3. Do not judge the severity of a wound by the size of the external wound. A piece of glass entering the hand through a 3–5 mm cut may yet totally divide major nerves or vessels, sometimes remote from the point of entry. Therefore explore all deep wounds under anaesthesia, using a tourniquet to obtain a bloodless field, in the operating theatre, with good lighting.

4. Since the physical signs of peripheral nerve injury may be initially indistinct, always explore when in doubt.

5. Always examine the function of each tendon individually. Separately examine flexor digitorum profundus (FDP) and flexor digitorum superficialis (FDS) for each individual finger. Remember that the profundus tendon is the sole flexor of the distal interphalangeal joints and that the superficial tendon is the sole flexor of the proximal interphalangeal joint in a finger when, and only when, the other three fingers are fully extended.

6. Do not expect peripheral nerve injuries to produce signs which conform to stereotyped anatomy. They do not.

7. Joint injuries are no less treacherous. When there is generalized pain and swelling, the deformity of a radiocarpal or carpal fracture, dislocation or fracture dislocation may not be obvious. Carefully study the X-rays, if necessary after taking comparable views of the other hand and wrist. In particular, inspect the congruity of the lines of the intercarpal and radiocarpal joints: they should be smooth, nearly concentric semicircles on anteroposterior views.

**Problems**

1. Oedema (swelling) should ideally be prevented but when it develops or is developing it is an indication for immediate treatment. Admit the patient to hospital; elevate the arm with a suspended roller towel. Apply a 'boxing glove' bandage with the interphalangeal joints extended (the Edinburgh position). Place a large ball of fluffed gauze or good-quality cotton wool in the concavity of the hand, with dressing gauze separating the fingers, held in place with a few firm but not tight turns of bandage. Following release from the bandage, institute active, supervised physiotherapy.

2. Skin loss is not a cause for immediate worry. Never stitch wounds under tension. Many, especially those in the palm, are better left open. Strive to save thumb skin but do not strive to save crushed skin on the finger tips.

3. Wounds must be thoroughly debrided, i.e. all dead tissue and foreign material must be removed. Excise ragged and non-viable wound edges.

4. Digital amputation. Thumb and multiple finger amputations should be considered for microsurgical reimplantation.

5. Fractures of the hand form a complex subject. Unstable carpal injuries require fixation. Carpometacarpal dislocations or fracture dislocations occur as Bennett's fracture at the base of the thumb and also at the base of the ring and little fingers. Metacarpal fractures may develop a rotational as well as an angular deformity. Phalangeal fractures involving joint surfaces or with angular or rotational displacement require accurate reduction and fixation.

6. Extensor tendons may be ruptured, avulsed or lacerated.

7. Flexor tendon repair is in the province of experts in hand surgery. Particularly difficult are those lying between the distal palmar crease and the distal interphalangeal joint crease.

## Rehabilitation

Excellent early assessment and subsequent surgery is wasted unless safe splintage and bandaging, early physiotherapy and occupational therapy are instituted.

1. Splintage ensures that joint capsules and ligaments are stretched and prevented from developing secondary contracture when the metacarpophalangeal joints are flexed and the interphalangeal joints are extended.

2. Physiotherapy is intended to reduce swelling, and facilitate active or assisted active movement. Forced passive movements may be damaging.

3. Splints that are dynamic counteract deformity and assist weakened movement. Static splints worn overnight or between treatments rest and immobilize the hand and prevent secondary deformities developing.

---

PART 5.15
# MANAGEMENT OF BURNS
*S. Watson*

---

## THE BURN WOUND

### Depth of burn and cause of burn

*Superficial burns*

These are typically wet, pink and blister; there can be white areas among the pink. They are always sensitive to pin-prick. Superficial burns epithelialize in 14 days from the epithelial producing elements (hair follicles and sweat glands) and from the edges of the wound; they heal with normal-quality skin, although there can be some pigmentation changes. Superficial burns include: scalds by non-boiling liquids; some chemical burns; the edges of areas of flame burn; flash burns.

*Deep dermal burns*

This is an important depth of burn to diagnose

(see below). They are pink but do not blanch on pressure (called the zone of stasis), there are more areas of whiteness, they can blister. They are dull to pin-prick. These burns struggle to heal in three to four weeks. Healing is by epithelialization from the reduced number of epithelial producing elements and from the edge of the wound; there is also wound contraction. The final result of healing is either poor-quality skin or hypertrophic scar. There is some degree of wound contraction and marked pigmentation change: either hyper- or hypo-pigmentation. Deep dermal burns include scalds; contact burns and flame burns in areas of thick skin, e.g. the back; chemical burns; flame burns in concave areas.

*Full-thickness burns*

These are usually obvious and have no sensation to pin-prick. The diagnosis between deep dermal and full thickness can be difficult and sometimes is only made at surgery. They can only heal naturally by epithelialization from the wound edge and by wound contraction, leaving contracted poor-quality scars. Full-thickness burns are caused by many scald injuries with near-boiling water, especially in the thin skin of the elderly or young patient; even tea or coffee with milk can produce burns that fall into the deep dermal and full-thickness range. Also included are chemical burns like hydrofluoric acid, most flame burns, and virtually all electrical burns with a voltage of 220–240 V or higher. Most contact burns are full thickness in unconscious patients, e.g. post-epilepsy or from alcohol or drugs; they occur in denervated skin, e.g. diabetes and neuropathies.

Burns below the deep fascia do occur, e.g. some contact burns, scalds in non-accidental injury in children. High-voltage electrical burns can destroy muscle groups.

### Diagnosis of the depth of burn

This is not always easy. If doubtful, reassess at 24 hours using only non-stick dressings between examinations. The history may be a guide to depth; the best clinical test is sensitivity to pin-prick. Once silver sulphadiazine or betadine has been put on the burn, diagnosis of depth becomes much harder.

## Escharotomy

Circumferential full-thickness burns around limbs act as tourniquets. An escharotomy is performed by incising through the full-thickness burn to the mid-fat level. The incision must go from normal skin right through the burn to either normal skin distally or the end of the limb. In this way complete release of the tourniquet effect is achieved. No part of the burn must be left uncut otherwise a tourniquet will persist. Full-thickness burns around the chest will also have to be released. Escharotomy is not a minor procedure; it can cause considerable venous haemorrhage.

## INITIAL ASSESSMENT OF THE PATIENT

### Non-burn factors

A full medical history and examination are required but these may have to wait until after the start of treatment. In electrical burns an ECG is essential. Associated injuries have to be treated also.

### Pulmonary injuries

Burn to the lungs and the respiratory tract is of major importance. Any flame burn, especially in confined spaces, may produce a lung injury from heat, chemicals or blast. The lungs are damaged by the toxic products of combustion from burning furniture, upholstery and insulation materials. Carbon monoxide binds with haemoglobin to form carboxyhaemoglobin, preventing oxygen transport. Examine the nose, mouth and larynx for damage; examine the chest repeatedly over the next three days. Watch for signs of respiratory distress, including restlessness, and take a chest X-ray and measure blood gases. The treatment for pulmonary burns is to give oxygen in high concentration; do not treat them like chronic bronchitics. Plan the airway; oedema of the mouth and larynx develops rapidly and can cause obstruction within an hour. Early endotracheal intubation is essential.

### Size of the burn

The size of the burn is estimated on the percentage of body surface area burnt using the rule of nines. Head and neck 9%; front of trunk 18%; back of trunk 18%; each arm 9%; each leg 18%. The palm of the patient's hand is 1% of body surface area. In children, amend the head and neck percentage up to 18% and the legs down to 12% (when dealing with children it is best to consult specialist charts).

*Do not forget to examine the patient's back.* Record the size of burn and map the areas of superficial, deep dermal and full-thickness burns; record erythema separately. If you are not sure of your estimated percentage area of burn then calculate the percentage area of non-burn skin and subtract from 100 — it should give the same figure.

### Staphylococcal toxic shock syndrome

This can occur in children even with relatively small superficial burns (Frame et al 1985, Cole & Shakespeare 1990). If a child with even a 1% burn becomes unwell, toxic shock syndrome must be considered and the specific treatment — fresh frozen plasma and antistaphylococcal antibiotics — started immediately. Do not hesitate to start this treatment — it will be life saving.

## SHOCK PHASE

### Physiology and general principles

During the first 24–48 hours after a major burn the patient goes into hypovolaemic shock. There is no loss of fluid from the body but plasma volume passes out through the porous capillary bed into the intercellular space. This is initially into the area of burned tissue but subsequently all dependent areas become oedematous and oedema will develop in the lungs and brain. In the shock phase the circulation does not behave like other forms of hypovolaemic shock. It is not possible to keep the circulating volume within normal limits. The shock phase ends between 24 and 48 hours after the burn when the patient starts diuresis. Fluid balance then is more like that of a normal patient.

## Principles of resuscitation

The aim of treatment is to produce a circulation adequate to perfuse vital organs, even if it is not possible to keep the plasma volume normal. The large quantities of fluid that have to be given can cause concern in the elderly or those with respiratory problems. Resuscitation can be very much a compromise between maintaining circulation and not causing pulmonary oedema or, in children, cerebral oedema. There is controversy over which fluid and how much should be given. A practical account is given by Settle (1986). Successful resuscitation requires water and sodium, usually given intravenously in adult burns over 15% and children's burns over 10%. Resuscitation cannot be done with water alone and even with small burns free water should be restricted and the patient should drink balanced electrolyte solutions. There is a danger of hypernatraemia from too much sodium administration or too little sodium-free water. There is a danger of hyponatraemia if too much sodium-free water is given or drunk. This danger is greatest in children. When the burn wound is dressed the evaporative water loss is usually restricted to 1.5–2 ml kg/hr (a minimum of 30 ml $h^{-1}$ in children) and this can be given as salt-free water or intravenous 5% dextrose. Quantities of fluid above this should be given in the form of balanced electrolyte solutions. If the burn wound is managed exposed there is considerably more evaporative water loss.

Start a good intravenous line and catheterize the patient. Successful resuscitation requires repeated examination of the patient and alteration of the rate of infusion. This should be done hourly initially and then dropped to 4 and then 6-hourly periods. Resuscitation is monitored by clinical examination of the patient, in particular looking for good peripheral perfusion, with warm feet and filled veins; there should be a urine output ideally over 50 ml $h^{-1}$ but in severe burns 30–40 ml $h^{-1}$ can be accepted at least for several hours. Recording the haematocrit provides a good measure of the plasma volume and the changes in haematocrit from hour to hour provide a good estimate of whether the fluid infusion rate should be increased or decreased.

Red blood cells can be replaced in large full-thickness burns in the second 24-hour period. For full-thickness burns over 10% of body surface area whole blood is given, equal to 1% of the patient's normal blood volume for each 1% of burn (Muir et al 1986).

### Standard UK resuscitation

The fluid used is HPPF or albumin solutions isotonic for sodium, using the Muir and Barkley formula. A volume is calculated, equal to body weight in kilograms × percentage area burnt × 1/2 ml. This volume is given in the first, second and third 4-hour periods, from the time of the burn, then the next two 6-hour periods and the subsequent 12-hour periods until the shock phase ends. Fluid rates are greatest in the first 4-hourly periods. If a patient's treatment has been delayed higher rates of infusion are given until a good urine output is started. It must be emphasized that the formula is only a guide and the fluid given is frequently different from the formula. Oral non-sodium water is given as discussed and additional oral fluids must be of balanced salt solutions.

### Other resuscitation regimes

Many burns units use only normal saline, Ringer's or Hartman's solution to resuscitate (Demling & Lalande 1986). The Baxter and Shires regime advocates 4 ml of Ringer's lactate per kilogram per percentage of body burn in the first 24 hours, of which half is given in the first 8 hours. Other units resuscitate with dextran.

### Oral resuscitation

This can be done successfully in burns up to 30% of body surface area, possibly with the help of a nasogastric tube. Balanced salt solutions are required. A suitable solution is Moyer's solution, which contains 4 g sodium chloride (NaCl) and 1.5 g sodium bicarbonate $NaHCO_3$ per litre. It can be approximated by mixing 1 litre of normal saline with 1 litre of tap water and adding 100 ml of isotonic (1.25%) sodium bicarbonate solution (Settle 1986). For mass casualties a simpler regime has been suggested by Sørensen, who advocated patients to drink every hour 0.25 litres of water with a 1 g table salt, repeated for 48 hours.

## PLAN FOR THE BURNED WOUND

### Dressing policy

Small superficial burns and those awaiting surgery in the next five days are dressed using simple dressings. Other wounds are dressed using topical antibacterial agent and then sterile dressings. The two commonest agents are 1% silver sulphadiazine cream (Flamazine) or aqueous Betadine solution. These are changed every one or two days.

### Surgical plan

If the patient is fit, the first skin-grafting operation is performed within five days. Up to 20% of the body surface area burn is excised and grafted. The donor sites are allowed to heal and a second skin grafting can be performed 14 days later. Excision of burn tissue and skin grafting is a major surgical procedure; it causes considerable bleeding and requires expert anaesthetic and nursing support.

#### Deep dermal burns

The technique of tangential excision was first described by Jancercovitz for this depth of burn. Using a skin-grafting knife the burn is shaved down in thin layers until pinpoint bleeding is obtained in the deep dermal layers. Once there is pinpoint bleeding then the skin grafts will take even though the deeper layers of dermis have been damaged or killed by the heat. This is dermis that would slough if it was not skin grafted, so this technique preserves dermis and produces better scars with less contraction.

#### Full-thickness burns

These are excised and skin grafted onto the deep fascia. This ensures a good take of the grafts. With life-threatening burns good skin graft take is essential. Skin grafting to the mid-fat level gives a better final appearance but graft take is often poor.

### Specialized areas

The face, because of its very high blood supply, has enormous powers of healing but the eyelids have to be watched very carefully. If ectropion develops the eyelids must be grafted. Superficial burns of the hands and the less deep dermal burns are treated by putting the hands in polythene bags, Flamazine can be added to the bag. Deep dermal burns and full-thickness burns of the hands should be treated as hand surgery problems, not as burns. They need to be splinted in the position of function and great care must be taken to prevent exposure of the extensor tendons and joints. Some hand burns require skin flaps to resurface tendons and joints.

### Electrical burns

These usually require early excision and skin flaps; high-tension electrical burns require muscle excision or amputation.

## COURSE IN HOSPITAL

### Day-to-day management

The burned patient tends to get more sick as the weeks go by and is not out of danger until the last area of burn has healed. Good burns management requires obsessive care and attention to detail. Frequent measurements are required of the haemoglobin, electrolytes, plasma proteins and urine electrolytes and osmolality. Potassium in particular must be carefully watched. Bacteriology swabs should be taken from the burned wound at every dressing change so that it is always known what organisms are growing on the burn. Antibiotics are given during surgery and to treat septicaemia. The organism that is most worrying is the β-haemolytic streptococcus Lancefield group A: this organism completely destroys skin grafts.

### Nutrition

Gastrointestinal feeding is started during the

shock phase. Good nutritional input is essential. Parenteral feeding is avoided if at all possible because of the added risks of septicaemia.

## Pain relief

Good pain relief is essential. Morphine and diamorphine are used frequently. Chlorpromazine is very useful. Dressings can be applied under Entonox (50% nitrous oxide and 50% oxygen) or even general anaesthetic.

## PHYSIOTHERAPY, REHABILITATION AND RECONSTRUCTION

Physiotherapy is an important part of care to the chest, limbs and hands. Burns care goes on for months, if not years, even after final healing. Initially, scars are very hypertrophic and typically take one to three years to flatten to papery scars. The scars can be considerably helped by pressure garment therapy.

## OTHER ASPECTS

### Prevention

The commonest burn injury to children is scalds from electric kettles, cooking stoves, cups of tea and coffee and hot baths. All of these should be preventable. The effects of house fires could be drastically reduced by the use of circuit breakers to cut off the electricity supply and by the fitting of smoke detectors. More needs to be done to use materials in the home which are non-combustible or which do not give off poisonous materials when burned.

### When not to treat

The chances of a patient's survival diminish with increasing age and size of burn and with associated injuries or medical conditions. Treatment should be given until a burns specialist has assessed the patient. Patients with non-survivable burns, if well transfused, can be conscious and talk to relatives for a few hours. Adequate analgesia must be given.

## Non-accidental injuries (NAI)

Burns in children can be NAI and this must always be considered.

## Major disasters

Burns require enormous amounts of hospital resources. With a major disaster and large numbers of burned patients, treatment by our normal standards is impossible. A guide to resuscitation has been given above. Early surgery in patients would not be possible and the mainstay of treatment would be adequate dressings with Flamazine or aqueous Betadine.

REFERENCES

Cole R P, Shakespeare P G 1990 Toxic shock syndrome in scalded children. Burns 16: 221–224
Demling R H, Lalonde C 1989 Burn trauma. Thieme, New York
Frame J D, Eve M D, Hackett M E J, Dowsett E G, Brain D T, Gault D T, Wilmshurst A D 1985 The toxic shock syndrome in burned children. Burns 11: 234–241
Muir I F K, Barclay T L 1962 Burns and their treatment. Lloyd-Luke, London
Muir I F K, Barclay T L, Settle J A D 1986 Burns and their treatment (3rd edn). Butterworths, London
Settle John A D 1986 Burns: the first five days. Smith and Nephew

## PART 5.16
# MANAGEMENT OF FRACTURES
*C. S. B. Galasko*

## BIOLOGY OF FRACTURE REPAIR

Bone is a unique tissue in that it heals with bone, whereas every other tissue heals with scarring. When a fracture occurs not only is the bone broken, but the surrounding tissues are also damaged. Initially the bone ends are surrounded by haematoma which includes the surrounding injured tissues. There is necrosis of the ends of the fractured bone and within hours an aseptic inflammatory response develops within the fracture haematoma, which becomes organized. There is initially infiltration of polymorphonuclear leucocytes, lymphocytes and macrophages, with infiltration of blood vessels, and the development of granulation tissue and infiltration with fibroblasts.

Within this tissue bone is then laid down. This may be preceded by the development of cartilage with endochondral ossification, or intramembranous ossification may develop primarily in the organized fracture haematoma. The bone may be laid down on the deep surfaces of any 'stripped' but intact periosteum, and if there is an intact periosteal sleeve around the fracture callus develops rapidly, bridging the gap between the bone ends. Endosteal callus arises from osteoblast progenitor cells within the medullary cavity. The response of the periosteum and endosteum to any insult or injury is to form bone. It is this ability of bone to heal with new bone that makes it such a unique tissue. Ossification may also occur, but very much more slowly, from osteoprogenitor cells lying within the organized fracture haematoma. At the same time osteoclasts develop and resorb the necrotic bone ends.

The initial bone that is laid down (callus) consists of immature woven bone. With consolidation of the fracture, this is gradually converted to stable lamellar bone.

Primary bone healing occurs when the bone ends are held rigidly together; resorption takes place within the bone trabeculae as recanalizing Haversian systems bridge the bone ends.

There are basically two types of callus. The first is the primary callus response, which is due to the proliferation of committed osteoprogenitor cells in periosteum and bone marrow. These cells directly produce membranous bone and is a once-only phenomenon limited in duration. The second is inductive or external callus, which is derived from the surrounding tissues. This callus is formed by pleuripotential cells. A variety of factors, including mechanical and humoral factors, may induce these mesenchymal cells to differentiate to cartilage/bone.

The mediators for callus formation are not fully understood, but it is likely that the fracture ends emit osteogenic substances such as bone morphogenetic protein into the fracture haematoma, in addition to those mediators (interleukin-1 and growth factors) which are released from the fracture haematoma as occurs in wound healing. Movement of the fragments increases the fracture exudate. Angiogenic factors probably play an important role in the vascularization of the fracture haematoma. Rigid fixation minimizes the granulation tissue and external callus. Rigid fixation may also retard the release of morphogens and growth factors from the bone end. Reaming of the intramedullary canal may cause additional bone damage. Weight bearing stimulates growth factors and prostaglandins which act as biochemical mediators.

## TYPES OF FRACTURE

### Following trauma

The fracture occurs in normal bone as a result of trauma. The type of fracture depends on the direction of the violence. A twisting injury will cause a spiral or oblique fracture, whereas a direct blow usually causes a transverse fracture. Axial compression frequently results in a comminuted or burst fracture.

### Stress fracture

The underlying bone is normal and the abnormal load placed upon the bone would not be sufficient to cause a fracture on its own. However, the load is repetitive. This type of fracture is most frequently seen in individuals undertaking increased amounts of unaccustomed exercise, such as the 'march' metatarsal fracture in army recruits.

### Pathological fracture

The underlying bone is weak, perhaps as a result of metastatic cancer or metabolic bone disease, and gives way under minimal trauma.

## DIAGNOSIS OF A FRACTURE

There are three aspects to the diagnosis of a fracture, all of which form an essential part of the diagnosis.

## Is there a fracture?

The presence of a fracture is suspected on the clinical findings and is confirmed on radiographs. Be alerted to the possibility of a fracture by the presence of tenderness, pain and swelling. Swelling and bruising may not occur immediately. If the fracture is displaced the limb will be deformed. Fracture of a major long bone results in loss of function, but this sign is not always present. Do not try to elicit abnormal mobility or crepitus at the fracture site. Trying to do so produces unnecessary pain. If a fracture is suspected, request radiographs. View them to determine the presence of a fracture, its location, type (transverse, oblique, spiral, comminuted and compression), and the amount of displacement and angular deformity. The radiographs should include the entire length of the injured bone. Occasionally a fracture may not be obvious on the initial radiograph (e.g. a stress fracture), and further radiographs may be required 10–14 days later.

## Is the fracture compound or closed?

A fracture is compound if the injury extends through the skin, even if it is only a puncture wound. Under these circumstances there is a significant risk of infection, the soft tissues and fracture require urgent debridement and the patient requires prophylactic antibiotics. The treatment of the fracture may be secondary to the treatment of the compound wound, e.g. grade three compound fractures usually require external fixation.

## Is there associated damage?

The diagnosis is not complete until this question can be answered as, frequently, it is the associated damage that determines the treatment. There may be vascular injury, increased pressure within closed compartments (compartment syndrome), and nerve, joint, tendon, child's growth plate or skin trauma.

### Vascular damage?

Palpate the peripheral pulses. If there is any sug-gestion of ischaemia arteriography is indicated. If there is associated vascular damage the fracture must be internally fixed before the artery is repaired or grafted.

### Compartment syndrome?

This implies that the pressure within a tight osseo-fascial compartment is elevated. A compartment syndrome develops if the pressure within the compartment is sufficient to obstruct the blood supply to the intra-compartmental muscles. This pressure is much less than arterial pressure and is estimated to be about 40 mm Hg, or less than 40 mm Hg below mean arterial pressure. The presence of pain, despite having immobilized the fracture, or muscle spasm indicates that a compartment syndrome might be developing and that compartment pressures should be measured. Look for the presence of a compartment syndrome, not only on admission, but also following reduction of the fracture and in the follow-up period. The common sites are in the forearm and lower leg. Inability to passively fully extend the fingers or the toes without pain is suggestive of an underlying compartment syndrome. Untreated, the ischaemic muscle necroses, fibroses and the patient develops an ischaemic contracture of varying severity, depending on the amount of damage.

### Nerve damage?

This may be early, late, or potential. Carry out a neurological examination prior to treatment and after treatment. It is possible that a nerve may be damaged as a result of treatment; for example, the ulnar nerve may be trapped within the elbow when a dislocation of the elbow is reduced. Delayed nerve damage may be caused by pressure on the ulnar nerve or lateral popliteal nerve by a splint or plaster cast. A nerve may become compressed by callus, by a plate or screws used to fix the fracture, or may become embedded in callus.

Patients with unstable but undisplaced spinal fractures or fracture dislocations are at risk of developing quadriplegia or paraplegia (depending on the site of fracture), if the fracture is allowed to displace during handling of the patient. Therefore, treat every patient with multiple injuries and every patient you suspect of having a cervical or spinal injury as if they have an unstable fracture or fracture dislocation of the spine until this is excluded.

### Visceral involvement?

An isolated fracture of a rib is usually a minor injury, unless it is associated with damage to the underlying lung with the development of a pneumothorax, or bronchopleural fistula. In patients with fractures of the pelvis exclude damage to the urinary tract.

### Skin damage?

The skin may be damaged without the fracture necessarily being compound. A shearing force to the overlying skin may damage its blood supply and result in necrosis of an extensive area of skin. Treat this injury as if it were a compound fracture.

### Joint involvement?

If the fracture involves a joint, anatomical reduction is required to minimize the risk of subsequent post-traumatic arthritis.

### In a child does the fracture involve the growth plate?

If so, an anatomical reduction is required, but if internal fixation is required screws and plates must not cross the physis.

## TREATMENT

### Emergency treatment

1. Avoid unnecessary death. Secure the airway, ensure the patient can breath, control haemorrhage and treat shock.

2. Reduce morbidity. Handle the patient carefully. This is particularly important where injuries of the spine are suspected (see above). Remove rings, bracelets and any other constrictive object from an injured limb which is likely to swell. Avoid restrictive bandages. Reduce a grossly displaced fracture that is compressing vessels.

3. Relieve pain. Splint the fracture before the patient is moved, including sending the patient for radiographs. Careful handling minimizes the amount of pain suffered. Give analgesics as required.

## Reduction

Reduction of a fracture is not always required. It is only indicated if the displacement is unacceptable, and this depends on the site of the fracture and the age and general fitness of the patient. Reduction is not required if there is no significant displacement; if the displacement that is present is unimportant, such as the fracture of a rib; if reduction is impossible, for example a compression fracture in an osteoporotic vertebra; if subsequent immobilization is contraindicated, for example a rib fracture; or if reduction may cause further fractures, as in a patient with osteogenesis imperfecta.

The methods of reduction include manipulation under anaesthesia, traction which may be skeletal or skin, or open reduction. If a manipulation is undertaken, obtain postreduction radiographs before ending the anaesthetic. If open reduction is considered, have you the necessary expertise to reduce the fracture without causing any further damage, and fix the fracture in the reduced position? Take radiographs before the operation is completed to ensure that the reduction is satisfactory.

## Immobilization

Immobilization is not always necessary. It is used to maintain reduction, prevent displacement and promote union; it helps relieve pain and promotes healing of soft tissues.

There are many methods of immobilizing a fracture, the type of immobilization depending on the fracture. They include a sling (which is used if the arm requires support), collar and cuff (which is used when the arm does not require support, or if gravity is being used to improve the position of a fracture, such as a fracture of the proximal humerus), bandages, plaster of Paris cast, cast braces, splints, traction, internal fixation and external fixation.

The majority of fractures are treated conservatively. Operative stabilization is used to avoid immobilization of a patient, to avoid immobilization of a joint, to allow care of the associated injuries, following failure of non-operative methods, for the treatment of many pathological fractures, and in patients with multiple injuries, including severe pelvic injury. There is some evidence to suggest that stabilization of these fractures is associated with a lower morbidity.

Intraoperative radiographs are taken to confirm that the fracture has been reduced and that the fixation is holding the fracture in the reduced position, but radiographs will not assess rotatory deformity. This is a clinical assessment.

External fixation is indicated for severe soft tissue injury, bone loss and infection.

### Rehabilitation

Rehabilitation is an essential part of the management of every fracture. There are two phases.

*Maintenance of function of uninjured parts*

For example, a patient with a Colles' fracture requires mobilizing exercises of the shoulder, elbow and fingers while the fracture is uniting, in order to prevent stiffening of the uninjured joints.

*Restoration of function of injured parts*

Once the fracture has united, rehabilitation of the injured part is required. For example, in a patient with a Colles' fracture the plaster cast is usually removed at four to six weeks and physiotherapy is aimed at restoring wrist function and forearm rotation.

## COMPLICATIONS

There are a host of potential complications which are not always avoidable, but careful attention to detail can minimize their risk.

## PART 5.17
## THE PHYSIOLOGICAL RESPONSES TO INJURY
*R. A. Little*

The response to injury can be usefully divided into three phases: the early, acute 'ebb' phase, which is followed by either the 'flow' phase if resuscitation and homoeostasis are able to overcome the initial insult, or by 'necrobiosis' if treatment fails and death ensues (Fig. 5.17.1).

### THE EBB PHASE

The ebb phase includes the pattern of physiological and metabolic changes associated with the preparation for fight or flight (the defence reaction) on which will be superimposed the responses elicited by the tissue damage and fluid loss from the circulation associated with injury. This phase is characterized by a mobilization of energy reserves and changes in cardiovascular reflex activity. A link between these is the increased activity of the sympathetic nervous system which is initiated by the appreciation of danger and sustained by afferent neural impulses arising from the site of injury and cardiovascular reflexes triggered by reductions in blood pressure and volume. The increase in sympathetic activity is reflected by rises in plasma catecholamine concentrations which are directly related to the severity of injury.

Increased sympathetic activity stimulates the breakdown of liver and muscle glycogen leading, either directly or indirectly, to increases in plasma glucose levels. This hyperglycaemia is potentiated by the reduction in glucose utilization by skeletal muscle due to an inhibition — by the raised adrenaline levels — of insulin secretion and the development of intracellular insulin resistance. The mechanism of insulin resistance is unclear although glucocorticoids may be involved.

The changes in carbohydrate metabolism in the ebb phase can be interpreted as defensive. In addition to providing a fuel for fight or flight the hyperglycaemia may also play a role in the com-

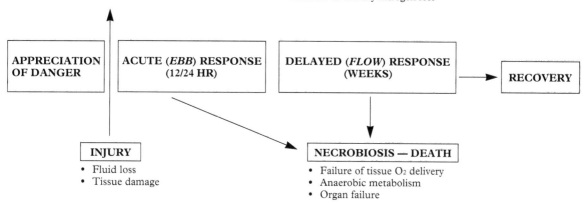

- Changes in homoeostatic reflex activity (themoregulatory and cardiovascular)
- Compensation of fluid loss
- Increase in plasma hormone levels (e.g. catecholamines)
- Mobilization of energy reserves
- Changes in fuel utilization
- Initiation of acute phase plasma protein response

- Increase in metabolic rate

- Insulin resistance
- Increase in skeletal muscle breakdown — loss of lean body mass
- Increase in urinary nitrogen loss

| APPRECIATION OF DANGER | ACUTE (*EBB*) RESPONSE (12/24 HR) | DELAYED (*FLOW*) RESPONSE (WEEKS) | RECOVERY |

INJURY
- Fluid loss
- Tissue damage

NECROBIOSIS — DEATH
- Failure of tissue $O_2$ delivery
- Anaerobic metabolism
- Organ failure

**Fig. 5.17.1**   Defence reaction.

pensation for post-traumatic fluid loss both through the mobilization of water associated with glycogen and through its osmotic effects. The decrease in glucose clearance associated with the development of insulin resistance can be considered as a mechanism for preventing the wasteful use of the mobilized carbohydrate, which is an essential fuel for the brain and the wound, at a time when the supply of nutrients may be limited.

The increases in sympathetic activity also cause mobilization of fat (triacylglycerol) in adipose tissue. Plasma concentrations of non-esterified fatty acids (NEFA) and glycerol are raised after accidental injury in man, although the relationship with injury severity is complex. For example, plasma NEFA is lower after severe than after moderate injuries; this may be related to metabolic (e.g. stimulation of reesterification within adipose tissue by the raised plasma lactate levels associated with severe injury) or circulatory (poor perfusion of adipose tissue) factors.

An increase in plasma cortisol, mediated by adrenocorticotrophic hormone (ACTH), occurs rapidly after all forms of injury although the relationship with severity is, once again, complex. Unexpectedly low cortisol concentrations have been found after severe injuries which cannot be related to a failure of the ACTH response. It has been suggested that an impairment of adrenocortical blood flow in the severely injured is responsible.

The original description of the ebb phase characterized it as a period of depressed metabolism and there is good evidence for this from experimental studies. The fall in metabolic rate following haemorrhage which is due to a reduction in tissue oxygen delivery can be reversed by transfusion; however, if hypovolaemia is accompanied by tissue damage transfusion is less effective. It seems that neural impulses, associated with tissue injury ascending to the brain via the spinal cord, cause the release of noradrenaline in the hypothalamus which, in turn, leads to an inhibition of thermoregulatory heat production and, at ambient temperatures below thermoneutral, a fall in oxygen consumption and body temperature.

The evidence for such an inhibition of thermo-regulatory heat production shortly after injury in man is, however, not nearly so clear. Indeed what evidence there is suggests that oxygen consumption is maintained at or, more commonly, above normal levels shortly after injury in man. There is, however, clinical evidence for changes in the control of thermoregulation at this time; for example, severely injured patients do not shiver, despite having body temperatures below the normal threshold for its onset, and also the selection of the ambient temperature for thermal comfort is modified.

In addition to modifying thermoregulation, nociceptive stimulation also modifies the cardiovascular response to fluid loss. For example, the heart rate response to simple haemorrhage is an initial tachycardia (mediated by the baroreflex) followed as the severity of haemorrhage increases by a bradycardia (mediated by the stimulation of neural afferents arising from the heart). This vagally induced bradycardia can be markedly attenuated, and blood pressure better maintained, if the blood loss is superimposed on a background of nociceptive stimulation. The sensitivity of the baroreflex is itself reduced by injury, although an increase is seen after haemorrhage. This impairment of the baroreflex, which can persist for several weeks after even quite modest injuries (e.g. fracture dislocation of the ankle), means that vasopressors such as vasopressin (ADH) released acutely after injury will be more effective in helping maintain blood pressure than normally, when the baroreflex will buffer their pressor effects. This complex interaction between the cardiovascular responses to haemorrhage and to injury may not be beneficial as it has been demonstrated that the ability to tolerate haemorrhage is reduced by concomitant tissue damage. Thus it seems that the better maintenance of blood pressure after haemorrhage and injury is achieved at the expense of intense vasoconstriction in peripheral vascular beds which may secondarily increase the severity of injury and increase the likelihood of the development of multiple organ failure.

If the magnitude of tissue damage and fluid loss from the circulation is so severe that endogenous homoeostatic mechanisms are overwhelmed and resuscitation is inadequate, the phase of *necrobiosis* is initiated. This is characterized by a progressive imbalance between oxygen demand and supply in the tissues such that a downward spiral of anaerobic metabolism and irreversible tissue damage is initiated, leading to death. However, if treatment is successful and tissue oxygen delivery is maintained, the ebb phase is followed by the flow phase.

## THE FLOW PHASE

The main features of the flow phase are increases in metabolic rate and in urinary nitrogen excretion, associated with weight loss and muscle wasting, which reach a maximum at seven to ten days after injury in uncomplicated cases. If sepsis and/or multiple organ failure supervene, this pattern of response may be prolonged for many weeks.

The increase in metabolic rate, which is directly related to the severity of injury, is due to a number of factors, probably the most important of which is an increased sympathetic drive secondary to an upward central resetting of metabolic activity. The wound, whether it is a fracture site or a burned surface, can be considered as an extra organ which is metabolically active and has a circulation which is not under neural control. It consumes large amounts of glucose which is converted to lactate; this in turn is carried to the liver, where it is reconverted to glucose. This is an energy-consuming process, which is reflected by an increase in hepatic oxygen consumption. Other factors which might contribute to the hypermetabolism are increases in cardiac output (needed to sustain a hyperdynamic circulation), the energy cost of the latent heat of evaporation of water from, for example, the surface of the burn, the energy costs of substrate cycling (metabolic processes which involve the expenditure of energy without any change in the amount of either substrate or product) and of increased protein turnover (although this is almost certainly less than thought previously).

Metabolic rates measured in the flow phase seldom exceed 3000–4000 kcal per day (twice normal resting metabolic expenditure), with the highest values noted after major burns. The levels of energy expenditure are often lower than expected and may be close to or even lower than values predicted from standard tables. The explanation for this is that the hypermetabolic stimulus of injury/sepsis is superimposed on a background of inadequate calorie intake, immobility and loss of muscle mass, all of which tend to reduce metabolic rate.

The hypermetabolism of the flow phase is fuelled by increases in the rates of turnover of both fat and glucose. Turnover of NEFAs is raised in relation to their plasma concentration, and the normal suppression of fat oxidation following the administration of exogenous glucose is not seen in these hypermetabolic patients. Both of these changes have been attributed to increased sympathetic activity, although plasma catecholamine concentrations are not always increased at this time. The rate of hepatic gluconeogenesis is increased from a number of precursors (e.g. lactate and pyruvate from the wound and muscle, amino acids from muscle protein breakdown and glycerol from fat mobilization). This increase in hepatic glucose production is not suppressed in patients with burns or sepsis by the infusion of large quantities of glucose. This apparent resistance to the effects of insulin is mirrored by the failure of peripheral glucose utilization to rise to the extent predicted from the raised plasma glucose and insulin concentrations. This insulin resistance in, for example, uninjured skeletal muscle seems to be an intracellular (postreceptor) change.

The balance between whole-body protein synthesis and breakdown is obviously disturbed in the flow phase. It seems that the changes observed represent the interaction between the degree of injury and the nutritional state: increasing severities of injury cause increasing rates of both synthesis and breakdown, while undernutrition tends to depress synthesis. Thus increasing nutritional intake ought to move a patient towards nitrogen balance; however, it seems that despite advances in techniques for administering nutrients and modifications to the type and composition of feeding regimes no amount of nitrogen is sufficient to produce positive balance after severe injuries. However, the use of anabolic agents, such as growth hormone,

and manipulations of ambient temperature may be of advantage as the patient moves from the catabolic flow phase into the anabolic convalescent phase.

A major site of net protein loss is skeletal muscle, both injured and distant from the site of injury. The loss can be sufficient to compromise mobility, especially in the elderly, whose reserves of muscle mass and strength are already reduced. Although the changes in skeletal muscle are very obvious, the liver is another tissue in which changes in protein synthesis are of particular interest after injury. The liver is the source of the acute-phase reactants (e.g. C-reactive protein, fibrinogen and $\alpha_1$-antitrypsin) whose concentrations rise in response to infection, inflammation and trauma.

These metabolic changes which cannot be attributed to starvation or immobility can be mimicked, to some extent, by the infusion of the counter-regulatory hormones glucagon, adrenaline and cortisol. However, the plasma concentrations required to elicit relatively modest increases in nitrogen excretion and metabolic rate and induce peripheral insulin resistance are much higher than those found in the flow phase, although they are similar to those noted in the ebb phase. It has been suggested that other factors must be involved and the cytokines, most probably interleukin-6, released by activated macrophages may have an important role.

FURTHER READING

Barton R N (ed) 1985 Trauma and its metabolic problems. British Medical Bulletin 41(3)

Barton R N 1987 The neuroendocrinology of physical injury. Baillière's Clinical Endocrinology and Metabolism 13(2) : 355–374.

Barton R N, Frayn K N, Little R A 1990 Trauma, burns and surgery. In: Cohen R D, Lewis B, Alberti K G M M, Denman A M (eds). The Metabolic and molecular basis of acquired disease. Baillière Tindall, London, pp 684–717

Bessey P Q, Wilmore D W 1988 The burned patient. In: Nutrition and metabolism in patient care. Kinney J M, Jeejeebhoy K N, Hill G L, Owen O E (eds) Saunders, Philadelphia, pp 672–700

Cuthbertson D P (1980) Alterations in metabolism following injury: part 1. Injury 11: 175–189

Fong Y, Moldawer L L, Shiners G T, Lowry S F 1990 The biologic characteristics of cytokines and their implication in surgical injury. Surgery, Gynecology and Obstetrics 170: 363–378

Frayn K N (1986) Hormonal control of metabolism in trauma and sepsis. Clinical Endocrinology 24: 577–599

Gann D S, Amaral J F 1989 Endocrine and metabolic responses to injury. In: Schwartz S I, Shires G T, Spence F T (eds) Principles of surgery (5th edn) McGraw-Hill, New York, pp 1–68

Irving M H, Stoner H B 1987 Metabolism and nutrition in trauma. In: Carter D, Polk H C Jr (eds) Butterworths international medical reviews: trauma surgery 1, pp 302–314

Stoner H B 1986 Metabolism after trauma and in sepsis. Circulatory Shock 19: 75–87

Wilmore D W 1977 The metabolic management of the critically ill. Plenum, New York

## PART 5.18
## ADULT RESPIRATORY DISTRESS SYNDROME
*R. Kishen*

Adult respiratory distress syndrome (ARDS) was first described in 1967. It refers to a rapid onset of respiratory difficulty and arterial hypoxaemia in patients suffering from a variety of critical illnesses. Until recently it was also commonly known as 'shock lung', 'post-perfusion lung', 'Danang lung', etc. Recently it has been suggested that the condition should be referred to as acute lung injury (ALI).

### DEFINITION AND DIAGNOSIS

Precise definition of ARDS is difficult because of its multiple causative factors and the absence of specific laboratory tests. Most clinicians define ARDS as a serious form of acute respiratory failure in patients with previously healthy lungs. It produces severe arterial hypoxaemia not corrected by conventional oxygen therapy. Stiffening of lungs makes their expansion difficult. Pulmonary compliance and functional residual capacity are reduced. These changes result in tachypnoea, dyspnoea, hypoxaemia, cyanosis and increased work of breathing. The chest X-ray (initially normal) shows diffuse bilateral irregular infiltrates in the lung fields and may be mistaken for pulmonary oedema due to left ventricular failure. Evidence of other organ failure like hypotension and oliguria is also usually present. The diagnosis of ARDS depends upon the presence of the

above signs and symptoms along with the presence of an initiating factor (see below).

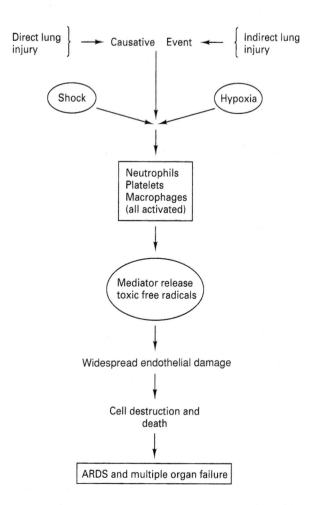

**Fig. 5.18.1**   A simplified flow chart illustrating the developments of ARDS.

### AETIOLOGY

ARDS is commonly associated with sepsis and multiple trauma, with an incidence of about 7% of all admissions to intensive therapy units in the UK. Aspiration of gastric contents into the lungs and multiple injuries in association with shock and soft tissue trauma increase its risk. ARDS may be caused by or is associated with the following conditions:

- direct lung injury due to lung trauma, i.e. blunt injury to the chest, resulting in pulmonary contusion, aspiration of gastric contents, near drowning, inhalation of toxic fumes and thermal injury to the respiratory tract and bacterial, viral or drug-induced (e.g. bleomycin) pneumonia, radiation injury and oxygen toxicity
- indirect causes (i.e. the primary insult is remote from the lungs) include sepsis, massive haemorrhage, multiple transfusions, 'shock' from any cause, disseminated intravascular coagulation, massive burns, major and multiple trauma, pre-eclampsia, amniotic fluid embolism, pancreatitis, head injuries and cardiopulmonary bypass.

The list is not exhaustive and it has been suggested that any critical illness that leads to inadequate cellular oxygenation can precipitate the syndrome.

## PATHOPHYSIOLOGY AND THE ROLE OF THE MEDIATORS OF LUNG INJURY

The factors that trigger this syndrome are not fully understood. Clinical conditions associated with ARDS are thought to initiate abnormal behaviour and movement of neutrophils, platelets and monocytes (macrophages), causing release of a wide variety of enzymes and factors. Neutrophils and platelets also attach themselves to capillary endothelium, damaging it and causing capillary leak. Abnormal macrophages release toxic oxygen radicals and further add to the existing capillary damage, thus causing widespread leakage of fluid into the tissues all over the body.

Despite diverse causative factors, the structural changes in the lungs follow a common pattern. Due to the capillary leak there is oedema of the lung tissue and movement of neutrophils and erythrocytes into the lung parenchyma. The lung lymph flow is increased and there is thickening of the alveolar capillary membrane. This results in impairment of oxygen diffusion and reduced lung compliance, as it is harder to distend an alveolus surrounded by fluid. Some of the fluid in the pulmonary parenchyma may leak into the alveoli, giving the characteristic appearance of a hyaline membrane. In the later stages of the disease fibrosis may be seen.

Clinical and experimental evidence suggests that generalized capillary leak and defects in peripheral tissue oxygenation lead to other organ failure simultaneously with the lung failure. It is therefore worth remembering that ARDS is merely the pulmonary manifestation of a generalized disease causing failure of multiple organ systems. Management therefore must be wide ranging and applied to the other organ systems as well (Fig 5.18.1).

## CLINICAL PRESENTATION

Not all patients presenting with sepsis and multiple trauma develop ARDS. The patients who develop ARDS have usually suffered hypoxia and/or hypotension at some stage in the management of their presenting problem. Untreated ARDS passes through four progressively worsening phases.

### Phase I:

This is the first stage in the development of ARDS and may start 16–24 hours after the onset of the presenting clinical condition. Apart from tachypnea and tachycardia, no other abnormalities may be present. Chest X-ray at this stage is normal.

### Phase II:

This phase develops up to 48 hours after the initial insult and 12–24 hours after phase I. The patient appears clinically stable but shows increasing dyspnoea with cyanosis. The skin may appear moist. The effort of breathing is greatly increased and hypoxaemia is present despite oxygen therapy. Clinically only minor chest signs (such as inspiratory ronchi) may be present.

### Phase III:

This follows phase II and there is now marked tachypnea and dyspnea, with increasing involvement of the accessory muscles of respiration. Auscultation of the lung fields reveals high-pitched ronchi. Chest X-ray shows bilateral diffuse pulmonary infiltration.

**Phase IV:**

This is the terminal phase of ARDS if effective treatment has not been started. The patient shows increasing lethargy and restlessness and may lapse into a coma. There is respiratory and metabolic acidosis with severe hypoxaemia and hypotension. Urine output is usually low (less than 0.5 ml/kg per hour). The prognosis at this stage is poor even if effective treatment is started as multiple organ failure has already set in.

Therapeutic intervention may alter many of these signs and phases, depending on when the treatment is started. Experience has shown that in phases I and II of ARDS the disease has a better prognosis if treated as the lungs show only mild to moderate injury. Therefore it must be emphasized that the syndrome should be recognized and treatment started, preferably early in the disease process.

## THERAPEUTIC CONSIDERATIONS

The current management of ARDS is entirely supportive in nature. The mortality of severe ARDS is about 60% and eventual outcome is due to setting in of multiple organ failure. Thus it is essential to consider the management of the patient as a whole, and any one supportive measure should not be considered in isolation. Patients exhibiting signs and symptoms of ARDS should be transferred to the intensive therapy unit without delay.

**Respiratory support**

Improving oxygenation of the blood is vital and all patients with ARDS should receive high concentrations of inspired oxygen. Increase in functional residual capacity of the lungs improves arterial hypoxaemia and in a spontaneously breathing patient this can be accomplished by the application of continuous positive airways pressure (CPAP). CPAP is administered using a tight-fitting face mask and appropriate apparatus. Usually, however, mechanical ventilation is almost always required. This involves endo-

tracheal intubation, intermittent positive pressure ventilation (IPPV) and in most cases some form of sedation to reduce the respiratory drive and increase the patient's acceptance of IPPV. Neuromuscular paralysis is frequently used but is not essential.

As physiological dead space (i.e. the portion of each breath not contributing to actual gas exchange in the lungs) is increased, large tidal volumes (12–15 ml kg$^{-1}$ per breath) may be needed to achieve reasonable carbon dioxide removal. With decreased pulmonary compliance (i.e. stiff lungs) it is possible that peak inspiratory pressure, i.e. pressure generated in the patient's airways by IPPV, may reach high levels, causing barotrauma such as pneumothorax, pneumomediastinum and pulmonary interstitial emphysema. Since increased intrapulmonary shunting (the proportion of cardiac output that passes through the lungs but does not take part in gas exchange) is the basic pathology, increasing concentration of inspired oxygen may not improve arterial hypoxaemia.

There is considerable debate about the toxicity of high concentrations of inspired oxygen and most clinicians attempt to keep inspired oxygen concentration below 60%. The strategy employed to improve arterial oxygenation at this or lower concentrations of inspired oxygen is the application of positive end-expiratory pressure (PEEP). This means that during expiration the airways pressure is maintained above atmospheric, usually in the range of 5–15 cm $H_2O$. PEEP is thought to work by 'recruiting' the alveoli that are 'closed' and not taking part in oxygenation of blood. PEEP is not without its deleterious effects and the resulting increase in intrathoracic pressure can decrease venous return and cardiac output, causing systemic hypotension and decrease of blood flow to the peripheral tissue. PEEP also causes overdistension of 'recruited' alveoli, interferes with right ventricular function and increases the risk of barotrauma.

**Circulatory support and fluid management**

Patients suffering from ARDS are generally hypovolaemic due to the capillary leak that shifts the fluid from the vascular compartment into the extravascular compartment. Hypovolaemia, especially in the presence of PEEP, reduces cardiac filling and causes a fall in cardiac output (normally 3–4 $l$ min$^{-1}$ m$^{-2}$ of the body surface area). Animal experiments and clinical experience have shown that these patients have a higher than normal tissue oxygen demand. Clinically, the only practical way of satisfying this increased oxygen demand is by increasing the flow of well oxygenated blood to the tissue. This is achieved by infusion of fluid (usually colloid), blood and cardiotonic drugs like dobutamine to increase the cardiac output. Fluid management in these patients can be difficult and is best judged by measuring left heart filling pressures. This can easily be measured by the bedside with a pulmonary artery flotation ( Swan Ganz) catheter, which also measures the cardiac output. Experience has shown that these patients require a higher than normal cardiac output (i.e. more than 4.5 $l^{-1}$ min$^{-1}$ m$^{-2}$ ) to satisfy the increased oxygen requirement of the tissue and to prevent multiple organ failure.

Other supportive measures necessary in ARDS include a thorough search for and elimination of infections. If the infection is surgically accessible then it must be drained and appropriate antibiotic therapy started. Nutritional support is necessary as it has been shown that malnutrition may contribute to organ failure. It is essential to realize that in conditions of sepsis and trauma lipids are preferentially utilized as the energy source. Besides this, lipid metabolism produces less carbon dioxide, which may be helpful in the management of ARDS. Only adequate calories are provided so that there is zero rather than positive caloric as well as nitrogen balance.

High-dose steroids have long been advocated as an adjunct to therapy of ARDS. There is very little scientific evidence to support this view. Recent studies have demonstrated that high-dose steroids have no proven value in the treatment of ARDS and may actually worsen the outcome of the disease besides further compromising the already deficient immune system of these desperately ill patients.

## CONCLUSION

ARDS is a serious complication of sepsis and trauma. Multiple trauma patients requiring prolonged multi-organ support because of the nature of their illness may sooner or later suffer from sepsis and may progress to ARDS and multiple organ failure. ARDS is the pulmonary manifestation of multiple organ failure syndrome. The mortality of severe ARDS is high. Hypoxia and shock in trauma and sepsis increase the risk of ARDS and organ failure. Thus prevention and early effective treatment of hypoxia and shock in trauma, sepsis and all critically ill patients is of the utmost importance.

### FURTHER READING

Bernard G R, Luce J M, Sprung C L et al 1987 High-dose corticosteroids in patients with adult respiratory distress syndrome. New England Journal of Medicine 317: 1565–1570
Bihari D, Kox W (eds) 1988 Shock and adult respiratory distress syndrome. Springer-Verlag, London
Bone R C, Fisher C J, Clemmer T P et al 1987 A controlled clinical trial of high-dose methylpredinisolone in the treatment of severe sepsis and septic shock. New England Journal of Medicine 317: 653–658
Hunter D N, Keogh B F, Morgan C J et al 1989 Management of adult respiratory distress syndrome: 1. British Journal of Hospital Medicine 42: 468–471
Matthay M A 1990 The adult respiratory distress syndrome: definition and prognosis. Clinics in Chest Medicine 11(4): 575–580
Murphy P G, Jones J G 1991 Acute lung injury. British Journal of Intensive Care 1(3): 110–117
Taylor R W, Norwood S H 1988 The adult respiratory distress syndrome. In Civetta J M, Taylor R W, Kirby R R (eds) Critical care. Lippincott, Philadelphia, pp 1057–1068.

PART 5.19
## COAGULOPATHY AND FAT EMBOLISM
*M. Y. A. Rady*

## COAGULOPATHY

Coagulopathy is defined as inappropriate intravascular activation of the coagulation and fibrinolytic systems causing depletion of platelets, coagulation and fibrinolytic factors. This is associated with the formation of platelet-fibrin thrombi in the microvasculature and raised fibrin degradation products in the plasma.

## Mechanisms

Several mechanisms can contribute to the incidence of coagulopathy and may include the following:

1. increased concentrations of activators of coagulation and fibrinolysis, e.g. serine-protease enzymes, thromboplastin or tissue factors from damaged tissues and endothelium
2. reduced concentrations of inhibitors, normally produced by vascular endothelium, e.g. antithrombin III, thrombomodulin, protein C and protein S, tissue plasminogen activator inhibitor type 1, plasmin inhibitors and prostacyclins
3. reduced hepatic synthesis of coagulation factors and release of platelets from megakaryocytes
4. reduced reticuloendothelial system (RES) clearance of intravascular fibrin, platelets and erythrocyte breakdown products.

## Initiation factors

The common action of initiation factors is injury and damage to the microvascular endothelium. Initiation factors may be produced during:

1. low tissue blood flow, e.g. hypoxia, thromboxanes, leukotrienes
2. high tissue blood flow, e.g. endotoxins, cytokines such as tumour necrosis factor, interleukins and free radicals.

## Manifestations

The clinical manifestations may involve:

1. vascular occlusion by platelet–fibrin thrombi producing end-organ ischaemia, infarction and failure
2. haemorrhage and uncontrolled bleeding at many sites, such as surgical wounds, pulmonary system, gastrointestinal tract, retroperitoneal and intracranial spaces.

## Therapy

Therapy should aim to:

1. prevent further insult and damage to the microvascular endothelium by restoring tissue oxygenation and appropriate operative treatment of localized crushed tissues or sepsis
2. replace deficient inhibitors such as antithrombin III, protein C and prostacyclin
3. replace depleted coagulation factors and platelets if haemorrhagic manifestations are present.

## Prevention

The incidence of coagulopathy may be reduced by:

1. *early* restoration of microcirculatory blood flow, and adequate tissue oxygenation during initial resuscitation
2. *early* operative treatment of injuries and localized sepsis.

## FAT EMBOLISM

Fat embolism is defined as thromboembolism of the pulmonary and systemic microvasculature, with lipid globules and fibrin–platelet thrombi. Lipid globules are formed mainly from circulating plasma triglycerides normally carried by very-low-density lipoproteins (VLDL).

## Mechanism

Plasma triglyceride concentration is raised because of:

1. increased peripheral mobilization of fatty acids and increased hepatic synthesis of triglycerides in stress conditions, as in post-trauma, sepsis and intravenous hyperalimentation
2. reduced peripheral uptake and clearance of plasma VLDL due to a reduced tissue lipoprotein lipase activity
3. release of lipid globules from damaged bone marrow adipocytes into the circulation.

## Site of action

Intravascular triglycerides interact with the cell membrane phospholipids present in the following cellular elements chart: (see Fig. 5.19.1):

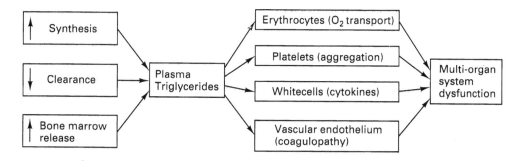

**Fig. 5.19.1** The mechanism of interaction between raised plasma triglycerides and the pathogenesis of multi-organ system dysfunction in fat embolism.

1. erythrocytes: this can reduce oxygen uptake by haemoglobin, increase blood viscosity and reduce microcirculatory blood flow
2. platelets: this facilitates platelet aggregation, activation of the coagulation pathways and the formation of fibrin
3. white cells: this can affect their chemotactic function, migration, phagocytosis, endothelial adherence and release of inflammatory mediators
4. microvascular endothelium: see Coagulopathy.

### Manifestation

Fat embolism usually manifests as multi-organ system dysfunction, such as:

1. pulmonary, e.g. ventilation–perfusion mismatch (increased pulmonary physiological shunt), impaired alveolar surfactant activity (reduced pulmonary compliance) and segmental hypoperfusion (increased physiological dead space)
2. cerebral, e.g. ischaemia/infarction, oedema (focal neurological deficit, confusion or seizures)
3. cardiac, e.g. reduced mechanical performance (compliance and contractility), arrhythmia
4. renal, e.g. lipiduria with tubular damage, ischaemic glomerular–tubular dysfunction (oliguric or polyuric renal failure)
5. cutaneous, e.g. capillary endothelial disruption and petechial haemorrhage.

### Diagnosis of fat embolism

The following criteria have to be fulfilled:

1. presence of fat globules in body fluids, e.g. sputum, urine, or lipid emboli in retinal vessels on fundoscopy
2. Histological demonstration of intracellular and intravascular aggregation of lipid globules (with Sudan black stain)
3. evidence of pulmonary and at least one other organ-system dysfunction.

### Therapy

Therapy should aim towards:

1. optimizing tissue oxygenation to meet increased metabolic demands
2. supporting the function of failing organ systems, e.g. respiratory, cardiac, renal
3. early operative intervention, e.g. internal fixation of long bone fractures, amputation of crushed limbs or drainage of localized infection.

### Prevention

*Early* optimal resuscitation and operative treatment of skeletal injuries should reduce the incidence of fat embolism.

FURTHER READING

Greenberg C S, Sane D C 1990 Coagulation problems in critical care medicine. Critical Care: State of the Art 11: 187

## PART 5.20
# REHABILITATION
*E. R. S. Ross*

The early meaning of rehabilitation was restoration of position, rank or possessions, and was the prerogative of the king. When used in a medical context it means the restoration of normal activity, independent living and reintegration into the community. *All* injured patients required rehabilitation. Four phases can be recognized during the period from injury to recovery when a variety of approaches to rehabilitate the patient are required.

### Restoration of normal activity

The human body is capable of a very wide range of activity but a few key functions govern that range. For example, standing without external support is dependent on the integrity of the lower limbs and nervous system. Injury to the lower limbs or nervous system may impair standing and thus all other activity secondary to that like walking, running, climbing stairs and so on. A further complication is the extent of damage which has occurred to any system. Some damage is permanent, e.g. a spinal cord transection. Rehabilitation still has the same aim but some permanent reduction in activity may have to be accepted. This contrasts with a fractured bone, where once healed full normal activity might be expected. A third group, such as a head injury, may at first have grossly impaired function but with the resolution of reversible damage startling improvement in function and thus activity may occur independent of an active rehabilitation programme.

### Restoration of independent living

Where full restoration of function is expected, only early dependence on others or aids will be necessary. A good example would be the temporary loss of independence following an isolated lower limb fracture, where initially crutches, a frame or a wheelchair may be necessary to regain some degree of independence. There are circumstances which will require substantial orthotic provision, e.g. following spinal injury, where a wheelchair, crutches, reciprocating gait orthosis or calipers may all be required to assist in the rehabilitation. Alongside this, modification of the home or working environment may need to be considered, like stair lifts, ramps or door widening.

### Reintegration into the community

Realistic goals have to be set following injury, bearing in mind recovery times and possible functional losses. A change of type of work may be required, either temporarily or permanently. This is part of the rehabilitation process and may involve employers, retraining schemes, the disablement resettlement officer, government assessment courses or sheltered working environments. Following trauma several phases may be considered.

### Phase one: Immediate post-injury period

This may be life threatening and, while little can be done in the active sense to rehabilitate, great care to prevent more damage must be taken. It is easier to rehabilitate an individual who has suffered a fracture of the cervical spine without neurological involvement. Creation of neurotrauma by failure to recognize the injury or protect the part is catastrophic.

Prevention is better than rehabilitation!

### Phase two: Perioperative

Stabilization of fractures by internal fixation, internal splinting (i.e. intramedullary rodding) or external fixation allows early recovery of the soft tissues. These techniques also allow early movement of joints and active use of muscles. Continuous passive motion machines encourage early joint motion, reducing stiffness, contracture and preserving articular cartilage. Physiotherapy is essential in the immediate postoperative period, to encourage active use of muscle to maintain its bulk, to prevent contractures and to encourage the patient to begin exercises and movements which will eventually culminate in walking or using the upper limb as normally as possible. Splintage may be required to prevent contracture, which can slow down or halt progress towards normal activity. This is vital in amputation surgery, where contracture of soft tissue can produce a flexion deformity in a nearby joint, thus preventing the fitting of the prosthesis.

## Phase 3: Early active

Here retraining to walk may require temporary or permanent aids. Fractures may be braced using 'functional braces' as popularized by Sarmiento. These braces allow weight bearing and joint motion while maintaining fracture alignment during the healing phase.

Temporary pylons may be provided for amputees until a permanent prosthesis is available. Simple walking sticks, crutches, rollators and frames all have a place in this phase. Also passive splinting of drop foot, preventing equinus deformity, may mean the difference between walking or not. Lively splints in the hand may substitute for muscle activity until a tendon repair is sound or a nerve repair has healed.

## Phase 4: Return to home and work

This phase probably requires the most help from outside agencies. Physiotherapists, occupational therapists, social workers, GPs, disablement resettlement officers and family members may all need to play their part here.

# 6. Resuscitation

*R. Touquet    J. Fothergill    R. M. Jones*

The cause of the collapse or coma (a symptom of a broad spectrum of life-threatening conditions that depress or injure the central nervous system) precipitating a patient's arrival in the resuscitation room is often unknown. Furthermore, there may be more than one pathology, for example the patient with hypoglycaemia who has fallen striking his head.

When a patient is brought into an accident and emergency (A&E) department with an altered level of consciousness, the resuscitation sequence described in the American College of Surgeons' Advanced Trauma Life Support Course is appropriate whether the cause is a medical or a surgical emergency. The initial sequence is known as the primary survey (ABCDE, see below). This is a systematic form of assessment which is carried out at the same time as any resuscitative procedures are undertaken. There is ongoing monitoring of the vital signs, and in particular monitoring of the vital signs in response to any procedure undertaken, such as the immediate infusion of 2 litres of cystalloid for the adult in hypovolaemic shock.

The standard sequence of the initial primary survey is as follows:

**A**irway, with cervical spine control
**B**reathing
**C**irculation
**D**isability — a brief neurological assessment
**E**xposure — undress the patient completely.

Due notice must be taken of the history from the ambulance crew. The ambulance transfer form must be signed by a member of the A&E staff. It is prudent to involve the ambulance crew in the inital resuscitation and to have that crew immediately available to give any further details about the history.

When the patient is stabilized, with clinically acceptable vital signs, the patient is examined from head to toe in order to prevent any pathology being missed. It is not infrequent that the A&E doctor is the last doctor to examine the patient in their totality. This systematic methodical examination is known as the secondary survey. However, if the patient has to be taken to theatre urgently then this secondary survey will have to be carried out later on the ward by the responsible admitting team.

## PART 1: PRIMARY SURVEY WITH INITIAL RESUSCITATION

Greet the conscious patient from the ambulance by talking to him and reassuring him that he is in the right place and that you know what to do. Do not treat the patient as an inanimate object.

### Airway

In all trauma victims apply an appropriately sized hard cervical collar. Steady the head — in-line cervical spine immobilization — to prevent those with unsuspected neck injury from sustaining an iatrogenic injury to the cervical spinal cord during manoeuvres on the airway. The neck is at particular risk during orotracheal intubation, when extreme vigilance is mandatory in those in whom a cervical spine injury has not been ruled out.

## Assessment

Assess the patency of the airway by talking to the patient, looking for signs of confusion or agitation which may indicate cerebral hypoxia. Listen for stridor or gurgling sounds from a compromised airway. Feel for warm air against your hand in a patient who is breathing. Following smoke inhalation there may be carbon deposits in the mouth or nostrils, raising the possibility of upper airway burns and associated carbon monoxide poisoning. In this situation call an anaesthetist, as early tracheal intubation will be required.

Look to see whether chest movements are adequate.

## Management

Keep the airway open and clear it. Remove any foreign bodies such as sweets, or vomit which is sucked out. Lift the chin forwards to bring the tongue off the back of the nasopharynx and if the gag reflex is diminished insert an oral (Guedel) airway. If a Guedel airway is not tolerated, but obstruction is still present, consider gently inserting a well-lubricated nasopharyngeal airway, ensuring that this is done atraumatically. Once the airway is secured deliver 10–15 $l$ min$^{-1}$ of oxygen via a face mask with a reservoir device, providing 85% oxygen.

None of these basic airway manoeuvres protects the lungs from aspiration of gastric contents or blood. In those unable to protect their own airway (absent gag reflex) a cuffed tracheal tube must be inserted via the oral or nasal route both to facilitate efficient ventilation and to protect the lungs.

If the airway cannot be secured by any of the above methods, urgently carry out a needle cricothyroidotomy followed if necessary by a surgical cricothyroidotomy.

## Breathing

### Assessment

Note any degree of cyanosis. Assess the neck veins and if they are engorged consider the possibility of a tension pneumothorax, cardiac tam-

ponade, air embolus, pulmonary embolus or myocardial contusion. Feel for the position of the trachea, and if it is deviated to one side decide whether it has been pushed over by a tension pneumothorax on the other side. Count the respiratory rate (normally 12–20 per minute) and expose, inspect and palpate the anterior chest wall. Assess air entry or the lack of it by auscultation. A severe asthmatic may present with collapse and have a silent chest because with extreme airway narrowing no air can move in or out of the lungs. In a flail chest there are three or more consecutive ribs each fractured in two or more places, with a segment of paradoxical chest wall motion; the underlying pulmonary contusion may cause acute respiratory failure. If there is any doubt about the adequacy of a patient's airway or breathing, urgently obtain expert help from physicians and anaesthetists.

### Management: control of ventilation

Preventing hypoventilation, hypercarbia, cerebral vasodilatation and a resultant increase in intracerebral pressure is vital in trauma patients, especially if they have suffered a head injury. Adults should have a tidal volume of 6 ml kg$^{-1}$, and children 10 ml kg$^{-1}$. If the patient is unable to sustain this then respiration must be assisted initially by bag valve mask positive pressure ventilation. Ventilate and oxygenate the hypoxic or apnoeic patient if possible for at least 3 minutes prior to attempted intubation, and do not prolong any attempt for more than 60 seconds before returning to bag valve mask ventilation. Any patient who is apnoeic obviously needs ventilation urgently.

The aim of assisted ventilation is to keep the arterial blood oxygen over 10 kPa (80 mmHg) and the carbon dioxide below 5.5 kPa (40 mmHg). A reduction of the arterial carbon dioxide tension (PaCO$_2$) to about 4 kPa (30 mmHg) will reduce cerebral oedema in a patient with a head injury and a decreased level of consciousness.

In those who are breathing spontaneously assume agitation, aggression or depressed level of consciousness is due to hypoxia, so these, and indeed all collapsed patients who are not likely to recover immediately must have arterial blood gases estimated urgently (also consider, where appropriate, a full bladder or tight plaster of Paris as causes of restlessness). Take the arterial blood into a heparinized syringe from the radial artery, or failing this the femoral artery.

The arterial oxygen tension ($PaO_2$) must be maintained at more than 10 kPa (80 mmHg) as cerebral function is impaired below this level. The exceptions are patients with chronic obstructive airways disease (COAD), who have a tendency to underbreathe when given added oxygen because their respiration is normally stimulated by a degree of hypoxia, rather than by any small increase in the $PaCO_2$ as in patients without COAD. With this caveat all collapsed patients should initially be given 85% oxygen as the problem of the patient whose respiration is driven by oxygen lack is uncommonly encountered in A&E.

Oxygen administration may also be necessary to produce a higher than normal $PaO_2$. This is indicated to correct a pathological state whose treatment is with an elevated $PaO_2$; some examples are carbon monoxide poisoning, elevated pulmonary vascular resistance, sickle cell crisis and anaerobic infections.

## Circulation

This is the third priority after **A**irway with cervical spine control, and **B**reathing.

### Assessment

Assessment of the patient for shock requires skill. Remember that the earliest signs of shock are anxiety, a tachycardia of 100–120 beats per minute, tachypnoea of 20–30 breaths per minute, skin mottling and a prolonged capillary refill time of more than 2 seconds, and postural hypotension. If there is postural hypotension with a fall of systolic blood pressure of 20 mmHg, a fall of diastolic blood pressure of 10 mmHg and a rise of pulse of 20 beats per minute — 20 : 10 : 20 rule — diagnose hypovolaemia due to an occult bleed until proved otherwise. Supine systolic blood pressure does not drop until an adult has lost around 1500–2000 ml of blood, or 30–40% of the blood volume of 70 ml $kg^{-1}$ body weight;

by this time the patient is ashen in colour because of blood-drained extremities.

The level of consciousness is also decreased because of inadequate cerebral circulation, particularly if blood loss was rapid. As a guide, a palpable peripheral pulse indicates a systemic blood pressure of at least 60 mmHg. If the carotid pulse is absent, initiate immediate basic cardiopulmonary resuscitation (CPR, see below).

### Management

Control haemorrhage from any external bleeding points by direct pressure with limb elevation where appropriate.

***Intravenous access.*** Poiseuille's law states that the rate of flow of fluid through a pipe is proportional to the fourth power of the radius, and inversely proportional to the length. In a severely traumatized or hypovolaemic patient, never fail to insert two short wide-bore cannulae of 14 gauge or larger, sited in peripheral veins, whether introduced percutaneously or by surgical cutdown.

Preferred sites for cutdown are the long saphenous vein anterior to the medial malleolus, or the basilic vein in the elbow crease. Cutdown is a safe, simple and quick procedure in which every surgical trainee should be skilled.

*Technique for venous cutdown.* Make a transverse 2 cm incision anterior to the medial malleolus or to the medial epicondyle of the humerus. By blunt dissection delineate the long saphenous vein or basilic vein. Ligate the vein distally with 2/0 black silk. Control the vein proximally with a similar loose ligature. Make a transverse incision for one third of the circumference of the vein, such that it is possible to insert a 14 to 12-gauge cannula into the vein. Secure the cannula in place by tightening the proximal suture. This technique is applicable for collapsed infants.

***Intraosseous infusion.*** An even simpler technique for children is to use an intraosseous trocar and cannula: these are specially designed to be inserted through the cortex of bone into the bone marrow. The site for introduction of the needle is two fingers distal to the tibial tuberosity on the anteromedial surface of the tibia. Clean the area thoroughly as osteomyelitis is a possible complication of the technique. Crystalloid and colloid may slowly be injected into the marrow (20 ml kg⁻¹ initially for the collapsed child) together with drugs used in resuscitation, with the exception of sodium bicarbonate and bretylium. The circulation time from here to the heart is only 20 seconds.

Central venous cannulation may be dangerous, even in experienced hands, for the trauma patient who is often restless. Such patients may not survive an iatrogenic pneumothorax or cervical spinal cord injury caused by the turning of an unsuspected neck injury, and as the above routes of access avoid the possibility of these complications they are to be preferred. Central venous pressure monitoring is useful in the stabilized patient, but these lines are not for resuscitation other than in patients with cardiac arrest, when drugs should be administered centrally.

Correct hypovolaemia with the rapid intravenous infusion of warmed crystalloid or colloid solution followed by blood. Rapid loss of greater than 40% of a patient's blood volume produces electromechanical dissociation leading to circulatory standstill unless immediate resuscitation is carried out. It is not possible to measure the blood volume of a patient in the resuscitation room. Therefore you must monitor the vital signs (delineated in Part 2) especially in response to treatment such as fluid replacement, and tailor your treatment accordingly.

If the carotid pulse is impalpable, the heart has become an ineffective pump and irreversible brain damage results unless immediate action is taken to correct the specific causes of electromechanical dissociation such as massive blood loss, tension pneumothorax or cardiac tamponade. If there is no improvement or these conditions are not present commence cardiac massage for cardiac arrest (Fig. 6.1A). Check the heart's electrical rhythm on the monitor. Place the leads in the correct positions as quickly as possible. If no rhythm shows ensure the gain knob is turned up on the monitor, and check for a rhythm in two different ECG leads; alternatively monitor through the paddles of a defibrillator, one placed just to the left of the expected position of the apex beat and one inferior to the right clavicle.

*External chest compression.* When the carotid pulse is not palpable after you have controlled ventilation, place one hand over the other on the sternum, the lower border of the hands being two fingers above the xiphisternal–sternal junction. If the hands are lower there is risk of damage to the liver. Keep the arms straight with the shoulders in a direct line over the hands in order that you do not tire. Depress the sternum in a smooth manner for 4–5 cm, at a rate of 80 per minute, with a ratio of one ventilation to about five compressions, both actions being carried out synchronously. Keep the compression rate regular so that the ventilation between compression five and the next compression runs from the fifth compression into the next first compression. In this way the pressure is increased generally in the chest both during part of compression five and compression one by that ventilation. In addition the expanding lungs drive the diaphragm down, leading to compression of the vena cava. This further facilitates blood being forced up the carotid arteries (the thoracic pump effect); feel for the carotid or femoral pulse every 2 minutes.

The correct cardiac rhythm must be diagnosed quickly. In a non-traumatic cardiac arrest patient the rhythm is ventricular fibrillation in 70% of cases, and the chances of a successful resuscitation are directly proportional to the speed of applying DC shock in the correct manner and sequence (Fig. 6.1B). Therefore there must be no delays from the time of arrest, and this is why ambulance crews are now being trained to use, and are issued with, defibrillators.

*Internal cardiac massage.* External chest compression does not effectively resuscitate an empty heart in cardiac arrest due to hypovolaemic shock. When there is not an appropriate response to prompt rapid transfusion, you should consider internal cardiac massage. This is the only indication for an emergency thoracotomy for internal cardiac massage in the A&E department by trained personnel. Internal cardiac massage is, in the hands of those with appropriate training, both safe and haemodynamically superior to external cardiac massage, although the latter can be initiated without delay and performed by non-surgeons. Open-chest cardiopulmonary resuscitation (CPR) enables direct palpation and observa-

**CARDIOPULMONARY RESUSCITATION**

| | | |
|---|---|---|
| Unresponsive | **AIRWAY** | Open airway |
| No breathing | **BREATHING** | Rescue breathing |
| No pulse | **CIRCULATION** | Cardiopulmonary resuscitation (CPR) |

**ECG**

**Electromechanical dissociation**

QRS without palpable pulse

Adrenaline 1mg/iv

Consider specific therapy for hypovolaemia
   pneumothorax
   cardiac tamponade
   pulmonary embolism

Consider calcium chloride (10mg of 10%)
for hyperkalaemia
   hypocalcaemia
   calcium antagonists

**Ventricular fibrillation (VF)**

Defibrillate 200J

Defibrillate 200J

Defibrillate 360J

Adrenaline 1mg/iv

Defibrillate 360J

Lignocaine 100mg/iv

Repeated defibrillations 360J
Consider:
different paddle
   positions
different defibrillator
other antiarrhythmic
   drugs

**Apparent asystole**

Iso-electric ECG

Defibrillate 200J

Defibrillate 200J

Defibrillate 360J

Adrenaline 1mg/iv

Atropine 2mg/iv

Consider pacing if P waves or any other electrical activity present

Continue CPR for up to 2 minutes after each drug. Do not interrupt CPR for more than 10 sec except for defibrillation. If an i/v line cannot be established, consider giving double doses of adrenaline, lignocaine, atropine via an endotracheal tube.

**Prolonged resuscitation**
Give 1mg adrenaline every 5 mins
Consider 50 mmol sodium bicarbonate
   (50 ml of 8.4%) or according to
   blood gas results

**Post-resuscitation care**
Check: Arterial blood gases
   Electrolytes
   Chest x-ray
Observe monitor and treat
   patient in an intensive care
   unit

A

**CARDIOPULMONARY RESUSCITATION**

Call for HELP
including Defibrillator
Airway adjuncts
Oxygen
Emergency kit

Consider
Precordial thump
in witnessed or
monitored arrest

If 2 rescuers,
simultaneous
cardiac massage
and
mouth to mouth
respiration
(1 : 5)

Place paddles correctly
if flat trace, check
switches, connections
and gain

Give oxygen

Secure airway
Intubate if necessary

Cannulate large vein

Continue CPR

B

**Fig. 6.1   A** Cardiopulmonary resuscitation. **B** Protocol for the treatment of cardiac arrest cases in hospitals. The Resuscitation Council (UK).

tion of the heart and direct electric defibrillation.

The technique for internal cardiac massage (by trained personnel) is as follows: make a left-sided thoracotomy through the fourth or fifth intercostal space once the patient is receiving intermittent positive pressure ventilation through a tracheal tube. Immediately compress the heart using the left hand, without at first opening the pericardial sac, by placing the thumb over the left ventricle posteriorly and the fingers anteriorly in front of the heart. The heart is compressed at the rate of 80 per minute, adjusting the compression force and rate to the filling of the heart. Open the pericardium, avoiding the phrenic and vagus nerves. Adrenaline, atropine and lignocaine, but not sodium bicarbonate, may be injected directly into the left ventricle, avoiding the coronary arteries. For internal defibrillation use internal 6 cm paddle electrodes with saline-soaked gauze pads and insulated handles. Place one paddle posteriorly over the left ventricle and one over the anterior surface of the heart (10–20 J).

**Drugs.** In a patient with cardiac arrest, drugs such as adrenaline should if possible be given centrally, and for this reason you must be proficient in at least one method of central venous cannulation. You should use the approach with which you are most familiar; however, the infraclavicular approach is often the most convenient and practical means of access for the surgeon.

*Technique for subclavian vein cannulation*

1. Preparation: clean the area with surgical antiseptic solution.
2. Position: use a 20° head-down tilt (in patients without head injury) to fill the vein and to reduce the risk of air embolus. For access to the right subclavian vein pull the right arm caudally, to place the vein in the most convenient position to the clavicle for cannulation. If the shoulder is obstructing access, place a sand bag below the upper thoracic spine so that the shoulders lie more posteriorly, unless there is any possibility of spinal injury.
3. Access: introduce the needle through the skin 2 cm inferior to the junction of the lateral and middle thirds of the clavicle. Advance the needle, aspirating continuously and snugging the inferior bony surface of the clavicle, aiming for the superior aspect of the right sternoclavicular joint for not more than 6 cm.
4. Technique: aspirate until blood freely appears, ensure the bevel of the needle is now directed caudally, remove the syringe and immediately insert the Seldinger wire, flexible end first, through the needle. Remove the needle, railroad the plastic cannula over the Seldinger wire, then remove the wire. Check that the cannula is in the central vein by briefly allowing retrograde blood flow into the attached intravenous giving set.
5. Aftercare: secure the line with a black silk suture through the skin and dress with sterile dressing. Return the patient to the horizontal position and obtain a chest X-ray to check the position of the central venous cannula and exclude a pneumothorax. Note that absence of a pneumothorax on this film does not exclude the possibility of one developing subsequently, possibly under tension.

If there is trauma to only one side of the chest then use this side for cannulation because there is already a risk of pneumothorax there.

If this direct venous access is not obtained during CPR for immediate drug therapy to the heart muscle, then drugs should be given via a peripheral venous line, with an infusion of 5% dextrose solution running after each drug to flush it into the central circulation. Certain drugs such as adrenaline, atropine, lignocaine and naloxone may be given via the tracheal tube route, in double the intravenous dosage diluted to 10 ml.

**Disability**

This term is used to signify a brief neurological assessment which must be carried out at this stage of the initial examination. The mnemonic used in the Advanced Trauma Life Support Course is useful:

A = **A**lert
V = responds to **V**erbal stimuli
P = responds to **P**ainful stimuli
U = **U**nresponsive.

In addition, now assess the presence or absence of orientation in time (knows day and month),

**Table 6.1** Pupil size and response to light in comatose patients

|  | One pupil | Both pupils |
|---|---|---|
| Dilated | Atropine in eye<br>3rd nerve lesion normal consensual light reflex, e.g. posterior communicating artery aneurysm<br>Enlarging mass lesion above the tentorium, causing a pressure cone<br><br>*Optic nerve lesion:*<br>Old: pale disc and afferent pupil<br>New: afferent pupil with normal disc, loss of direct light reflex, loss of consensual reflex in other eye — both constrict with light in other eye | Cerebral anoxia<br>Very poor outlook if increasing supratentorial pressure — if dilated pupils preceded by unilateral dilation or if due to diffuse cerebral damage<br><br>Overdose: e.g.   Amphetamines<br>                Carbon monoxide<br>                Phenothiazines<br>                Cocaine<br>                Glutethimide<br>                Antidepressants<br>Hypothermia |
| Constricted | Pilocarpine in eye<br>Horner's, e.g. brachial plexus lesion<br>Acute stroke uncommonly (brain stem occlusion or carotid artery ischaemia: small pupil opposite side to weakness) | Pilocarpine in both eyes (glaucoma treatment) Opiates, organophosphate insecticides and trichloroethanol (chloral)<br>Pontine haemorrhage or ischaemia (brisk tendon reflexes, and temperature increased: poor prognostic sign) |

If pupils normal in size, and reacting to light, consider metabolic, systemic non-cerebral causes
(N.B. Normal pupils do not exclude an overdose)

space (knows where he is) and person (knows who he is). These perceptions are usually lost in this sequence with lessening of consciousness. Defer delineation of the Glasgow Coma Scale until a more detailed head-to-toe examination can be carried out after the initial assessment is completed and resuscitation is underway.

Record the pupil size and response to light (Table 6.1). Bilateral small pupils denote opiate poisoning unless disproved by failure of naloxone to reverse the constriction. If necessary up to 2 mg of naloxone (i.e. five vials of 0.4 mg) are given.

If there is a response, more may have to be given because it has a short half-life; it may be given via an endotracheal tube if you do not have intravenous access. The other common cause of bilateral small pupils is a pontine haemorrhage, for which there is no specific treatment.

**Exposure**

In a severely traumatized patient always carry out a complete examination of all of the skin. This necessitates the removal of every scrap of clothing, being careful to protect the spine. Full examination includes log-rolling with a minimum of four trained personnel to examine the back. Perform this earlier if there is a specific indication (e.g. trauma to the posterior chest wall) or at the latest at the end of the secondary survey.

Consider inserting a nasogastric tube, or if there is a suspicion of a cribriform plate fracture an orogastric tube. Insert a urinary catheter after inspecting the perineum for bruising, and carrying out a rectal examination in an injured patient (see chapter on trauma).

## PART 2: MONITORING

Throughout this initial assessment, resuscitation proceeds with constant ongoing monitoring of vital signs and simple clinical measurements. You must constantly tailor your resuscitation according to results of your monitoring and keep an open mind to possible diagnoses and therefore appropriate treatment.

## Pulse

Remember that in an elderly or even middle-aged person a rate of more than 140 per minute is very unlikely to be sinus tachycardia as this is too fast for someone of that age. The atria flutter at around 300 beats per minute, and therefore if there is 2–1 atrioventricular block the ventricular rate is 150 per minute. The rate of supraventricular tachycardia is usually 160–220 beats per minute.

## Respiratory rate

The importance of this is all too easily forgotten. The normal range is 12–20 breaths per minute. It rises early with blood loss or hypoxia, and as well as being a very useful indication of the patient's clinical state is one of the physiological parameters that is mandatory for the calculation of the Revised Trauma Score.

## Blood pressure

With hypovolaemia this drops when the blood loss is greater than 1500–2000 ml. Fit young adults, and especially children, maintain their blood pressure resiliently, but then it falls precipitously when compensatory mechanisms are overwhelmed.

## Pulse pressure

This is the difference between systolic pressure and diastolic pressure. Initially with haemorrhage the diastolic pressure rises due to vasoconstriction from circulating catecholamines, while the systolic stays constant. Therefore the pulse pressure decreases. This is followed by a greater decrease in the pulse pressure as the systolic blood pressure falls once 30% of the patient's blood volume has been lost.

## Capillary refill time

This is the time it takes for blood to return to a compressed nail bed on release of pressure — the time can be longer because of hypothermia, peripheral microvascular disease and collagen diseases as well as in hypovolaemia. The normal value is 2 seconds, but this time increases early in shock, following a 15% loss of blood volume.

## Temperature

Quite apart from primary hypothermia, in a hypovolaemic patient a decreased temperature is an indication of the degree of blood loss. Blood volume must be restored adequately, because if the hypovolaemic patient is simply warmed the blood pressure falls further by virtue of the resulting vasodilation. The patient with primary hypothermia is usually hypovolaemic as well, which is why rapid rewarming results in a drop in blood pressure unless blood volume is replaced. Every resuscitation room should have a warming cabinet so that intravenous fluid can be immediately infused at 37°C to the hypovolaemic or hypothermic patient.

## Urinary output

The minimal normal obligatory output is 30 ml $h^{-1}$. In a child it is easily remembered as 1 ml $kg^{-1}$ $h^{-1}$.

## Central venous pressure (CVP)

This is measured in centimetres of water by positioning the manometer on a stand such that the zero point is level with the patient's right atrium. The normal pressure is around 5 $cmH_2O$ from the angle of Louis, with the patient at 45° to the horizontal.

With a normally functioning heart the measurement of CVP is an indirect indicator of the preload to the left ventricle (left ventricular end-diastolic pressure, LVEDP) or the state of filling of the systemic circulation. It does not give a direct measurement of LVEDP.

The CVP is low if the patient is hypovolaemic, and rises to normal with correction. The CVP is raised if the circulating volume is too large, as might happen with renal failure or with overtransfusion.

Overtransfusion not only precipitates heart failure, but in a patient with a head injury the resultant rise in intracranial pressure may cause irreversible damage to the already bruised brain. Monitoring the CVP in these circumstances is therefore crucial.

The CVP also rises if the right side of the heart is malfunctioning. The CVP cannot then be used as an indication of the filling of the systemic circulation. It may be raised for mechanical reasons such as a tension penumothorax or cardiac tamponade. It is raised in the presence of pulmonary embolism, or when the heart is failing for lack of muscular power due to contusion or infarction.

## Arterial blood gases

Normal values for $PaO_2$ and $PaCO_2$ are described above (see Breathing — Management). Arterial blood pH is normally between 7.36 and 7.42. This is dependent upon the arterial $PCO_2$ being 4.7–5.7 KPa and the plasma bicarbonate being 24–30 mmol$^{-1}$. Carbon dioxide is the largest generator of $H^+$ ions, ten times more than the production from lactic and other organic acid production or from urea synthesis (Table 6.2).

Patients in early hypovolaemic shock have a respiratory alkalosis due to tachypnoea. Respiratory alkalosis gives way to a mild metabolic acidosis which then becomes more severe if the inadequate organ perfusion is not successfully treated.

Most acid–base abnormalities are the result of an imbalance between the production and removal of $H^+$ ions, as demonstrated in Table 6.2. When the primary disturbance is due to abnormal carbon dioxide elimination it is respiratory, while all other primary disturbance — classes II and III — are termed metabolic. Interpretation of pH results may be facilitated by an acid–base diagram with pH on the $y$ axis and $PCO_2$ on the $x$ axis, as in Figure 6.2. The bands shown demonstrate the expected response to uncomplicated disorders of acid–base balance.

The central shaded area shows the normal limits. Thus the patient with uncomplicated metabolic acidosis has values above and to the left of the shaded area, while the patient with uncomplicated respiratory acidosis lies in the band above and to the right. A patient with a result in sector A or C probably has a combination of two primary conditions, while one in

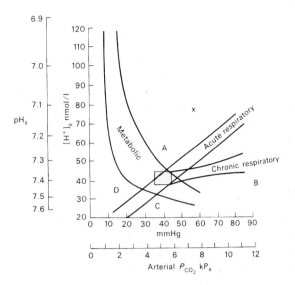

**Fig. 6.2** Blood gases. Reproduced from Cohen & Woods (1987), with permission.

sectors B or D would be the result of compensation of a primary abnormality. The diagram facilitates the plotting of response to treatment.

Treatment with sodium bicarbonate has in the past been over-enthusiastic and there are definite hazards in its uses, listed in Table 6.3. It is now recognized that bicarbonate should not be given during the first 15 minutes of a cardiac arrest in a previously healthy patient. The principal method of controlling acid–base status during a cardio-respiratory arrest is adequate ventilation. At 15 minutes give either 50 ml of 8.4% sodium bicarbonate (1 ml = 1 mmol) or calculate the amount of bicarbonate needed to correct the metabolic acidosis from the blood gas result. Multiply the base deficit by the estimated extracellular volume, i.e. divide the product of the patient's weight in kilograms and their base deficit by three. Base deficit is defined as the millimoles of alkali required to restore the pH of 1 litre of the patient's blood to normal at pCO$_2$ 5.33 kPa. In practice the initial amount to be given should seldom exceed 1 mmol kg$^{-1}$. In the traumatized patient what is of paramount importance, in addition to ventilation, is restoration of blood volume.

**Table 6.2**   Production and elimination of hydrogen ions

| Class | | Daily production (mol) | Source | Excreted in breath | Metabolic removal possible | Normal organ of elimination |
|---|---|---|---|---|---|---|
| I | $CO_2$ | 15 | Tissue respirtion | + | − | Lungs |
| II | *Organic acids and urea synthesis* | | | | | |
| | Lactic | 1.2 | Muscle, brain erythrocytes, skin, etc. | − | + | Liver (50%), kidneys, heart Many tissues (not liver) |
| | Hydroxybutyric and acetoacetic | 0.6* | Liver | − | + | |
| | Free fatty acids (FFA) | 0.7 | Adipose tissue | − | + | Most tissues |
| | $H^+$ generated during urea synthesis | 1.1† | Liver | − | + | Most tissues (see text), small fraction in urine |
| III | *'Fixed acids'* Sulphuric | ⎫ | | Dietary sulphur-containing amino acids | − | − | Urinary excretion (partly) |
| | Phosphoric | ⎬ 0.1 | | Organic phosphate metabolism | − | − | |

The daily production rates for the organic acids are calculated from results obtained in resting 70 kg man after an overnight fast, and are proportioned up to 24-hour values.
*Because of ingestion of food during daytime and consequent suppresion of FFA and ketone body production, the values for these acids may be considerable overestimates.
† On 100 g protein diet.

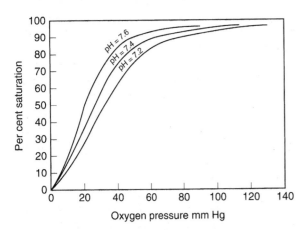

**Fig. 6.3**   Effect of pH on the oxyhaemoglobin dissociation curve of human blood at 38°C. From Roughton (1964).

Furthermore, because of the Bohr effect of pH on the oxygen dissociation curve (Fig. 6.3), acidosis increases ease of unloading oxygen from the blood into tissues. Increasing temperature and increasing partial pressure of carbon dioxide have the same effect, the latter not just because of an associated acidosis but also because carbon dioxide combines directly with haemoglobin to form carbamino compounds.

In summary, in cardiac arrest a lowered pH is desirable provided that it does not fall below 7.2. Below this, further acidosis lowers the threshold of the heart to ventricular fibrillation and inhibits normal cell metabolism, and should therefore be corrected.

### Blood sugar

Order an immediate blood glucose estimation using a reagent strip on every patient who has an altered level of consciousness, otherwise hypoglycaemia will be missed. This is followed by a laboratory estimation.

### PART 3: THE SECONDARY SURVEY: DETERMINING THE CAUSE OF THE PATIENT'S COLLAPSE

After carrying out the initial assessment (primary survey) and resuscitation of a collapsed patient

**Table 6.3**  Hazards of bicarbonate therapy

1. Inactivates simultaneously administered catecholamines
2. Shifts the oxyhaemoglobin dissociation curve to the left, inhibiting the release of oxygen to the tissues
3. Exacerbates central venous acidosis and may, by production of carbon dioxide, produce a paradoxical acidosis
4. Induces hypernatraemia, hyperosmolarity and an extracellular alkalosis; the latter causes an acute intracellular shift of potassium and a decreased plasma ionized calcium

presenting to the A&E department with no history, a deceptively incomplete history or, worse, an incorrect history, you must now go on to make a full head-to-toe examination. This is the secondary survey, during which you aim to gain a clearer picture of the cause of the patient's collapse.

Ensure that there is no occult injury. Examine all the skin, including the mouth and throat, the external auditory meatuses and the perineum. Always remember the possibility of non-accidental injury in children, and in the elderly. Consider all the forensic possibilities, noting needle marks, pressure blisters and the presence of any visible soft tissue injuries. Remember that bruising may appear at a distance from the site of injury.

You must:

1. keep an open mind to all diagnostic possibilities while both collecting the clinical evidence and monitoring the response of the vital signs to treatment
2. actively consider the common causes of collapse. This is especially important when there is a problem of communication, perhaps because of language, or when obvious initial clinical signs deflect you from finding the hidden life-threatening pathology. An example is a patient found by the police smelling of alcohol but developing an acute intracranial haematoma after a relatively trivial head injury. Beware!

It is wise to leave on the cervical collar in all trauma patients while they are in the resuscitation room. This is mandatory for all patients who have evidence of trauma above the level of the clavicle and have any decrease in their level of consciousness, whether it be from the trauma itself or from drugs, especially alcohol.

A synopsis of the main causes of collapse are best considered under systems in order that sins of omission are not committed in the frenetic atmosphere of the resuscitation room of the A&E department (Table 6.4). The synopsis is not comprehensive, but does include the common causes, together with less common causes that are easily missed, with dire consequences for the patient (Table 6.5).

If the gag reflex is depressed the patient cannot protect his own airway. Provided he is breathing spontaneously place the patient in the recovery position on his side (ensure first there is no evidence whatever of a spinal injury). Otherwise intubate the trachea in order to protect the lungs. This applies if the patient is to receive gastric lavage and cannot protect his own airway with complete certainty. If gastric contents are aspirated into the lungs they must be promptly sucked out because they produce a chemical pneumonitis and bacterial pneumonia. The clinical picture may well develop into adult respiratory distress syndrome.

Rhabdomyolysis and myoglobinuria may develop in any comatose patient after prolonged tissue pressure and muscle ischaemia, which is then relieved. Local swelling of muscles may be evident and compartment syndromes can develop because of positional obstruction of the circulation. Muscle death starts after 4 hours of complete ischaemia.

Look for the early symptoms and signs of pain and paraesthesia in a pallid, cool weak limb. Passively extend the fingers or flex the foot to test for a developing compartment syndrome (anterior tibial compartment syndrome is the commonest). Loss of distal pulses, numbness, paralysis and development of a flexion contracture are all late signs.

With myoglobinuria ensure that the urinary output is maintained at over 100 ml $h^{-1}$ in an adult, or 2 ml $kg^{-1}$ $h^{-1}$ in a child. Alkalinization of the urine increases the excretion of myoglobin, and will help prevent renal failure.

**Table 6.4**   Synopsis of causes of collapse to be considered during secondary survey

| System | Diagnosis | Notes |
|---|---|---|
| Respiratory | Upper airway obstruction | Inhaled foreign body (try Heimlich manoeuvre)<br>Infection such as epiglottitis (occurs in adults although commoner in children)<br>Call help urgently<br>Trauma including respiratory burns |
|  | Ventilatory failure | Asthma<br>Chest trauma such as sucking open wound<br>Paralysis such as in Guillain–Barré Syndrome |
|  | Failure of alveolar gas exchange | Pneumonia<br>Pulmonary contusions<br>Cardiogenic pulmonary oedema<br>Adult respiratory distress syndrome |
|  | Tension pneumothorax | From trauma (including iatrogenic)<br>ruptured emphysematous bulla |
| Cardiac | Ventricular fibrillation<br>Asystole<br>Electromechanical dissociation | Follow Resuscitation Council (UK) guidelines for treatment of cardiac arrest<br>Look for treatable cause: tension pneumothorax, cardiac tamponade, hypoxia or hypovolaemia, drug overdose |
|  | Cardiogenic shock or failure | Acute myocardial infarct<br>Arrhythmia<br>Pulmonary embolism<br>Cardiac contusions after blunt chest trauma<br>Valve rupture |
| Vascular | Hypovolaemic shock | Revealed or concealed haemorrhage<br>Diarrhoea and vomiting<br>Fistulae<br>Heat exhaustion |
|  | Anaphylactic shock | From stings and bites, drugs or iodine-containing contrast used for radiological investigation |
|  | Dissecting thoracic aorta | Usually in previously hypertensive patients, pain radiates to back |
|  | Leaking abdominal aortic aneurysm | Always check femoral pulses so that you consider aortic pathology (although pulses may not be lost) |
|  | Septic shock | Initially massive peripheral vasodilation: 'warm shock'. Temperature may be normal |
|  | Neurogenic shock | From loss of sympathetic vascular tone in cervical or high thoracic spinal cord injury |
| Gastrointestinal | Haemorrhage<br>Perforated peptic ulcer<br>Pancreatitis<br>Mesenteric embolism | <br><br>Always check serum amylase<br>Abdominal signs may be absent initially |
| Gynaecological | Ruptured ectopic pregnancy | Usually at 4-6 weeks' gestation..Always think of diagnosis in collapsed young woman. |
| Obstetric | Supine hypotension | The gravid uterus obstructs venous return from the vena cava unless the pregnant woman is turned onto her left side |
|  | Eclampsia<br>Pulmonary embolism<br>Amniotic fluid embolism | |

**Table 6.4** (con't)

| System | Diagnosis | Notes |
|---|---|---|
| Neurological | Head injury | Isolated head injuries do not cause shock in adults. Look for sites of blood loss elsewhere |
| | Infection | Meningitis in children (often meningococcal in UK), tetanus, botulism, poliomyelitis, rabies |
| | Cerebrovascular | Intracranial embolism or haemorrhage<br>Subarachnoid haemorrhage may present solely as a severe headache |
| | Epilepsy | Including the postictal state |
| | Poisoning | see Table 6.5 |
| Haematological | Sickle cell crisis | May lead to respiratory failure |
| | Malaria | Cerebral malaria causes coma |
| | Coagulopathy | Thrombocytopenia may present with bleeding |
| Metabolic | Hypoglycaemia | Check blood glucose in *every* patient |
| | Hyperglycaemia | Coma may be first presentation of diabetes melitus |
| | Hyponatraemia | May be Addisonian crisis |
| | Hypocalcaemia | May present with fits |
| | Hepatic failure | Precipitated by paracetamol overdose in previously fit people, and by intestinal haemorrhage, drugs, or high-protein diet in those with chronic liver disease |
| | Renal failure | Pre-renal from dehydration<br>Renal, e.g. from crush syndrome and myoglobinuria<br>Post-renal from ureteric obstruction (dangerous hyperkalaemia causes tall tented T waves and widening of the QRS complexes) |
| | Hypothermia | Resuscitation must include passive or active core rewarming<br>Sepsis and hypovolaemia often coexist |
| Endocrine | Addisonian crisis | Give 200 mg hydrocortisone i.v. (hypotension, low serum sodium, raised serum potassium) |
| | Myxoedemia | Always consider in hypothermic patients |

## CONCLUSION

Patients are often brought into the resuscitation room in a physical condition which is very alarming to the inexperienced trainee. Unless the patient is rapidly transported to the operating theatre, adhere to the methodical sequence of Primary Survey with Initial Resuscitation (see Part 1), Monitoring (see Part 2), Secondary Survey (see Part 3) while the patient is in the resuscitation room of the A&E department. By having a known sequence of procedures to go through you and the nurse will gain confidence as the resuscitation continues, and you will not miss pathology. The patient then has the best chance of survival and also the least chance of morbidity.

Keep an open mind as to the cause of the clinical signs. Monitor the vital signs and level of consciousness, and do not jump to preconceived conclusions — this is all too easy to do under pressure. If there is any clinical deterioration return to the basic initial sequence of the primary survey and recheck AIRWAY, BREATHING, CIRCULATION yet again.

Do not allow the patient to leave the A&E department without stable vital signs, appropriate intravenous lines in place, and having been thoroughly examined, unless there is an acceptable reason. A patient may all too easily deteriorate clinically in the X-ray room or, even more dangerously by reasons of secluded space, in the computed tomography (CT) scanner.

**Table 6.5**    Common drugs and poisons

| Drug | Symptoms and signs | Treatment |
|------|--------------------|-----------|
| Paracetamol | Liver and renal failure, hypoglycaemia<br>May be asymptomatic initially | Lavage Charcoal or methionine<br>Acetylcysteine |
| Salicylates | Tinnitus, abdominal pain<br>Vomiting, hypoglycaemia, hyperthermia, sweating<br>Acid-base disturbances | Lavage and charcoal<br>Rehydration<br>Diuresis |
| Tricyclic antidepressants | Arrhythmias and hypotension<br>Dilated pupils, convulsions<br>Coma | Lavage and charcoal<br>Cardiopulmonary support |
| Benzodiazepines | Respiratory depression | Flumazenil if acute iatrogenic |
| Opiates | Pinpoint pupils<br>Loss of consciousness<br>Respiratory depression<br>Needle marks | Naloxone |
| Phenothiazines | Dyskinesia, torticollis | Procyclidine |
| Lignocaine | Tingling tongue<br>Perioral paraesthesia<br>Ventricular fibrillation<br>Convulsions | Cardiopulmonary support<br>Diazepam |
| Carbon monoxide | 33% of fatal poisoning in UK<br>insidious from inefficient gas fires<br>Nausea and vomiting<br>Headache, drowsiness<br>Hallucinations, convulsions | 100% or hyperbaric oxygen |
| Cyanide | Headache, vomiting, weakness<br>Tachypnoea, convulsions<br>Coma | Dicobalt edetate |
| Iron | Hypotension, vasodilatation<br>Gastric haemorrhage | Lavage<br>Desferrioxamine |
| Organophosphates<br>(pesticides, nerve gases) | Nausea, vomiting, diarrhoea<br>Salivation, pulmonary oedema<br>Pinpoint pupils, convulsions, coma | Lavage<br>Atropine |

Patients with a diminished level of consciousness must be seen by an anaesthetist, at the very latest before they leave the A&E department. Patients must be in the best possible clinically supported condition for transportation, whether their journey is to the CT scanner, a ward or to another hospital. If necessary the patient must be ventilated, depending on the length of journey and vehicle employed, and must be accompanied by appropriate attendants such as an anaesthetist.

Strictly adhere to standard guidelines for protection of medical and nursing staff from contamination with body fluids: wear gloves, waterproof gowns and masks with visors. Staff must be immunized against hepatitis B virus.

Keep clear, precise medical records of any

resuscitation sequence, remembering that from 1st November 1991 patients or their relatives have the legal right to see medical records. This record keeping is the responsibility of the senior doctor present. Take appropriate care with forensic evidence, especially from terrorist incidents — anything removed from victims must be removed by a named person and be handed to a named person who personally seals the item in a labelled bag.

There must be at the very least a doctor of registrar grade in command of the resuscitation team. For an A&E department to receive patients who need immediate resuscitation from a 'blue-light' ambulance, the hospital must have a minimum of an anaesthetic registrar, medical registrar and surgical registrar 'living in' on site 24 hours a day. Even if the patient does not survive you will be able to tell the relatives truthfully that everything possible was done.

Both medical audit and medicolegal considerations dictate the above minimal adequate standards of care. All doctors who are expected to resuscitate the collapsed patient as part of their work practice are expected to be trained in the above. This is your responsibility, but more especially of the supervising consultant and above all of the employing authority.

FURTHER READING

Advanced Trauma Life Support Course Manual 1989. American College of Surgeons
Cohen RD, Woods HF 1987 Disturbances of acid–base homeostasis. In: Weatherall DJ, Ledingham JGG, Warrell DA (eds) Oxford textbook of medicine. Oxford University Press, Oxford, pp 9.164–9.175
Don H 1987 Oxygen therapy. In Callam M L (ed) Current therapy in emergency medicine. B C Decker Inc, pp 345–348
Evans TR 1990 ABC of Resuscitation. British Medical Association, London
Henry J, Volans G 1984 ABC of poisoning. British Medical Association, London
Jones RM 1989 Drug therapy in cardiopulmonary resuscitation. In: Baskett PJF (ed) Cardiopulmonary resuscitation, p 101.
Roughton FJW 1964 Transport of oxygen and carbon dioxide. In: Fenn WO, Rahn H (eds) Handbook of physiology (Vol 1), p 776

Royal College of Physicians of London 1991 Some aspects of the medical management of casualties of the Gulf War. February
Safar P, Bircher NG 1988 Cardiopulmonary cerebral resuscitation (3rd edn) Saunders, Philadelphia, pp 212–219
Skinner D, Driscoll P, Earlam R 1991 ABC of major trauma. British Medical Journal, London

## APPENDIX: Chemical Weapons

In the 1990–91 Gulf War it was considered possible that the chemical weapons of nerve gases and mustard gas would be used.

### Nerve gases (e.g. Tabun)

These agents are organophosphorus compounds which act by inhibiting the enzyme acetylcholinesterase and therefore prevent the breakdown of acetylcholine at motor end plates. The symptoms and signs are the same as for organophosphorus insecticide poisoning, i.e. overactivity of the parasympathetic system and paralysis of the muscles of respiration. Early treatment involves the reversal of the effects of acetylcholine at muscurinic receptors by atropine, 2 mg being given intravenously every 10–15 minutes in severe poisoning. Management also involves the support of respiration, the reactivation of inhibited acetylcholinesterase by oximes (pralidoxime mesylate) and the suppression of convulsions by diazepam. Pretreatment with pyridostigmine (reversible inhibitor of acetylcholinesterase) protects a proportion of the total quantity of enzyme present against subsequent attack by nerve gas.

### Mustard gas (sulphur mustard)

Exposure to the liquid or vapour produces blistering of the skin and damage to the cornea and conjunctiva. Classically there is an asymptomatic latent period of up to 6 hours, before reddening of the skin, leading to blistering. Burns are initially superficial, and blister fluid does not contain free sulphur mustard.

Eye damage usually resolves over a number of weeks but treat with saline irrigations, mydriatrics, vaseline to prevent sticking of the eyelids, dark glasses and antibiotic drops.

Inhalation produces damage to the upper respiratory tract, with sloughing of the epithelium of the airways and nasal passages. The most severely affected patients need assisted ventilation with oxygen. Absorption leads to depression of the bone marrow and a fall in the white count, with a maximum effect at about two weeks' post-exposure.

In the First World War the death rate from mustard gas was 2% of those exposed, resulting from burns, respiratory damage and bone marrow depression.

# 7. Preoperative preparation for surgery

*T. Cooke   G. Keogh*

## INTRODUCTION

A meticulous approach to the preparation of patients for surgery is important if morbidity and mortality of the procedures are to be kept to a minimum. In the preoperative period assessment of risk factors which may compromise recovery from surgery can be made and steps taken to correct them. Also it is the time to implement preventative measures to prophylact against commonly occurring complications. Until recently it has been traditional in the United Kingdom to admit patients undergoing major surgery to hospital for varying periods to undergo preoperative 'work-up'. Due to increasing financial constraints this period is now being decreased, although as yet it has not reached the stage practised commonly in the United States where patients, even for major surgery, are admitted only a few hours prior to their procedure. However, in future the tendency will be for a minimal preoperative admission period. The implication of this is that assessment will have to be carried out as an outpatient and this would most efficiently be performed in joint preoperative clinics with anaesthetic colleagues.

## PREOPERATIVE ASSESSMENT OF RISK

An accurate definition of risk for an individual patient is obviously important. Firstly, it would enable patients and their families to be counselled more precisely on the outcome from the surgical procedure. In some cases this knowledge could lead to a decision by surgeon and patient not to carry out surgery because the risk outweighs possible benefit of treating underlying disease. Secondly, measures to improve the level of

risk could be initiated and supportive measures for the peri- and postoperative periods planned. For example, the need for postoperative intensive care could be predicted, availability of beds sought in advance and patients introduced to the units and be briefed on what they might expect on admission there.

Over the last two decades there has been a continuing interest in evaluating surgical risk. Prognostic scoring systems have been proposed especially in the field of intensive care. An example of this is the APACHE II system. However, these are designed to predict mortality in critically ill patients and are not necessarily useful for preoperative evaluation of patients undergoing elective procedures. Attempts to adapt these scoring systems, which take into account such factors as nutritional, anthropomorphic and immunity assessment, are still under investigation and not yet proven for use in routine clinical practice. The factors which contribute to these scoring systems often reflect the underlying disease process for which the patient is being treated. However, other intercurrent medical problems particularly relating to the cardiovascular and respiratory systems may have an impact on both patient fitness to undergo surgery and on the eventual outcome. On top of the magnitude of the operative procedure, the underlying pathology, the anaesthetic and technical ability of the surgeon also play a part in determining morbidity and mortality. Some of these factors will be discussed in more detail.

The other form of scoring which is easier to use and more recognizable is that of ASA physical status (Table 7.1). This classification of preoperative status is not meant to be a multifactorial index or predictor of outcome, but it enables clinicians to facilitate communication. It also seems to correlate well with total operative mortality.

**Table 7.1**

| Category | Description |
| --- | --- |
| I | Healthy patient |
| II | Mild systemic disease<br>No functional limitations |
| III | Severe systemic disease with definite functional limitation |
| IV | Severe systemic disease that is a constant threat to life |
| V | Moribund patients not expected to survive 24 hours with or without operation |

## Nutritional assessment

There have been claims that assessment of nutritional state can identify groups of patients at high risk of postoperative complications. It has been further proposed that preoperative nutritional support might be used for those at high risk. Whilst there is a large body of evidence to support the first claim there is still doubt as to whether the risk can be decreased with active treatment. Weight loss, anthropomorphic measurements, assessment of muscle function and biochemical factors such as plasma proteins and transferrin levels have all been used either singly or as part of a scoring system to predict outcome. Of these, the most consistent association with poor risk appears to be depletion of plasma proteins which in a number of studies is correlated with poor wound healing, the development of sepsis and increased mortality.

The reason why nutritional support in the preoperative phase fails in many incidences to prevent complication in the postoperative period is that derangement of plasma proteins may reflect causative factors other than malnutrition. Underlying sepsis is the principal one of these and should be excluded in all patients with a low serum albumin. The assessment of cutaneous delayed hypersensitivity using the measurement of recall antigens and plasma fibronectin estimations also may reflect deep seated sepsis. However, if sepsis can be excluded as a cause of a low serum albumin there may be some logic in preoperative nutritional support.

## Cardiovascular Assessment

Of the five million patients per year in the United Kingdom undergoing surgery, approximately 500,000 have or may develop coronary artery disease. The increasing ageing of the population means that, with time this proportion will continue to rise as these older patients have a perioperative myocardial infarction rate of up to 15%. There has been a large number of studies both retrospective and prospective, analysing outcome for patients with cardiovascular disease following surgery. Only recent myocardial infarction and heart failure are proven risk factors for perioperative cardiac morbidity and it is less clear whether other factors such as hypertension and arrhythmias constitute an adverse risk.

One third of patients undergoing anaesthesia within three months of myocardial infarct will have a further episode. This risk reduces to 10% between three and six months and to 5% after this time. Clearly elective surgery should be deferred until risk is minimal. The choice of anaesthetic does not alter the perioperative cardiac morbidity and avoidance of general anaesthesia will not reduce the likelihood of re-infarction. Emergency vascular and abdominal or thoracic surgery lasting longer than three hours are all compounding risk factors.

Identification of the patient at risk of myocardial disease is therefore of paramount importance, if the risk of surgery is to be assessed. The most important indicators of ischaemic heart disease can be identified from the patient's history with a high degree of accuracy. The history obtained either provides a clear indication of myocardial disease or may provide a clue to asymptomatic disease. The patients who should be suspected of having myocardial disease are those who have significant risk factors, for example diabetes, hypertension, smoking or hypercholesterolaemia, who manifest signs of other vascular disease or who have poor exercise tolerance. Further evidence may be obtained on physical examination by the presence of signs of cardiac failure or by ECG evidence of left ventricular hypertrophy or rhythm disturbances. Up to 44% of patients with normal ECGs and peripheral vascular disease may have a 50% stenosis in one or more coronary arteries, and 30% may have a stenosis of 75%.

Exercise stress ECG may be helpful in preoperative prediction of patients with significant myocardial disease. More sophisticated testing such as echocardiography, radionuclear imaging with technetium or dipyridamole thallium to detect areas of infarction or coronary artery stenosis are not for routine use and their role in predicting outcome for high risk patients is still controversial.

Well controlled hypertension does not appear to be an adverse factor in predicting peri- and postoperative myocardial risk. In the past, antihypertensive therapy was withdrawn prior to general anaesthesia but this now appears not to be necessary except for monoamine oxidase inhibitors. Likewise, patients being treated for arrhythmias should continue with therapy. Untreated hypertensive patients should probably be controlled prior to the undertaking of elective surgery. It is also important to take into account that there may be end-organ damage in response to long-standing hypertension and this could increase the risk of general anaesthesia. The areas which may be involved include the cerebral circulation, the peripheral arteries, the renal vascular bed as well as the coronary arteries.

## Respiratory assessment

A good history and physical examination of the respiratory system are the most important methods of assessment. The commonest problems seen are chronic obstructive airways disease, with or without a reversible bronchospastic element, and asthma. Many surgical patients develop postoperative pulmonary dysfunction and the spectrum of disease ranges from atelectasis to severe respiratory failure requiring ventilatory support. It is therefore important to identify the patients with pre-existing respiratory disease as the common postoperative complications may be exaggerated, and preoperative therapy may ensure survival of an at risk patient.

Chest X-ray, peak expiratory flow rate (PEFR), vital capacity (VC) and forced expiratory volume in one second (FEV1) will be able to distinguish between restrictive and obstructive patterns of airways disease. Repetition of the tests with a bronchodilator will detect a useful reversible element. Abnormalities on spirometry correlate with the incidence of postoperative respiratory complications, but the severity of these complications does not directly correlate with the severity of preoperative lung disease. Additional factors such as smoking, the site of the incision, obesity and age are probably as important in assessing risk.

Sophisticated pulmonary function tests are useful in assessing the parameters of lung dysfunction but are seldom performed. Preanaesthetic blood gas estimation will help in quantifying the severity of pulmonary dysfunction and serve as a base line with which to compare peri- and postoperative measurements.

Having identified respiratory dysfunction preoperatively, it is advisable to correct any reversible component. Cessation of smoking should preferably occur six to eight weeks prior to elective surgery in order to diminish postoperative complications. Smoking produces carbon monoxide and the subsequent formation of carboxyhaemoglobin interferes with oxygen delivery in the periphery. Smoking is also responsible for increased airway reactivity to anaesthetic gases and impairs tracheo-bronchial clearance of more viscous secretions. There is also evidence that smoking can result in immunodepressive effect by producing a decrease in immunoglobulin levels, pulmonary macrophage and natural killer cell activity.

Other measures which may help in improving preoperative respiratory dysfunction are chest physiotherapy and addition of bronchodilators. An important part of preoperative management is the education of the patient in the problems associated with smoking and the need for postoperative deep breathing and coughing. This can be achieved by the ward physiotherapist using devices such as incentive spirometers which encourage sustained deep breathing. Sputum should be cultured and any significant infection treated with the appropriate antibiotics.

## Anaemia

Preoperative anaemia below 10 gm/dL should be corrected before major surgery where bleeding might be expected. However, the use of blood products is becoming increasingly controversial not only because of possible risk of transmission of infection but also because of the suggestion that immunodepression induced by blood transfusion may have an adverse effect on survival in patients with malignant disease. Although this is not yet proven and the evidence is conflicting, blood transfusion should only be given with significant anaemia and, where possible, two to three days preoperatively to maximise its oxygen carrying capacity.

## Obesity

Obesity poses significant risks for operation and anaesthesia. An increase in ideal weight of thirty percent results in a forty percent increase in the chance of dying from heart disease and in a fifty percent increase in the chance of dying from stroke, and these risks may be compounded by the stresses induced by anaesthesia and surgery. Morbidly obese patients may also exhibit carbon dioxide retention (the so called *Pickwickian syndrome*) due to alveolar hypoventilation. They may also have significant hypertension, airway obstruction, as well as increased volume and acidity of gastric secretions. The postoperative recovery may also be complicated by the increased incidence of venous thromboembolism and wound infection.

## Renal Disease

Although the perioperative management of patients with end-stage renal failure or chronically insufficient kidneys is in the realm of nephrologists, the surgeon must be aware of the principles of management. The timing of dialysis must be coordinated with the timing of surgery so that uraemia and electrolyte abnormalities, especially hyperkalaemia can be corrected. In patients with insufficient kidneys the principle is one of preservation of existing renal function. This is achieved by avoidance of dehydration and hypovolaemia in the preoperative fasting period by administration of intravenous fluids and by avoidance of drugs which may have an adverse effect on the kidneys. Patients who have a functioning transplant are also managed with these principles in mind and may present special difficulties since they are chronically immunosuppressed. Patients with renal disease may also have abnormal haemostasis due to a functional platelet disorder.

## Jaundice

The jaundiced patient requires special preoperative evaluation and treatment. Apart from the need for diagnostic testing, Vitamin K should be given to reverse the clotting disorders consequent upon liver dysfunction. Patients with chronic liver disease should be assessed for clotting disturbances, albumin levels, degree of encephalopathy, presence of ascites and level of jaundice as the degree of liver dysfunction directly correlates with perioperative morbidity and mortality (Pugh modification of Child's classification).

The presence of cholestatic jaundice also conveys the special risk of hepato-renal syndrome so that adequate preoperative hydration and prophylactic antibiotics should be instituted.

## Diabetes

This common endocrine disorder is important to the surgeon because of its complications and the special preparation required for the insulin-dependent patient. Diabetes renders the patient more susceptible to infection and protein depletion. In addition, microangiopathy may affect the renal, peripheral and coronary circulations; ischaemic heart disease is the commonest cause of death in long standing diabetics. The preoperative preparation of these patients includes scheduling the operation as early as possible in the operating sessions and commencement of insulin/dextrose infusions, either continuously or on a sliding scale basis, starting, for example at 06.00, for a morning operating session. The dose of insulin should be titrated to blood sugar estimations.

## Drugs

An adequate drug history must be taken prior to

surgery being undertaken. Most medications should be continued in the peri-operative period with the exception of monoamine oxidase inhibitors, lithium, tricyclic antidepressants and phenothiazines, which may interfere with the action of anaesthetic agents. Modification of dosage may be required as in the case of steroids, and different routes of administration could also be required, especially in the fasting patient, for example with insulin and digoxin. Anticoagulants such as warfarin will have to be reversed several days preoperatively and substituted with a heparin infusion.

Whether the oral contraceptive pill should be stopped is a controversial issue. The associated thrombotic tendency relates to the oestrogen content and the high dose preparations are associated with significant changes in coagulation. The risk of postoperative thromboembolism in patients on oral contraceptives is 0.96 percent; this risk diminishes to 0.5 percent for non-users. However, it has generally been accepted that patients on oestrogen based oral contraceptives should, where possible, discontinue the pill four weeks prior to major elective surgery. In the young patient undergoing a minor procedure it is probably safe to continue the pill prior to surgery in the absence of other risk factors. Obviously, advice should be given as to alternative contraception if the decision to stop the pill has been made.

The possibility of illicit drug abuse should also be explored since the requirements of narcotics may be increased and acute withdrawal of a number of substances may add significantly to perioperative morbidity. These patients also present a potential infective risk to medical and nursing staff and should be assumed to carry viruses if screening cannot be carried out prior to surgery.

## Routine preoperative testing

### Biochemical tests

Unexpected abnormalities are found on routine biochemical testing in 2 to 10% of patients. The incidence of significant abnormalities is closer to 5 percent and of these, 70 percent relate to blood sugar or urea levels. Under fifty years of age the incidence of abnormal findings is even lower for asymptomatic patients, apart from the incidence of diabetes. It is therefore reasonable for minimised preoperative biochemical tests in asymptomatic patients under fifty years of age with normal urinalysis and blood sugar.

### Chest X-rays

Abnormalities on chest X-ray are present in approximately ten percent of patients. This incidence increases with age, to 35 percent in patients over 60 years of age. The findings on chest X-ray do not necessarily influence management since over 90 percent of patients with both normal and abnormal chest X-rays still proceed to operation. Preoperative chest X-rays are therefore justified in patients over 50 years of age or in those with respiratory symptoms. They may also be useful in screening for pulmonary metastases in oncology patients, in those individuals who reside in areas which have a high incidence of tuberculosis, or as a baseline investigation when postoperative pulmonary complications are expected.

### Electrocardiograms

The ECG findings of altered rhythm or conduction, myocardial ischaemia, left ventricular hypertrophy or tall peaked T waves may alter management in the preoperative period. Abnormalities on ECG are not uncommon: the incidence is around 10 percent in patients of 40 years of age and increases to 25 percent at the age of 60. However, very few studies have examined the incidence of abnormal ECG findings in asymptomatic individuals but the incidence appears to be less than 1 percent. Therefore, in asymptomatic patients under the arbitrary age of 40 with no risk factors of ischaemic heart disease and a normal physical examination, preoperative ECG screening is not justified.

### Full blood count

Very little data exists to determine the optimal level of haemoglobin necessary in order to avoid perioperative morbidity. Anaemia of 10 g/dL should be corrected as discussed previously but care must be exercised in the elderly patient with cardiac failure in order to avoid circulatory overload. All patients undergoing major surgery should undergo a full blood count, as should all women undergoing all but minor procedures. The detection and treatment of polycythaemia markedly reduces perioperative morbidity and mortality.

### HIV testing

Testing asymptomatic patients for HIV infection has a low yield and consent is usually required. A more reasonable approach is to identify high risk groups by careful history taking. If a patient in a high risk group is HIV negative, it is still possible that HIV infection is present, since sero-conversion may not have occurred. Universal precautions are beyond the budgets of most institutions, but it is reasonable to exercise care in the high-risk patient undergoing surgery, in the absence of sero-positivity.

## RISKS OF EMERGENCY SURGERY

Emergency surgery is particularly high risk because there is a shorter period of time to fully assess the patient and implement corrective therapy. As well as the risk factors discussed above, shock, sepsis and fluid imbalance may play a significant part in the clinical presentation. Therefore, emergency surgery, particularly out of hours, should be avoided as far as possible. Appropriate resuscitation and antibiotic therapy may allow one to buy time in order to optimise the patient for urgent surgery. In patients with particularly high risks such as recent myocardial infarction or those in heart failure, a non-surgical approach to the treatment of conditions such as peritonitis should be considered. Recent studies using modern antibiotics and aggressive fluid replacement have demonstrated the effectiveness of this non-operative approach.

## IMPLEMENTATION OF PREVENTATIVE MEASURES

In the preoperative phase, measures to prevent thromboembolic and septic complications should be considered for all patients undergoing major surgery.

### Thromboembolism prophylaxis

Thromboembolism remains a significant cause of postoperative morbidity and mortality. Pulmonary emboli account for 10 percent of inpatient deaths in the United Kingdom and the majority of these emboli arise from asymptomatic lower limb deep venous thromboses. Screening for these thromboses is not cost effective. The simplest method of preventing fatal and non-fatal thromboembolism is in using appropriate prophylaxis in patients of moderate and high risk groups. This approach is cost effective if one takes into account the investigation, treatment and increased hospital stay of those with non-fatal thromboembolism.

The risk of developing thromboembolic complications varies with the patient, the operation and the underlying disease. Epidemiological, necropsy and screening studies all observe an increase in risk with age; this risk rises appreciably after 40 years and this age forms the boundary in identifying higher risk groups. Other risk factors include surgery to the lower limb, pelvis, trauma, malignant disease, obesity, varicose veins and prolonged immobility. Medical conditions such as recent myocardial infarction, heart failure as well as high dose oestrogen therapy and previous thromboembolic episodes should also be considered (Table 7.2).

If patient and operative risk factors are combined, the risk of thromboembolism can be predicted (Table 7.3). Routine prophylaxis for moderate and high risk groups is cost effective and admisable.

Prophylaxis for DVT includes mechanical and pharmacological measures. Mechanical methods include graduated stockings and intraoperative pneumatic compression. Neither increases the risk of bleeding and both are effective in moderate risk patients. They also convey benefit in high risk groups in combination with subcutaneous heparin. Pharmacological means include twice daily low dose subcutaneous heparin and the more recently introduced low molecular weight

**Table 7.2**

| Patient factors | Disease or surgical procedure |
|---|---|
| Age | Trauma or surgery, especially of |
| Obesity | pelvis, hip, lower limb |
| Varicose veins | Malignancy, especially pelvic, |
| Immobility (bed rest over | abdominal, metastatic |
| 4 days) | Heart failure |
| Pregnancy | Recent myocardial infarction |
| Puerperium | Paralysis of lower limb(s) |
| High dose oestrogen therapy | Infection |
| Previous deep vein | Inflammatory bowel disease |
| thrombosis or pulmonary | Nephrotic syndrome |
| embolism | Polycythaemia |
| Thrombophilia | Paraproteinaemia |
| Deficiency of anti- | Paroxysmal nocturnal haemoglobinuria |
| thrombin III, protein C | Behcet's disease |
| or protein S | Homocystinaemia |
| Antiphospholipid antibody | |
| or lupus anticoagulant | |

**Table 7.3**

| | Deep vein thrombosis | Proximal vein thrombosis | Fatal pulmonary embolism |
|---|---|---|---|
| Low risk groups | <10% | <1% | 0.01% |
| Moderate risk groups | 10–40% | 1–10% | 0.1–1% |
| High risk groups | 40–80% | 10–30% | 1–10% |

| Low risk groups | Minor surgery (<30 min); no risk factors other than age |
|---|---|
| | Major surgery (>30 min); age < 40; no other risk factors* |
| | Minor trauma or medical illness |
| Moderate risk groups | Major general, urological, gynaecological, cardiothoracic, vascular, or neurological surgery; age ≥ 40 or other risk factor* |
| | Major medical illness; heart or lung disease, cancer, inflammatory bowel disease |
| | Major trauma or burns |
| | Minor surgery, trauma, or illness in patients with previous deep vein thrombosis, pulmonary embolism, or thrombophilia |
| High risk groups | Fracture or major orthopaedic surgery of pelvis, hip, or lower limb |
| | Major pelvic or abdominal surgery for cancer |
| | Major surgery, trauma, or illness in patients with previous deep vein thrombosis, pulmonary embolism, or thrombophilia |
| | Lower limb paralysis (for example, hemiplegic stroke, paraplegia) |
| | Major lower limb amputation |

heparins. Intravenous Dextrans may also convey benefit in patients after surgery for hip fractures but not with the efficacy of subcutaneous heparin in general surgical patients.

*Low dose subcutaneous heparin in general surgical patients*

Low dose subcutaneous heparin is effective in the prevention of about two-thirds of DVTs and fatal pulmonary emboli. In general surgical usage it can be given with a minimum of side-effects although the incidence of wound haematomas is marginally increased, especially if the injection is given adjacent to the operative incision. There has also been the occasional report of skin necrosis at the injection site and rarely, thrombocytosis may be induced. In the main, changes in coagulation cause no real problems in abdominal surgery although this may not be the case for some orthopaedic and urological procedures where excessive bleeding may give rise to major complications. In orthopaedic patients, low molecular weight heparins are probably more effective than conventional heparin in preventing thromboembolic complications and reducing these coagulation side-effects. At present there is no clear evidence that they are superior in general surgical patients and the convenience of a once daily dose must be weighed against their greater cost.

## Sepsis prophylaxis

The use of prophylactic antibiotics in the perioperative period is now widely recognised to reduce septic complications for some types of operation. However, their use should be judicious because of possible harmful effects such as toxic and allergic reactions and the overgrowth of resistant organisms which may give rise to conditions such as antibiotic related colitis. Prophylactic antibiotics are unnecessary when the expected infection rate is below 2 percent which includes all clean operations and clean–contaminated operations such as cholecystectomy when there has been no biliary stasis. They should be used in clean operations in which foreign material, for example, vascular grafts and joint prostheses are implanted. In operations where contamination is expected antibiotics should be administered at a time prior to surgery either with the premedication or on induction of anaesthesia. It is important to have a significant tissue level of the drug before the operative procedure begins. One dose treatment is all that is required for most clean–contaminated procedures extending to three postoperative doses for contaminated operations such as those on the colon or for gastric carcinoma.

The choice of antibiotic depends on the site of operation. For the clean–contaminated operations on the biliary tract and stomach and for vascular and orthopaedic operations single dose cephalosporin would be appropriate. For the heavily contaminated colonic procedures where there is a heavy growth of both gram negative and anerobic bacteria antibiotic therapy should include drugs that will be effective against this range of organisms with the use, for example, of a combination of a cephalosporin and metranidazole. Operations on the obstructed biliary tract and stomach and for gastric carcinoma should be considered to be contaminated and the use of antibiotics similar to that for colonic surgery is indicated.

## Preparation of the gastrointestinal tract

Another method of reducing postoperative infection is the mechanical cleansing of the gastrointestinal tract. This includes gastric washout using a wide bore nasogastric tube in patients with pyloric stenosis and bowel preparation prior to colonic surgery. The latter can be achieved using purgatives of two to three days combined with colonic washouts. Alternatively hyper-osmolar liquids such as mannitol given via a nasogastric tube or taken orally by the patient may be used on the evening prior to surgery. For emergency surgery on the colon the use of on-table colonic washouts have been proposed. There is some danger in all of these methods particularly in the elderly and those with sub-acute colonic obstruction and electrolyte imbalance, especially hypokalaemia, should be monitored. Some surgeons have abandoned the use of mechanical bowel preparation and advocate the use of intra-operative peritoneal lavage to reduce septic complications. However, these views are still in a minority.

## Preparation of the operation site

Numerous studies have now demonstrated that preoperative shaving significantly increases postoperative wound infection. When the operation site is heavily overgrown with hair this should be removed with barber's clippers or depilatory creams. If shaving is unavoidable it should be carried out as close to the operation time as possible preferably following induction of anaesthesia.

## Consent to operation

The preoperative period is the time when the

operative procedure and its results and possible side-effects are discussed with the patients. It is important that this should be carried out by the most senior member of the surgical team. Informed consent is not only an ethical necessity: it has been demonstrated that good communications will reduce patients' dissatisfaction with the outcome of surgery. When procedures are being carried out which will produce a loss of function, will result in a stoma formation or have a high complication rate, this should be discussed at length, with a witness present such as a senior member of the ward nursing staff. It is essential that this discussion is recorded in the patients' case notes. When informed consent is impossible or difficult because of mental impairment the patient's family should be involved in the decision making.

Consent for operation for minors up to the age of 16 years should come from the parent or guardian. If this is refused for what is considered to be a life saving procedure then permission will have to be sought through the courts by making the child a Ward of Court. If it is considered that treatment is required with urgency the opinion of at least one further senior doctor should be sought and the result of the discussions recorded in full in the case notes. Emergency treatment for unconscious patients should be carried out after consent from a relative, but in the absence of such a person surgery should be performed preferably after the recorded opinion of an independent surgeon has been obtained.

FURTHER READING

Miller R D 1990 Anaesthesia. 3E Churchill Livingstone, New York
Thromboembolic Risk Factors (THRIFT) Consensus Group 1992 Risk of Prophylaxis for venous thromboembolism in hospital patients. British Medical Journal 305: 567–574 (108 references)
Cuschieri A, Giles G R, Moosa A R 1988 Essential Surgical Practice. 2E Butterworth Heinemann, London

# 8. Premedication and anaesthesia

*M. W. Platt*

## PREMEDICATION

Premedication is the prescribing of drugs to be administered preoperatively. These are usually agents prescribed by the anaesthetist, at the preoperative visit, to allay anxiety, relieve pain, to dry saliva, and to maintain the dosage of intercurrent medication. After a brief discussion of intercurrent medication, the broad topic of anaesthetic premedication will be considered.

### Intercurrent medication

Many patients coming to surgery have other medical problems which are treated by a variety of different drugs. Refer to the section on medical problems for detailed notes.

Some patients who need special consideration include those on antihypertensive therapy; antiarrhythmic therapy; anticoagulated patients; patients on diabetic therapy (oral hypoglycaemics or insulin); those on endocrine replacement therapy (particularly thyroxine); those on adrenocortical replacement or augmentation therapy; those patients undergoing treatment for asthma or chronic obstructive airways disease with bronchodilators and allied treatments; and those having cardiac failure therapy and diuretics.

Because of fasting, and sometimes the surgical problem itself, it is not always possible for this medication to be continued. However, many drugs need to be continued up to the time of surgery. Sometimes, a parenteral form of the agent can be substituted.

### Anaesthetic premedication

1. Anxiolysis
2. Drying secretions
3. Analgesia

*Anxiolysis* (Table 8.1)

Patients attending for surgery are normally anxious about the outcome. They may have a fear of the unknown, of pain, of dying, of cancer, or non-specific fears. Although the preoperative visit by the anaesthetist does much to allay anxiety by reducing the unknown element, waiting for an operation may be unpleasant. Anxiolytics calm the patient and help to reduce time spent 'dwelling' on fears. Agents specifically used for anxiolysis are the benzodiazepines, particularly the shorter-acting agents such as temazepam, usually given orally 2 hours preoperatively. For major operations such as cardiopulmonary bypass, a long-acting drug such as lorazepam may be used. Opioid analgesics calm and sedate the patient and are often used, especially if analgesia is required (see below).

Phenothiazines may also be used, usually in combination with an opioid. Promethazine is frequently combined with pethidine. These agents are useful especially in the elderly, since they calm the patient without too much sedation. Phenothiazines are also appropriate in atopic individuals (e.g. asthmatics), where their antihistaminic action may be useful. Prochlorperazine is used for its combined sedative and anti-emetic properties.

Butyrophenones, such as droperidol, are now no longer used for sedation since they cause dysphoria and the so-called 'locked-in syndrome'. The latter is a state of fear elicited in the patient by a feeling of not being able to communicate

**Table 8.1**  Anxiolytic agents in common use

| Agent | Dose | | Approx. duration(h) |
|---|---|---|---|
| *Benzodiazepines* | | | |
| Diazepam | 0.05–0.3 | mg kg$^{-1}$ | 36–200 |
| Temazepam | 0.15–0.5 | mg kg$^{-1}$ | 5–20 |
| Lorazepam | 0.015–0.06 | μg kg$^{-1}$ | 10–20 |
| Midazolam | 0.07–0.08 | mg kg$^{-1}$ | 0.5–2 |
| *Phenothiazines* | | | |
| Promethazine | 0.2–0.5 | mg kg$^{-1}$ | 8–12 |
| Prochlorperazine | 0.1–0.2 | mg kg$^{-1}$ | |

with the outside world, although they appear very calm. In very low doses, however, e.g. 0.01 mg kg$^{-1}$ of droperidol, these agents are very potent antiemetics.

## Drying secretions (Table 8.2)

In the days of ether anaesthesia, it was particularly important to dry oral secretions, because ether stimulates salivary secretions on induction, potentiating the possibility of laryngospasm. With modern anaesthesia it is less of a requirement, although it may be useful to dry secretions prior to dental surgery, bronchoscopy or surgery on the lung and for paediatric patients in whom salivation can be a problem. In addition to drying secretions, muscarinic receptor antagonists also prevent bradycardia, a common side-effect of general anaesthesia, especially in very young children.

Hyoscine, in contrast to atropine, contributes to the sedative properties of premedication. Glycopyrrolate does not cross the blood–brain barrier, and is a more potent inhibitor of salivary secretions, with less effect on the vagus nerve and hence on the heart rate. Atropine has also been shown to have a small antiemetic effect, presumably through inhibition of the vagus nerve, as well as a slight bronchodilator effect.

**Table 8.2**  Drying agents in common use

| Agent | Dose (mg kg$^{-1}$) | Approx. duration | |
|---|---|---|---|
| | | i.v. | i.m. |
| Atropine | 0.02 | 15–30 min | 2–4 h |
| Hyoscine | 0.008 | 30–60 min | 4–6 h |
| Glycopyrrolate | 0.01 | 2–4h | 6–8 h |

## Analgesia

There are two main reasons for using opioid analgesia as part of the anaesthetic premedication, apart from the excellent sedative properties. Primarily, patients with painful conditions such as fractured hips and other types of trauma need analgesia for a comfortable transfer to theatre. Opioid analgesics are also used preoperatively to provide a continuous background of analgesia to aid the anaesthetic and extend analgesia into the postoperative period. Premedication with an opioid is usually combined with anticholinergic agents, such as glycopyrrolate, to dry secretions and (in the case of hyoscine) to potentiate sedation.

Generally speaking, the choice of premedication depends very much on the individual patient. For example, a moribund patient will not benefit, and may indeed suffer from such side-effects as respiratory or cardiovascular depression, whereas a young, fit, anxious patient could perhaps benefit from anxiolysis or sedation, besides possible analgesic requirements, especially in trauma.

**Table 8.3**  Analgesic agents in common use

| Agent | Dose (mg kg$^{-1}$) | Approx. duration i.m. (h) |
|---|---|---|
| Morphine | 0.1–0.2 | 4 |
| Papaveretum | 0.2–0.4 | 3 |
| Pethidine | 1.0–1.5 | 3–4 |

Notes:
1.  Papaveretum is a mixture of alkaloids which contains morphine (45–55% dry weight), codeine, papaverine, thebaine and noscopine. It should not be used in women of child-bearing age, because noscopine has been shown to be a gene toxin.
Papaveretum is most commonly used as a premedication in combination with hyoscine, and comes in a premixed ampoule containing papaveretum 20 mg ml$^{-1}$ and hyoscine 0.4 mg ml$^{-1)}$.
2.  Pethidine is often premixed with promethazine as pethidine 50 mg ml$^{-1}$ and promethazine 25 mg ml$^{-1}$. Atropine is sometimes given in addition.
3.  Morphine, often used alone for both its sedative and analgesic properties, is usually combined with a drying agent such as atropine (also useful to prevent bradycardia), or in combination with an antiemetic drug.

## GENERAL ANAESTHESIA

General anaesthesia is a reversible, drug-induced

state of unresponsiveness to outside stimuli, characterized by non-awareness, analgesia and relaxation of striated muscle. Older agents such as ether need to be given in large amounts to achieve these aims, and they take a long time for induction and recovery.

With the advent of newer, more specifically acting agents such as the muscle relaxants, modern general anaesthesia is a balance between the triad of 'relaxation', 'analgesia', and 'hypnosis' (lack of awareness).

A general anaesthetic may be considered in three phases, analogous to an aircraft flight:

'take-off' = 'induction'
'cruising' = 'maintenance'
'landing' = 'reversal and recovery'

Each part of the triad of general anaesthesia will be considered separately, under the heading of each phase of the anaesthetic.

## Induction of anaesthesia

### Hypnosis at induction of anaesthesia

In the anaesthetic room, patients are induced using one or other of several intravenous anaesthetics. In approximate order of frequency, those shown in Table 8.4 are the most commonly used agents.

When drugs are taken up in the bloodstream, initial distribution is to 'vessel-rich' tissues and those taking a large fraction of the cardiac output. Thus the brain, which is vessel rich and also taking a large fraction of the cardiac output, receives a considerable portion of intravenous anaesthetic given as a bolus. Subsequently, drugs diffuse out of the brain, down a concentration gradient formed by the falling blood concentration, and are redistributed to other vessel-poor

tissues. This results in an initial short redistribution half-life. The longer elimination half-life of a drug represents its metabolism and elimination from the body. In some instances, for example propofol and midazolam, this can appear to take a long time, due to the slow leaching out of drug from vessel-poor fat tissues.

*Thiopentone*, a very short-acting barbiturate, was the first widely used intravenous induction agent. It was first used to great effect on casualties from the bombing of Pearl Harbour in 1942. However, the ability of thiopentone to depress the myocardium was tragically evident in the deaths of young sailors already shocked from hypovolaemia. It was soon learned to reduce the dose and only give enough thiopentone to cause sleep (a 'sleep dose'), titrating carefully with each patient — especially those with a low cardiac reserve.

*Propofol* has a very short half-life, and tends to be used particularly in day-case surgery, where rapid recovery is indicated. It is also used to abate the effects of procedures which occasionally cause laryngospasm, such as laryngeal mask placement and anal stretching. Propofol is sometimes infused intravenously to maintain anaesthesia, because of its short half-life. The initial bolus of propofol sometimes causes a profound fall in blood pressure and inhibits compensatory increases in heart rate. Preinduction administration of glycopyrrolate or atropine may attenuate this.

*Etomidate* is indicated only for induction of anaesthesia. As a side-effect, it causes a reversible suppression of an enzyme in the adrenal cortex, leading to inhibition of cortisol secretion — especially important if it is used as an infusion. Etomidate is indicated in patients with poor cardiac reserve, or other patients in whom a fall in cardiac output could prove catastrophic, because it tends to maintain cardiac output. It is relatively long acting.

*Ketamine* is used in shocked patients, because it stimulates the sympathetic nervous system and prevents a fall in cardiac output. However, patients already on full sympathetic drive will suffer a reduction in output. Ketamine produces a state known as 'dissociative anaesthesia' with profound analgesia. It is structurally related to LSD.

**Table 8.4** Anaesthetic agents

| Drug | Dose (mg kg$^{-1}$) | Distribution half-life (min) | Elimination half-life (h) |
| --- | --- | --- | --- |
| Thiopentone | 3–5 | 3–14 | 5–17 |
| Propofol | 1–3 | 2–4 | 4–5 |
| Etomidate | 0.3 | 2–6 | 1–5 |
| Ketamine | | | |
| i.v. | 1–2 | 10 | 2–3 |
| i.m. | 5–10 | 15 | 2–3 |
| Methohexitone | 1–3 | 3–8 | 26 |
| Midazolam | 0.03–0.3 | 6–20 | 1–4 |

*Benzodiazepines* given intravenously, particularly midazolam (the most efficacious in this respect), are occasionally used to induce or assist induction of anaesthesia.

*Opoids* in very high doses are used to induce anaesthesia in some situations. The most commonly used agents for this are the highly potent synthetic derivatives fentanyl, alfentanil and sufentanil. Fentanyl is used in a dosage of up to 1.0 mg kg$^{-1}$, particularly in cardiac anaesthesia, since it avoids hypotension and maintains cardiac output. Without other agents, awareness may occur, however, and chest rigidity, preventing adequate ventilation, occasionally occurs (easily reversed with the use of muscle relaxants).

Generally, with the exceptions outlined above, all intravenous anaesthetic agents depress the myocardium.

### Relaxation at induction

On induction, muscle relaxation is necessary to facilitate (tracheal) intubation. Relaxation during maintenance of anaesthesia is discussed in the next section.

*Suxamethonium* is a depolarizing relaxant used primarily for difficult intubation and crash induction. It only lasts approximately 5 minutes, after a dose of 1.5 mg kg$^{-1}$. Suxamethonium is essentially two acetylcholine molecules joined together. Its great similarity to acetylcholine results in activation of the receptor and depolarization of the muscle membrane. However, this depolarization lasts some 5–10 minutes, and muscles become unresponsive to acetylcholine. As it lasts some 5–10 minutes, suxamethonium is useful, apart form intubation, for very short surgical procedures.

Side-effects of suxamethonium include:

1. *Histamine release.* 'Scoline rash' is very common following intravenous administration of suxamethonium. An erythematous rash is seen spreading over the upper trunk and lower neck anteriorly. Very occasionally, suxamethomium will cause bronchospasm and other more severe sequelae.

2. *Bradycardia.* This is seen particularly if a second or subsequent dose is given, especially in children. Atropine is given to prevent or reverse this effect.

3. *Generalized somatic pain.* The actual cause of this is unknown, but may be a result of widespread fleeting muscle contractions, termed 'fasciculations', caused by the depolarization of muscle fascicles.

4. *Hyperkalaemia.* Suxamethonium causes the release of potassium from muscle cells. This may be accentuated in acute denervating injuries such as spinal cord trauma or burns and can lead to cardiac arrest.

5. *Persistent neuromuscular blockade.* Some patients may have deficient or abnormal plasma pseudocholinesterase, resulting in prolonged action of suxamethonium, sometimes called 'scoline apnea'. This is genetically related. The completely silent gene is rare, occurring in approximately 1 : 7000 of the population.

6. *Malignant hyperthermia.* This is a condition occurring in some 1 : 100 000 of the population. It occurs as a reaction to certain anaesthetic drugs, of which suxamethonium and halothane are the commonest. Muscle metabolism becomes uncontrolled because of an abnormality of intracellular calcium flux. Body temperature rapidly rises at the rate of at least 2 deg. C every 15 minutes and PaCO$_2$, reflecting the massively raised metabolic rate, also increases with alacrity. Treatment is with ventilation and surface cooling and intravenous dantrium given promptly before death ensues.

### 'Crash Induction'

This consists of a rapid-sequence intravenous induction, cricoid pressure and tracheal intubation, with the aim of preventing regurgitation and aspiration of stomach contents. The patient is given a precalculated dose of thiopentone (3–5 mg kg$^{-1}$), immediately followed by suxamethonium (1.5 mg kg$^{-1}$), currently the fastest-acting muscle relaxant, acting within one circulation time. A trained assistant applies pressure to the cricoid cartilage simultaneously, compressing the oesophagus between cricoid ring and vertebral column. The trachea is intubated with a cuffed tracheal tube, and the cuff inflated. Only when the anaesthetic circuit is attached and cuff seal confirmed, is cricoid pressure relaxed at the request of the anaesthetist.

The following patients are at risk of aspiration of stomach contents on induction of anaesthesia:

1. all nonfasted patients
2. patients with a history suggestive of hiatus hernia
3. any emergency trauma patient (trauma slows stomach emptying)
4. intestinal or gastric obstruction or stasis
5. pregnancy (stomach emptying slowed and cardiac sphincter relaxed)
6. any other intra-abdominal tumours that may cause slowing of gastric emptying.

## Maintenance of anaesthesia

### Hypnosis during anaesthesia

Anaesthesia is usually maintained with *volatile agents*, which are hydrocarbons, liquid at room temperature, with high saturated vapour pressures and lipid solubility. Diethyl ether was the earliest agent used, and is still used commonly in other parts of the world. Ether is inflammable and explosive. By adding fluoride and other halogens, however, the hydrocarbon molecule becomes much more stable. Modern agents are non-inflammable, non-explosive, and much more potent than ether. Being less soluble in blood (as indicated by the blood/gas partition coefficient), they also have a much faster uptake and elimination time than diethyl ether. Table 8.5 shows the most commonly used anaesthetic volatile agents (with ether as a comparison)

***Halothane.*** A hydrocarbon with fluorine, chlorine and bromine atoms. This was the first modern volatile anaesthetic agent which was not explosive or inflammable. Synthesized in 1951 and first used clinically in 1956, it was the most commonly used anaesthetic agent for thirty years. Halothane is a potent anaesthetic which allows a smooth induction (important especially for gaseous induction of children), and relatively rapid onset of anaesthesia. In the body, up to 20% is metabolized by the liver, the majority being eliminated unchanged via the lungs. The recovery time from halothane anaesthesia is also brisk and smooth. The most common side-effects of halothane are secondary to its effects on the heart. Halothane slows the SA node, slowing heart rate and causing variations in the p–q interval. It reduces

**Table 8.5** Anaesthetic volatile agents

| Agent | Structure | MAC | Blood/Gas Partition Coefficient |
|---|---|---|---|
| Diethyl ether | $CH_3CH_2$-O-$CH_2CH_3$ | 1.92 | 12 |
| Halothane | $CF_3CHClBr$ | 0.75 | 2.3 |
| Enflurane | $CHF_2$O-$CF_2CHFCl$ | 1.68 | 1.9 |
| Isoflurane | $CHF_2$O-$CHClCF_3$ | 1.05 | 1.4 |

Notes:

1. MAC: the minimum alveolar concentration of a gas or vapour in oxygen required to keep 50% of the population unresponsive to a standard surgical stimulus (opening of the abdomen). MAC is expressed as a percentage concentration.

2. Blood/gas partition coefficient: indicates how rapidly a gas or vapour is taken up from the lungs. The higher the blood solubility, the longer it takes for the brain to gain adequate anaesthetic concentrations.

3. Summary of effects of modern vapours on organ systems:

   a. *Heart*: generally cause depressed contractility: halothane > enflurane > isoflurane (halothane causes more arrhythmias)

   b. *Blood vessels*: generally cause vasodilation: isoflurane > enflurane > halothane

   c. *Respiration*: depressed by all agents: enflurane > isoflurane > halothane

   d. *Brain*: All may cause vasodilation and raised intracranial pressure: halothane > enflurane > isoflurane (isoflurane safe up to 1 MAC)

myocardial workload. Like verapamil, halothane produces these effects by blocking calcium channels in the heart. However, it also sensitizes the heart to catecholamines and may precipitate arrhythmias (especially important in the presence of adrenaline-supplemented local anaesthesia and if arterial carbon dioxide tension $PaCO_2$ is elevated). By reducing cardiac output, halothane attenuates splanchnic blood flow, diminishing hepatic blood flow and possibly aggravating its effects on the liver. Using very fine indicators of hepatic performance, it has now been shown that even the briefest exposure to halothane will cause some degree of liver dysfunction. This is probably related to the large amount of halothane that is metabolized (up to 20%). There is also an idiosyncratic reaction which occurs after halothane exposure in some patients, known as 'halothane hepatitis'. The latter is a fulminant centrilobular necrosis of the liver which appears two to five days postoperatively. The incidence is 1 : 35 000 of the population (from the National Halothane Study, USA, 1966), with a mortality of over

50%. Halothane is now used in only 10% of anaesthetics given in the UK, the majority of these being for paediatric anaesthesia.

***Enflurane.*** Enflurane is an ether synthesized in 1963 and first used in 1966. It is halogenated with fluorine and chlorine atoms to render it non-explosive and non-inflammable. Enflurane is more efficacious in reducing peripheral vascular resistance and is less likely to cause cardiac arrhythmias, nor does it sensitize the heart to catecholamines. Its pungent odour makes it unsuitable for gaseous induction in children, however. Enflurane causes greater respiratory depression than halothane or isoflurane, so is less suitable for maintaining anaesthesia in the spontaneously breathing patient. Enflurane is only slightly metabolized by the liver (up to 2.5%), and appears not to cause hepatitis.

***Isoflurane.*** Isoflurane is the most recent volatile agent in common use. It was synthesized in 1965 and first used in 1971. It is actually a structural isomer of enflurane, but with different properties. Isoflurane tends to act on the peripheral vasculature as a calcium antagonist, causing a reduction in peripheral vascular resistance. Although it has minimal effects on the heart, isoflurane may cause 'coronary steal', a phenomenon whereby blood is diverted from stenosed coronary arteries to dilated unblocked coronary arteries, possibly compromising ischaemic areas of myocardium. This is still a controversial area, however, and isoflurane generally causes minimal depression of contractility. In the brain, isoflurane has the least effect on cerebral blood flow, causing no significant increase up to 1 MAC. Isoflurane causes least respiratory depression and is suited to the spontaneously breathing patient. Only up to 0.2% of isoflurane is metabolized by the liver and no cases of hepatitis have been reported.

***New volatile agents.*** *Desflurane* and *sevoflurane* are currently being evaluated in clinical trials. Both are characterized by remarkable molecular stability, with very little hepatic metabolism. They also have a very low blood gas solubility coefficient, resulting in very rapid onset and recovery. Desflurane is more pungent than sevoflurane, the latter being potentially more useful for gaseous induction of children. We await the introduction of these agents with interest.

***Nitrous Oxide.*** Nitrous oxide $N_2O$, unlike the volatile agents, is a gas at atmospheric pressure and room temperature. It has a MAC value of 103% at sea level. The requirements of keeping the patient well oxygenated mean that it can never be relied upon to provide anaesthesia in its own right. It is, however, a very potent analgesic agent. Fifty per cent $N_2O$ is equivalent in efficacy to approximately 10 mg of morphine sulphate. It continues to enjoy popularity as the main background anaesthetic gas, usually given as 70% in oxygen. In concentrations greater than 50% it causes amnesia and contributes significantly to the overall anaesthetic.

### Relaxation during anaesthesia

To allow the surgeon access to intra-abdominal contents, or to allow artificial ventilation of the patient, for example in chest surgery, muscle relaxation (paralysis) is required.

Agents used specifically to relax muscles are called relaxants. Relaxants are agents which block acetylcholine receptors on muscle end plates. There are two types of relaxants: *depolarizing* and *non-depolarizing*.

***Depolarizing muscle relaxants.*** Only one depolarizing relaxant is still in common use, *suxamethonium*, which is described above in relation to induction.

***Non-depolarizing muscle relaxants.*** There are many different relaxants available today. Due to the side-effects of suxamethonium, research continues to find a non-depolarizing relaxant with a very rapid onset and very short half-life. Non-depolarizing relaxants have an onset time of the order of 2–3 minutes, and last from 20 minutes to 1 hour. They are competitive inhibitors of the acetylcholine receptors on muscle end plates, preventing access of acetylcholine to receptor, resulting in non-transmission of nerve impulse to muscle. Curare was the first relaxant of this class, developed from an arrow poison used by Amazonian tribesmen to kill animals for food. Only the dextrorotatory isomer is active; the term 'tubo-' refers to the bamboo tubes in which it is carried by the Amazonian tribesmen — hence '*d*-tubocurare'. Modern relaxants tend to be shorter acting, with fewer side-effects (Table 8.6).

*Analgesia during anaesthesia*

The final part of the triad of general anaesthesia during its maintenance consists of analgesia. The anaesthetized patient derives analgesia from three potential sources: the premedication, anaesthesia supplementation with opioids, and from the analgesic properties of volatile and gaseous agents.

*Premedication*. Opioids used in premedication, as discussed earlier, will tend to last intra-operatively and into the postoperative period. In this way, premedication affects both the anaesthetic and postoperative analgesia.

*Anaesthetic opioid supplementation*. Intra-operatively, opioids are often administered to deepen the effect of the anaesthetic, or to reduce the amount of volatile agent used (often because of their side-effects such as hypotension). To limit the effects of opioids to the perioperative period, anaesthetists often use highly potent short-acting agents such as fentanyl, alfentanil or sufentanil. These agents are all much more potent than morphine, and much shorter acting, of the order 20–30 minutes. They may need to be reversed at the end of the operation, to facilitate spontaneous respiration. However, this is at the expense of analgesia. Longer-acting opioids such as morphine, papaveretum, or pethidine may also be used — especially if postoperative analgesia may be a problem.

*Analgesic properties of volatile agents*. Modern volatile anaesthetic agents have poor analgesic properties and contribute little to this part of the anaesthetic. However, $N_2O$ is a very good analgesic, as described earlier, and is also used for analgesia during labour (as a 50% mixture with oxygen, known as 'Entonox').

## Recovery from anaesthesia

At the end of surgery, anaesthesia is terminated. Volatile agents and nitrous oxide are turned off on the anaesthetic machine and oxygen alone administered. Anaesthetic gases and vapours diffuse down concentration gradients from the tissues to alveoli of the lungs and out via the airway.

*Reversal of muscle relaxation*

Competitive muscle relaxants usually need to be reversed to ensure full return of muscle power. The degree of neuromuscular blockade can be monitored with a peripheral nerve stimulator.

*Neostigmine* (0.05 mg kg$^{-1}$) or *edrophonium* (0.5 mg kg$^{-1}$) is given intravenously. These agents block acetylcholinesterase in the neuromuscular junction, resulting in accumulation of acetylcholine. This overcomes the competitive blockade of the relaxant molecules in favour of acetylcholine.

However, both neostigmine and edrophonium cause acetylcholine accumulation at both muscarinic and nicotinic sites. Muscarinic receptors are those cholinergic receptors in the heart, gut, sweat glands etc. Therefore, to prevent bradycardia, profuse sweating, and gut over-activity, *atropine* (0.02 mg kg$^{-1}$) or *glycopyrrolate* (0.01 mg

**Table 8.6** Non-depolarizing muscle relaxants

| Agent | Dose mg kg$^{-1}$ | Duration of effect (min) | Side-effects |
|---|---|---|---|
| *d*-Tubocurare | 0.5 | 30–60 | Sympathetic ganglion blockade, histamine release, hypotension |
| Alcuronium | 0.3 | 20–40 | As above |
| Pancuronium | 0.01 | 45–120 | Vagolytic: tachycardia, increase BP |
| Vecuronium | 0.01 | 30–45 | Bradycardia |
| Atracurium | 0.06 | 15–40 | Histamine release |

*Notes:*

1. With the exception of atracurium, all these agents require renal and hepatic function for their clearance.

2. Atracurium is excreted by two mechanisms: Hofmann elimination (up to 40%) and hepatic metabolism. Hofmann elimination results in breakdown of the atracurium molecule as a result of pH and temperature. It is used in those patients with renal failure.

3. The histamine release associated with atracurium is only a quarter of that associated with tubocurare, and tends not to cause the hypotension seen with the latter agent.

4. The duration of effect with each agent varies slightly according to anaesthetic technique. The use of volatile agents, particularly enflurane and isoflurane, potentiates the effect of non-depolarizing muscle relaxants. Hypothermia also potentiates non-depolarizing relaxants.

5. The shorter-acting agents atracurium and vecuronium are often used as infusions for long cases and in intensive care.

6. Muscle relaxants have no intrinsic anaesthetic effect.

kg⁻¹) must be given with the anticholinesterase.

Full reversal of muscle relaxation is only apparent by appropriate neuromuscular monitoring, or when the patient is able to maintain head lifting. This aspect of recovery from anaesthesia is crucial, since full muscular control is necessary for coughing and for good control of the airway. Indeed it highlights the importance of adequate recovery facilities in the theatre suite.

## REGIONAL ANAESTHESIA

### Definition

Regional (local) anaesthesia is the reversible blockade of nerve conduction by regionally applied agents, for the purpose of sensory ablation, either of traumatised tissue, or to enable minor surgery. These agents are referred to as 'local anaesthetics'. Both motor and sensory nerves may be blocked, depending on the agent used and the anatomical region where the agent is applied.

Nerves may be blocked anywhere between the central nervous system and the site of required sensory loss. Local anaesthetics are used to block pain fibres as they enter the spinal cord: epidural, spinal and paravertebral techniques. They may also be blocked along their anatomical route in the neurovascular bundles: field blocks, or specific nerve blocks. Finally, local infiltration around the required site may be performed (for example, skin and subcutaneous infiltration), to block conduction at the nerve endings.

### Types of nerve fibre

The speed with which local anaesthetic agents are taken up by nerve fibres depends on their size and whether they are myelinated. Nerve fibres are classified according to their size and speed of conduction (Table 8.7).

### Sensitivity to local anaesthetics

The smaller fibres are more sensitive to local anaesthetic agents than the larger fibres. Hence, 'C' fibres conducting pain are more sensitive than motor fibres in the 'A' group. This is why patients may still be able to move limbs, even during

**Table 8.7**   Types of nerve fibre

| Fibre | Type | Function | Cond. vel. (ms) | dia. (μm) |
|---|---|---|---|---|
| A: | α | Motor, prop'eption | 70 – 120 | 12 – 20 |
| | β | Touch, pressure | 30 – 70 | 5 – 12 |
| | γ | Motor (spindles) | 15 – 30 | 3 – 6 |
| | ∂ | Pain, temp., touch | 12 – 30 | 2 – 5 |
| B: | | Pregang. autonomic | 3 – 15 | < 3 |
| C: | | D. root: Pain, reflexes | 0.5 – 2 | 0.4 – 1.2 |
| | | sympathetic: Post-gang. | 0.7 – 2.3 | 0.3 – 1.3 |

regional anaesthesia.

The reason for the differential is most likely due to more rapid absorption and uptake of local anaesthetic into the smaller fibres within neurovascular bundles.

### Local anaesthetic agents

Drugs used as local anaesthetics all tend to have 'membrane stabilising' properties.

Local anaesthetic agents act by inducing a blockade of nerve transmission in peripheral nerve impulses. This occurs as a result of obstruction to sodium channels in the axon membrane, preventing ingress of sodium ions necessary for propagation of an action potential.

Local anaesthetic agents belong to one of two chemical classes according to their structure, which consists of an amide or ester linkage separating an aromatic group and an amine:

| Aromatic group | >————< Amide or ester | Amine group |
|---|---|---|

### ESTER CLASS

The only ester still in frequent is **cocaine**, which is an ester of benzoic acid. It is used generally only for topical anaesthesia of mucous membranes in the nose and sinuses.

Amethocaine is still used occasionally as a topical agent, as is benzocaine.

# AMIDE CLASS

The first amide to be synthesized was **lignocaine**. This was shown to be safer than cocaine and has remained a mainstay for local anaesthetic practice. **Prilocaine** has the highest therapeutic index, and is considered the safest agent for intravenous blockade. Other amides in common usage include **bupivacaine, mepivacaine** and **etidocaine.** Bupivacaine is longer acting than lignocaine and is commonly used in epidural analgesia.

**Table 8.8** Amide class

| Drug | Maximum Dose (mg) | Side-effects |
| --- | --- | --- |
| Lignocaine | 300 (500+adr) | No unusual features CNS excitation with toxicity |
| Prilocaine | 600 | Least toxic Methaemoglobinaemia > 600 mg |
| Bupivacaine | 175 (225+adr) | Sudden cardiovascular collapse Not indicated for intravenous blockade |
| Cocaine | 150 | Cardiac arrhythmias CNS excitation Topical use only |

*Notes*

1. Above table includes only those agents currently in common use and maximal doses relate to adult size (70 kg body weight). The bracketed dosages refer to maximal doses in the presence of adrenalin.

2. All local anaesthetic agents have membrane stabilizing properties. Their toxic effects therefore relate to this property and involve mainly the cardiovascular and central nervous systems.

Toxic effects on the central nervous system include fitting and coma, leading to death from hypoxia without adequate resuscitation. Cardiovascular effects from toxicity include hypotension, cardiac arrhythmias and acute cardiovascular collapse.

Bupivacaine has a high affinity for cardiac muscle cells – a property which is thought to be responsible for the high incidence of cardiovascular collapse associated with its use for intravenous blockade (Bier's block), for which it is no longer recommended.

3. Toxic effects may also occur with the accidental intravascular injection of drug.

4. Concentration of local anaesthetic agents varies. Bupivacaine comes as 0.5% or 0.25%, with or without adrenaline. Lignocaine generally comes as 0.5, 1.0, 2.0 % concentrations, again plus or minus adrenaline. The higher concentrations obviously have lower maximum safe volumes (1% = 10 mg/ml, 2% = 20 mg/ml).

5. Local anaesthesia techniques should always be performed where adequate resuscitation facilities are present.

6. Adrenaline and other vasoconstricting agents, such as felypressin, allow higher doses of local anaesthetic to be used, the vasoconstriction resulting in reduced absorption.

## Clinical application

1. Local infiltration is used for surgery alone or in combination with general anaesthesia. Used with adrenaline, it reduces bleeding at the operative site. It also produces good post-operative analgesia.

2. 'Field' blocks and nerve blocks are useful for producing wider areas of anaesthesia and analgesia, for example in inguinal hernia repair, brachial plexus blockade for the upper limb and femoral and sciatic blocks of the lower limb.

3. Spinal, epidural and paravertebral blockade produces widespread anaesthesia and analgesia. The pain of labour and childbirth involves nerve roots of lower thoracic, lumbar and sacral regions of the spinal cord. Epidural techniques, involving the epidural placement of a catheter allow continuous analgesia or anaesthesia, alleviating pain from all these groups of fibres. Regional anaesthesia such as this is frequently employed for urological and other surgery in the lower half of the body. It should be noted, however, that spinal and epidural techniques also block sympathetic ganglia at the appropriate levels. Hypotension will occur unless adequate precautions are taken.

BIBLIOGRAPHY

The following books are useful for further reading and reference:

Atkinson R S, Rushman G B, Lee A 1987 A synopsis of anaesthesia. 10E Wright, London

Barash P G, Cuplen B F, Stoelting R K 1989 Clinical anaesthesia. Lippincott, Philadelphia

Gilman A G, Goodman L S, Rall T W, Murad F 1985 Goodman and Gilman's pharmacological basis of therapeutics. 7E Macmillan, London

Miller R D 1990 Anesthesia 3E Vols I–II. Churchill Livingstone, Edinburgh

Nimmo W S, Smith G 1989 Anaesthesia Vols I–II. Blackwell Scientific Publications, Oxford

Stoelting R K 1987 Pharmacology and physiology in anesthetic practice. Lippincolt, Philadelphia

Vickers M D, Morgan M, Spencer P S J 1991 Drugs in anaesthetic practice. 7E Butterworths, Oxford

# 9. Infection

*A. M. Emmerson*

PART 9.1
## ASEPSIS AND ANTISEPSIS
*A. M. Emmerson*

## THEATRE CLOTHING

### Gowns

When conventional cotton theatre wear is used in a theatre in which the air is ventilated in a conventional way, i.e. high-level input, the airborne counts depend on the number of people present and their degree of activity. Normal cotton clothing does little to prevent the passage of bacteria, especially when present on large skin scales, as the diameter of the holes at the interstices of the cloth is normally greater than 80 μm. Materials are available which reduce the dispersion of skin scales and bacteria but these may be restrictive in nature. 'A surgeon who is comfortably dressed in light, cool theatre clothing is less likely to make an error of judgement than one who is perspiring in a heavy, airless gown.' A compromise has to be reached and clothing made from *disposable nonwoven fabric*, e.g. Sontara (Fabric '450') is suitable. However, these disposable materials are expensive, especially since the whole team has to wear them to reap the benefit. Special attention has to be made to the design so that bacteria are not lost or pumped out at the neck or at the ankles. *Breathable membrane fabrics* are available, e.g. Gore-Tex, which consists of a fabric in which a layer of PTFE is laminated to one or two layers of a polyester. Other materials such as *tightly woven washable* poly cottons are also effective but require careful laundering. The most effective reduction of airborne bacteria is obtained by using the Charnley exhaust gown. However, to obtain maximum benefit this protective barrier has to be used in conjunction with a unidirectional air flow system and owing to its restrictive nature it is rarely used by general surgeons.

In a conventional operating theatre air is prefiltered and delivered to the theatre in a turbulent fashion but is free of known pathogens such as *Staphylococcus aureus* and *Clostridium perfringens*. Almost all of the airborne bacteria present in theatres are derived from people in the room; airborne contamination can be decreased by restricting the entry of non-essential personnel. Once the surgical operation has commenced, movements (excessive activity) should be controlled. This kind of discipline is still required even when verticle laminar flow (unidirectional) systems are used. Such systems are expensive to install in existing theatres and may only be of significant value in clean implant surgery (Lidwell et al 1982). However, it must be borne in mind that low infection rates can also be achieved by good surgical technique, theatre discipline, purpose-designed occlusive clothing (Whyte et al 1990) and the propitious use of single-dose prophylactic antibiotics.

### Masks

Face masks are worn for many and varied procedures but their use is seriously questioned. Few bacteria are dispersed from the mouth during normal breathing and quiet conversations and it is argued that for general abdominal operations masks are not required. They are certainly not required for members of staff not directly assisting in the operating theatre. If it is decided that masks should be worn, e.g. in implant surgery, then a fresh mask must be worn for each operation and discarded with care at the end of each operation. Reuse or manipulation of the mask during use will simply contaminate the outside of the mask and the hands with skin commensals, including staphylococci.

An efficient mask must be capable of arresting low-momentum droplets which contaminate the front of the operator's gown, gloves and subsequently the wound. Paper masks have no place in operating theatres as they become wet within a few minutes and lose their barrier qualities. As with clothing, the frequency of wet strike-through correlates well with the length of operation and the degree of wetness. Disposable masks made out of synthetic fibres are tolerable and contain filters made of polyester, e.g. Bard Vigilon, or polypropylene, e.g. Filtron. Surgical anti-fog masks with flexible nosebands are available which follow facial contours and yet retain a high efficiency of filtration.

### Eye protection

Masks and protective eyewear or face shields should be worn during procedures that are likely to generate droplets of blood or other body fluids, to prevent exposure of mucous membranes of the mouth, nose and eyes. A variety of anti-fog goggles, wrap-around spectacles and face shields are now available which are efficient, easy to wear and pleasant in appearance. They are light-weight, adjustable and do not obstruct vision. An educational programme is necessary to introduce surgeons to these new barriers.

### Hair/beard cover

All members of staff entering into the theatre area must wear their hair in a neat style. Long hair should be tied back in such a way that when the head is bent forward hair does not fall forward, occlude vision or at worst fall into a surgical wound. Hair must be completely covered by a close-fitting cap made of synthetic material. Once the head cover is in place it must not be adjusted or manipulated as this facilitates the

dispersal of many bacteria-carrying particles. Beards should be fully covered by a mask and a hood of the balaclava type which is tied securely at the neck.

### Footwear

There is little evidence to show that the floor plays a significant role in the spread of infection in hospital, and expensive efforts to minimize bacterial contamination of feet are unnecessary. Staff should wear clean, comfortable, antislip and antistatic shoes. If there is a real risk of fluid spillage, e.g. in genitourinary surgery, then ankle-length antistatic boots should be worn. These should be cleaned when required, with warm soapy water and stored dry. A variety of styles of shoes and clogs is available which allows choice with style. They should fit snugly and must not be allowed to produce a bellows effect. If sufficient shoes or half wellingtons are not available then freshly laundered socks should be provided as hygienic inserts.

### Gloves

It is now commonplace for all surgeons to wear gloves in order to reduce the risk of contaminating operation wounds. Nowadays, it is equally important to wear gloves in order to prevent the transmission of blood-borne viruses, e.g. hepatitis B (HBV) and HIV, from surgeon to patient and patient to surgeon. However, it is a sobering thought that between 20% and 30% of gloves develop holes during surgery through which bacteria can escape. Often, the wearer of the glove is unaware of the fact that the glove has been punctured. Worse still, many gloves have been found to have pre-existing holes prior to use as a result of poor manufacture and inadequate quality-control procedures.

Some surgeons have attempted double gloving and additional protection is achieved but at the expense of possible discomfort, reduced sensitivity and dexterity. Others have tried covering the first pair of gloves with glutaraldehyde cream and then covering the cream with a second pair of gloves. Unfortunately, even this 'sandwich' technique will not stop a determined assistant from puncturing the latex gloves. It is important to purchase sterilized (by irradiation) single-use, surgical rubber gloves from a reputable source and bearing the kite mark (BS 4005; 1984).

Surgical gloves made from natural rubber (latex) are increasingly reported to cause cutaneous and sy90stemic hypersensitivity reactions. Non-latex gloves without glove powder are available.

### Protective Clothing

There are occasions when operations have to be performed on patients known to be carriers of, or infected with, notifiable diseases. Under these circumstances and where it is known that heavy aerial dispersal of microorganisms is inevitable and blood soak through is commonplace, protective clothing is required. Some gowns are made entirely of impermeable materials (double-layered polyester fabric or laminated plastic films) while others have these materials in key areas, such as in the front and on the sleeves. Surgical staff may get uncomfortably hot in gowns made only of these materials unless the room temperature is lowered or ventilation turnover is increased. If these costly fabrics are not available then disposable long-sleeve gowns can be used together with disposable plastic aprons. All skin must be covered, including face, eyes and hair.

## PREPARATION OF THE SURGEON

In Sweden it is considered unethical to perform high-risk surgery without preoperative whole-body disinfection with chlorhexidine. The microbiologist who made this statement was in fact referring to the preoperative preparation of the patient. What about the preoperative preparation of the surgeon? Surgeons have to be physically fit to sustain the rigours of surgical activities. Some operations last hours and require intense concentration and intricate surgery, while others are short, physical and crude. Theatres are not the place for the faint hearted and the below-par surgeon. Surgeons must not operate when they are suffering from skin infections or are in the prodromal period of viral infections. Most theatre-acquired infections are of endogenous origin but

a surgeon who is actively disseminating staphylococci from active skin lesions is a menace.

Surgeons should begin the day with socially clean hands; they should scrub dirt off the nails and hands with nail-brushes before entering the operating department in the morning.

### Showering

The Swedish experience points to the benefits obtained by patients using 4% chlorhexidine gluconate soap solution (Hibiscrub) during two preoperative whole-body showers. These results have been challenged by a European Working Party on the Control of Hospital Infection but there is sufficient evidence to show that showering is preferable to bathing in terms of removal of skin bacteria, and chlorhexidine has a greater effect than non-medicated soap. It would seem reasonable that surgeons could safely shower between long operations or between sessions using Hibiscrub followed by non-perfumed body oils to all accessible skin. The benefits of a refreshing 'top-to-toe' shower outweigh any theoretical disadvantages.

### Scrubbing up

Repeated hand disinfection with scrubbing brushes between operations results in skin abrasions and result in more bacteria being brought to the surface. A surgeon's hands must be socially clean before he or she enters the operating theatre. If scrubbing brushes are used at all they should be sterile, single use and made of polypropylene. Wooden brushes with bristles should not be used. An initial scrub of 3–5 minutes at the beginning of an operating list is all that is required. Modern-day skin antiseptics act rapidly and often show a cumulative effect. Repeated scrubbing is counter-productive but the term 'scrubbing up' is unlikely to disappear from surgical practice; 'washing up' doesn't have the same impact or mystique! Hexachlorophane (pHisoHex) is effective against Gram-positive bacteria only and is slow activating but has a cumulative effect even under rubber gloves. Povidone–iodine (Betadine/Disadine) acts more rapidly than hexachlorophane and has a broader spectrum but does not have a prolonged effect. Chlorhexidine gluconate 4% w/v (Hibiscrub) is rapidly active, broad spectrum and persists. It is easy to use and requires constant running water to wash off the detergent-like effect. Patients allergic to chlorhexidine can use either povidone–iodine or hexachlorophane.

Hands should be thoroughly dried using single-use sterile towels. Hot-air drying machines have been tested but are not recommended for this purpose. Disinfection of the surgeon's hands is important because gloves, which often develop small holes during use, are an imperfect barrier against contamination of operation wounds.

## PREPARATION OF THE PATIENT

The longer the patient stays in hospital before an operation, the greater is the likelihood of a subsequent wound infection (Cruse & Foord 1980). The hospital stay before the operation should be as short as possible; in particular, tests and therapeutic measures that will prolong the pre-operative stay beyond one day should be performed in the out-patient department where possible. Cultures from postoperative wound infections often suggest that organisms are transferred from other areas of the patient to the operative site (endogenous transfer) despite the use of antiseptics. A preoperative shower using hexachlorophane for washing has value in reducing wound infection. The programme practised in Sweden for whole-body disinfection involves three 'top-to-toe' (including the hair) sessions — one the day before admission, one the evening before the operation and one on the operative day. Hibiscrub is used. Not all countries in Europe practise this procedure.

All signs of skin infection in the patient should be identified and pretreated or covered with waterproof dressings.

### Shaving

Hair adjacent to the operative site is often removed to prevent the wound from becoming entangled with hair during the operation. However, hair removal often causes injury to the skin and wound infection rates have been shown to be higher when skin is shaved. If hair removal is necessary, clippers should be used and it should be performed as near to the time of the operation as possible and preferably by the surgeon. If clippers are not available depilatory cream can be used.

### Preoperative screening

Preoperative screening of nasal or skin areas is of little value and is not cost effective. In general the mere presence of potentially pathogenic bacteria is not commensurate with subsequent infections.

### Transport of the patient to theatre

After the patient has been prepared for operation and has been changed into a clean operating gown he or she can be transferred directly from the ward to the operating room in a bed, provided ward bedding is removed before entering the theatre. There is little advantage in having a transfer area and changing trolleys or putting on overshoes. Trolleys are exposed to some degree of contamination during the journeys to and from the wards and require cleaning on a daily basis. Passing the trolley wheels over a sticky mat has doubtful benefits and the cost does not justify their use.

### Preparation of the patient's skin

The area around and including the operative site should be scrubbed with a detergent-impregnated sponge or swab. No benefit is to be gained by preparing the skin the night before operation, as was performed with povidone–iodine for lower limb amputations. After the skin has been cleaned and degreased antiseptic solutions should be used. Application of alcohol or of alcoholic solution of chlorhexidine or povidone–iodine gives better disinfection when the antiseptic is rubbed on until the skin is dry. This can be achieved by using a double-gloved hand or sponge forceps. To obtain maximum reduction of transient skin flora the alcohol must be allowed to dry. Care must be taken when using alcoholic solutions with diathermy. Alcohol must not be allowed to pool in the umbilicus and under the perineum. For vaginal and perineal disinfection it is advised that a solution of chlorhexidine and cetrimide (Savlon) should be used.

## Drapes

Part of the ritual of preparing the patient for surgery includes protecting the periphery of the proposed incisional site with sterilized cotton drapes. Because these cotton drapes become wet very quickly and their protective properties are diminished, the use of incisional plastic drapes has been advocated. Early work by Cruse & Foord (1980) demonstrated that wound infections are not decreased by applying adhesive plastic skin drapes to the operative area. More recent work has confirmed this finding in a study of Caeserian section.

## STERILIZATION

This is a process usually defined as the complete destruction or removal of all microorganisms, including spores and viruses. In practice this is difficult to establish and the definition is often couched in the probability of a single viable organism or virus being present in one million items (i.e. equal to or less than $10^{-6}$). This definition meets the requirement of the European Pharmacopoeia and will probably be accepted in Europe.

The term sterilization is applied to inanimate objects, e.g. instruments and equipment, but *not* to the skin as the process is a tissue-damaging one.

## Sterilization by steam

Steam under pressure attains a temperature higher than boiling water and the final temperature is directly related to pressure. Instruments can be sterilized reliably by steam under pressure using autoclaves. Steam transfers its latent heat of condensation to microorganisms on the surface of previously cleaned instruments. Both vegetative bacteria (including TB) viruses (e.g. HBV and HIV) and heat-resistant spores (e.g. *Clostridium tetani* and *Clostridium perfringens)* treated in steam pressure vessels are rendered non-infectious and non-viable (i.e. killed).

The recommended combination of time and temperature varies and for instruments which can withstand moist heat under pressure the following cycles are recommended:

1. 134°C (30 lb/sq. in.) for a hold time of 3 minutes
2. 121°C (15 lb/sq. in.) for a hold time of 15 minutes

The higher temperature of 134°C for 3 minutes is preferred. It is important to remember that these times are the 'hold time' at the stated temperature and that the entire cycle time, i.e. heating up/cooling down, is much longer; the cycle time at 134°C is approximately 30 minutes. In the past flash autoclaves operating at 147°C (40 lb/sq. in.) were used but these are no longer recommended or available, for safety reasons.

All steam sterilizers should comply with the requirements of BS 3970, British Standard for Sterilizing and Disinfecting Equipment for Medical Products. All sterilizers should have a preset automatic cycle which cannot be interrupted until the cycle is completed. Most large autoclaves are centralized in specialized units, e.g. Central Sterile Service Departments (CSSD) or Theatre Sterile Service Units (TSSU) and are subject to close scrutiny and maintenance by highly trained personnel.

### Wrapped instruments/packs

All pre-packed materials/instruments are processed through a porous load autoclave which includes a pre-vacuum cycle, necessary to extract air. Unless the trapped air is removed, dry saturated steam cannot penetrate efficiently and the sterilization process will be hindered.

### Unwrapped instruments

A convenient method to sterilize small numbers of surgical instruments is to use a portable steam sterilizer, e.g. Little Sister II. Instruments should be thoroughly cleaned and dried and placed on a perforated stainless steel tray that slides into the autoclave. When the autoclave cycle is completed, the instruments should be left to cool down (often down to 80°C) and can be used straight away or stored dry on a trolley laid with sterile paper (BS 6255). This is a convenient way to deal with dropped (or thrown!) instruments.

### Monitoring

The sterilizer must be maintained according to the manufacturer's instructions. In addition, maintenance requirements and routine and commissioning performance tests are strictly controlled (HTM10).

*Porous load* autoclaves are checked daily using the steam penetration test (e.g. Bowie–Dick test), and cycle performance is recorded on a temperature chart. Biological indicators are *not* appropriate but there is a limited role for chemical indicators (e.g. Browne's tubes no. II) which provide visual indication that a particular time/temperature relationship has been achieved.

*Bowel and instrument autoclaves* employ fixed automatic cycles and tend not to have temperature chart recorders attached. Browne's tubes no. I can be used to verify that the cycle is completed.

Much reliance is placed on process control and autoclaving at high temperatures (e.g. 134°C) will usually meet the required standard with a very large safety margin.

### Sterilization of fluids

Fluids for parenteral or topical use are generally prepared by industry or by specialized pharmacy production units. Fluids are prepared aseptically and appropriately labelled in sealed containers (bags or bottles) and sterilized in bottle autoclaves at 121°C for 15 minutes or 115°C for 30 minutes.

## Sterilization by hot air

The efficiency of dry heat sterilization depends on the initial moisture of the microbial cells, but *all* microorganisms are killed at 160°C for a hold time of 2 hours. Compared with moist steam sterilization, dry heat sterilization is inefficient.

The main *advantages* of dry heat sterilization are its ability to treat solids, non-aqueous liquids, grease/ointments and to process closed (airtight) containers. Lack of corrosion is important in the sterilization of non-stainless metals and surgical instruments with fine cutting edges (e.g. ophthalmic instruments).

The process is *not* to be used for aqueous fluids or materials that are denatured or damaged at 160°C for 2 hours (e.g. rubber, plastics, i.v. fluids).

It is essential that all items are thoroughly cleaned, dried and packed before they are placed inside a hot-air oven. The chamber must be fitted with perforated shelves and the oven must be fitted with an electrical heater and fan unit with an independent adjustable thermostat.

Hot-air ovens should meet the specification for Performance of Electrically Heated Sterilizing Ovens in BS 3421. It is *not* appropriate to use converted catering equipment! Door seals must be maintained routinely and all instrumentation and charts checked.

### Monitoring

The duration of the sterilization cycle is governed mainly by the penetration and holding times. Temperatures are checked using thermocouples.

Biological indicators such as *spores* are *not* used routinely. Chemical indicators (e.g. Browne's tubes no. III) may be used to demonstrate that the packages have been processed.

## Sterilization by ethylene oxide

Ethylene oxide (EO) is a highly penetrative, non-corrosive agent which has a broad-spectrum cidal action against vegetative bacteria, spores and viruses under optimal conditions of concentration, relative humidity, temperature and exposure time. At ambient temperatures and pressures, EO vaporizes rapidly and is flammable in mixtures containing more than 3% vapour in air. It is also toxic, irritant, mutagenic and potentially carcinogenic. Nevertheless, under strictly controlled conditions it is an extremely valuable sterilization process. It is not to be used where heat sterilization of an item is possible.

## Preferred uses

Sterilization by EO is restricted to wrapped and unwrapped heat-sensitive materials. It is ideal for delicate items such as electrical equipment, flexible-fibre endoscopes, photographic equipment and for reuse or resterilization of single use-items, e.g. cardiac catheters. This practice is *not* condoned by the Department of Health but it is recognized that recycling occurs.

EO is predominantly an industrial process used, for example, for single-use medical devices constructed of plastics. Limited NHS regional units process predominantly cardiovascular items.

The process is *not* recommended for ventilatory and respiratory equipment and is inappropriate for soiled items. Organic debris, oil, serum, etc. exhibit a marked adverse effect. The preferred wrapping is spun-bodied polyotefin (Tyvek) or sterilization paper (BS 6255).

EO sterilization is usually carried out within the temperature range 20–60°C and with operating cycles from 2 to 24 hours.

*High-pressure* sterilizers (6 bar) operate with a mixture of inert gases such as carbon dioxide. This greatly reduces the risk of flammability but increases the risk of leaks. Gas cylinders require replacement after one to four cycles, which makes the process expensive. The cycle time is 1.5–2.5 hours.

*Sub-atmospheric* sterilizers are operated by single-shot canisters situated inside the chamber and punctured automatically during the cycle. Pure EO is used to maintain an optimal concentration. The chamber capacity is small (115 litres) and the cycle time long (3.5–5 hours).

## Monitoring

It is imperative that the purpose-designed cabinet is operated according to the manufacturer's instructions. Physical parameters such as humidity, pressure, temperature and EO concentration are monitored. Since these measurements do not guarantee sterility, rigorous monitoring by biological indicators (e.g. *Bacillus subtilis* var. *niger* spore strips) and chemical indicators is essential.

EO sterilization is an expensive and potentially dangerous process and must be carefully controlled. A major disadvantage is that the gas takes a long time to elute. Prolonged aeration requirements make for long turn-round times for processed items. This means that contaminated items, e.g. endoscopes, may not be returned to the user (owner) for five to seven days. However, the Health and Safety Commission have taken a particular interest in EO usage and it is unlikely that short cuts in safety measures will be taken.

## Sterilization by low-temperature steam and formaldehyde (LTSF)

This is a physicochemical method which uses a combination of dry saturated steam and formaldehyde to kill vegetative bacteria, bacterial spores and most viruses. The main advantage of this process is that sterilization is achieved at a low temperature (73°C) and is suitable for heat-sensitive materials and items of equipment with integral plastic components susceptible to damage by other processes.

LTSF is *not* recommended for sealed, oily or greasy items or those with retained air. Other items are excluded where chemical reactions between the steam/chemical atmosphere and the material/object concerned may produce damage. Reversible absorption by some plastics and fabrics may lead to delayed elution of formaldehyde and subsequent hypersensitivity. All items contaminated with body fluids are excluded because hardened fixed protein deposits will be produced by this process. Narrow-bore tubing is likely to contain condensed water with trapped formaldehyde which will be hazardous to patients. This consideration excludes endoscopes as well as tubing.

LTSF is carried out in a purpose-built sterilizer and undergoes an automatic control system similar to that of other sterilizers. The cycle includes air removal and the introduction of dry saturated steam at 73°C (under vacuum) into which formaldehyde is introduced in a pulsing fashion. Prior to removal of sterilized objects all formaldehyde must be removed to provide a dry, sterile, formalin-free load.

## Monitoring

Monitoring requires the recording of process time,

temperature and steam pressure, the amounts of formaldehyde introduced into the chamber, and the duration of the various stages. In addition, biological indicators are used to confirm the effectiveness of the process. These are standard test objects bearing a known number of the spores of *Bacillus stearothermophilus* NCTC 10003. The Line Pickerill helix is employed as a standard test carrier for these biological monitors.

## Sterilization by irradiation

Sterilization by irradiation employs γ-rays or accelerated electrons. Sterilization by ionizing radiation is an industrial process and is unsuited to the constraints of the NHS. It is particularly suited to the sterilization of large batches of similar products, e.g. single-use items such as catheters, syringes, I.V.Is etc.

The delivery of irradiation dose in excess of 25kGy (2.5 Mrad) is accepted as providing adequate sterility assurance. When packaging of any sterile product has been damaged, the sterility of the contents cannot be guaranteed.

### Monitoring

The dose delivered at any point within a product container can be measured by the use of dosimeters. The validation and routine monitoring of sterilization by irradiation is under the control of the UK Panel on Gamma and Electron Irradiation.

*NB:* irradiation can cause serious physical deterioration of materials and therefore the resterilization of γ-irradiated items by any other method may further damage the item and jeapordize its function.

## Disposal by incineration

This is the preferred method of disposal for all combustible material of an infective nature, e.g. contaminated needles, plastic syringes and clinical waste. In purpose-designed incinerators immediate combustion occurs in furnaces with a secondary combustion zone exit gas temperature in excess of 850°C. This temperature should exceed 1000°C if cytotoxic drugs are in the waste stream.

Careful separation of clinical waste must occur before colour coded (e.g. yellow) plastic bags and boxes are incinerated. This process is *not* to be used for metal instruments or equipment. Disposable linen and infected protective clothing and drapes should be incinerated. There is no need to incinerate equipment, instruments or reusable linen as advice on the decontamination of such materials does not include incineration.

FURTHER READING

A code of practice for sterilization of instruments and control of cross infection. Published by the BMA, ISBN 0 7279 0274 1. Price £4.95
Guidance for Clinical Care Workers: protection against infection with HIV and hepatitis viruses. Published by HMSO, ISBN 0 11 321249 6. Price £4.80
A code of practice for the safe use and disposal of sharps. Published by the BMA, ISBN 0 7279 0294 6. Price £4.95
Ayliffe GAJ, Collins BJ, Taylor LJ Hospital-acquired infection: principles and prevention (2nd edn). Published by Wright ISBN 0 7236 1259-5. Price £12.95

# DISINFECTION

Disinfection is a process used to reduce the number of viable microorganisms and which may not necessarily inactivate some viruses and bacterial spores. Cleaning is a process which physically removes contamination but does not necessarily destroy microorganisms. The reduction of microbial contamination cannot be defined and will depend on many factors, including the efficiency of the cleaning process and the initial bioburden. Cleaning is a necessary prerequisite of equipment decontamination to ensure effective disinfection or sterilization.

## Disinfection with low-temperature steam (LTS)

This disinfection pasteurizing process kills most vegetative microorganisms and viruses by exposure to moist heat.

Typical conditions are exposure to dry saturated steam at a temperature of 73°C for a period of 20 minutes at below atmospheric pressure. Items and materials not damaged by the conditions of the process are suitable, provided that air removal and subsequent steam penetration are assured. This is a useful process which can be used to render safe to handle 'dirty returns' from operating theatres and clinics which may be contaminated with protein from bodily secretions and microorganisms. Following LTS instruments can be readily cleaned as the coagulated protein residues are readily removable, unlike the 'baked on' residues produced following autoclaving.

The process requires a disinfector, which is most likely kept in TSSU. Instruments can be replaced on the tray on the 'set-up' trolley or can be transferred to TSSU in impermeable plastic bags and transported in leak-proof polypropylene or metal boxes. These boxes can subsequently be cleaned and disinfected.

## Disinfection with boiling water

Boiling water is an efficient disinfection process which kills vegetative bacteria (including TB), some viruses (including HBV and HIV) and some spores. It is *not* a sterilizing process. Water is non-toxic but at high temperature causes tissue damage. Soft water at 100°C at normal pressure for 5 minutes or more forms the disinfection cycle. All items for disinfection must be thoroughly cleaned and totally immersed in boiling water in a safe manner. Suitable items include metal instruments such as speculae, proctoscopes and sigmoidoscopes. Care should be taken to ensure that air is not trapped in tubing, etc.

A purpose-designed water boiler should be used which should be electrically heated and incorporate an overheating cut-out. The machine should have a hinged lid and a perforated tray with a raising/lowering lever. The unit should be designed to operate at temperatures such that the contained water will continue to boil when instruments are lowered into it.

### Monitoring

It is not possible to monitor this process satisfactorily. A temperature gauge is fitted but a record is not kept. A time-lock should be fitted to prevent cycle disruption.

A major disadvantage of the process is that it leaves the article wet and unfit for storage. Items should be stored dry and covered prior to use.

## Disinfection with formaldehyde

Formaldehyde gas is a broad-spectrum antimicrobial agent which under optimal conditions of concentration, exposure time and relative humidity can be used as a disinfecting agent. This process is quite distinct from LTSF. At atmospheric pressure and temperatures up to 50°C the gas has limited sporicidal action.

The formaldehyde cabinet comprises a large airtight cabinet and a control console which automatically dispenses and circulates gaseous formaldehyde up to 50°C. Following an appropriate exposure time for disinfection, ammonia gas is released to neutralize residual formaldehyde. The cabinet and its contents are flushed through with fresh air.

Formaldehyde is a hazardous substance; it is a flammable and explosive gas, irritant to the eyes, respiratory tract and skin. Such properties require careful control and monitoring of the process and consideration of possible adverse effects to staff, equipment and patients.

This process can be used to provide terminal disinfection of large thermolabile items such as ventilators, suction pumps and incubators. If ventilators can be protected by bacterial filters this process is not required. Paper, rubber and some plastic materials are excluded from this process because formaldehyde residues may persist or be trapped within the product.

Two main types of formaldehyde cabinet are currently used in the UK:

1. The *Draeger Aseptor Unit* offers a short cycle (3.5 hours) or a long cycle (10 hours).

2. The *Vickers Formalaire* is a smaller machine and can accommodate only a single item; cycle time is 3 hours.

### Monitoring

There is limited process control directly monitoring the item to be processed. Formaldehyde-sensitive indicator paper may be used to indicate that the gas has reached a particular part in the load but will not confirm disinfection. Biological indicators for this process are available but require careful evaluation as to their applicability to the process.

## REFERENCES

Cruse P J E, Foord R 1980. The epidemiology of wound infection: a 10-year prospective study of 62,939 wounds. Surgical Clinics of North America 60: 1.

Lidwell O M, Lowbury E J L, Whyte W, Blowers R, Stanley S J, Lowe D 1982. Effects of ultra clean air in operating rooms on deep sepsis in the joints after total hip or knee replacement: a randomized study. British Medical Journal 285: 10–14.

Whyte W, Hamblen D L, Kelly I G, Hambraeus A, Laurell G 1990. An investigation of occlusive polyester surgical clothing. Journal of Hospital Infections 15: 363–374.

## PART 9.2
# THE RISKS TO SURGEONS OF NOSOCOMIAL VIRUS TRANSMISSION
*C. Wastell*

Since the inspirational work of Semmelveiss we have been progressively more aware of the dangers of transmission of microorganisms from patient to patient, patient to surgeon and surgeon to patient. Jenner was perhaps the first experimental worker, however, to manipulate the pox virus with his classical studies on the prevention of smallpox by means of immunization. With this eighteenth and nineteenth century background and all the great works of the microbiologists, it appears extraordinary that practising surgeons in the late twentieth century accept both contamination of themselves by the blood and body fluids of their patients and the contamination of the patients with their own blood when a sharps injury occurs during an invasive procedure. It is perhaps the advent of the human immunodeficiency virus (HIV) that has resulted in a sharpened perception of the dangers inherent in this contamination. In the UK the majority of surgeons still insist on wearing linen gowns, which offer absolutely no protection against anything at all, except perhaps the sensibilities surrounding nakedness.

This chapter will consider briefly the main viruses which may be transmitted either way, that is from surgeon to patient or patient to surgeon, and then provide guidelines for a safe system of practice.

## VIRAL HEPATITIS

### Hepatitis A

The precise prevalence of hepatitis A is unknown but it is likely to be almost universally present in most countries. It is likely that the incidence is decreasing in industrialized and developed countries. Infection is generally via the faecal–oral route and the incubation period is between three and five weeks. There is no known carrier state and subclinical and subjaundice infections are common. Although transmission of the virus can occur by means of sharps injuries this is unusual and the presence of hepatitis A virus cannot be demonstrated by immune electron microscopy in the stool after the first week of illness.

### Hepatitis B

The hepatitis B virus (HBV) may be transmitted by inoculation via sharps injuries from blood or products derived from blood, by droplet transmission, for example in association with open systems of renal dialysis, and also by sexual and oral contact. The prevalence of the virus is much higher in less well developed countries including those of Eastern Europe, the Middle East, Asia and South America. In the UK the prevalence is relatively low, being only between 1%–2% except for certain selected groups of workers, and these include health care workers, particularly those involved in invasive procedures, those working in geriatric and psychiatric institutions, dentists and personnel employed in pathological laboratories. The incubation period of HBV is between six weeks and six months, although it may occasionally be longer. Between 5% and 10% of infected patients will develop a carrier state and awareness of this possibility is important for surgeons. The onset of the clinical disease may be insidious but in a small proportion of those infected fulminant hepatitis may develop. Also in a small proportion of patients hepatitis B carrier state is associated with chronic active hepatitis and eventually cirrhosis.

There are a number of antigen–antibody systems relating to HBV.

### HBsAg

Detection of the surface antigen to hepatitis B is

the first manifestation of infection before other evidence of liver disease. The surface antigen persists throughout the clinical disease and in the majority of those infected will develop an antibody to this surface antigen. The demonstration of the antibody to HBs is associated with protection from infection from further inoculations of the virus and non-infectivity from the patient.

### HBcAg

The c antigen is detected by the development of an antibody to it which appears shortly after the surface antigen to hepatitis B is detected. It may persist for between one and two years. Its significance is that in donors infectivity has been demonstrated where HBsAg has been negative but HBc antigen is present. With the development of antibodies, infectivity becomes absent.

### HBeAg

The e antigen is found only in HBsAg-positive sera and appears during the incubation period. The importance of this antigen is that it is an index of infectivity. Carriers with a persistence of this antigen are many times more likely to infect others. Surgeons have been shown to infect their patients during operative procedures, particularly in the pelvis when they have carried this antigen (Welch et al 1989).

## DNA polymerase

DNA polymerase activity is first detectable in serum when the titre for HBsAg is rising. It is suggested that this enzyme indicates the presence of virions in the serum and is associated with viral replication. Its presence is usually transient but it may persist for years in the patient who is a carrier and it may therefore be associated with continuing infectivity.

## Delta agent

This is a defective viral RNA genome and has only been demonstrated in association with hepatitis B infection. It has only been demonstrated in the presence of HBsAg. It is usually associated with more severe forms of HBV infections and has been reported to be present in half those patients who develop fulminant hepatitis.

## Hepatitis C

The hepatitis C virus appears to be responsible for the majority of hepatitis infections occurring as a result of contaminated transfusion. It would seem likely that vertical transmission is a possibility.

## Other viral causes of hepatitis

Hepatitis may be associated with infection with the Epstein–Barr virus and the cytomegalovirus.

## Treatment

### Hepatitis A

Human normal immunoglobulin is available which protects if given during the incubation period. It should be given to all close personal contacts of patients who are known to have developed hepatitis A and to persons who are travelling to areas of high endemicity (all countries except northern Europe, North America, New Zealand and Australia) and will protect for a period of up to five months.

### Hepatitis B

1. Hyperimmune globulin may protect an infected individual if given within seven days of exposure. A second dose is required 21–23 days later and is recommended for individuals who are at risk of having received contamination via mucous membranes or implantation. In addition vaccination with the hepatitis B vaccine should be commenced at the same time.

2. Hepatitis B vaccine is now available from a monoclonal source and is appropriate for individuals who are HBsAg and HBcAb negative. It should be given to individuals at high risk of developing the infection, and these include patients on renal dialysis, renal dialysis technicians, patients receiving repeated transfusions and the partners of HBsAg-positive patients, male homosexuals and the neonates of HBsAg-positive mothers. All

individuals entering nursing or the medical professions, depending upon the indications above, should receive immunization against hepatitis B. The development of a fulminant hepatitis or a carrier state is no longer an acceptable risk. If a surgeon becomes HBeAg positive he will be unable to perform invasive procedures until such time as this state can be reversed.

## HUMAN IMMUNODEFICIENCY VIRUS (HIV)

The first report in the world implicating the virus was in 1981 by Gottlieb et al, who reported five patients with pneumocystis pneumonia who also had profound depression of cellular immunity. Since that time the virus has been identified as being a retrovirus containing a reverse transcriptase. Certain anti-retroviral drugs acting by the inhibition of this enzyme system have been developed, such as Zidovudine (AZT). The use of AZT even in the asymptomatic but infected patient has been shown both to reduce morbidity and to prolong survival. However, acquisition of HIV in the vast majority of patients eventually results in death from profound depression of cellular immunity.

The virus is acquired sexually, most commonly by sexual intercourse between men but to an increasing degree during heterosexual intercourse, by implantation of the virus following contamination with the blood, body fluids or transplanted tissues of an infected person, and by babies from infected mothers which may occur in utero or possibly during delivery (European Collaborative Study 1992). From this may be derived a list of groups of high-risk individuals:

- homosexual males
- intravenous drug abusers
- haemophiliacs before October 1985
- residents from areas of high endemicity
- sexual partners of the above
- children of infective mothers.

Following infection with the virus there is a period of up to 6–12 weeks during which no detectable antibody response occurs, but there is a rising titre of antigen and the patient is presumably capable of passing on the infection. At 12 weeks approximately 85% of patients have mounted an antibody response that is detectable in serum, the antigenaemia falls to undetectable levels and, though HIV antibody positive, the patient is not infective. There are a small number of individuals in whom an antibody response takes longer to develop and has even been reported as taking two years. The second stage of the infection is not associated with any symptoms at all and is detectable only by antibody testing. At some time, usually between three and 12 years, the antibody response diminishes, antigen becomes detectable in serum and body fluids and the patient moves into the next stage of the disease process and eventually AIDS. The virus has been isolated from blood, semen, saliva, tears, urine and cervical secretion. Up until the 31 December 1991 there were 16 828 people in the UK who had HIV antibodies; 5451 cases of AIDS had been reported, of whom 3391 were known to have died (Report of a working group at the Royal College of Pathologists 1992). The greatest risk of HIV acquisition for the health care worker relates to lifestyle. However, there are currently reports of 60 health care workers who would appear to have acquired HIV 1 by virtue of their occupation, and these are summarized in Table 9.2.1.

**Table 9.2.1**   The number of health care workers who are HIV positive as a result of occupationally transmitted infection (Report of a working group of the Royal College of Pathologists 1992)

|  | USA | Rest of World | Total |
|---|---|---|---|
| Definitely occupationally acquired infections | 23 | 9 | 32 |
| Presumptive occupationally acquired infections | 17 | 7 | 24 |
| Others, e.g. home care | 1 | 3 | 4 |
| Total | 41 | 19 | 60 |

The majority of occupationally acquired HIV infection occurs as a result of a sharps injury. It is clear that such an injury from a hollow needle carries greater risk than from a solid needle, particularly where the source of the infection is a patient with AIDS rather than a pre-AIDS infection. The risk of transmission following a sharps injury was reviewed by Gill et at (1991), who found that of 2475 percutaneous exposures nine resulted in seroconversion, giving a transmission rate of 0.36%.

Contamination of the surface of the skin is more common in more junior grades of surgeons and in operations where larger quantities of blood are lost. Since it is known that it is possible to become infected with the hepatitis B virus by contamination of the conjunctiva, great anxiety has been expressed about blood droplet aerosol created by power tools such as used by orthopaedic and ENT surgeons. However, to date no case of seroconversion has occurred by this route.

## Treatment

The question as to what should be done following either a needle stick injury, mucosal or contamination of non-intact skin surface from a high-risk patient has been considered exhaustively. There would seem to be no good evidence that post-exposure chemoprophylaxis with Zidovudine is effective. There are of course enormous pressures on physicians expert in this area to treat a health care worker who has been hazarded in this way but there is really no evidence for the efficacy of Zidovudine. Hospitals have tended to develop their own policies and to offer the health care worker this drug with appropriate speed; that is, within a period of 6 hours and at an appropriate dose. Unfortunately symptoms of nausea, malaise and fatigue, headache and vomiting have been reported in a high proportion of cases taking the drug.

## HERPES VIRUSES

### Herpes simplex type 1, Type 2

These members of this group of DNA viruses are mainly important because of the possibility in the health care worker of greater contact with direct cutaneous or mucocutaneous lesions produced by the virus. These herpetic sores may become widespread and extragenital, for example affecting the anal canal in patients who are immunosuppressed.

### Treatment

Several drugs are effective in inhibiting replication of herpes viruses and these include acyclovir, which may be given intravenously, 15 mg kg$^{-1}$ per 24 hours, which is effective in symptomatic primary genital infections and in disseminating herpetic mucocutaneous lesions in patients with AIDS. In addition, oral acyclovir 200 mg five times daily can also be effective. Topical acyclovir in a 5% concentration will help to reduce viral shedding.

### Cytomegalovirus

This is the human herpes virus 5 and is acquired by mucocutaneous contact. It is present in up to one quarter of healthy individuals and in up to 95% of homosexual men, in whom it is sexually transmitted.

Because of its ubiquitous nature it is not especially important in relation to the transmission of the disease from patient to surgeon or vice versa. In patients with AIDS it can produce a wide variety of symptoms but amongst the most troublesome is included retinitis, for which treatment with gancyclovir or foscarnet may be required.

## PAPILLOMA VIRUSES

There are over 40 types of human papilloma virus and their importance apart from the enormous clinical load that is provided by cutaneous juvenile warts relates to their ability to stimulate neoplasia. Types 6, 16 and 18 are associated with uterine and cervical carcinomas.

Fifty per cent of all surgical referrals in patients who are HIV 1 positive are for anorectal complaints. Of these, anogenital warts form a high proportion. Ninety per cent of patients presenting to a rectal clinic with warts were found to be in a high-risk group.

The significance to surgeons treating anogenital warts is that the smoke resulting from laser destruction has been shown to contain viable virus particles. These particles can become implanted in the nasopharynx of the surgeon.

## PREVENTION OF INFECTION

The principles of the prevention of infection of

health care workers from virus diseases in patients are to maintain an effective barrier between patient and surgeon and to ensure that all the usual measures to prevent cross-infection are undertaken.

### Identification of high-risk patients

The term 'high-risk patient' means a patient who is at a high risk of being HIV or hepatitis B positive. It is possible that a patient who is so infected may also harbour the human papilloma virus and types 1 and 2 herpes virus. Debate exists as to whether detection of high-risk patients is either desirable or possible. However, many surgeons feel that if they know they are operating on high-risk patients their technique is modified so as to avoid sharps injuries.

The history is helpful and if skilfully taken often provides knowledge as to risk behaviour. Identification of the significant physical signs is also important; for example, the multiple injection marks associated with drug addiction or the likely association between anogenital warts and homosexuality.

### Testing for HIV and hepatitis B

If it appears that a patient may be in a high-risk category the patient is advised to accept antibody testing for the above viruses. This is always only carried out with the express permission of the patient, and after counselling in the case of the HIV test. It is important even in asymptomatic patients to know the HIV antibody status, since current evidence would suggest that AZT even in the asymptomatic patient is effective in prolonging life. This can then be added to the benefit to the surgeon of knowing the HIV antibody status of the patient.

## All patients

### The operating theatre

The provisions necessary within the operating theatre are those necessary to prevent cross-infection. The table top is covered with an impervious sheet so that the mattress is not contaminated with blood or body fluids. The surgeon scrubs up in the normal way and wears a completely *impervious gown*. Currently it is sometimes necessary to wear a plastic apron beneath the gown, particularly if heavy contamination is expected. A particular area of risk is the forearm, and contamination tends to seep between the top of the glove and the elasticated cuff. The bottom of the gown should be lower than the top of impervious footwear. A mask is worn and this should be a special impervious mask if warts are being treated by either diathermy or laser.

The skin of the patient is cleaned in the usual way and impervious drapes are used so that neither blood nor fluid seeps around the patient's body.

During the operative procedure no sharps are passed hand to hand between the scrub person and the surgeon. Knives and needles are conveyed from one to the other in a transit dish. After use, all sharps are disposed of in a self-locking disposal carrier or an appropriate bin which is not filled to more than half its capacity. In no circumstances is the finger used as a guide for a needle, particularly in body cavities such as the pelvis.

## High-risk patients

### Before operation

High-risk patients are not placed at the end of the operating list unless this is appropriate for other reasons. Such placement is discriminatory if it occurs and is associated with a greater tendency for cancellation because of lack of time. The patient is transported to the anaesthetic room in the normal manner and the anaesthetic is induced in the usual way before transfer to the operating room. Anaesthetists should wear gloves and eye protection.

### The operating theatre

The procedures are exactly similar to those outlined above and used for all patients.

### Recovery room

By the time the patient leaves the operating theatre all wounds should be dressed and not leaking.

Any spills of blood or tissue fluids are covered with a suitable antiseptic such as hyperchlorite solution. The disposable drapes and the gowns are placed in a yellow viscose bag for incineration.

The patient is recovered in the usual way in the recovery room.

*Extra precautions to be taken for high-risk patients*

1. Double gloving: two pairs of gloves are worn as there is good evidence to show that the likelihood of glove perforation is reduced by this practice. It is usual to wear one of the pairs of gloves a half size larger than the surgeon's usual size.

2. Eye protection: eye protection should be worn at all times when power tools are being employed, but it should also be used by the surgeon and those immediately around the operating table when high-risk patients are being operated on. Splash contamination of the conjunctiva is not uncommon and should be avoided particularly from the point of view of transmission of hepatitis B.

3. Overshoes: these are worn to prevent contamination of footwear.

## CONCLUSION

It is impossible to know accurately the existence or otherwise of hepatitis B and/or HIV in all patients. In principle anyhow, we should assume that all patients may contain a potentially dangerous infective organism. Therefore when handling all patients much stricter attention must be paid to the barrier that should exist between patient and surgeon. This barrier, though in fact mechanical and composed of impervious materials of one sort or another, is also the barrier of good practice.

It is important to identify so far as possible those patients who carry a higher risk of harbouring the hepatitis virus or HIV. Obviously when operations are carried out on these patients the precautions dictated by good practice and an impervious barrier must also be employed, but these must be added to by the use of double-gloves, eye protection and overshoes. Unfortunately no satisfactory treatment or prophylaxis exists for HIV but there is now absolutely no excuse for health care personnel not to be immunized and protected against hepatitis B.

REFERENCES

European Collaborative Study 1992 Risk factors for mother-to-child transmission of HIV1. Lancet 339: 1007–1012

Gill O N, Heptonstall J, Porter K 1991 Occupational transmission of HIV: summary of published report to September. Internal publication of the Public Health Laboratory Service

Gottlieb M S, Schanker H M, Fann P F et al 1981 Pneumocystis pneumonia: Los Angeles. Morbidity and Mortality Weekly Report 30: 250–252

Report of a working group at the Royal College of Pathologists 1992 HIV infection: hazards of transmission to patients and health-care workers during invasive procedures.

Welch J, Webster M. Tilsey A J, Noah N D, Banatvala J E 1989. Hepatitis B infections after surgery. Lancet i: 205–207.

# 10. Operating theatres and special equipment

*M. K. H. Crumplin*

## OPERATING THEATRE DESIGN AND ENVIRONMENT

### Introduction

The operating theatre environment must provide a safe, efficient, user-friendly environment that is as free from bacterial contamination as possible. Operating theatre suites should be sited near to each other for efficient flexibility of staff movement. The theatres should preferably be situated on the first floor, away from the main hospital traffic. Ideally, operating rooms should be on the same level and adjacent to intensive care units and surgical wards. The suite should incorporate the theatre sterile supply unit. There should be minimum distance between operating rooms and the accident and emergency unit and X-ray facilities, which will both be sited on the ground floor.

All district general hospitals should now have a multi-disciplinary user committee to optimize efficiency and safety. This should be composed of surgeons, anaesthetists, operating theatre and anaesthetic nurses, microbiologists, a manager and a finance officer in line with recent Department of Health recommendations. This committee should meet on a regular basis.

Although there is no such entity as a standard operating theatre, an attempt was made by the DHSS in 1978 to introduce the nucleus concept, which at least provided hospitals with theatre suites appropriate to the average district general hospital requirements. Naturally with orthopaedic, cardiac, neurosurgical, laser and other specialist requirements, there would have to be adjustments to the standard design, for example the Charnley tent, controlled areas for laser therapy and the provision of a pump preparation room off a cardiac bypass theatre.

### Construction, design and environment

The basic construction of theatre units is usually of reinforced concrete or metal frames with reinforced concrete floors cast in situ. The ideal height of an operating theatre room should be about 3 m and, where possible, the wall and floor construction should be jointless. Wall construction is usually of plaster and plastic paint which must be easy to clean and of mellow tones. Flooring material should be antistatic and is usually made of polyvinyl chloride or terrazzo which is laid on a screed. Electrical power points should be numerous, antispark and waterproof. Each dedicated area within the suite must provide freedom for movement of staff, patients and supplies, each to serve its particular purpose with a minimum of interference to another group. The shape of an operating room is ideally square and requires a floor area of approximately 50 m$^2$. The anaesthetic room should measure approximately 17 m$^2$, and gowning-up room should be 10 m$^2$. Unfortunately in many present-day operating theatres such dimensions are not achieved. Likewise there is often under-provision for storage space within theatre suites and it is important that many items such as image intensifiers, spare tables, etc., do not clutter corridors. The anaesthetic room should have adequate cupboard and bench space. The recovery area must be adjacent to the operating theatre and the usual allocation is 1.5 recovery beds for each operating room, with a space of 9.3 m$^2$ per bed. There needs to be electrical wall facilities, monitoring equipment, piped gases and vacuum for each bed. In any operating theatre suite an attempt should be made to minimize bacterial contamination, especially in the vicinity of the operating table; thus the concept of zones is necessary:

1. an outer zone — e.g. patient reception area
2. clean zone — the area between the reception bay and theatre suite
3. aseptic zone — the operating theatre
4. dirty zone — e.g. disposal areas and dirty corridors.

## The antiseptic environment

To provide a minimally contaminated environment for surgeons and patients, various principles must be employed.

### Air flow

Directional air flow (laminar air flow) may be vertical or horizontal. Here, in addition to normal turbulent air flow through theatre which is necessary to maintain humidity, temperature and air circulation, an increased rate of air change is necessary to reduce the number of contaminated particles over the patient. Air is pumped into the room through filters and passed out of vents in the periphery of the operating room and does not return into the operating suite. Most theatres have air changes of 20 – 40 per hour but this rate may increase to 400 an hour in the vertical laminar flow system of a Charnley tent.

### Wearing of disposable, non-woven fabrics

This obviously reduces dispersal of bacteria-laden particles which may emanate from the operating or nursing staff. Optimally, everybody would have to wear these gowns, which might prove costly.

### Body exhaust suits

Here personal air circulation takes place within a specially designed operating suit and helmet so that exhaust air is removed from the suit by a pipe.

### The operating tent environment

There is a high vertical laminar flow within the tent, and clean air from above the table is expelled down to floor level in a funnel shape,

thereby reducing contamination. By using suitable exhaust suits and such tents, infection in hip replacement may be kept as low as 0.5%.

### Behaviour in theatre

It is desirable that the minimum number of people should be in the operating theatre to provide for the patient's safe and efficient management. The bacteriological count in theatre is related to the number of persons and their movement in the operating room.

### Temperature and humidity control

A steady level of temperature and humidity during surgery is desirable for comfort and may be varied to individual preference. The temperature in the operating theatre will need to be higher for neonates, children, elderly patients and for prolonged surgery. The usual comfortable temperature range in the operating room would be 20 – 22° C (68 –71.6°F).

Temperature and humidity control should be integral to the air-conditioning system which, while maintaining a constant working milieu, will require approximately 20 – 40 air changes per hour. Patients will become hypothermic if the temperature is below 21°C (69.8°F) during prolonged procedures. Loss of heat may be reduced by using warming blankets placed on the sorbo-rubber table surface and by infusing warmed intravenous fluids. This is achieved by passing the blood, crystalloid or colloids through a coiled plastic infusion pipe in a heated water-bath. Postoperatively heat loss may also be minimized by wrapping the patient in aluminium foil.

### Lighting

Apart from a comfortable background general theatre lighting which should provide about 400 lux intensity, every operating theatre should contain a ceiling-mounted lamp which is capable of a satisfactory range of movements and tilt. These in general consist of powerful radial light sources, usually arranged in a circular fashion, thus avoiding heads and hands getting in the way of a focused beam. There is often a centre beam to the light in addition to the radially placed lamps. These lights should be of high intensity, giving up to 40 000–50 000 lux at the focused area of surgery and 8000–10 000 lux in the depth of a wound. Each theatre should carry a separate ceiling-mounted swivel satellite lamp of similar characteristics to the main lamp, though smaller in size. It is desirable, also, for there to be a mobile spotlight which can be wheeled around theatre for throwing a beam of light at a lower level into deep cavities. The alternative to this would be a headlamp worn by the surgeon.

### Gas supply and extraction

Essential to every anaesthetic and operating room and recovery suite is the provision of piped services, namely oxygen and nitrous oxide and suction facilities. Gas and vacuum fixtures should be available on the wall in the induction room and there are various modes of delivery within the operating room; often an overhead boom is used from which the piped services are delivered. If wall fixtures are used in the operating room then they should be placed at a height of approximately 1.8 m.

Contamination by anaesthetic waste gases should be avoided in the operating environment as far as possible. If these waste gases are not scavenged, a cloud of exhaled or leaked gas will linger around the operating table. It is said that 0.5 parts per million of halothane and 25 parts per million of nitrous oxide are considered safe, acceptable levels of contamination.

The general principle of scavenging exhaled gases is that there is, connected to the anaesthetic circuit, a system of light tubing which feeds waste to a high-volume, low-pressure extraction apparatus (i.e. -0.5 cm of water pressure extracting 150 litres of gas per minute). During recovery 100 000 parts per million of nitrous oxide may be exhaled, making extraction facilities equally important in the recovery area. This may be achieved by placing a plastic funnel near to the patient's face with a similar extraction apparatus. The waste gases are fed to the roof of the hospital, preferably through different ports, so that if there is failure in one system others may still function.

## Noise

Extraneous noise in operating theatres is obviously to be kept to a minimum, and door and cupboard fittings should be quiet.

## Staff facilities

Requirements in theatre suites vary but the provision of a rest and coffee room, changing rooms, lockers, washing and toilet facilities, and office accommodation for the secretarial staff are mandatory. There may need to be seminar and interview rooms and laboratory facilities.

## OPERATING TABLES

Operating tables need to be heavy and stable, easily manoeuvrable, comfortable for the patient and highly adjustable in terms of positioning the patient correctly for a particular operative procedure. There are two basic types of operating table. First, and most common, are those which are completely mobile, thus allowing replacement if necessary. The second type of table is one which has a fixed and permanently installed column in the centre of the operating room with a variety of table tops which can be mounted on the column. These tables are usually expensive and have remote control for their various movements. The problem is that if a fault develops with the table that theatre will be out of service. The advantage of the fixed base system is that there is efficiency of patient handling and flexibility in operating room scheduling using interchangeable table tops.

## Essential characteristics of operating tables

It is important that the surface upon which the patient is placed is sympathetic to the contours of the patient. This is generally achieved by soft sorbo-rubber padding, which moulds to the patient to a certain degree. These pads are removable and easily cleaned. The sorbo padding will lift the patient above the metal table, for it is imperative that no part of the patient should come into contact with the metallic structure of the table. There should be easily accessible table controls, which may be motorized or hand operated. The table should be capable of two-way tilt, and breaking at its centre so that positions such as the lateral nephrectomy or jack-knife position may be used. The bottom half of the table must be easily removed so that various types of leg support and stirrups may be employed for gynaecological, urological, orthopaedic and pelvic surgery. With these leg supports it is important that joints are not over-stressed and undue pressure does not fall upon any point of the patient's lower limb. Tables for general surgery and urology should have a radiolucent section so that static X-ray films or image intensifier may be used. A variety of arm-rests, screen support bars, shoulder and pelvic supports should be available.

## Safety and position on the operating table

In addition to the soft cushion support surfaces which line the hard surface of the operating table, it may be desirable to have built-in lumbar supports which are adjustable. Alternatively, partially filled intravenous fluid infusion bags can be placed under the patient's lumbar lordosis. When patients' arms are positioned either by their side, over their head or at right angles to the body, care must be taken that joints, ligaments and nerves are not over-stressed. Various nerves are at risk from injury or pressure due to inappropriate position on the table. The brachial plexus may be stretched during arm movements, the ulnar nerve damaged at the elbow during pole insertion into the canvas sheet before transfer of a patient, and the lateral popliteal nerve may be damaged by pressure against a leg support bar. If the patient has osteoarthrosis this may be aggravated either by rough handling during transfer or excessive joint movement or distortion during the operative procedure. Should a patient have spinal or joint disorders it is perfectly reasonable to rehearse the position on the table with the patient prior to anaesthesia to make sure this is comfortable, e.g. cervical extension during thyroid surgery. Great care must be taken moving patients on and off the operating table, and ensuring that all tubing attached to the patient is not dislodged during transfer.

## Operating table fixtures for specialist procedures

### Orthopaedic surgery

There are a great variety of limb attachments to an operating table to enable circumferential access to a limb, manoeuvrability and also allowing the surgical team to use the image intensifier following fixation or reconstructive procedures.

### Neurosurgical procedures

Access to the cranial cavity may be optimized by having the patient sitting up and an appropriate padded head support placed opposite the surgical field to keep the head in a comfortable and safe position.

## SPECIAL EQUIPMENT IN THE OPERATING THEATRE

### Diathermy

#### Principles and effects

Surgical diathermy involves the passage of high-frequency alternating current through body tissue: where the current is locally concentrated (a high current density) heat is produced, resulting in temperatures up to 1000°C.

Low-frequency alternating current such as mains electricity (50 Hz) causes stimulation of neuromuscular tissue. The severity of the 'electrocution' depends on the current (amps) and its pathway through the body. Five to ten milliamps can cause painful muscle contractions, while 80-100mA passing through the heart will cause ventricular fibrillation. However, if the current frequency is increased there is a reduction in the neuromuscular response; at current frequencies above 50 000 Hz (50 KHz) the response disappears.

Surgical diathermy involves current frequencies in the range 400 KHz to 10 MHz. Currents up to 500 mA may then be safely passed through the patient. Heat will be produced wherever the current is locally concentrated.

#### Monopolar and bipolar diathermy

Monopolar diathermy is the most common

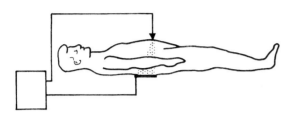

**Fig. 10.1**   Monopolar diathermy.

configuration (Fig. 10.1). High-frequency current from the diathermy generator (or 'machine') is delivered to an active electrode held by the surgeon. Current density is high where this electrode touches body tissue and a pronounced local heating effect occurs. Current then spreads out through the body and returns to the diathermy generator via the patient plate electrode (often incorrectly called the 'earth plate'). This plate should be in good contact with the patient over at least 70 cm² (preferably twice this or more). This ensures that current density at the plate is so low as to cause minimal heating. Misapplication of the patient plate is by far the most common cause of inadvertent diathermy burns.

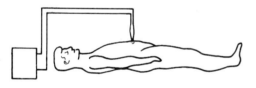

**Fig. 10.2**   Bipolar diathermy.

Bipolar diathermy (Fig. 10.2) avoids the need for a plate and uses considerably less power. The surgeon holds a pair of forceps connected to the diathermy generator. Diathermy current passes down one limb of the forceps through a small piece of tissue to be coagulated, and then back to the generator via the other limb of the forceps. This inherently safer system has not gained wide use for two main reasons:

1. It cannot be used for 'cutting' (see below): cutting involves a continuous arc (spark) between the active electrode and the tissue involved. In bipolar diathermy an arc could only be struck between the limbs of the forceps.

2. It will not work with the common surgical practice of holding bleeding vessels with ordinary surgical forceps and 'buzzing' them with the active diathermy electrode. No current will pass through the tissue held by the surgical forceps. Bipolar current will only pass directly from one diathermy forceps limb to the other.

### Cutting, coagulating and blend

Cutting diathermy involves the generator producing a continuous output, causing an arc to be struck between the active electrode and tissue. Temperatures up to 1000°C are produced. Cell water is instantly vaporized, causing tissue disruption with some coagulation of bleeding vessels.

Coagulating diathermy involves a pulsed output. This results in desiccation and the sealing of blood vessels with the minimum of tissue disruption.

Most diathermy generators have a 'blend' facility. This only functions when in cutting mode, and allows a combination of cutting and coagulation waveforms to increase the degree of haemostasis during cutting.

### Earth referenced and isolated diathermy generators

**Earth referenced generators.** Older diathermy generators, many of which are still in everyday use, have valves and spark-gaps to generate high-frequency current. These unsophisticated circuits produce a wide frequency range which includes frequencies above 1 MHz, and large earth leakage currents are unavoidable. The patient plate on these generators is earthed via a capacitor. The capacitor allows easy passage of high-frequency current such as diathermy, but presents a large resistance to low-frequency currents such as mains electricity. (The patient is therefore not earthed for mains (50 Hz) current to reduce the risk of electrocution.)

As long as the patient plate is correctly applied, the patient is kept at earth (zero) potential for alternate sites such as ECG electrodes or a drip stand accidentally touching the patient's skin. Unfortunately, if the patient plate is omitted, diathermy current will still flow (though a higher setting may be required) using the ECG electrodes or drip stand for the return pathway. An ECG electrode or drip stand presents skin contact of only $1 - 5$ cm$^2$, so a severe burn is inevitable.

**Isolated generators.** The more modern, often smaller, generators use transistors and 'solid-state' circuitry to produce the high-frequency current. Sophisticated electronics result in a much tighter frequency range ($400 - 600$ KHz) and a considerable reduction in earth leakage currents. Some of these solid-state generators (but by no means all) are designated 'isolated': the diathermy circuit is not earthed. This type of generator is inherently safer than an earth-referenced machine. Diathermy current can only pass back to the generator via the patient plate; there is no pathway back via earth. If the plate is omitted no current will flow.

## Safety

*General safety.* Whenever electrical equipment is to be used on patients it is vital that the equipment meets the required safety standards and is properly maintained. Everyone using the equipment should be properly trained in its use.
At the very least, read the user's manual: all diathermy machines are supplied with one.

*Responsibility.* The thorny problem of exactly who has overall responsibility for surgical diathermy is often not considered until a diathermy disaster occurs. In many operating theatres the diathermy is set up by nurses, or ODAs, and the anaesthetist is often the only doctor present when the patient plate is applied. Few surgeons check the diathermy prior to use. The surgeon using the diathermy must realize his overall responsibility, and check the alarm wiring and patient plate before use.

*Alarms.* Monopolar diathermy depends on the patient plate for its safety. All diathermy machines in use will alarm when switched on if the plate is not connected to the machine (plate continuity alarm), but only a few possess any alarm system that will ensure the plate is attached to the patient. Safe practice demands rigid adherence to correct procedures: first the patient plate is connected to the patient; the return lead is connected to the plate; the diathermy machine is switched on and the plate continuity alarm will sound; only then is the return lead connected to the diathermy machine, thus silencing the continuity alarm. Never do this in the reverse order. At the end of every case all these connections must be undone and the diathermy machine switched off. If the continuity alarm fails to silence change the patient plate and lead first, not the machine. Some modern diathermy generators (e.g. Eschmann and Valleylab) possess systems that monitor the patient – plate interface. These systems will be explained in the user's manual. Never disregard these alarms: check the patient plate contact carefully.

*The patient plate.* The most common cause of accidental diathermy burns is incorrect application of the patient plate. It may not be applied at all. More often there is a failure to follow guidelines. The plate should be sited close to the operation while ensuring that diathermy current is moving away from ECG and other monitoring electrodes. The area under the plate should have a good blood supply to remove any heat generated: avoid bony prominences and scar tissue. All the plate must have good skin contact: shave hairy skin and ensure the plate is not kinked or crinkled. Do not let skin preparation fluids seep under the plate.

*The patient.* The second most common cause of diathermy burns is the patient touching earthed metal objects such as drip stands, uninsulated 'screens', and parts of the operating table. These small skin contacts can become alternative return pathways for the diathermy current, and the local current densities may be enough to cause a burn.

*Sensible diathermy.* The third most common cause of diathermy burns is careless technique. For safe diathermy:

- Check the dial settings before use.
- If a spirit-based skin preparation fluid is used, ensure it has all evaporated or been wiped away before starting or the diathermy may set it alight.
- Only the surgeon wielding the active electrode should activate the machine.

- Always replace the electrode in an insulated quiver after use.
- If diathermy performance is poor, carefully check the patient plate and lead rather than increase the dial settings.
- Beware of using diathermy on or inside the gut. Intestinal gas contains hydrogen and methane and the result is often inflammable and explosive.
- Beware of using diathermy on appendages (salpinx, penis) or isolated tissue (testis). In these circumstances a high current density can persist beyond the operative site.

*If a burn occurs.* Diathermy burns are often poorly investigated and remain unexplained. Other skin lesions such as chemical burns from preparation solutions or pressure sores may masquerade as diathermy burns. Definite electrothermal burns are rarely due to a fault in the diathermy machine, but usually due to lapses in procedure. The operating theatre record for all patients subjected to diathermy should include the site of the patient plate, and when the plate and monitoring electrodes are removed the underlying skin should be inspected. If a possible burn is discovered at the end of a surgical case, the patient and all attached equipment should remain in the operating theatre and the electro-medical safety officer summoned. If the alleged burn is discovered after the patient has left theatre, all personnel involved in the case should be contacted: the precise arrangement of equipment and patient plate should be determined. Then *all* electrical equipment used should be tested, including the patient plate lead. Diathermy burns are usually full thickness and will require excision. The patient should be informed of the misadventure.

*Diathermy and pacemakers.* There are two possible dangers:

1. The high-frequency diathermy current may interact with pacemaker logic circuits to alter pacemaker function, resulting in serious arrhythmias, even cardiac arrest.

2. Diathermy close to the pacemaker box may result in current travelling down the pacemaker wire, causing a myocardial burn. The result will range from a rise in pacemaker threshold to cardiac arrest.

For safe use of diathermy with pacemakers:

1. Contact a cardiologist. Information required includes the type of pacemaker, why and when it was put in, whether it is functioning properly, what is the patient's underlying rhythm (i.e. what happens if the pacemaker stops?).

2. Avoid diathermy completely if possible. If not, consider bipolar diathermy .

3. If monopolar diathermy has to be used, place the patient plate so that diathermy current flows away from the pacemaker system. Use only short bursts, and stop all diathermy if any arrhythmias occur.

## Lasers

The Laser is a device for producing a highly directional beam of coherent (monochromatic and in phase) electromagnetic radiation, which may or may not be visible, over a wide range of power outputs.

LASER is an acronym for Light Amplification by the Stimulated Emission of Radiation.

This describes the principle of operation of a laser. Energy is pumped into the lasing medium to excite the atoms into a higher energy state to achieve a population inversion in which most of the atoms are in the excited state. A photon emitted as a result of an electron spontaneously falling from the excited to the ground state, stimulates more photons to be emitted and lasing action starts. After reflection back and forth many times from a pair of mirrors at opposite ends of the resonant optical cavity containing the lasing medium, the number of photons is amplified i.e. the light intensity or power is increased. One of the mirrors is only partially reflecting and allows a small part of the laser light to emerge as the laser beam.

The lasing medium is commonly gaseous, e.g. Argon, $CO_2$ but may be crystalline e.g. Neodymium Yttrium Aluminium Garnet (NdYAG).

It is the lasing medium which determines the wavelength emitted. It is mainly the wavelength of the laser which determines the degree of absorption in tissue. However the surgical applications also depend on the power density and exposure duration being just sufficient to produce the effect required and the design of delivery systems to allow the laser beam to be transported, aimed and focused onto the treatment site.

For example, Argon and NdYAG lasers are transmitted down fibre-optics to a slit lamp or into an endoscope. Carbon dioxide laser light is usually routed via a series of mirrors through an 'articulated arm', thereafter through a micromanipulator attached to a microscope or colposcope.

### Types of laser

1. Carbon dioxide infra red laser light has a wavelength of 10.6 μm. It is invisible and is rapidly absorbed by water in tissue and has very little penetration. It is therefore useful for vaporizing the surface of tissue and water or wet drapes can be used as a safety barrier. There is a very small margin of damaged tissue and healing is rapid, with minimal scarring. Treatment is relatively pain free.

2. The Nd-YAG laser penetrates more deeply, to 3 – 5 mm. The wavelength is 1.06 μm and is in the invisible infra red light range. It is useful for coagulating larger tissue volumes and leaves behind an eschar of damaged tissue.

Both the above types mentioned require a visible guiding beam which is usually a red helium/neon beam.

3. Argon laser light is blue/green and hence absorbed by red pigment. The principal wavelengths are 0.49 and 0.51 μm. It is used principally in ophthalmology and dermatology.

### Clinical applications

**Gastrointestinal tract.** The Nd-YAG laser is frequently used in the treatment of gastrointestinal problems. It can be employed for vaporizing and debulking recurrent or untreated advanced oesophageal carcinoma. Its use is predominantly in fairly short malignant strictures and may be superior to intubation. It is labour intensive and requires treatments every six to eight weeks. This laser can be used for controlling gastrointestinal haemorrhage from the stomach, oesophagus and duodenum, and for laparoscopic surgery, e.g.

cholecystectomy, destruction of small ampullary tumours in the duodenum and palliative resection of advanced rectal carcinomas. In the future photosensitization may prove to be of value.

**Urology** The Nd-YAG laser can be used to treat low-grade, low-stage transitional cell lesions in the bladder and is suitable for treating outpatients under local anaesthetic. Here again, photosensitizing agents such as haematoporphorin (Hpd) may be used in conjunction with a laser light wavelength of 630 nm. The beam is directed at sensitized tissues which are then more easily destroyed.

**Ophthalmology.** The Nd-YAG laser can be used to destroy an opaque posterior capsule during extracapsular cataract extraction. The argon laser may be employed for trabeculoplasty, to decrease intraocular pressure in patients with open-angled glaucoma. Laser photocoagulation has become standard treatment for patients with various retinal diseases such as diabetic retinopathy, and as a prophylactic measure in patients at risk from retinal detachment. Most ophthalmic photocoagulators are argon lasers.

**Otolaryngology.** A carbon dioxide laser may be used for haemostasis, removal of benign tumours and pre-malignant conditons. The argon laser has been used in middle ear surgery.

**Vascular surgery.** Laser angioplasty (carbon dioxide, Nd-YAG and argon) has been used to vaporize atheromatous plaques. Only approximately 50% of patients benefit, and significant complications are reported (e.g. perforation of vessel wall).

**Plastic surgery.** Pulsed ruby lasers may be used to remove tattoos, and port wine stains selectively absorb the argon laser beam. The carbon dioxide laser may be employed to resect atretic bony plates in congenital bony coanal atresia.

**Gynaecology.** There are several uses in gynaecology. Perhaps the most frequent is the treatment with a $CO_2$ laser of cervical and vulval precancerous lesions which are identified by colposcopy.

### Classification

Lasers are classified according to the degree of hazard.

*Class 1 (low risk).* These are of low power and are safe. The maximum permissible exposure (MPE) can not be exceeded.

*Class 2 (low risk).* These are of low power, emitting visible radiation. They have a maximum power level of (1 mW). Safety is normally afforded by natural aversion responses, e.g. the blink reflex.

*Class 3a (low risk).* These emit visible radiation, with an output of up to 5 mW. Eye protection is afforded by natural aversion. There may be a hazard if the beam is focused to a point, e.g. through an optical system.

*Class 3b (medium risk).* These emit in any part of the spectrum and have a maximum output of 0.5 W. Direct viewing may be dangerous.

*Class 4 (high risk)* These are high-power devices with output in any part of the spectrum. A diffusely reflected beam may be dangerous and there is also a potential fire hazard. Their use requires caution. Most medical lasers are in this class.

The manufacturers are required to classify and label the product according to hazard level.

*Hazards*

1. To the patient: inevitably burning of normal tissue or perforation of a hollow viscus may occur with increasing depth of treatment, e.g. perforation of oesophagus, or damage to trachea or lungs during ENT procedures.

2. Operator hazard: usually the operator is not exposed to laser beams, but should accidental exposure occur it is frequently the eyes or skin that are damaged. Eye protection is important as some laser beams will penetrate and be focused on to the retina. Also corneal burns or cataract formation have occurred with less penetrating beams.

## Safety measures

1. There should be a laser protection advisor (LPA) to consult on the use of the instruments throughout the hospital and to draft local rules.

2. A laser safety officer (LSO) should be appointed from the staff of the appropriate department using each laser. This person may well be, for example, a senior nurse and will have custody of the laser key.

3. All persons using the laser should be adequately trained in its use and be fully cognizant with all safety precautions.

4. There should be a list of nominated users.

5. A laser controlled area (LCA) should be established around the laser while it is in use. There should be control of personnel allowed to enter that area and the entrance should be marked with an appropriate warning sign, usually incorporating a light which illuminates while the laser is functioning.

6. While in the laser controlled area adequate eye protection should be worn. This must be appropriate to the type of laser used. The laser should not be fired until it is aimed at a target and usually there will be an audible signal during laser firing.

7. The laser should be labelled according to its classification. Lasers in classes 3a, 3b and 4 should be fitted with a key switch and the key should be kept by a specified person. The panels which constitute the side of the laser unit should have an interlocking device so that the laser cannot be used if the panels are damaged.

There are various safety features which are required by way of shutter devices and emergency shut-off switches. Foot-operated pedals should be shrouded to prevent accidental activation. Medical lasers require a visible low-power aiming beam which may be an attenuated beam of the main laser, should this be visible, or a separate class 1 or 2 laser, e.g. helium/neon. The laser must be regularly maintained and calibrated.

8. Environment: reflective surfaces should be avoided in the laser controlled area. However, matt black surfaces are not necessary. Adequate ventilation must be provided and should include an extraction system to vent the fumes produced. These fumes are known as the laser plume.

Attention should be paid to the avoidance of fire as class 4 lasers will cause dry material, e.g. drapes, swabs, to ignite. Thus, damp drapes will provide an effective stop, e.g. for a carbon dioxide laser beam.

## Fibreoptics in theatre

### Flexible instruments

The advent of fibre-optics has undoubtedly made an immense impact on the management of patients. There is little evidence, however, that the use of instruments which incorporate fibre-optics necessarily reduces mortality. Hollow viscera may be carefully inspected and both diagnostic and therapeutic procedures can be performed under clear vision. Fibre-optic instruments are integral to the development of minimal access surgery (e.g. ureteric or bile duct stone retrieval).

In the 1950s Professor Harold Hopkins of Reading University, UK, developed the earlier work of John Logie Baird (the inventor of television) to further design fibre-optic bundles which not only could transmit a powerful light beam but also, when suitably arranged, deliver an accurate image to the viewer. In the 1960s urological instruments were developed incorporating multiple flexible glass-fibre rods. Each fine fibre rod is constructed of high-quality optical glass and transmits the image (or light beam) by the process of total internal reflection. This principle allows light to travel around bends in the fibre. Each fibre is small ( 8–10 μm in diameter) and to achieve the principle of total internal reflection must be covered by a coating of glass of low refractive index to prevent light dispersion. Many such coated fibres are bound together in bundles which can bend. For light transmission, fibres may be arranged in a haphazard manner (non-coherent) but for clear image transmission the fibres must be arranged in a coaxial way (coherent) (Fig. 10.3). The following are examples of flexible endoscopes currently available utilizing fibre-optic light bundles:

1. oblique (for endoscopic, retrograde, cholangiopancreatography ERCP) and end-viewing gastroscopes
2. laryngoscope
3. bronchoscope
4. fibre-optic sigmoidoscope and colonoscope
5. cystoscope (pyeloscope)
6. choledochoscope
7. arterioscope.

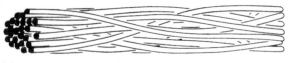

(a)

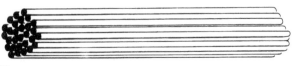

(b)

**Fig. 10.3** **(a)** Non-coherent fibre bundles for light transmission. **(b)** Coherent fibre bundles for viewing. Reproduced from Ravenscroft & Swan (1984) by permission of Chapman and Hall.

Each instrument has similar design principles incorporating the following:

1. coherent fibre bundles for high-quality visual image transmission
2. non-coherent fibre-optic bundles for light transmission
3. a lens system at the tip and near the eyepiece of the instrument
4. a proximal control system to manoeuvre the tip of the instrument and also to control suction and air/water flow
5. channels for blowing air or carbon dioxide and water down the instrument; and for suction — this latter doubles as a biopsy channel
6. a wire guide incorporated to control tip movement, which takes place in four directions, each usually allowing a deformity of greater than 180° movement
7. a cladding, consisting of a flexible, jointed construction, covered by a tough outer vinyl sheath.

Figures 10.4 and 10.5 show the basic structure of a typical endoscope, and Figure 10.6 shows the tip of an instrument, illustrating the lenses for light transmission and viewing, a suction channel (which should be large for use in the presence of gastrointestinal haemorrhage) and a small nipple directed over the lens, to enable the wash solution to clear the lens of debris.

Light sources should emit a powerful beam and the intensity is usually 150 W. Many light sources employ a halogen bulb which needs to be fan cooled.

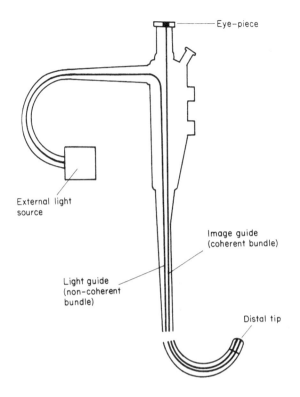

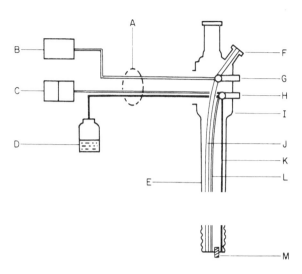

Fig. 10.5    Further details of basic design. A, endoscopic 'umbilicus'; B, suction pump; C, air pump; D, water reservoir; E, endoscopic insertion tube (cladding); F, biopsy port; G, suction button; H, air/wash button; I, endoscope control head; J, combined suction biopsy channel; K, water channel; L, air channel; M, combined air/water port. Reproduced from Ravenscroft & Swan (1984) by permission of Chapman and Hall.

Fig. 10.4    Basic design of fibre-optic endoscope. Reproduced from Ravenscroft & Swan (1984) by permission of Chapman and Hall.

## Rigid endoscopes

Optical systems in rigid endoscopes also employ the principle of total internal reflection but there are several lens systems in addition. The objective lens systems are nearest the image and the relay lens systems nearer the eyepiece of the rigid instrument, through which the observer views a rectified and magnified image. A light cable (non-coherent fibres or liquid electrolyte solution) is employed and the fibres direct the light coaxially with the lens systems in the rigid tube. Some of the longer lenses are made of high-quality optical glass and act as a single large optical fibre for image transmission. Examples of rigid instruments are:

1. cystoscope, urethroscope, pyeloscope, ureteroscope
2. choledochoscope
3. laparoscopes.

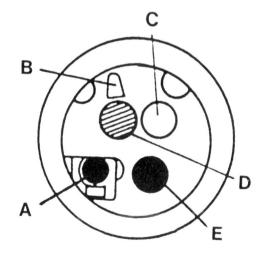

Fig. 10.6    The tip of an end-viewing fibre-optic instrument. A, forceps raiser; B, wash jet; C, image guide; D, light guide; E, biopsy/suction channel. Reproduced from Ravenscroft & Swan (1984) by permission of Chapman and Hall.

The lenses at the far end of the instruments will vary to allow differing fields of view and minimize peripheral field distortion.

*Care of fibre-optic instruments*

1. Instruments must be properly cleaned and disinfected before use. Debris may block channels and make suction and insufflation of air and liquid difficult. After use, the instruments should be cleaned internally by utilizing one of several automatic cleansing machines and externally with a suitable detergent solution. 'Q' tips may be employed to clean lenses. Instruments should be soaked for at least 5–10 minutes between patients and a 2% gluteraldehyde solution is frequently used, though 70% alcohol and low-molecular-weight providone–iodine are alternatives.

2. Avoidance of damage to the instrument: in most district hospitals endoscopies are performed in dedicated units where the care is certainly superior. When a variety of people handle and clean the instrument, damage is more likely to occur. Forcible distortion, dropping and particularly crushing of the instruments, e.g. by patients' teeth, must be prevented. In the latter instance biting may be prevented by insertion of a suitable mouth gag. Individual fibres may break and become opaque, appearing as black dots down the instrument.

## Cryosurgery (syn. cryotherapy or cryocautery)

Cryosurgery is the freezing of tissue to destruction. Although cells are destroyed at –20°C they may recover at higher temperatures than this. After freezing, the destroyed tissue sloughs off and reveals a clean, granulating base. The treatment is relatively pain free and minimizes blood loss. The object is to destroy abnormal tissue growth and preserve adjacent, healthy areas. This is achieved by the production of an ice ball at the tip of a cryoprobe (Fig. 10.7). To control the volume of tissue destroyed the size of the ice ball produced may be watched. The size of the lesion produced by cryosurgery depends on the temperature at the tip of the ice probe, the size of the tip and the number of freeze/thaw sequences. The size of the iceball will increase until the heat loss at the edge of the iceball is too small to permit further freezing of adjacent tissues. The size of an iceball and the extent of destruction can then be increased by a further freezing sequence. It is

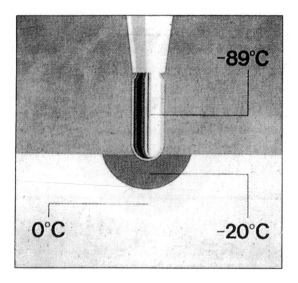

**Fig. 10.7**  Ice ball at the tip of a cryoprobe. Reproduced by permission of Eugene A. Felmar, Santa Monica Hospital Medical Center, USA.

usually recommended to allow spread of the ice-ball 2–3 mm into healthy tissue to ensure adequate destruction of the diseased area. Inevitably freezing a wart on the sole of the foot is less critical than re-attaching a retina, and for all the tasks demanded of cryosurgery there are various probe tips available.

*Principles of therapy*

The Joule–Thompson principle is that when gas expands heat is absorbed from the surrounding matter. The simplest example of this is spraying ethyl chloride on skin which subsequently freezes. With a cryoprobe, however, the liquid gas (ususaly nitrogen or carbon dioxide) is sprayed against the inside of a hollow metal probe. The gas then expands in the tip and freezes the tissue on contact (Fig. 10.8).

*Cell injury with cryotherapy*

1. Immediate phase: rupture of the cell membrane caused by formation of ice crystals in the cell (most effective with rapid freezing, e.g. greater than $5°C \, s^{-1}$.

2. Intracellular dehydration: this will result in increased and toxic levels of intracellular electrolytes.

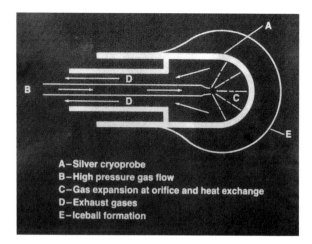

A—Silver cryoprobe
B—High pressure gas flow
C—Gas expansion at orifice and heat exchange
D—Exhaust gases
E—Iceball formation

**Fig. 10.8**   Cross-section of cryoprobe tip, illustrating the Joule–Thompson principle. Reproduced by permission of Eugene A. Felmar, Santa Monica Hospital Medical Center, USA.

3. Protein denaturation: this occurs to the liporotein structure of the cell membrane, nucleus and mitochondria.

4. Cellular hypometabolism: this results in enzyme inhibition.

Later in the course of injury there is also a loss of blood supply which causes tissues necrosis, and the resultant slough, before separation, will protect the tissues deeper to the injury so that when the slough separates it will leave a clean ulcer.

As nerve endings are susceptible to cold injury, painful lesions can be rendered insensitive. Also the treatment is not particularly painful to the patient and local analgesia is usually unnecessary. Adjacent neurovascular structures are relatively safe as collagen and elastic tissue resist freezing. Thus, the advantages of cryotherapy are that it is a relatively pain-free and simple method of destroying tissue, usually leaving clean wounds, often with a reasonable scar. The disadvantages of the technique are that frozen tissue cannot be histologically analysed, thus this method of treatment is unsuitable for any lesion requiring microscopic examination. It may sometimes be difficult to gauge the exact penetration in the depth of the tissues treated. Thus, its use may be limited in curative treatment of malignancy but obviously is of value in palliation. There may also occasionally be some bleeding and discharge after the

slough separates, e.g. in the cryosurgical treatment of haemorrhoids.

*Clinical applications*

Given the various shapes of probe tips a reasonable variety of therapeutic applications is available. When placing the probe tip, freezing must occur through a wet contact to ensure proper thermal conductivity. Two to three freeze/thaw cycles may be applied with overlap of areas treated if necessary.

*Examples*

1. proctology: haemorrhoids and warts
2. gynaecology: cervical erosions and warts
3. dermatology: warts, low-grade skin cancers, herpetic lesions.
4. ENT: pharyngeal tonsillar remnants, carcinoma of the trachea, hypophysectomy
5. ophthalmology: cataract extraction, glaucoma, detached retina
6. neurosurgery: Parkinson's disease and cerebral tumors.

**X-rays in theatre**

*Preoperative work-up*

Normally completed prior to surgery, the preoperative work-up should address details of diagnosis and, where appropriate, anatomical or physiological factors which could affect the conduct or outcome of surgery. It should go without saying that appropriately labelled radiographs must be available in theatre at the time of operation.

The preoperative chest X-ray is generally unhelpful in the absence of cardiothoracic symptoms and should be reserved for older patients or those with specific indications.

*Perioperative procedures performed in X-ray*

***Example: needle localization for impalpable breast lesions.*** Coordination between the surgeon and radiologist is vital and both need to understand what the other is doing. Premedication can make the procedure very difficult, e.g. the patient may faint while sitting upright for mammography. It is imperative for the surgeon to inspect the post localization mammogram for the relationship between the wire and the suspected abnormality. Remember that mammograms are performed with the patient sitting and the breast subsequently compressed. The breast usually adopts a different configuration when supine. The excised specimen should be radiographed to confirm a satisfactory biopsy before the patient is wakened.

***Example: retrograde pyelogram.*** This examination can be performed in theatre at the time of cystoscopy using fluoroscopy or subsequently in the X-ray department, where the radiologist has the advantage of being able to turn the patient and obtain films.

### Intraoperative procedures

These fall into two categories. The first is purely diagnostic.

***Example: on-table cholangiography.*** Use sufficiently dilute contrast medium to allow one to 'see through' the common bile duct on the film. The biliary tree should be adequately filled to show the main intrahepatic ducts as well as the common bile duct. Contrast medium is heavier than bile and tends to gravitate to dependent ducts. If the ampulla is patent, contrast medium flows into the duodenum, which is clearly recognizable by its mucosal pattern. Remember to put a 20° lateral tilt on the table to eliminate the overlap of contrast on the vertebral column.

***Example: intraoperative angiography.*** Films may be exposed following a steady intra-arterial injection in theatre and adequate results obtained. Adverse reactions to modern contrast media while under general anaesthetic are very rare.

The second category consists of procedures where imaging is used to facilitate a therapeutic procedure. They require fluoroscopy and range from simple procedures such as reducing fractures to the sophisticated techniques of interventional uroradiology. Many of these techniques can be performed either in the operating room or in the X-ray department but it is fair to say that facilities for fluoroscopy are usually better in X-

ray while asepsis is better in theatre. X-ray machines are difficult to clean and a potential source of cross-infection. Specialist centres may have dedicated complex X-ray rooms which are organized in a fashion similar to operating theatres (or vice versa).

### Equipment

This may be static or mobile, and it is the latter which is usually found in the operating theatre. Image intensification allows 'screening' without having to dark-adapt your eyes first! A mobile image intensifier for use in theatre will be mounted on a small 'C' arm. The table top must be radiolucent and there must be space under as well as over the table for the X-ray tube and the image intensifier. If films only are required, the table top will need a 'tunnel' to admit the X-ray cassette under the patient. Alternatively, the cassette may be draped in sterile towels. This would be necessary, for example, if intraoperative mesenteric angiography was to be performed on bowel lifted out of the abdomen at laparotomy. For a small field, the X-ray cassette can be placed on the image intensifier itself, and film obtained. Some modern machines can produce dry sliver images directly from the TV monitor.

Biplane screening is a luxury not usually available in the operating theatre. The mobile 'C' arm is nevertheless quite versatile and the effect of 'parallax' can help to judge 'depth'.

Mobile X-ray sets operate from designated 13 A sockets which are on a separate ring main from other essential equipment. Modern 'mobiles' use 'sparkless' switching and should not therefore ignite inflammable gases. It is desirable to keep the mobile X-ray machine in the operating suite.

### X-rays and the law

X-rays (and scalpels) can be weapons of assault if not used with care and a prospect of benefit to the patient. Medical staff clinically directing examinations employing ionizing radiation are required to have obtained a certificate demonstrating that they have received some training in radiation protection. It is hoped that eventually this will be included in the undergraduate curriculum. Staff physically directing exposure must be either a radiologist, radiographer, or hold an approved qualification.

Equipment must be regularly serviced and calibrated, and 'local rules' applied. the radiation protection supervisor in the hospital is the point of contact if in any doubt.

*Safety*

Look after yourself, other staff in the theatre, and the patient. Use the lead aprons. Remember that the patient 'scatters' the X-ray beam. The inverse square law applies, so staff should not be unnecessarily close. Be aware of the screening time and record it.

The abdomen of pregnant patients should be X-rayed only if absolutely necessary. The last menstrual period should be established before the patient is anaesthetized.

*Sundry points*

1. Maintain a close relationship with the department of radiology.
2. Discuss problems before surgery. Radiologists (generally) will want to know the outcome. Remember that this includes anatomical details as well as the diagnosis.
3. Give the radiographer as much notice as possible.
4. Dim the theatre lights when using fluoroscopy and use viewing boxes to view films.
5. Take an interest in imaging, as 'a picture is worth a thousand words'.

## Microscopes in the operating theatre

Microscopes have had a very gradual introduction to the operating theatre; however, they have now become indispensable in a wide variety of surgical fields.

*Advantages*

The microscope offers an improved view of the surgical field, more precision, greater flexibility and less trauma to delicate tissues. It provides good stereoscopic appreciation of depth, through a narrow surgical approach, much smaller than the unaided surgeon's own interpupillary distance would allow.

*Historical*

Spectacles have been available for nearly 700 years and the compound microscope for about 300 years, but it was only 70 years ago that a microscope was used in theatre and only 30 years ago that its usage became more widespread.

A Swedish otolaryngologist, Nylen, introduced his monocular microscope in the surgical treatment of otosclerosis in 1921. A year later his chief, Professor Holmgren, used a binocular microscope for the same condition. In 1925 Hinselman used a microscope for colposcopy but aside from this otolaryngologists alone continued its use for three decades.

In Chicago, Perritt used a microscope for ophthalmic surgery in 1950, Zeiss started to mass-produce their MiI surgical microscope in 1953. Clinical applications then expanded: Jacobson in vascular surgery in 1960, Kurle in neurosurgery and Burke in plastic surgery in 1962.

*Features of an Operating microscope*

**Eyepieces.** There is an adjustment for interpupillary distance and each eyepiece has a range of 5 dioptres.

**Binocular tube.** This can be straight or inclined.

**Beam splitter.** This is for connection of extra viewing tubes for observation and assistance. It also makes the use of still and video cameras possible as teaching aids.

**Magnification system.** Magnification is available as a Galilean system, variable in steps, e.g. $\times 6$, $\times 10$, $\times 25$, $\times 40$, or as a zoom system.

**Objective lens.** This affects working distance by changing lenses with variable focal lengths. For example:

| | |
|---|---|
| $f = 150, 175, 200$ | for ophthalmology and plastic surgery |
| $f = 250$ | for otology and vascular surgery |
| $f = 250$ or $300$ | for tubal surgery (gynaecology) |
| $f = 300$ or $400$ | for neurosurgery |
| $f = 400$ | for laryngoscopy |

**Depth of field.** Stereoscopic depth of field is less at higher magnification. It is best to focus at higher magnification first, then to reduce to working magnification so as to have the best focus at the centre of the depth of field.

**Light.** A powerful coaxial halogen light is incorporated in the body of the microscope. Oblique light is available for eye surgery.

*Instruments used with microscopes*

Each specialty has developed microsurgical instruments for its own needs. However, the following basic instruments are common to many specialities.

**Spring-handled needle holder.** Needle holders such as Borraquer or Castrovieso, ophthalmic, are available.

**Spring-handled microscissors.** These can be straight or curved. The straight are for cutting vessels and the curved for cutting tissue and thread.

**Jewellers' or watchmakers' forceps.** A wide variety of these are available.

**Microsurgical clips.** Scoville–Lewis microsurgical clips or a fine Heifetzs neurosurgical clips can be used for vessel anastomosis.

**Micro-electrode.** Monopolar or bipolar cautery is necessary.

**Suture material.** (a) Blood vessel anastomosis: 9.0 or 10.0 nylon on a 3–6 mm needle with a tapered end. (b) Nerve anastamosis: as above but the needle needs a cutting point. (c) Fallopian tube work: no. 7.0 or 8.0 absorbable non-reactive suture with a 4 mm or 6 mm reverse cutting needle.

**Sterilization.** Sterile rubber cups or drapes are available to cover the controls.

**Adjustment.** Versatility in position needs several interlocking arms, counterbalanced vertical movement as well as a geared angled coupling between the microscope carriage arm and body. This will enable the microscope to swing from side to side while mounted in an oblique axis.

**Mounting.** This can be on a solid, well-balanced mobile floor stand, or a fixed ceiling mounting. Wall-mounted microscopes are also available.

*Control of tremor*

Counteracting surgical tremor is of vital importance. The key is that the instrument or the limb on which it is held must be firmly supported as close to the point of work as possible.

**The future**

The combination of the laser with a micromanipulator to the objective lens of the microscope will enhance the use of both instruments in the future.

## ACKNOWLEDGEMENTS

I am deeply grateful for help with writing this paper to Mr John Barcroft for the diathermy section; Dr David Parker for the section on X-rays in theatre; Mr Derry Coakley for the section on microscopes; and to my wife for her help in the section on lasers. I should also like to thank Miss Sharon Langford for typing the manuscript.

REFERENCES

Brigoem R J 1988 Operating theatre technique, 5th edn. Churchill Livingstone, Edinburgh

Douglas D M (ed) 1972 Surgical departments in hospitals: the surgeons's view. Butterworth, London

Johnston I D A, Hunter A R (eds) 1984 The design and utilization of operating theatres. Edward Arnold, London

**Diathermy**

Editorial 1979 Surgical diathermy is still not foolproof. British Medical Journal 12: 755–758

Dobbie A K 1974 Accidental lesions in the operating theatre. NAT news. December edition.

Earnshaw J J, Keene T K 1989 Gastric explosion: a cautionary tale. British Medical Journal 293: 93–94

Pearce J A 1986 Electro surgery. Chapman and Hall

**Laser**

1983 Guidance on the safe use of lasers in medical practice. HMSO, London

1982 General guidance on lasers in hospitals. Medical physics and bioengineering working group. Welsh Scientific Advisory Committee (WSAC)

Murray A, Mitchell D C, Wood R F M 1992 Lasers in surgery — a review. British Journal of Surgery 79: 21–26

**Fibreoptics**

Ravenscroft M M, Swan C M J 1984 Gastrointestinal endoscopy and related procedures — a handbook for nurses and assistants. Chapman and Hall

**X-rays**

Mould R F Radiation protection in hospitals (Medical Sciences Series), Adam Hilger Ltd, Bristol and Boston. Ionising radiation regulations, 1985, 1988

**Microscopes**

Taylor S 1977 Microscopy. Recent Advances in Surgery. Churchill Livingstone, Edinburgh, Ch. 8

# 11. Surgical access, incisions and the management of wounds

*D. J. Leaper*

There are records describing successful wound management as long ago as the time of the Assyrians and the ancient Egyptian empire. Techniques using sutures and threads, linen adhesive strips and skin 'clips' of soldier ant heads have all been described historically. Dressings have been equally diverse, their value often being based on erroneous principles, but in the last 30 years there has been increasing interest resulting in many, tailor-made and improved, types of dressing.

The scourge of successful wound healing is infection, which was well recognized by Hippocrates and Galen, although some of their remedies were far from adequate. Microscopic confirmation of Celsian hypotheses and observations was slow in coming but the understanding of the physiology of wound healing has advanced greatly over the last two to three decades and is continuing to do so. The correct concepts and control of infection became established with the introduction of antisepsis through Semmelweis and Lister, associated with the work of Pasteur. Aseptic techniques were adopted at the turn of this century. Antibiotics are an integral part of surgical management, particularly in prophylaxis, and again we have seen continuing advances since the days of Ehrlich, Fleming, and Florey and Chain.

In retrospect our surgical repertoire seems to have found no bounds or restrictions. Operative surgery and anaesthesia allow procedures such as heart–lung transplantation to be undertaken safely. Our forebears would not believe what is now possible but the natural processes of wound healing must not be forgotten. The aphorism of 'cut well, sew well, get well' depends on a knowledge of these wound-healing mechanisms and adverse effects which may influence them.

## SURGICAL ACCESS AND INCISIONS

Laparotomy incisions reflect the requirements for any type of operative approach. To be useful they must allow adequate access or allow extension if necessary for an operative procedure or a full staging assessment, for example. Most abdominal incisions can be planned for a specific operation as surgical diagnosis is near to perfect, particularly with the availability of modalities such as computed tomography (CT) scanning and ultrasound. An upper right transverse abdominal incision allows access to explore the common bile duct and a Lanz incision allows appendicectomy but neither wound allows a full laparotomy. It is unusual, except occasionally in management of the acute abdomen, to need an exploratory midline or right paramedian (the 'registrar's' incision) to make or confirm a presumptive diagnosis (Fig. 11.1).

There must be no wound failures on closing an incision. Insecurity following an abdominal incision may result in burst abdomen or incisional hernia. Complications such as infection (including knots and wound sinuses) must be minimal. Finally our patients expect an acceptable cosmetic appearance of their healed wounds, without excessive or persistent pain.

*Requirements of a laparotomy incision*

- Allow access
- Be secure
- Low complication rate
- Be pain free
- Cosmetic appearance.

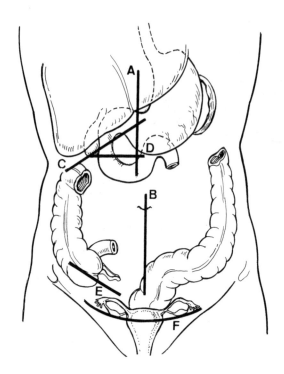

**Fig. 11.1** Favoured laparotomy incisions: **A** paramedian, **B** midline, **C** Kocher, **D** tranverse, **E** Lanz, **F** Pflannenstiel.

## OPERATIVE DRAPES

Following skin preparation, usually with 0.5% chlorhexidine or 1% povidone–iodine in 70% alcohol, the operative field needs to be delineated with operative drapes. Conventionally these are resterilized double-thickness linen sheets which are held with towel clips. These need substantial care for further use, as well as the need for steam sterilization, and they have the drawback of allowing permeation related to the weave. Disposable fabrics do not allow penetration by body fluids and their waterproofing is a benefit when operating in the face of contamination or when there is a risk of HIV or hepatitis infections. They are expensive.

Incise drapes of adhesive polyurethene film were introduced over 30 years ago. They are widely used in prosthetic or vascular surgery when there is an increased risk of opportunist infection by skin organisms such as *Staphylococcus epidermidis*. There is no definite indication that they reduce infection and in fact the wound bacterial count increases during their use. Antiseptic impregnation has little protective effect. However, in general surgical operations incise drapes avoid the need for towel clips and can isolate stomas or an infected nearby focus (such as an infected separate wound). Wound guards can be placed into the wound but do not reduce the risk of wound infection although they reduce bacterial contamination during open viscus surgery.

## TYPES OF LAPAROTOMY INCISION

Laparotomy incisions can be broadly categorized as vertical or transverse, or as muscle cutting or muscle splitting. Many incisions used in the past with eponymous names have disappeared from modern use and there is a trend to use incisions placed cosmetically in Langer's lines which are usually transverse in type. There will never be a replacement for midline incisions, nor paramedian, particularly the lateral paramedian which is associated with a low wound failure rate.

### Vertical incisions

Midline incisions allow rapid access to the abdominal cavity and are easily extended when necessary. When placed accurately through the linea alba they are associated with minimal bleeding and are quickly closed in a single layer using a mass technique. The peritoneum does not require closure. The skin incision may be placed through the umbilicus or curved around the umbilicus (banana incision). Undercutting the periumbilical skin should be avoided as it makes cosmetic closure more difficult.

Paramedian incisions are time honoured and have been recently popularized as a lateral variant which appears to give sound wounds and a low incisional hernia rate relating to the shutter mechanism (Fig. 11.2). They take longer to make and to close, and blood loss is more than in midline incisions although probably not appreciably so.

### Transverse incisions

These may be muscle cutting in type (e.g. the

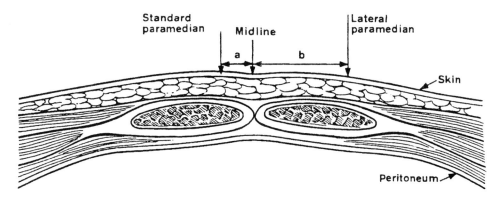

**Fig. 11.2**  Lateral and standard paramedian incisions: a = 2 cm; b = two-thirds from midline to lateral rectus sheath.

Kocher incision for cholecystectomy) or muscle splitting (e.g. the Lanz incision for appendicectomy). There is some evidence that they are associated with wound failures and less postoperative pain. Muscle-cutting incisions take more time to make and close, with more blood loss than midline incisions.

**Complex incisions**

These incisions afford access to specific sites for major procedures. They may be muscle cutting (the gable or roof-top incision for pancreatic operations), be extended into the chest (the left abdominothoracic incision for lower third oesophagectomy) or be partly muscle splitting (the extraperitoneal approach to the infrarenal abdominal aorta).

Retraction must be adequate during laparotomy. Conventional retractors in abdominal surgery are the Deavers, eyballs and Morris types, or the St Marks retractor for pelvic dissection, which require extra skilled assistants for most benefit. Specialized ring retractors (favoured for gynaecological and pelvic surgery) and sternal retractors (for mediastinal approaches to the heart) allow hands to be free. Self-retaining retractors are useful in more superficial surgery, such as the Joll for thyroid surgery, or the many types of clawed retractors, such as the Travers, useful in inguinal surgery.

Theatre lighting based on ceiling mounts offers focused, well-directed light for all procedures, particularly when experienced operating department assistants are available. Sterile handles allow placement of satellite lighting by the operating surgeon. Head lighting or cold light sources are necessary for procedures when access is limited.

LAPAROTOMY CLOSURE

The success of laparotomy closure depends on adequate technique, materials and avoidance of adverse factors, particularly infection. The closure of the musculoaponeurotic layers is traditionally performed in layers. Such closure is still necessary for closing paramedian incisions and some surgeons prefer it for transverse incisions, but it is unnecessary (and not easily performed) for closing midline incisions. Mass closure has been shown to have a low incidence of burst adbomen and can be undertaken for all midline and transverse incisions, but there appears to be no benefit in reducing the incidence of incisional hernia. The earliest described mass closures employed a far-and-near or figure-of-eight technique using interrupted sutures but simple over-and-over continuous sutures are easier to place, avoid excessive numbers of knots and are secure (Figs 11.3 and 11.4). Jenkins has shown that a wound length : suture length ratio of 1:4 should avoid wound dehiscence. This allows for the increased tension and increased effective length of vertical abdominal incisions during healing. This requires sutures to be placed 1 cm apart with at least 1 cm tissue bites, but is not so easy to achieve in layered closure without risking entering the perito-

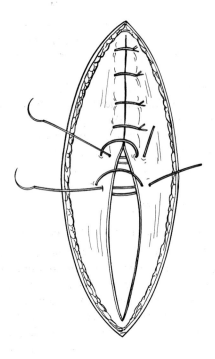

**Fig. 11.3**  Interrupted far-and-near mass closure: 1 cm bites, 1 cm apart.

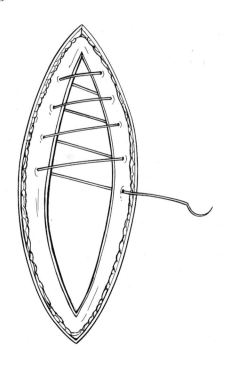

**Fig. 11.4**  Continous over-and-over mass closure: 1 cm bites, 1 cm apart.

neal cavity with a second layer and the risk of damage to underlying viscera. Using mass closure the viscera can be seen and protected with the non-dominant hand during suture. Cadaveric studies have reinforced that 1 cm bites are secure. There is also biochemical evidence that a 1 cm bite affords security because there is a zone of activity around a wound where collagen lysis prior to repair reduces the tissue integrity. Sutures placed within this zone (which widens with infection) are insecure. The tightness of abdominal wall closure has been shown to be important: too much risks later incisional hernias; too little risks burst abdomen. Tension sutures cause cosmetically unacceptable scars and make the siting of stomas difficult. There is some evidence that they are associated with more pain but no evidence that wound closure is more secure with their use.

Skin closure should be cosmetically acceptable, with avoidance of inversion of the edges, and avoid infection, hypertrophic scars or keloid formation. Several techniques are available: continuous or interrupted, simple or mattress and subcuticular. All are acceptable but the latter gives the best results. Tape closure and clip sutures are associated with a low infection rate and also give good cosmetic results. The use of a polyurethene adhesive sheet dressing (Bioclusive, Opsite) over a sutured wound acts as a large tape closure, allowing easy inspection. Cyanoacrylate skin adhesives are expensive and demand near-perfect haemostasis. There is no definite evidence that reducing dead space with subcuticular sutures or drains is either effective or prevents wound infection. Undue tension must be avoided to allow postoperative swelling. Sutures require removal as a working rule at 3–5 days (head and neck), 7 days (inguinal and upper limb), 10 days (other abdominal incisions, lower limb) and up to 14 days for dorsal incisions. Knots placed well to the side of the incision facilitate removal. Special instruments allow painless removal of clips (rapidly if necessary after thyroidectomy).

Langer's lines are low-tension lines in the skin and correspond to natural skin creases. If an incision crosses them at right angles then there is a risk that resultant scars become hypertrophic and cosmetically unacceptable. Whenever possible therefore, Langer's lines should be followed for incisions. When these lines have to be crossed for surgical access, particularly in operations on small joints, for example, then skin crease lines should be crossed obliquely or incisions employing Z-plasties or an S-shape should be planned.

Hypertrophic skin scars follow the proliferation of scar tissue which stays within the boundaries of the wound and not beyond it as keloids do. They tend to occur in scars around joints and in areas of skin tension. With the passage of time they become avascular and may regress to form a white, stretched, widened scar.

Contractures should not be confused with the normal process of wound contraction. Contractures follow delayed wound healing and occur after infection and inadequate treatment of burns in particular. Deep burns which are not excised are prone to contracture. Established contractures can be released by plasty incisions, excised and covered with split-thickness grafts or with transposition flaps.

Keloids are formed by abnormal collagen metabolism and result in proliferation of scar tissue beyond the boundaries of the original wound. They occur in dorsal areas of the body and over the face and deltopectoral region. Keloids occur in dark-skinned people and may be encouraged to form as a cultural body decoration. Excision of keloids is almost always followed by a more exuberant recurrence. X-rays have been used but topical steroid creams or steroid injections are more definitely effective. Pressure on an excised keloid can prevent recurrence, a useful example being the use of a clip or peg on an earlobe that has developed a keloid after piercing for earrings.

## HAIR REMOVAL

Body hair is conventionally removed from a proposed operative field the day before surgery. This is done for aesthetic reasons and also to allow painless removal of dressings, particularly the currently popular polymeric transparent sheet dressings (such as Op site or Bioclusive). It has been shown, however, that the time of shaving is critical: when performed over 12 hours before surgery clean wound sepsis rates increase from 1–2% up to more than 5%. Inexpert or unsupervised shaving by patients worsens these rates.

Minor skin abrasions and cuts which are exuding by the time of surgery allow emergence of skin commensals to the surface and colonization by pathogens.

Clipping of hair or the use of depilatory creams reduces infection rates down to a tenth of those following shaving. Shaving, if it is necessary, should be undertaken shortly prior to surgery. Avoidance of shaving altogether does not increase wound infection rates.

## CHEST INCISIONS

There are three principal routes into the chest:

1. The lateral thoracotomy may be anterior or posterior in approach or a combination. An anterior approach, through the 4th rib space, allows access for transaxillary sympathectomy, and a posterior approach, through the 6th rib space, allows access to the lung; a combination gives access to the whole pleural cavity for pulmonary or on the left side oesophageal surgery. This latter incision is made in the 6th or 7th rib interspace or the rib bed starting medial to the nipple, passing 2–3 cm under the scapula, then turning superiorly between the scapula and midline. Muscles are divided using diathermy, the pectoralis major anteriorly then latissimus dorsi, serratus anterior and the rhomboids. Once the scapula is raised the periosteum of the selected rib can be incised with diathermy, then elevated. There is no need to remove the rib but division at the neck facilitates insertion of a rib-spreader to give access. Chest closure requires pleural drainage with an apical chest drain connected to an underwater seal. A basal drain may be added. Drains should be removed as soon as the pneumothorax is evacuated (after transaxillary sympathectomy) or after a few days, depending on the amount of drainage or need to ensure pleurodesis. Chest closure is effected in layers using a rib approximator using 00 non-absorbable (Prolene) or absorbable (Vicryl) material. The intercostals are approximated and the serratus anterior and latissimus dorsi are closed separately. Skin closure is the same as for laparotomy closure.

2. The thoracoabdominal incision is used when access is needed urgently following trauma, and electively for wide exposure of the liver and

kidney (on the right) or spleen, oesophagogastric junction and kidney (on the left). Access may be allowed to the great vessels between chest and abdomen. The incision runs obliquely from the midline in the epigastrium in line with the 9th or 10th rib. The incision is muscle cutting in the abdomen, the muscles being divided over the ribs, and is extended to the anterior or mid-axillary line.

3. Median sternotomy allows access to the pericardium, the heart and great vessels in the chest. It is made strictly in the midline from the suprasternal notch to the xiphoid. The sternal periosteum is divided with diathermy and the rectus muscles split in the midline before inserting a finger into the mediastinum, above and below, and behind the sternum. The anaesthetist should keep the lungs in expiration while the sternum is divided using a power or Gigli saw. Closure requires strong monofilament non-absorbable sutures (stainless steel wire or Nylon) together with drainage of the pericardium and deep to the sternum.

## MATERIALS FOR WOUND CLOSURE
(Table 11.1)

The time-honoured use of natural sutures such as catgut and silk are slowly giving way to synthetic absorbable and non-absorbable polymers. Certainly catgut should not be used for abdominal wall closure as it is accompanied by an unacceptable wound failure rate, probably related to the tissue reaction it excites. Equally, although silk handles well and is easily and securely tied, it causes a tissue reaction which leaves cosmetically

**Table 11.1**  Suture materials for wound closure

| Suture type | Example (trade name) | Presentation |
|---|---|---|
| Natural — absorbable | Plain catgut | Monofilament twist collagen |
| | Chromic catgut | Monofilament twist collagen — chromicization delays absorption |

Comments: Highly irritant in tissues. May predispose to infection in contaminated wounds. Useless in deep wound closure (abdominal wall) with high suture failure rate and infection. Still popular for bowel anastomosis and ties. 21-day catgut can disrupt with a few days in infected wounds.

| | | |
|---|---|---|
| Non-absorbable | Silk (silicone coat) | Twist or braid for best handling and knotting |

Comments: Biodegradeable and irritant. No use for long-term security. Should not be used in contaminated wounds. Braids risk capillarity and may increase infection.

| | | |
|---|---|---|
| Non-absorbable | Cotton, linen | Braided |

Comments: Used for tying ligatures — being replaced by modern polymeric absorbables.

| | | |
|---|---|---|
| Non-absorbable | Stainless steet wire | Monofilament |

Comments: Used for strength, closing abdominal and chest wounds with low infective risk but difficult to tie. Safe in contaminated wounds.

| | | |
|---|---|---|
| Synthetic — absorbable | Polyglycolic acid (Dexon) | Braided with final coat for handling and knotting |
| | Polyglactin (Vicryl) | Braided |
| | Polydioxanone (PDS) | Monofilament |
| | Polyglyconate (Maxon) | Monofilament |

Comments: Replacing catgut as resorption rates are predicable and irritative effect in tissues is lessened. Some (PDS) have long-life tissue integrity and may be used for wound deep layers and skin closure. Shorter-life sutures may relate to wound irritation but subcuticular sutures do not require removal. Braids ideal for ligature ties.

| | | |
|---|---|---|
| Non-absorbables | Polyamide (Nylon, Nuralon) | Extruded polymers as a monofilaments or braids which |
| | Polyester (Dacron) | may be coated for easier handling and knotting |
| | Polypropylene (Prolene) | |
| | Polyethylene | |
| | Polybutester (Novafil) | |
| | Polytetrafluoroethylene (PTFE) | |

Comments: Nylon is biodegradeable and should not be used in vascular surgery. Prolene, Polybutester or PTFE monofilaments are used for vascular surgery. As monofilaments they may be used for wound closure with low infection rates. No irritation in tissues unless knots become infected by contamination. Subcuticular sutures require removal. Give the best cosmetic results in skin because of no irritation (if braids not used) and very fine sutures have high tensile strength. Braided forms used for deep tissue apposition (hernia repair) with low infection rates.

unacceptable scars in the skin. The capillarity of the braid in silk encourages the spread of bacteria and the formation of suture abscesses. The new synthetic absorbables (polyglycolic acid, polyglactin, polydioxanone) have been used successfully for closure of the abdominal wall and subcuticular skin. They do not require removal from skin but excite a tissue reaction, which monofilament synthetic non-absorbables do not. Their use for subcutaneous closure to lessen dead space is debatable. Wire affords secure closure but is difficult to tie. The author's preference is a looped monofilament BP 1 polyamide (Nylon) suture for abdominal wall closure, using a mass technique starting at each end of the wound with a single buried knot at the wound centre. Similarly, a subcuticular closure with BP 2/0 or 3/0 monofilament polypropylene (Prolene) on a cutting linear needle is preferred without subcutaneous closure. For minor operative surgery, particularly on the face, BP 5/0 or 6/0 closure with interrupted sutures results in cosmetically acceptable scars.

## THE USE OF DRAINS

The indications for postsurgical drainage are nebulous. Drainage of an anastomosis after low anterior resection may allow the surgeon to feel more secure in the belief that any bleeding, leakage or infection will be lessened, or that a fistulous track is encouraged should a failure of anastomotic healing occur. On the contrary, there is ample evidence to show that drains soon block or are walled off and probably have little effect within 48 hours of surgery. In addition drains may be a source of secondary infection and secondary haemorrhage, and may promote increased collagenase at the site of an anastomosis with the attendant risk of leakage. The use of suction drains may even enhance leakage through an anastomosis. It seems pointless to drain the peritoneum after dealing with generalized peritonitis but there is adequate evidence to show that drains are efficient in reducing infection after localized peritonitis, such as that associated with perforated appendicitis.

Drains are also widely used for the theoretical reduction of dead space. While they are probably better than the overuse of sutures to close dead space, there is little evidence that they prevent effusions or collections, after mastectomy for example. Postoperative drainage will continue to be widely used but it seems more logical when there is a risk of opportunistic infection, particularly after prosthetic surgery or when there is a large raw surface area after incisional hernia repair. Closed system suction drains prevent the risk of exogenous infection.

Drains may be classified as being active or passive, the former employing some kind of suction. There are many active suction drains available with a closed system — most are disposable and expensive. Reusable systems usually incorporate a glass bottle but they are cumbersome for the patient and the cost of repackaging and sterilization is not insubstantial. The sump drain is an open system suction drain and can be useful in protecting skin when, for example, there is an upper gastrointestinal–cutaneous fistula.

Passive drains do not usually incorporate a non-return valve, so that exogenous organisms can migrate along the drain if it is left in place for too long a time. They work by siphonage, gravity or increases in abdominal pressure. Open drainage, using Penrose or corrugated rubber drains, have largely been replaced by closed system drainage.

The tubing attached to a drainage system which is inserted under skin or into body cavities may be made of latex (when a track is encouraged to form, as in T-tube drainage of the common bile duct) or of plastic materials, particularly Silastic (when minimal reaction is wanted, as in multiple drainage of necrosing pancreatitis by large-bore Robinson drains). Smaller drains incorporate many holes in their distal end to permit suction drainage over a wider area, whereas larger drains have their single open end which permits lavage if necessary as well as drainage. Drains may break or become knotted within cavities, so that simple traction cannot remove them and an open operation is required. The advantages of their use should be carefully considered for each patient.

## SURGICAL DRESSINGS

The last 30 years have seen an increased depth of understanding of wound-healing processes and many dressings are being manufactured to provide the requirements of the ideal wound environment. There is no clear-cut evidence, however, that wounds should be left open with a dry surface and a fibrinous coagulum, which seals the wound, or whether they should be covered

**Table 11.2** The ideal surgical dressing (which does not exist)

---

Absorbent and able to remove excess exudate
Maintain moist environment and aid own tissues to debride necrotic material and promote healing
Prevent trauma to underlying healing granulation tissue or to prevent shed of foreign particles into the wound
Be leakproof and prevent strike-through and secondary infection
Maintain temperature and gaseous change
Allow simple dressing changes, easy, less frequent application and removal, and be pain free
Be odourless, cosmetically acceptable and comfortable
Not be expensive

---

(and hidden from view). Exuding wounds are at risk of secondary infection and may not be protected by a dressing. If covered by an absorptive dressing pathogenic organisms can track through a soiled wet dressing from its surface (strike-through). The requirements of an ideal surgical dressing are listed in Table 11.2. Some of their requirements are theoretical but many are based on sound experimental evidence. The armamentarium of modern surgical dressings is mainly directed at management of chronic open wounds such as venous leg ulcers.

Polyurethane incise drapes have become popularized as a primary wound dressing for sutured wounds and skin donor sites. They maintain moisture which enhances epithelial closure, and allow easy inspection and aspiration of excessive exudate. On donor sites they are claimed to relieve pain. They are gas and water vapour permeable but excessive maceration risks secondary infection although the dressings are impermeable to organisms. More traditional wound dressings include Melolin or non-adherent sheet dressings which require a secondary pad dressing if there is excessive exudate.

For open wounds such as a healing pilonidal sinus cavity or a superficially dehisced, infected abdominal wound we are spoilt for choice. The moulded polymeric Silastic form dressing is ideal, allowing pain-free wound care, by the patient if necessary. Other bead and powder dressings may be equally useful which absorb exudate and maintain the moist environment (examples are Debrisan, Iodosorb and Scherisorb). Sheet polymeric dressings are reserved for more superficial open wounds. They may be fully occlusive (Comfeel Ulcer Dressing or Granuflex) or semi-occlusive (Geliperm) or with a biological source (the alginates Kaltostat or Sorbsan). The list of dressings increases and satisfactory trials are required to show their merit and comparative relative worth.

## FURTHER READING

Anonymous 1986 Dressings for ulcers. Drug and Therapeutics Bulletin 24: 9–12
Cox P J, Ausobsky J R, Ellis H, Pollock A V 1986 Towards no incisional hernias: lateral paramedian versus midline incisions. Journal of the Royal Society of Medicine 79: 711–712
Harland R N L, Irving M H 1988 Surgical drains. Surgery 1: 1360–1362
Jenkins T P N 1976 The burst abdominal wound: a mechanical approach. British Journal of Surgery 63: 873–876
Leaper D J 1985 Laparotomy closure. British Journal of Hospital Medicine 33: 317–322
Leaper D J 1991a Local effects of trauma and wound healing. In: Burnand K G, Young A E (eds) Ian Airds Companion to Surgical Studies. Churchill Livingstone, Edinburgh, in press
Leaper D J 1991b Surgical factors influencing infection. In: Taylor E W (ed) Infection in surgical practice. Oxford University Press, Oxford, in press
Leaper D J, Foster M E 1990 Wound healing and abdominal wound closure. In: Taylor I (ed) Progress in surgery 3. Churchill Livingstone, Edinburgh, Ch 2, pp 19–31
Lucarotti M E, Billings P J, Leaper D J 1991 Laparotomy, wound closure and repair of incisional hernia. Surgery. In press
Wadstrom J, Gerdin B 1990 Closure of the abdominal wall: how and why. Acta Chirurgica Scandinavica 156: 75–82

# 12. Wound healing

## N. Woolf

The biological objectives of wound healing are twofold. They are:

1. to restore the integrity of epithelial surfaces should this have been lost. In this way, the underlying tissue are protected against
   a. an abnormal environmental milieu, e.g. abnormal drying or wetting of the exposed surface
   b. infection
   c. the ingress of non-living foreign material
2. to restore the tensile strength of the subepithelial tissue.

### Healing by primary and secondary 'intention'

Whatever the type of wound, the basic mechanisms involved in healing are the same, and the differences described are largely those of degree rather than of kind. However, almost by convention, the healing of cleanly incised wounds, where the edges are in close apposition, tends to be considered separately from those in which there is extensive loss of epithelium, a large subepithelial tissue defect which has to be filled in by scar tissue and where the edges cannot be brought together with sutures. These two circumstances are described in archaic terminology as being 'healing by first intention' or 'healing by second intention', these terms first appearing in a surgical treatise published in 1543, though Thomson (1813) in 'Lectures on Inflammation' gives the credit for introducing these terms to Galen.

### The healing of an incised wound

Incision involves the division of:

- epidermis
- dermal connective tissue fibres and matrix
- subcutaneous tissue
- blood vessels.

Severing of blood vessels obviously leads to haemorrhage with the resulting accumulation within the tissue defect of platelets and pre-eminently among the plasma proteins, *fibrinogen* and *fibronectin*. Clotting mechanisms are activated and the former becomes converted to a clot consisting of polymerized fibrin, which is stabilized by fibronectin binding to it by means of a glutaminase bridge. Fibronectin is the term used for a set of large, extracellular matrix glycoproteins, and the gel formed by fibrin and fibronectin acts in the early stages of healing as a 'glue' which helps to keep the severed edges of the tissue apposed. It has a number of other possible roles in wound healing and, indeed, is one of the key substances involved in healing, but these can be best considered after the morphological events which make up the healing process have been described.

Purely as a matter of convenience, these events can be considered under two headings: those which concern the *epidermis*; those taking place within the *dermis*.

## EPIDERMAL EVENTS

Within a few hours of wounding, a single layer of epidermal cells starts to migrate from the wound edges to form a delicate covering over the raw area exposed by the loss of epidermis. This migratory process can be studied in vitro by observing the behaviour of epidermal cells when small cubes of excised skin are cultured at 37°C in appropriate nutrient media. Under these circumstances, the epidermal cells begin to spread over the five raw dermal faces, and eventually the whole cube of dermal tissue is enclosed by epidermis like a small parcel. The jargon term applied to this spreading process is *epiboly*. The idea that cell movement plays a significant part in this is supported by the fact that substances such as cytochalasin B, which are known to interfere with cell migration, inhibit epiboly.

## Mechanisms involved in cell migration

Epidermal cell migration across the area of epithelial loss depends on interaction between the keratinocytes at or near the wound edges and the extracellular matrix glycoprotein fibronectin. The fibronectins are large two-chained glycoproteins which are present both within plasma and within tissues. Originally they were thought to be cell surface proteins but it is now realized that instead they constitute part of the extracellular matrix and exert much of their effect by providing sites which act as ligands for receptors on a wide variety of cell types. This ligand-receptor binding mediates cell-matrix adhesion. The binding sites often include the tripeptide arginine-glycine-aspartate (colloquially known as RGD sites). The receptors on cells, which serve as ligands for the RGD sequence, belong to what is known as the integrin family of receptors; this includes those surface molecules on phagocytic cells which mediate adhesion to the endothelial cells in the microcirculation. Differences between plasma and tissue fibronectins appear to be mediated by post-translational modifications, differences in splicing being particularly important. In relation to the epidermis in wounds, the type of splicing of fibronectin mRNA resembles that which is found in early embryogenesis. Keratinocytes from normal, *unwounded skin* do *not* possess receptors which bind to fibronectin, being tightly attached to basement membrane which contains laminin and collagen type IV. Those derived from wounds, however, express a fibronectin receptor which is very similar to a fibronectin receptor expressed on fibroblasts. As already stated, the wound is infiltrated by a gel rich in fibronectin and the activated keratinocytes preferentially adhere to the RGD sequences on the fibronectin and thus migrate across and, indeed, through this matrix.

## Epithelial cell proliferation

Epidermal cell movement can provide an initial covering for very small wounds, but in most instances epithelial re-covering cannot be accomplished without proliferation of epidermal cells, the new cells being derived from the stem-cell compartment of the epidermal cell population which is made up of the basal cells just above the dermal–epidermal junction. From about 12 hours after wounding, there is a marked increase in mitotic activity in the basal cells about three to five cells from the cut edges. This is preceded by an increase in DNA synthesis of about 30% over normal, and similar cycles of increased DNA synthesis and mitosis follow. The new epidermal cells grow under the surface fibrin/fibronectin clot and for a little distance down the gap between the cut edges to form a small 'spur' of epithelium, which afterwards regresses. If the wound has been sutured, a similar downgrowth of new epidermis occurs in relation to the suture tracks and, on occasion, these may form the basis of keratin-forming cysts within the dermis — so-called 'implantation dermoid cysts'.

## DERMAL EVENTS

Within the first few hours after wounding a mild acute inflammatory reaction takes place with the usual influx of neutrophils into and around the wound (up to day 1 after wounding). This is followed by migration of macrophages into this area (one to two days after wounding)—a key event since it is these cells that orchestrate the complex interplay of chemical signals which now takes place.

Viewed in an operational sense the objectives of this phase of the healing process are:

1. demolition and removal of any inflammatory exudate and tissue debris
2. restoration of the tensile strength of the sub-epithelial connective tissue. This involves
   a. chemoattraction of cells which synthesize and secrete collagen and other connective tissue proteins, i.e. fibroblasts

b. expansion of the existing small fibroblast population by stimulating the cells to proliferate
c. stimulation of these new fibroblasts to secrete extracellular connective tissue proteins
3. causing the ingrowth of new small blood vessels into the area undergoing repair; this is particularly important where there has been a substantial degree of tissue loss, leaving a large defect to be filled in with scar tissue. This involves
   a. budding of new endothelial cells from small intact blood vessels at the edges of the wound
   b. chemoattraction of these new endothelial cells into the fibrin/fibronectin gel within the wounded area.

In a surgical wound, fibroblasts and myofibroblasts appear in the wound between two and four days after wounding, and endothelial cells follow about one day later. The infiltration of macrophages and fibroblast proliferation are followed, as stated above, by the ingrowth of new capillary buds which are derived from intact dermal vessels at the margins of the wound. Initially these buds consist of solid ingrowths of endothelial cells but these soon acquire a lumen. An essential starting step for the ingrowth of new vessels is local degradation of the basement membrane of the existing capillary, this local defect permitting the budding of new endothelial cells. At this stage newly formed capillaries have little basement membrane substance and, compared with a normal capillary, are extremely leaky. This combination of a richly vascularized gel in which both inflammatory cells and collagen-producing fibroblasts are present is known as *granulation tissue*.

This name, which in biological terms is meaningless, derives from the fact that when the raw surface of a large wound is inspected it shows a granular appearance rather like that seen on the surface of a strawberry. Each of these granules contains a loop of capillaries and hence bleeds easily if traumatized.

## Collagen production

The ultimate development of tensile strength in a wound depends on the production of adequate amounts of collagen and on the final orientation of that collagen. Collagen is the only protein which contains large amounts of the amino acids hydroxyproline and hyroxylysine. Within 24 hours of wounding, protein-bound hydroxyproline appears within the damaged area and within two to three days some fibrillar material may be seen though, as yet, it lacks the dimensions and the typical 64 nm banding of polymerized collagen. Within a few weeks of the infliction of a surgical wound the amount of collagen in the wounded area is normal, though preoperative tensile strength is not regained for some months. This suggests that replacement and remodelling of the collagen formed early in wound healing is an important part of the whole process.

Each type of collagen (there are about ten, of which types I, II and III are the chief fibrillar collagens) consists of three peptide α chains which are wound round each other in a helical pattern. These chains are synthesized in the rough endoplasmic reticulum of the fibroblast following translation of the mRNA for each chain. They then undergo post-translational hydroxylation of their proline and lysine moieties and the hydroxylysine is then glycosylated. Linkage of the three chains is accomplished through the medium of disulphide bonds. The three chains then become twisted into a helix and the molecule passes to the Golgi zone. Assisted by the microtubules, the soluble procollagen molecules are secreted into the extracellular environment. Solubility is conferred by the presence of an extra peptide. This is removed by a peptidase, and the cleaved molecules then assemble into fibres which gain tensile strength by cross-linking. The typical periodicity of the collagen fibres is due to the assembled molecules having a staggered arrangement. On some occasions, the control mechanisms which determine an appropriate amount of new collagen for healing a given wound are faulty and excess collagen may be formed, leading to the formation of a bulky scar which stands proud of the surrounding surface. This is known as a keloid.

## Healing of wounds associated with a large tissue defect

A large volume of tissue loss can occur in cases of

severe trauma or extensive burns, or, much less frequently, in relation to certain surgical procedures. Qualitatively there are few differences between the healing of such a wound and that of an incised wound, though of course there are quantitative differences, since the formation of granulation tissue and ultimately of scar tissue must be on a far larger scale. One feature of the healing process in large tissue defects which is not seen in relation to healing of incised wounds is wound contraction.

### Wound contraction

Two or three days after the formation of large open wounds, the area of raw tissue starts to decrease. This is the expression of a real movement of the wound margins and is quite independent of the rate at which covering by a new epithelial layer can take place. In some fur-bearing animals the raw area may decrease in size by as much as 80% in two weeks, and, sometimes, the degree of contraction may be so great as virtually to close the wound.

The wound contraction occurs at a time when relatively little new collagen is being formed in the dermis and subcutaneous tissue, and it seems therefore unlikely that shortening of collagen fibres at the wound margins is responsible for the contraction. Indeed, inhibition of collagen formation does not interfere with the process of wound contraction.

A currently favoured hypotesis is that the contraction is brought about by the action of cells which appear at the margins of the wound in the first few days and which, on electron microscopy, show features suggesting both fibroblast and smooth muscle differentiation. This has led to the term *myofibroblast* being applied to them. Use of appropriation antibodies shows that these cells contain actin, but no smooth muscle type myosin has been found within their cytoplasm. In any circumstances, for a pulling force to be exerted there must be a connection between the object being pulled and whatever is applying the force. In wound contraction the connection is provided by fibronectin molecules which form bridges between collagen fibres on the one hand and receptors on the myofibroblasts on the other.

Thus strips of granulation tissue from healing wounds can be made to shorten in vitro by any pharmacological agents which cause actin fibrils to contract. It has been postulated that a similar mechanism is responsible for the contracture of dermal connective tissue seen in such conditions as Dupuytren's contracture.

## GROWTH FACTORS AND CYTOKINES IN WOUND HEALING

It is clear from what has been said in the previous sections that the cellular events in wound healing must depend on a series of 'instructions' which:

1. cause the cells concerned in repair, e.g. fibro-blasts and endothelial cells, to *migrate* into the wound
2. cause these cells and also the epithelial cells which must cover the raw surface to *proliferate*.

These instructions consist of a set of chemical signals derived from a number of sources. Some, which have as their principal function a mitogenic effect on the cells to which they bind, are known as growth factors. The other, chiefly derived from inflammatory cells, are known as cytokines.

### Growth factors

Growth factors are peptides which may reach their specific targets via one or more of three pathways.
These are:

● *The endocrine pathway,* where the growth factors are synthesized at some considerable distance from their targets and are delivered to them via the bloodstream
● *The paracrine pathway,* where the growth factors are synthesized and released by cells which are in the close neighbourhood of their targets
● *The autocrine pathway,* in which the same cells both synthesize and use the growth factor.

Growth factors can be divided into two groups depending on the phase in the life of a stem cell during which they operate.

A *competence* growth factor is capable of moving a cell out of the $G_0$ phase back into cycle, while a *progression* growth factor has a mitogenic effect only on cells which are not in the $G_0$ phase.

Typical competence growth factors, which are likely to be involved in the healing process as well as in a number of other pathological situations such as atherogenesis, interstitial fibrosis within the lung and the formation of fibrous tissue stroma in relation to tumours, are platelet-derived growth factor and fibroblast growth factor, while the progression growth factors are represented by such molecules as insulin-like growth factors 1 and 2 (the somatomedins) and epidermal growth factor.

### Platelet-derived growth factor

Platelet-derived growth factor (PDGF) is a basic protein which has a molecular weight of about 30 000. It consists of two peptides (an A chain and a B chain) which are bound by disulphide bridges. Reduction of the disulphide bridges causes the mitogenic activity of the growth factor to be lost. The B chain is the gene product of the cellular proto-oncogene *c-sis*.

The name platelet-derived growth factor is somewhat misleading in two senses. First, while it is certainly stored in the α granules of platelets and released from them when the platelets are activated, the growth factor is synthesized and secreted from other cells as well. These include:

- endothelial cells
- macrophages
- arterial smooth muscle cells
- cells from certain tumours.

Second, PDGF has a number of functions apart from its undoubted powerful, mitogenic effect. These include the following:
- PDGE is chemotactic for the same cells for which it is a mitogen.
- It increases intracellular synthesis of cholesterol and also increases binding of low-density lipoprotein (LDL) by increasing the number of LDL receptors expressed on the plasma membrane of the target cell.
- It increases prostaglandin secretion, initially by making more of the starting material (arachidonic acid) available and later, by stimulating the synthesis of cyclooxygenase.
- PDGF induces changes in cell shape accompanied by a reorganization of actin filaments within the cells.
- It induces increased synthesis of RNA and protein.
- It is a potent vasoconstrictor.

Thus PDGF can carry out both tasks which were outlined at the beginning of this section. It can attract mesenchymal cells into the wound (with the exception of endothelial cells which do not possess the PDGF receptor) and it acts as a mitogen and stimulator of protein production.

PDGF and other growth factors bind to receptors which, after ligand–receptor interaction, act as tyrosine kinases.

The binding of PDGF to its receptor produces a conformational change in the latter which induces it to act as tyrosine kinase. The phosphorylation of tyrosine residues which follows affects at least two proteins which may have an important part to play in the signal transduction pathway triggered by tyrosine kinases.

The first of these is a novel lipid kinase which phosphorylates phosphatidylinositol at the 3-position to yield metabolites such as 1, 3-PIP and 1, 3, 4-PIP$_2$ which have been found in cultured cells transformed by oncogenes.

The second is a cytoplasmic serine–threonine kinase which is believed to be involved in the transmission of signals from cell plasma membranes to the cytoplasm and possibly to the nucleus. This kinase is the gene product of the proto-oncogene *c-raf*. The *c-raf* kinase can also be activated via protein kinase-C in cells which have been rated with phorbol ester.

The transduction of the mitogenic signal from the cell membrane is followed within a few minutes by activation of the protooncogenes c-*fos* and c-*myc* and also by the activation of the genes which code for the production of the contractile protein actin and for the production of β-interferon.

### Epidermal growth factor and transforming growth factor alpha

Epidermal growth factor (EGF) is a 53-amino-acid polypeptide which is cleaved from a larger precursor protein. It was discovered by the Nobel laureate Cohen in the course of experiments in which he was engaged in a search for a nerve growth stimulating factor in the salivary glands of baby mice, such a factor having been discovered previously in the salivary glands of snakes. However, extracts of these glands when injected into baby mice caused their eyes to open prematurely and their incisor teeth to grow faster, these effects being due to a stimulation of epidermally derived tissues. The factor was purified and is now known as epidermal growth factor, though it stimulates mitogenesis in connective tissue as well as in epithelial cells. The salivary glands and, as shown recently, the lacrimal glands also, are storage sites for EGF which can be released in saliva and tears. Thus, licking one's wounds in the literal rather than in the metaphorical sense may be of definite biological advantage, as may be the irrigation of the cornea by tears in corneal abrasion or ulceration. EGF, or a molecule with considerable homology, is also produced in the Brunner's glands in the duodenum and its metabolite, urogastrone, may be measured in the urine. In rodents EGF may be found in the plasma but in humans blood-borne EGF is concentrated within platelets, for the most part in the $\alpha$ granules. Since EGF protein can also be found in the bone marrow in the cytoplasm of megakaryocytes, it seems almost certain that platelet EGF is derived from synthesis within the megakaryocytes rather than by uptake from the plasma.

In experimental wounds the application of EGF has been found to accelerate significantly the rate of epidermal regeneration. EGF has also been shown to have a beneficial effect on the dermal component of healing in experimental wounds, causing an increase in proliferation of dermal connective tissue and an increase in the tensile strength of incised wounds. In humans, also, topical application of EGF accelerates the healing of donor sites for skin grafts.

There is no evidence that EGF is produced by any of the cells taking part in the healing process, though, as already stated, platelets store EGF. However, there is another factor, known as transforming growth factor alpha (TGF$\alpha$), which shows a considerable degree of homology with EGF and which can be produced by both epidermal cells and by macrophages in healing wounds. TGF$\alpha$ binds to the same receptor on target cells as does EGF and has the same mitogenic effect. In this way TGF$\alpha$ may be a direct mediator of wound healing.

### Transforming growth factor beta

Transforming growth factor beta (TGF$_\beta$) is a polypeptide, first discovered in culture media conditioned by transformed cells, but is produced by almost all cell lines in culture. In the presence of EGF it acts as a mitogen, but in some assays has also been found to inhibit growth. It is possible that these contradictory actions may be a reflection of the different types of assay used and may not tell us much about what is happening in vivo. There is, however, good evidence that macrophages in healing wounds express mRNA for TGF$_\beta$ as well as for TGF$_\alpha$. TGF$_\beta$ has also been shown to be a powerful chemoattractant for monocytes and its release from the first wave of inflammatory cells migrating into the wound may act as a mechanism for recruiting additional monocytes/macrophages.

The pattern of expression of growth factors in healing wounds supports the idea that the macrophage plays a leading role in the healing process, as does some other evidence such as the observations that:

1. Wound fluid stimulates cell division and promotes the ingrowth of new vessels.

2. Ablation of macrophages in animals slows the process of wound healing.

3. Macrophages in wounds also express other growth factors such as insulin-like growth factor 1.

## CYTOKINES

*Cytokine* is the term used for a group of protein cell regulators which includes such members as:

- lymphokines
- monokines
- interleukins
- interferons.

Growth factors could also, with some justification, be called cytokines and treating them as a separate class of regulator, as has been done here, is somewhat artificial, if convenient.

The four classes referred to above are low-molecular-weight proteins (usually less than 80 kDa). They tend to be produced rapidly and locally and can act in either an autocrine or a paracrine fashion. They are produced by a wide range of cells and have many overlapping actions which are mediated by their binding to high-affinity receptors on their target cells. The response of an individual cell to a given cytokine is dependent on the cell type, what other chemical signals are being received at the same time, and the local concentration of the cytokine. Two cytokines which play a significant role in wound healing are inter-leukin-1 (IL-1) and tumour necrosis factor alpha ($TNF_\alpha$) (syn. cachectin).

IL-1 (formerly known as endogenous pyrogen) is a small (17 kDa) protein which is produced by a wide variety of cell types, those having relevance for healing being macrophages and epidermal cells. IL-1 has many biological actions, which in relation to healing include a proliferative effect on dermal fibroblasts and up-regulation of collagen synthesis by the fibroblasts. It also increases collagenase production and this may be one of the ways in which the collagen in wounds is remodelled so as to achieve maximal tensile strength.

$TNF_\alpha$ is another monocyte/macrophage product which is released following tissue injury or infection. It is the main factor responsible for macrophage-mediated tumour cell killing and is also responsible for the wasting (cachexia) which is seen in certain chronic bacterial and parasitic infections. Its biological activity has a remarkable overlap with that of IL-1, though it does not appear to have the immunoregulatory functions of that molecule. Its receptors, however, are quite distinct from those of IL-1 and presumably the similarities in their actions indicate that they stimulate the same 'second messenger' systems. The expression of $TNF\alpha$ by monocytes and macrophages requires activation of these cells. This may be brought about in a number of ways, such as:

- interacting with fibrin (which is always present in wounds)
- binding of transforming growth factor beta
- the action of $\alpha$–interferon
- the action of endotoxin.

$TNF_\alpha$ is a potent stimulus for the ingrowth of new blood vessels in healing wounds, being not only chemotactic for endothelial cells but also being the agent responsible for the focal degradation of capillary basement membranes which precedes the migration of endothelial cells into a healing wound.

## Can cell proliferation in healing occur because of *loss* of some factor which restrains cell division? — the chalone theory

The foregoing sections dealing with growth factors and cytokines presupposes a model of epithelial proliferation in which cell division is *driven* by binding of mitogenic signals to their specific receptors on fibroblasts, endothelium and epidermal cells. Another model put forward before the discovery of growth factors, suggests that the cell proliferation occurring in healing is due to the loss of some normal restraint that controls the rate of cells turnover in labile cells and, for most of the time, represses cell division in stable cells during postnatal life. The hypothesis in this model is that repression of mitosis is mediated by a group of substances which have been extracted, but never purified, from a number of cells types, of which the epidermis is one. These substances, which appear to be glycoproteins, have been called *chalones* — a term derived from the Greek *chalinoeion* which means to bridle or restrain. It is postulated that normal numbers of a given cell population are maintained as a result of the secretion of chalones from fully differentiated cells, the result being a 'damping down' of cell division in the stem cell compartment of the cell population. When, for example, epidermal cells reach the end of their natural term, become keratinized and are shed, the chalone level would fall slightly and new epidermal cells would be recruited as a result of decreased repression of stem cell division. If cell loss on a large scale were to occur (as in wounding), there would be a sudden marked drop in chalone concentration locally and a corresponding wave of mitotic activity which would persist until the original cell mass had been restored. The model is a neat and attractive one but is lacking in hard evidence. Until this is forthcoming it deserves the Scottish verdict: 'not proven'.

## FACTORS WHICH MAY INTERFERE WITH WOUND HEALING

Failure to heal satisfactorily can be the result of either systemic or local factors.

### Systemic factors

*Nutrition*

**Protein**. The state of nutrition of the patient is a potent factor in determining the success or failure of the healing process. There may be at least two explanations for this. First, the under-nourished patient shows evidence of depression of the immune system and wound infection, and the inflammatory response to this may delay healing. Second, a deficient protein intake may inhibit collagen formation and so inhibit the regaining of tensile strength. In this regard, sulphur-containing amino acids such as methionine seem to be particularly important, and increasing the intake of this amino acid alone can partially offset the effects of a low protein intake on wound healing.

**The role of vitamin C**. Vitamin C holds the most prominent place among the individual dietary factors which can affect healing. It has been known since the seventeenth century that scurvy is associated with poor healing of wounds and fractures. Indeed, there are colourful descriptions of old wounds, acquired honourably or otherwise in combat, breaking down after the onset of scurvy. While we owe our knowledge of how to avoid scurvy to the maritime founders of our once far-flung Empire, it was not until well into this century that vitamin C was discovered by Szent-Gyorgy. Once this was done it was possible to examine the effects of vitamin C deficiency on experimental wounds. Vitamin C lack was found to inhibit the secretion of collagen fibres by fibroblasts and this was due to a failure of hydroxylation of proline in the endoplasmic reticulum of the fibroblast. In addition Vitamin C concentrations in biological fluids appear to affect the production of galactosamine and hence the deposition of chondroitin sulphate in the extracellular matrix of granulation tissue.

**Vitamin A**. Vitamin A has important functions in relation to morphogenesis, epithelial proliferation and epithelial differentiation. Data relating to its effect in the context of wound healing are scanty but it is believed to promote the epithelial component of the process.

**Zinc**. A role for zinc in wound healing was discovered more or less by accident. In the course of a study on the effects of certain amino acids on wound healing, a phenylalanine analogue which had expected to impair healing instead accelerated it. Careful study of this analogue revealed that the sample used had been contaminated by zinc. Further studies showed that zinc does indeed accelerate the healing of experimental wounds. Zinc deficiency, such as is found in patients who have been on parenteral nutrition for long periods and in patients with severe burns, is associated with poor healing and this is reversed by the administration of zinc.

*Steroid hormones*

Many studies show that glucocorticoids have an inhibitory effect on the healing process and on the production of fibrous tissue. Indeed advantage is taken of this by administering steroids in situations where inappropriate scarring is taking place, such as in interstitial fibrosis in the lung. It is still not clear whether steriods exert their effect indirectly by damping down the inflammatory process or whether they directly affect one or more of the mechanisms which have been outlined in the foregoing sections.

### Local factors

*The presence of foreign bodies or infection*

The presence of infection or of a foreign body will increase the intensity and prolong the duration of the inflammatory response to injury and will inhibit a satisfactory conclusion to the healing process. It is worth remembering that fragments of dead tissue, such as bone, and other elements of the patients' own tissues which have become misplaced, such as hair or keratin, act as foreign bodies.

*Excess mobility*

Even the least observant will have noticed that a cut across a joint, such as an interphalangeal joint, will take longer to heal than one which is not subjected to frequent movement. Excess mobility in a wound will, inevitably, increase the time taken for a wound to heal. This is of particular significance in relation to fracture healing (which is why the severed ends of the bone are immobilized) but applies in other tissues as well.

### Perfusion and venous drainage

The degree of arterial perfusion and the efficacy of venous drainage play key roles in the healing of injured tissues. Where the arterial perfusion is compromised by stenosis or occlusion of the supplying vessel, a quite trivial injury may give rise to a disproportionate degree of tissue damage and healing may be delayed or even completely inhibited. Adequate venous drainage is also important, and impairment of this may play a part in the genesis of chronic ulcers, which often occur on the anterior surface of the legs in elderly patients. Histological examination of the margins of these lesions suggests that drainage is compromised by the presence of cuffs of polymerized fibrin round the venules. This can, in part, be prevented by administration of the synthetic steroid stanazolol. Sub-oxygenation of normally perfused tissue such as may occur in the presence of severe anaemia will also lead to defective healing.

The presence of diabetes mellitus, especially if this is of long standing, will also impair healing. This is particularly noticeable on the soles of the feet, where quite trivial injuries may develop into very chronic, non-healing ulcers. Blood vessel disease affecting both the large muscular arteries of the lower limb (atherosclerosis and its complications) and changes in the walls of arterioles and capillaries probably makes the major contribution to failures of healing in diabetics, but these patients show increased susceptibility to infection (particularly if their diabetes is badly controlled) and may have a sensory neuropathy as well which makes them more liable to sustain injuries to their extremities.

## REPAIR IN SOME SPECIALIZED TISSUES

### Bone

The processes involved in the early stages of fracture healing are basically the same as those which have been described in the foregoing sections. Thus the tissue defect created by the fracture is, in the first instance, made good by well-vascularized connective tissue in a manner similar to what occurs in the healing of large open wounds.

Once this stage has passed, important new features are imposed on the basic model of healing. These are necessary because bone, unlike soft tissues, requires mechanical and weight-bearing efficiency of a high order. These needs are met through the operation of two types of specialized cell:

1. the *osteoblast*, which lays down seams of uncalcified new bone (osteoid)
2. the *osteoclast*, a multinucleated cell probably of macrophage lineage which resorbs bone and which, therefore, plays a key part in the remodelling of the new bone formed in the course of fracture healing.

### Stages of fracture healing

1. When a bone is fractured, tearing of blood vessels takes place, *haemorrhage* results and the defect between the fractured ends of the bone becomes filled with blood clot and other plasma-derived proteins.

2. As in any other tissue, the injury elicits an *acute inflammatory reaction*, though the degree of neutrophil infiltration is mild. The combined effect of the haemorrhage and the inflammatory oedema causes loosening of the periosteum from the underlying bone ends and this results in a fusiform swelling at the fracture site.

3. Some degree of bone necrosis is almost inevitable and is due to cutting off the blood supply to some areas as a result of damage to blood vessels. It takes 24–48 hours for the first morphological evidence of bone necrosis to become apparent, the marrow being the site of the first changes. Fat necrosis is seen, and if haemopoietic marrow is involved the cells lose their nuclear staining. So far as the bony tissue itself is concerned, the extent of necrosis depends on the anatomy of the local blood supply, and some sites such as the talus, the carpal scaphoid and the head of the femur are particularly likely to show significant ischaemic necrosis after fracture. Empty

lacunae, the dead osteocytes having disappeared, are a reliable indication of bone necrosis.

4. *Macrophages* now invade the fracture site and commence the process of demolition. This is followed by the formation of granulation tissue, and about four days after fracturing the bone the mass of blood clot has been replaced by granulation tissue which also extends upwards and downwards within the marrow cavity for a considerable distance from the fracture site. Within the granulation tissue small groups of cartilage cells are beginning to differentiate from connective tissue stem cells.

5. *The formation of provisional callus.* Provisional callus is the term used to describe a cuff of woven bone admixed with islands of cartilage which serves to unite the severed portions of bone on their external aspect but not across the gap between the bone ends. The origin of the callus is from two sources, and the relative proportions of these vary depending on a number of factors. The first and more important is the periosteum. The cells on its inner aspects proliferate and begin to lay down woven bone (i.e. bone in which the collagenous osteoid tissue is not deposited in a lamellar or 'onion skin' fashion but in series of short bundles of parallel fibres, each bundle having a different orientation). Where the periosteum has been raised from the external surface of the bone (see above) the new woven bone fills the gap so that there are two cuffs of new bone around the periosteal aspect of the separated fragments. These cuffs then extend upwards and downwards until they meet, though there is, as yet *no* direct union across the gap between the separated bone ends. The degree of efficiency with which this external callus formation occurs depends on the adequacy or otherwise of the blood supply around the fracture site. Some of the new blood vessels are derived from the periosteum itself, while others come from the muscle and other soft tissues which abut on the fractured bone. The amount of cartilage admixed with this periosteal new bone is small in human fractures which are healing well, but tends to be greater in cases where the local blood supply is poor or where the fractured bone ends have not been properly immobilized. The second source of provisional callus is the medullary cavity where, following on the forma-

tion of granulation tissue, fibroblasts and osteoblasts start to proliferate and lay down bone matrix. Some of this is deposited on trabeculae of dead bone while the remainder forms new trabeculae.

6. *Healing across the fracture gap.* The provisional callus, as stated above, extends round the separated ends of the fractured bone but does not bridge the actual gap *between* the separated portions of bone. Well after the provisional callus has been formed the clot which fills the gap between the fragments is invaded, first by granulation tissue capillaries and then by osteoblasts. Ossification within this gap may occur as a primary event, the osteoblasts being derived from the provisional callus. In some cases the bone ends are united by fibrous tissue and over a period of time this is replaced by woven bone. This takes far longer than direct ossification and is more likely to occur if the fracture has not been properly immobilized or if there is any other factor present which is likely to inhibit healing (e.g. infection or extensive and severe periosteal damage). Occasionally the fibrous tissue filling the gap is not replaced by bone (non-union) and weight bearing by the affected limb is not possible. In cases of delayed or non-union, some improvement may be brought about by electrical stimulation, which appears to accelerate ossification at fracture sites.

7. *Remodelling.* Once union has occurred and the patient is bearing weight, the lumpy new cortical bone gradually becomes resorbed and smoothed out and the excess medullary new bone is similarly removed, with restoration of a normal medullary cavity. Woven bone, which is quite rapidly formed and which is much less efficient at weight bearing, is resorbed completely and is replaced by lamellar bone. This is a lengthy process and restoration to normal may take up to a year.

## Nervous tissue

### The central nervous system

Most neurones cannot be replaced once they have been lost, though there is some evidence to suggest that a limited degree of regeneration can take place in the hypothalamic–neorohypophyseal system. In contrast to the peripheral nerves where injury is not associated with any marked tendency towards scarring, necrosis within the central nervous system elicits the proliferation of glial cells and the formation of new glial fibres which, together with the ingrowth of capillaries, may constitute a physical barrier to the regeneration of new neuronal fibres.

### Peripheral nerves

When an axon is severed, the nerve cell shows chromatolysis (i.e. it swells and the Nissl granules which represent zones of the endoplasmic reticulum studded with many ribosomes disappear). The axon swells and becomes irregular, and its lipid-rich myelin sheath splits and later breaks up. The surrounding Schwann cells proliferate and accumulate some of the lipid released from the damaged myelin.

Soon new neurofibrils start to sprout from the proximal end of the severed axon and these invaginate the Schwann cells, which act as a guide or template for the new fibrils. The neurofibrils push their way down through the Schwann cells at a rate of about 1 mm per day. Eventually they may reach the appropriate end organ and their myelin sheaths are reformed as a result of the secretory activity of the Schwann cells and, in this way, a degree of functional recovery is attained. In some instances neurofibril sprouting takes place but the fibrils do not grow down existing endoneurial channels, and grow instead in a haphazard fashion. The end result may thus be a tangle of new nerve fibres embedded in a mass of scar tissue, the whole being called a traumatic or 'stump' neuroma.

# 13. Minimal access surgery

*A. Cuschieri*

Conventional open surgery entails open access to the diseased organ. In this respect, adequate exposure is essential for the safe and expeditious conduct of surgical operations. In addition to the wound, retraction of the parietes, often forceful, is required. This open conventional approach has certain intrinsic disadvantages which, to a large measure, influence the immediate postoperative course and delay patient recovery following treatment:

1. In the first instance, open exposure incurs additional trauma. In functional and some ablative operations, this exceeds the tissue damage inherent to the procedure itself and is reflected by the severity of the postoperative catabolic response. In addition to the well-documented physical and biochemical changes, poorly understood neuropsychological symptoms, e.g. asthenia, lethargy and mental debility, are often encountered and these may persist for several weeks.

2. Postoperative pain is largely caused by the parietal wound. The pain limits mobility and respiratory excursion and thereby contributes in a significant fashion to the common postoperative complications associated with surgery such as pulmonary collapse and infection and deep vein thrombosis. The opiate analgesia required routinely in the postoperative period carries its own respiratory morbidity and delays the return of bowel function.

3. The breach of the 'milieu interior' results in cooling of the patient and the internal organs, which lose water by evaporation. The cooling effect is especially important in children and the elderly. The desiccation of intestinal loops, particularly during long procedures, if unchecked, delays recovery of intestinal function and may jeopar-

dize the integrity of gastrointestinal anastomosis.

4. Retraction by metal implements is responsible for a number of iatrogenic injuries particularly to solid organs during abdominal surgery. Aside from this, prolonged retraction by metal retractors impairs tissue perfusion of the compressed tissue. Handling of the intestinal loops disturbs the intrinsic myoelectric activity of the gut.

5. The breach of the delicate serosal lining together with the gross manipulations lead to adhesion formation, particularly in relation to the laparotomy or thoracotomy wounds. Some patients are particulary prone to adhesion formation, which in the abdomen may lead to long-term intractable problems with recurrent intestinal obstructions.

6. Finally the operative parietal wound is itself the source of significant morbidity in terms of infection, dehiscence and subsequent incisional hernia formation. Despite prophylactic measures, including the use of antibiotics, postoperative wound infection remains common, prolongs hospital stay and adds significantly to the costs of surgical treatment.

## NATURE OF MINIMAL ACCESS SURGERY

The hallmark of minimal access surgery is the reduction of the trauma of access without compromise of the exposure of the operative field. Surgical operations are conducted by remote surgical manipulations carried out within the closed confines of body cavities or lumen of hollow organs under visual control via telescopes which incorporate the Hopkins rod lens system linked to CCD (charge couple device) cameras such that the surgeon can operate across the television screen. In addition to avoidance of large painful access wounds, the instruments used for dissection are small and fine and thus the tissue trauma inherent to surgical dissection is reduced further. The operation is thus carried out with minimum trauma inside the closed confines of the respective body cavity with avoidance of exposure, cooling, desiccation, handling and forced retraction of internal organs. Thus the overall traumatic assault on the patient is curtailed drastically, and as a result of this recovery to full activity is markedly accelerated. This is the most important benefit of the new approach and far outweighs the diminished cost of hospital treatment of minimal access surgery.

There are additional advantages which impart undoubted benefit. Thus there is virtual abolition of all wound related complications, early and late. When one considers that the average extra cost of an infected laparotomy wound is £1500, the cost saving, aside from diminished morbidity, by the avoidance of significant abdominal wounds is substantial. Likewise, the abolition of postoperative wound dehiscence (burst abdomen) and large incisional hernias particularly in obese patients constitutes a real and significant advance.

Another important advantage of minimal access surgery is the significantly reduced contact with the patient's blood during the course of the operative procedure. The importance of this in relation to diminished risk of transmission of viral disease such as hepatitis B and AIDS is both real and timely.

There are other perceived benefits of minimal access surgery. These include a reduction of the common postoperative complications associated with recumbency and pain, such as postoperative pulmonary collapse, chest infections and deep vein thrombosis. Although probable, the reduction in the incidence of these postoperative complications remains to be confirmed by prospective clinical trials. There is also a distinct impression among many endoscopic surgeons that adhesion formation is greatly reduced by minimal access surgery. The factors, other than the avoidance of a large wound, responsible for this effect remain unknown at present and indeed the clinical observation requires confirmation by prospective studies.

## NOMENCLATURE

Buess (1990) has advocated the term 'endoscopic microsurgery' to differentiate the new surgical techniques from other endoscopic procedures, such as snare resections of pedunculated polyps. This terminology, although accurate, has failed to gain acceptance. The term 'minimally invasive surgery' (MIS) coined by Wickham & Fitzpatrick (1990) has met with widespread approval and usage.

In the author's view, this terminology is inappropriate because it conveys the wrong meaning. In the first instance it carries connotations of increased safety, which is incorrect because there is no correlation between 'invasiveness' and risk, aside from the fact that 'to invade' is absolute and thus cannot be qualified. Semantic considerations apart, the most important argument against the use of this terminology is that it fails to convey the essential attribute of the new approach — the reduction of the trauma of access. The alternative terminology 'minimal access surgery' (MAS) is more accurate and descriptive (Cuschieri 1990).

## SCOPE OF MINIMAL ACCESS SURGERY

Minimal access surgery spans a wide spectrum of the existing surgical specialties and involves several approaches:

1. laparoscopic
2. thoracoscopic
3. endoluminal
4. perivisceral endoscopic
5. intra-articular joint surgery
6. combined.

### Laparoscopic surgery

This has been the most significant advance in general surgery in recent years. There is little doubt that laparoscopic cholecystectomy is rapidly becoming the standard method of treatment of gallstone disease, applicable to over 90% of patients (Cuschieri et al 1991, Southern Surgical Club 1991). Several other abdominal procedures can be performed laparoscopically (Table 13.1). No doubt, with improvement in instrumentation

**Table 13.1** Laparoscopic operations

Cholecystostomy
Cholecystectomy
Common duct exploration
Cholecystojejunostomy for malignant jaundice
Deroofing of hepatic cysts
Appendicectomy
Femoral/inguinal hernia repair
Cardiomyotomy
Ligamentum teres cardiopexy
Partial (Toupet, Dor) fundoplication
Crural repair and total fundoplication
Suture toilet of perforated duodenal ulcer
Vagotomy: truncal, HSV (highly selective vagotomy), others
Varicocele
Rectopexy
Nephrectomy

and ancillary technology, the scope of laparoscopic surgery will be extended further. It seems likely that all abdominal functional procedures and ablative operations for benign disease will be performed endoscopically. Some excisions for malignant disease pose problems in terms of the radicality of the procedure and the extraction of the specimen in such a manner as to permit accurate histopathological staging. Currently there are justifiable fears that the morcellation of malignant tissue (to permit extraction) is violating established principles of safe cancer surgery.

**Table 13.2** Thoracoscopic operations

Thoracodorsal sympathectomy
Ligature of bullae and pleurectomy/pleurodesis
Pulmonary wedge lobar, total resections
Pericardiectomy
Long oesophageal myotomy
Oesophagectomy

## Thoracoscopic surgery

The benefits accruing from the avoidance of a thoracotomy by the established thoracoscopic procedures are even greater that those derived by laparoscopic surgery. The various thoracoscopic procedures which are currently performed in a number of centres are outlined in Table 13.2. It seems likely that all operations on the oesophagus, resective or otherwise, will be conducted thoracoscopically in the near future. Likewise, open surgery for patients with recurrent pneumo-

thorax will be superseded by the new approach. Presently, a number of centres are developing techniques which will permit safe pulmonary resections, such as removal of specific bronchopulmonary segments, lobectomy and even pneumonectomy.

## Endoluminal surgery

Endoluminal surgery is applicable to the upper and lower reaches of the gastrointestinal tract, which are accessible to the endoscopic approach. Both fibre-optic and rigid telescopic approaches can be used. Examples of the former include endoscopic sphincterotomy and, more recently, endoscopic mucosectomy for early gastric cancer. Transanal endoscopic microsurgery, pioneered by Buess et al, has opened new therapeutic possibilities for the treatment of rectal tumours (large adenomas, early carcinomas) and rectal prolapse.

## Perivisceral endoscopic dissection

This approach differs from the previous ones in that dissection is conducted within loose areolar tissue planes in the absence of a natural cavity. The dissection entails creating the space for visualization of the organ, which is then mobilized under vision from the surrounding structures and organs. Examples of this technique include retroperitoneal surgery for denervation procedures such as lumbar sympathectomy, nephrectomy, and mediastinal endoscopic dissection of the oesophagus.

**Table 13.3** Combined approaches

1. *Endoscopic — open access*
   Right hemicolectomy
   Left hemicolectomy

2. *Combined endoscopic*
   Oesophagogastrectomy with cervical anastomosis
   Endoscopic left colectomy

## Combined approaches (Table 13.3)

There is little doubt that the future lies in the use of combined approaches: minimal access combined with open surgery and combined minimal access interventions. Currently the former is used to perform oesophagectomy with cervical anastomosis and laparoscopic assisted colectomy. In the latter situation the dissection and mobilization are carried out endoscopically but the resection and anastomosis are performed extracorporeally after exteriorization of the colon. Endoscopic oesophagectomy entails dissection of the gullet either via the mediastinal route through a cervical incision using the operating mediastinoscope of Buess or thoracoscopically through the right pleural cavity, as practised in Dundee. The gastric mobilization is undertaken using the standard open abdominal approach. Following resection and removal of the oesophagus and tumour, the stomach or gastric tube is pulled up into the neck by a guiding tube and the cervical anastomosis between the proximal oesophagus and the stomach is then performed.

As an indication of the potential scope of the combined minimal access, the equivalent of a standard three-stage oesophagectomy has been undertaken endoscopically in the pig. The development of the sheathed proctoscopic cannula, which permits delivery of the colon through the rectal stump and the maintenance of the pneumoperitoneum when the rectum is transected, allows the performance of a left colectomy under total endoscopic control.

## DISADVANTAGES AND LIMITATIONS OF MINIMAL ACCESS SURGERY

It is appropriate to consider the limitations and hazards of the new approach, since like all advances in clinical practice minimal access surgery has created new problems which have to be addressed by the profession.

Some emanate from the remote nature of the surgical manipulations. In this context the lack of direct handling of tissues, with the loss of tactile feedback so important to the surgeon in the evaluation of the local pathology and orientation, is obvious. There are ways around this problem, such as the development of 'tactile' exploratory ultrasound probes. It is difficult to predict to what extent this will redress this basic disadvantage. Another problem is the control of bleeding, which is undoubtedly more difficult to achieve endoscopically as the bleeding point often retracts within surrounding tissues. As an index of its significance, bleeding was found to be the commonest cause for conversion to the open procedure during laparoscopic cholecystectomy in a recent audit from several major European centres (Cuschieri et al 1991). Aside from the risks of hypovolaemia, bleeding during minimal access surgery considerably obscures the field of vision, due largely to light absorption by the extravasated blood.

In general, procedures performed by the new approach require more technical expertise and are slower to perform, especially when one takes into consideration the setting-up time. This has important consequences on our routine practice in terms of operating sessions and scheduling of cases. The longer operating time relates, in particular, to the execution of difficult cases. Thus, for example, although the extra time needed to execute a straightforward laparoscopic cholecystectomy may be inconsequential, a difficult gallbladder (contracted organ with foreshortened cystic pedicle) often takes twice as long to complete laparoscopically when compared to the standard open operation. There is obviously a need for preoperative tests which predict the ease of performance or otherwise of a particular endoscopic operation.

There is another consequence of the execution of 'difficult endoscopic operations' — increased iatrogenic intraoperative injury. This is exemplified by the higher incidence of bile duct damage during laparoscopic cholecystectomy which in some countries has risen to four to sixfold higher than that following open cholecystectomy. It is difficult to be certain of the exact reasons for this unsatisfactory state but it seems likely that different factors have operated in different centres. One suspects, however, that lack of training, poor clinical judgement and the use of inappropriate technology such as laser to cut the cystic duct and dissect the gallbladder have been foremost amongst the causative factors. In embracing the new approach, surgeons must accept the principle that the elective conversion to the equivalent open procedure must not be regarded as 'failure' but as an indication that in that particular patient open surgical intervention was the appropriate form of treatment. The outcome of such positive common-sense deliberations is far better than that which follows persistence with the endoscopic approach in the face of technical difficulties, which often dictate open intervention several hours later when iatrogenic damage has been enacted, or worse still when it declares itself in the postoperative period.

One of the real problems intrinsic to extirpative surgery by the minimal access approach is organ extraction. In some instances use is made of natural pathways such as the mediastinum for the oesophagus and rectum for the colon. In all other situations, however, the problem remains unresolved. Some are advocating methods designed to 'morcellate, mince or liquidize' the organ to enable removal. In the case of malignant disease this practice violates some of the fundamental principles of surgical management since detailed examination of the resected specimen is essential for prognosis and subsequent treatment of the patient. In the context of cancer treatment, this practice, by precluding histological staging of the tumour, is unacceptable. Organ retrieval is one of the most important limitations of minimal access surgery.

## FUTURE DEVELOPMENTAL NEEDS

There are three major developmental needs (Cuschieri 1991). The first concerns the future practice of minimal access surgery. Some operations such as laparoscopic cholecystectomy and appendicectomy will probably be performed by most general surgeons after suitable training. More complex and exacting endoscopic procedures are, however, best performed within specialist centres and in our view there is a need for the recognition of a new surgical specialty of minimal access/invasive surgery. How this would interact with the existing major specialties is the key problem. The most sensible approach would be its integration within these major specialties, e.g. thoracic and thoracoscopic surgery.

Following from the above, there is a need for training programmes both for general surgeons and for experts in the new specialty. Finally, the present endotelevision imaging systems, instrumentation and ancillary technology require development to facilitate and improve the safety of remote surgical manipulations carried out under endoscopic vision.

REFERENCES

Buess G (ed) 1990 Endoskopie: von der diagnostik bis zur neuen Chirurgie. Deutscher Artze-Verlag, Koln
Cuschieri A 1990 Minimal access surgery: the birth of a new era. Journal of the Royal College of Surgeons of Edinburgh 35: 345–347
Cuschieri A 1991 Minimal access surgery and the future of interventional laparoscopy. American Journal of Surgery 161: 404–407
Cuschieri A, Dubois F, Mouiel J et al 1991 The European experience with laparoscopic cholecystectomy. American Journal of Surgery 161: 385–387
Southern Surgical Club 1991 A prospective analysis of 1518 laparoscopic cholecystectomies. New England Journal of Medicine 324: 1073–1078
Wickham J, Fitzpatrick J M 1990 Minimally invasive surgery (editorial). British Journal of Surgery 77: 721

# 14. Adjuncts to surgery

*A. L. G. Peel*

In health service economics an operating suite requires large capital and revenue budgets and this will be favourably influenced by careful management of utilities—thus good care of quality instruments will ensure their long use, appropriate ordering and stocking means the shelf life of equipment is not exceeded, wastage due to change in practice is reduced to a minimum, storage space is efficiently used and the avoidance of an unnecessarily wide range of equipment and materials allows better use of capital. From the medicolegal aspect, the establishment of simple protocols aids efficient management within the theatre complex and helps to reduce errors, such as breakdowns in sterility or retention of swabs or instruments in the patients.

A practical example of the rapidly changing scene in surgical practice is illustrated by orthopaedic surgery where considerable expansion, particularly in prosthetic joint replacement, has occurred and in this field infection can result in very costly failure in terms of patient morbidity and financial implications to the health service. In the attempt to 'abolish' infection in elective orthopaedic surgery the following factors are considered important:

1. Patient screening for occult infection, especially urinary tract infection in females, and rejection of patients with positive carrier status until corrected.

2. Theatre management:

a. A theatre dedicated to orthopaedics in which no dirty or contaminated orthopaedic surgery is carried out and no general surgery whatsoever.

b. The routine use of clean air enclosures. This has resulted in the infection rate in prosthetic joint surgery (hip and knee) falling from 1.5% in the conventionally ventilated theatre to 0.6% (Lidwell et al 1982). Unidirectional air systems, especially with a downflow direction, will reduce bacteria carrying particles from between 400 and 500 m$^{-3}$ down to 30–40 m$^{-3}$. Power tools produce additional problems since they produce an aerosol spray which effectively disseminates bacteria and viral particles.

c. Airborne bacterial dispersion can be further reduced by the use of appropriate fabric clothing. It is not widely appreciated that in either conventional or unidirectional airflow theatres the use of disposable fabric gowns alone in lieu of cotton gowns has not achieved a significant reduction in bacteria-carrying particles. The drawbacks to conventional sterile cotton clothing and gowns are not always appreciated and they fail to prevent:

(i) bacteria being pumped by air through or out of the clothing into the room air

(ii) bacteria being drawn through the clothing by capillary action when wet and thence, by contact transfer, to the wound

(iii) contamination of the surgical team with the patient's fluids.

In addition to fabric gowns the following garments are currently available:

(i) Charnley total-body exhaust gowns
(ii) disposable, non-woven clothing
(iii) breathable plastic membrane fabrics
(iv) close-woven polyester or polycotton fabrics.

Of these, the use of the first is well established in clean orthopaedic surgery; the second, Sonta (manufactured by Du Pont Ltd), has been shown to be effective; the third requires seals at the neck and trouser opening, with the result that the wearer soon becomes hot and uncomfortable. The fourth option is expensive, but represents a significant improvement over conventional garments. Although the cost to the health service would appear to be high, this must be equated with the significant costs of morbidity due to infection. It has been stated that pharmaceutical manufacturing areas would be closed down if they used clothing currently worn in the majority of operating rooms (Whyte, 1991).

3. Theatre technique:

a. Appropriate disinfection of hands in scrubbing up.

b. Closed gloving and routine double gloving in joint replacement and when power tools, wire saws, chisels, etc., are used.

c. Prophylactic antibiotics at induction of anaesthesia and incorporated into the cement.

d. Occlusive dressings to orthopaedic wounds with no disturbance until the wound is healed; transparent dressings allow for inspection of wounds.

## INSTRUMENTS

Surgeons and instrument makers have combined to produce a wide range of instruments. Some, such as certain scissors, forceps and retractors, may be of use in several different fields of surgery. Others are more specific; for instance, those used in anal surgery (Park's anal retractor and Lockhart–Mummery fistula probes) and, although involving modest additional expenditure, their use in conjunction with the inventing surgeon's contributions to both surgical pathology and operative technique have improved the results of surgery in this field. It is important for surgeons, trained or in training, to consider their requirements for instruments and to appreciate the range and potential of different instruments. One advantage of a training rotation scheme is that it allows experience to be gained in a number of surgical disciplines and permits the surgeon to observe the use of instruments in different surgical disciplines; this knowledge can be reapplied to particular problems in whatever field the surgeon subsequently works.

Instruments are a sound investment and, whenever possible, the highest quality should be purchased, but of equal importance is the investment in maintenance care, not forgetting the basics of mechanical and chemical cleansing of the instruments, particularly their hinge joints, adjustment of misalignment and regular sharpening in the case of cutting instruments. In this context the surgeon has a very important role in avoiding trauma to the instruments, an obvious example being to drop them on the theatre floor, and the more subtle, such as avoiding their inappropriate use, e.g. cutting sutures with fine dissecting scissors, or using fine artery forceps to clip bulky 'bites' of tissue or to draw drains through tissues during their insertion or using fine-pointed needle holders to hold large needles, which will irreversibly damage both the points and strain the hinge.

### Sterilization

The majority of instruments are autoclaved (moist heat under pressure for a prescribed time) and this process needs constant monitoring, with care in the packing of the autoclave and verification that the temperature, pressure and time are correct. Where standard autoclaving is impracticable and may cause damage alternatives include:

1. Formaldehyde autoclaving.
2. Ethylene oxide gas sterilization.
3. Prolonged immersion in 2% gluteraldehyde (due to toxicity attention to avoidance of skin contact and adequate ventilation must be ensured). Replacements are currently being researched and an expensive alternative, Steris (Rimmer Bros.), is under evaluation.
4. γ-Irradiation is widely used commercially for non-metallic utilities.

### Instrument sets

It is of considerable advantage to have the instruments required for a particular surgical procedure packed and sterilized in a single set and within this set, as far as possible, each type of instrument should be in multiples of five. Thus each separate design or size of artery forceps may be grouped in separate fives or tens, whereas scissors of differing size and design will be grouped in fives, etc.. A standardized typed list of contents and numbers for each particular tray is routinely retained in the sterilized set. This reduces the number of single packed instruments that require to be opened and, more importantly, simplifies the instrument count at the beginning and end of each procedure.

A suggested instrument plan for a district general hospital theatre complex would be:

1. Basic sets:
   a. minor (70 instruments)
   b. intermediate
   c. major (85 instruments).
2. Supplementary sets, eg thoracotomy, vascular, gastrointestinal, urological and orthopaedic — in the latter the number is large, reflecting the complexity of joint replacement surgery (33 special sets in general surgery, including vascular and urology, compared with 64 in orthopaedic surgery at North Tees District General Hospital in north-east England).
3. Individually packed instruments, e.g. long Nelson scissors or deep Kelly retractor for use in the obese patient.

A close liaison between the Central Sterile Supply Department (CSSD) and theatre management is vital in the provision of adequate supplies of trays to meet the demand of a full schedule of operating lists, particularly when many minor procedures with a quick turnover are carried out.

## LIGATURES, SUTURES, STAPLES AND CLIPS

When selecting a ligature or suture a surgeon may consider several factors with regard to the material itself:

1. whether the material is to be absorbed
2. the tensile strength
3. the thickness
4. the handling and knotting properties
5. the intensity of the body's inflammatory reaction to the material.

A fine, absorbable suture is frequently selected for anastomoses in the gastrointestinal tract, and catgut is being replaced by the more reliable and less reactive synthetic monofilament polydioxanone (PDS, PDS II) or polyglactin 910 (coated Vicryl — the coating comprising glycolide, lactide and calcium steorate). When longer-lasting, maintained tensile strength is required, polymers, such as polyamide (Nylon), polypropylene (Prolene) or polytetrafluoroethylene (PTFE, Goretex) have proved to be of considerable value in, for example, abdominal wound closure and vascular anastomoses.

The majority of sutures are now atraumatic, which facilitates passage through the tissues and also relieves the scrub nurse of the arduous and tedious job of threading needles — the older practice of adding a half hitch at the needle eye to prevent unthreading of the suture is especially traumatic to tissues. Having considered the suture material the surgeon will then make his choice of needle according to:

1. shape — straight or curved and, if the latter, the extent of the circle
2. the tip — round-bodied suitable for suturing viscera or fascia, or cutting for skin suture, or taper cut for penetration of a considerable thickness of tissue or for tissues of different density, e.g. the approximation of intestine and skin at the time of the creation of an ileostomy
3. size and thickness — a knowledge of the requirement is important, thus a slim-blade needle is suitable for subcuticular sutures, but delicate needles may break when suturing more fibrous tissue, e.g. breast.

Steristrips and staples may be used in skin closure and are preferred by many surgeons. The introduction of a variety of staples for use in visceral tissues has also involved a number of changes in practice. The surgeon needs to be aware of the range, the indications and contraindications with each type of instrument, including staple size, differences in design between manufacturers and particularly in those instances where surgical technique needs to be adapted as compared with that for the standard suture procedure. In the author's view staples should be used in preference to sutures only when:

1. the procedure can be carried out with greater immediate safety, e.g. avoiding anastomotic leak, and with no significant increase in later postoperative complications, e.g. stenosis

2. the procedure can be performed more quickly but with equal safety and the surgeon considers that the time factor is of clinical importance, e.g. in the elderly patient undergoing a major procedure, such as oesophagectomy, total cystectomy with creation of an ileal conduit, low anterior resection or a Duhamel procedure, etc..

## SWABS AND PACKS

All cotton or fabric swabs and packs used during surgery must have radio-opaque marking. The size must be appropriate to the procedure and purpose must be defined, e.g. small 'patty' swabs for neurosurgical procedures, narrow swabs for tonsillar surgery for removing blood, large packs or gauze rolls for keeping abdominal viscera out of the operative field or for limiting gross contamination or for haemostatic purposes, such as the raw area after proctocolectomy.

Although haemostasis is usually achieved by electrocoagulation, ligation, undersewing or the use of clips, it is invaluable in certain situations to use certain manufactured haemostatic agents in the presence of a slow ooze. There is a choice between Surgicel® Oxycel® or Sterispon® and, again, experience of the particular properties of each of the above is important, thus the application of Surgicel to the gallbladder bed with overlying pressure from a warm, moist swab controls a slow persistent ooze and allows subsequent removal of the swab, leaving the haemostatic agent undisturbed, whereas in neurosurgery the use of the more delicate Sterispon may be preferred.

## DISPOSABLE ACCESSORIES

Included in this category are accessories that remain on the surface of the body, skin or epithelial lining or those that attain access to the interior of the body usually for a limited time period. It is important to remember that they cause tissue irritation and create a break in the body's defence system:

1. Vascular cannulae and catheters for the administration of intravenous fluids and drugs, central venous and arterial access lines for use in pressure monitoring or biochemical analysis, and parenteral feeding catheters; adjuncts to arterial surgery, such as Fogarty embolectomy catheters.

2. Urological catheters and stents.

3. Oesophageal stents for strictures; nasogastric and the less commonly used intestinal decompression tubes; fine-bore enteral feeding tubes and hepatobiliary/pancreatic tubes and stents.

4. Stoma appliances.

5. Neurological valved shunts.

6. Drains which are most frequently manufactured from polyvinyl chloride and designed to transmit fluid from the operative area, or a body cavity or compartment to the exterior either as an open system, which is more liable to bacterial contamination, or a closed system with a reduced pressure within the container that not only encourages effective drainage but reduces contamination. The reader may consider the following points in relation to the use of drains:

a. evidence that a drain is helpful to the patient rather than making the surgeon feel more comfortable

b. the material of the drain, e.g. the danger of polyvinyl chloride drains when used as a biliary T-tube for a relatively short time (ten days) that does not allow the formation of an adequate 'walled-off' tract. The latter is important in limiting the intraperitoneal dispersal of any bile on withdrawal of the tube; red rubber tubes, now rarely used, cause severe local inflammation

c. the particular purpose of the drain and consequently the size and design that will be most efffective, e.g. if escape of pancreatic enzymes is anticipated a tube drain would have considerable advantage over a Yeate's or corrugated drain

d. care in the insertion of the drain:

(i) the avoidance of visceral or vascular injury during passage through the patient's tissues or parietes

(ii) the avoidance of injury to the surgeon or assistant.

## ENDOSCOPES

The development of endoscopes and their application in diagnosis and therapy continues to advance — instruments are applicable to the upper and lower respiratory tracts, the upper and lower alimentary tracts (including the biliary tree and pancreas), the upper and lower urinary tracts, the female genital tract, the peritoneum and arteries. Design modifications have resulted in a wide range of instruments with considerable therapeutic capabilities, but nevertheless require a large number of specialized accessories such as laparoscopic surgery, and both space and expertise are necessary for storage and maintenance. Cleaning, decontamination and disinfection of flexible fibre-optic endoscopes are essential to avoid transmission of infection, particularly viral, e.g. hepatitis B, HIV. Problems with gluteraldehyde and duration of immersion (20 minutes) need consideration. Modern cystoscopes, for instance, may now be autoclaved.

It should not be forgotten, however, that a knowledge of the simple instruments, such as a proctoscope and anal retractor, e.g. Park's or Eisenheimer, will also benefit the general surgeon and his patient.

## PRECAUTIONS AGAINST LOSS OF INSTRUMENTS OR SWABS

The following precautionary measures are essential:

1. The correct organization of instrument trays, with the limitation of the number of individually packed instruments as far as possible.

2. The arrangement of swabs and packs in 'fives' bound together with red cotton or, if small, carefully packaged, e.g. on a safety pin.

3. Checking the number of instruments on trays against printed lists incorporated in each pack.

4. Record all sutures, swabs, packs, needles and extras clearly and legibly on a board in the theatre.

5. The use of special swab racks, including the modern disposable wallets, facilitates the count after long complex operations where many swabs are used and staff become fatigued.

6. The radio-opaque marking of non-implantable non-metallic equipment could be usefully marked in this way, but is variable, e.g. drains, laporomat.

7. The theatre record book is signed by the scrubbed and assistant nurses.

8. The surgeon should record and sign that the count was correct at the end of the operation note in the patient's records.

The way to reduce errors is to establish a simple, well-disciplined routine of accountability, including a permanent and accurately maintained record.

## IMPLANT MATERIALS

Prosthetic surgery continues to expand and perhaps the greatest impact has been in orthopaedic surgery, where successful joint replacement is well established in the hip, knee and interphalangeal joints and to a more limited extent in the shoulder and elbow joints. Prosthetic implants are also used widely in general, vascular, cardiac, urological, plastic and other branches of surgery and there is wide variation in the materials used. Basic considerations and principles apply:

1. Ease and reliability of manufacture and cost.

2. Appropriate tensile strength and durability, e.g. some joint replacements need revision after a number of years due to wear and tear, causing fragmentation.

3. Reaction between prosthetic materials themselves or the body tissues, e.g. the metal and plastic components of certain artificial hip replacements or between the joint prosthesis, cement and the bone.

4. Platelet aggregation and plasma protein precipitation that occur around intravascular prostheses.

5. The degree of incorporation into the body. Both metallic and silicone implants are surrounded by a collagen capsule but PTFE (Goretex) allows the ingrowth of fibroblasts.

### Implant materials in orthopaedic surgery

1. Surgical-grade stainless steel is used for joint replacement bearing surfaces, plates, screws and wires.

2. Alloys, including Vitallium, are also used in joint replacement surfaces, wires and, less frequently now, in plates, owing to the preference for compression steel plating for internal fixation.

3. High-density polyethylene (ultra-high molecular weight) is used for joint replacement bear-

ing surfaces to articulate with steel or Vitallium.

4. Silicone is used for hinge-type joint replacement, but not in bearing surfaces where debris produces a synovitis. It has been very successful in metacarpophalangeal and proximal interphalangeal joints.

5. Dacron and PTFE are materials that can be used under tension, e.g. synthetic ligament repair. Carbon fibre has been abandoned due to fragmentation and foreign body reaction.

## The risk of infection

This is one of the most serious complications of prosthetic surgery and the following risk factors must be considered:

1. immune compromised host
2. active infection present elsewhere in the host or in contacts
3. positive carrier state in patient or staff
4. cross-infection in hospital
5. failure of sterilization and/or packaging
6. inadequate air ventilation in the operating theatre and ineffectual operating theatre clothing
7. poor operative technique with contamination, poor haemostasis or ischaemic tissue.

The time-scale of presentation is of significance, and this is one of the areas where late infection up to a year or more after surgery may occur, particularly with the deep insertion of a prosthesis. The implant itself can be of significance: whereas a smooth surface is bacteriostatic and non-wettable, a textured surface allows the entrapment of blood, serum, particles and bacteria in the crevices.

In deep infection occurring late around implants, e.g. hip, the bacteria may produce changes: *Staphylococcus aureus* produces a thickening of the capsule and *Staphylococcus epidermidis* produces a polysaccharide slime. The prosthesis becomes loose, causes pain and may need removal.

When considering the use of an implant the surgeon should first be convinced that there is not a natural alternative. Thus in vascular surgery vein grafts are preferred for certain lower limb arterial bypass surgery, infra-inguinal bypass (especially below-knee femoropopliteal bypass).

Synthetic materials, Dacron (collagen-coated knitted Dacron) or Goretex (PTFE) may be used, particularly where large vessels need to be bypassed or replaced.

## Tissue response to foreign material

Tissue reaction varies according to the material and the roughness of the surface — thus marked inflammatory response with micro-abscess formation occurs around a buried silk or linen knot, but by comparison minimal response occurs around polypropylene, with not only a reduced likelihood of bacterial infection but also increased tensile strength dependent on the material and the lack of surrounding tissue inflammatory infiltrate.

Silicone forms a capsule — fibroblasts orientate themselves to the surface of the foreign material and the collagen is formed in mirror image to the specific surface. Fibroblasts cease to secrete collagen when they are in contact with other fibroblasts, but not when in contact with other cells. Thus over a smooth surface sheets of collagen are produced with increased contractile force of the capsule. Gradually, fibroblastic activity on the free surface subsides, collagen deposition is completed and moulding takes place, producing a mature capsule at approximately three months after surgery. Collagen production against the smooth inner capsular surface continues due to the fibroblasts not being in contact with each other and as a result the cavity diameter decreases and contractile force increases. By comparison roughened surfaces allow fibroblasts to conform to the crevices; the fibres of collagen are then orientated at random with counteracting contractile forces and the fibroblasts lie in different planes and directions, which allows a greater chance of contact with each other, thus reducing the collagen deposition and resulting in a thinner capsule. Silicone particles are found in phagocytes in the capsule wall adjacent to lymphatic vessels, in the outer layer of capsules, and may reach the lumen of lymphatic vessels since they are found in regional lymph nodes.

Metal-on-metal joint replacement produces small particulate debris which is incorporated into the synovium, producing foreign body giant cells.

Acrylic cement, polymethylmethacrylate, used in fixation of prostheses, becomes encapsulated by fibrous tissue, the inner layer of which is sometimes hyaline and acellular and sometimes contains histiocytes and multinucleate giant cells. No evidence for malignant transformation or chronic inflammatory reaction with sinus formation exists (Charnley 1970). Revisional surgery of the cemented prosthesis is difficult. Alternatives under trial are based on isoelastic or mesh coating of the prosthesis to allow fibrous tissue to grow in.

## TISSUE GLUES

Research into new methods of surgical tissue repair has yielded the prospect of using tissue glues. One such method is fibrin adhesion, based on the conversion of fibrinogen into fibrin on a tissue surface by the action of thrombin. The fibrin is then cross-linked by factor XIIIA to create a firm stable fibrin network with good adhesive properties.

The indications are for tissue adhesion, haemostasis and suture support. In general and abdominal surgery it may be used in patients where there has been trauma or surgical resection of either the liver, spleen or pancreas, after cholecystectomy to aid haemostasis and healing of the gallbladder bed, to support difficult anastomoses such as pancreaticojejunostomy after Whipple's operation (pancreaticoduodenectomy) and anastomoses of the small and large bowel. In the specialties it has been particularly useful in neurosurgery for repair of dural tears, thus sealing leakage of cerebrospinal fluid, and in securing haemostasis when there is bleeding from the cerebral surface. It is also useful in peripheral neural anastomoses. In orthopaedic and trauma surgery it is useful for reattachment of osteochondral fragments, in acetabuloplasty when using cement-free hip joint prostheses and in certain tendon and ligament repairs. In cardio-vascular surgery it has also proved useful for sealing anastomotic suture lines and in the placement of patches, in bypass surgery, valve replacement surgery and prosthetic implantation. It has been used with success in sealing accidental injury to the thoracic duct. It is also applicable in ophthalmic surgery, in cataract operations and in ear, nose and throat surgery, again for sealing CSF leaks and in plastic operations on the tympanic membrane. It is undergoing assessment in urology for suture support and also for haemostasis, particularly after transurethral resection of the prostate. In plastic surgery it has found considerable application in securing skin grafts.

There has been concern that the use of human fibrinogen and factor XIII might allow the transmission of viral agents such as hepatitis B, hepatitis C or HIV. Commercial inactiviation of a virus is achieved by pasteurization with purification of the proteins and then heating the solution for 10 hours at 60°C. Laboratory studies have demonstrated that this process not only inactivates the hepatitis B virus, HIV virus, but also herpes simplex and cytomegalovirus.

Marked arterial or venous bleeding renders the system ineffective. Hypersensitivity reactions have been described. The process is under evaluation in the UK.

### ACKNOWLEDGEMENTS

My gratitude to Sister J Knott SRN for extracting current data relating to usage and costs and to Mr John Stothard FRCS for his help with regard to orthopaedic surgery.

### REFERENCES

Charnley J 1970 Acrylic cement in orthopaedic surgery. E and S Livingstone, Edinburgh
Lidwell O H, Lowbury E J L, Whyte W et al 1982 Effect of ultraclean air in operating rooms in deep sepsis in the joint after total hip or knee replacement: a randomised study. British Medical Journal 285: 10–14
Whyte W 1991 Operating theatre clothing: a review. Surgical Infection 3: 14–17

# 15. Transplantation

*P. McMaster    L. J. Buist*

## BASIC PRINCIPLES

Early Christian legends attest to the attempts by man to replace diseased or destroyed organs or tissues by the transfer from another individual. The father of modern surgery, John Hunter, carried out extensive experiments on the 'transposition of tissues' and concluded what he thought were successful experiments on the transposition of teeth! However, it was not until the dawn of the twentieth century that the practical technical realities of organ transfer were combined with sufficient understanding of the immunological mechanisms involved to allow transplantation to become a practical reality.

While it had long been recognized that successful blood transfusion was in large measure dependent on matching donor and recipient cells, it was only in the 1950s that Mitchison (1953) demonstrated that while cell-mediated immunity was responsible for early destruction and rejection, it was the humoral mechanism with cytotoxic antibodies that was primarily involved in the host response to foreign tissue.

It became increasingly recognized that all tissue and fluid transfer was governed by basic immunomechanisms (Table 15.1)

**Table 15.1** Forms of tissue transfer

| Transfer of tissue | Transfer of solid organ |
| --- | --- |
| Blood | Skin |
| Bone marrow | Cornea |
| | Kidney |
| | Heart |
| | Liver |
| | Pancreas |

The need in the Second World War to find improved ways of treating badly burned pilots led Gibson & Medawar (1943) to carry out a series of classic experiments on skin transplantation. They were able to conclude that the transfer of skin from one part of the body to another in the same individual — an autograft — survived indefinitely, whereas the transfer of skin from another individual — an allograft — was in due course destroyed and that the recipient retained memory of the donor tissue and further transfers or allografts were destroyed in an accelerated mechanism. Thus the wider recognition of the universal acceptance of autografts became realized, whereas the failure of an allograft was recognized as part of an immune response.

An alternative source of organs is, of course, the animal world and the transfer from another species is known as a xenograft.

## FIRST CLINICAL PROGRAMMES

The recognition that an autograft would be universally acceptable led to the first successful attempts at organ grafting in man. Murray et al (1955) at the Peter Bent Brigham Hospital in Boston in the early 1950s was able to demonstrate the successful transfer of a kidney graft from an identical twin with acceptance and successful function, and to develop a programme of renal transplantation between monozygotic twins. Living related organ transfer continues to be the most successful form of grafting without the need to alter the recipient's immune mechanism, as it fails to recognize the donor tissue as 'foreign'.

Some of the recipients of kidney transplants

from identical twins remained well more than 30 years after grafting. However, grafts between un- related living individuals performed by this same group invariably failed, although not as quickly as experimental studies might have suggested.

## RESPONSE

The other major human source of organs, other than from living relatives, is from individuals who have died as a result of road traffic accidents or cerebral injuries. Cadaveric organ grafting from non-related individuals is now the major source of organs. Within Europe more than 90% of all organs transplanted are from brain-dead donors.

Thus, although technical consideration pre- sented the initial formidable barrier to organ transfer, it was increasingly the understanding of the immune response causing organ destruction by rejection which led to clinical schedules per- mitting practical transplantation services to be established.

The body's immune response to destroy the 'invading' organ we now recognize as rejection.

## REJECTION

Early experimental studies involving tissue trans- fer suggested genetic regulation of the rejection process. It was suggested in the 1930s that rejec- tion was a response to specific foreign antigens (alloantigens) and that they were similar to blood groups of other species. The development of inbred lines of experimental animal models allowed the demonstration of antigens present on red blood cells and the concept of histocompatability. This suggestion of an immunological theory of tissue transplantation stimulated Medawar's (1944) work in rabbits and later in mice and led to simi- lar studies in man with the discovery of the human leucocyte antigen (HLA) system.

Further experimental studies defined the con- cept of rejection into three primary categories: hyper-acute rejection, which can occur in a matter of hours due to preformed antibodies in a sensitized recipient; acute rejection, which takes place in a few days or weeks and is usually caused by cellular mechanisms; and finally chronic rejec- tion, which occurs over months or years and

remains largely undefined, but involves primarily humoral antibodies. A detailed review of experi- mental and modern transplantation biology is quite beyond the scope of such a monograph, but increasing understanding of this area will allow more refined changes in rejection management and increasingly successful organ grafting.

## AVOIDING REJECTION

The degree of disparity between donor and recip- ient is an important key element in the severity of the immune rejection response. In xenografting (transfer between species) the presence of pre- formed antibodies leads to rapid endothelial dam- age, causing vascular thrombosis, gross interstitial swelling and necrosis of the graft, all within a matter, usually, of hours.

Similarly, when transfer occurs between human beings, the degree of compatability between donor and recipient is important to the success or otherwise of the graft.

As indicated earlier, transfer between identical twins is associated with universal success without the need to modulate the immune mechanism. However, transfer between non-identical relatives or using cadaveric organs produces the recogni- tion of 'non-self' by the recipient and the mount- ing of an immune response. It is the avoidance or modification of this immune response which has been the main target over the last 25 years and the avoidance of overwhelming rejection a prime goal.

Two approaches have been taken to the problem: *tissue typing*, and *reduction of immune response*.

### Tissue Typing

In the method to match the donor and recipient more closely the concept of typing has become widely developed. Early work demonstrating that blood transfusion was dependent on matching between donor and recipient was extended into experimental and then clinical transplantation studies in the 1960s and 1970s.

The human chromosome 6 contains the genet- ically determined major histocompatability com- plex (MHC), i.e. the HLA-A, HLA-B, HLA-C (class 1) and HLA-DR (D-related; class 2) loci.

A whole series of additional genetic regions have been linked to the HLA complex, although in clinical terms these are probably less significant.

Thus it has become increasingly possible, using serological studies, to genetically map an individual on the basis of the HLA region of this chromosome. Since one chromosome is inherited from each parent and each individual has two HLA haplotypes there is a 25% chance that two siblings will share both haplotypes (i.e. identical) and by standard and Mendelian inheritance a 50% chance that they will share one haplotype. Thus in first-degree relatives when the donor and recipient are matched for HLA-A and B antigens there is an excellent likelihood of graft success, whereas because of the complexity of the MHC allele, the wide divergence of antigens and random cadaveric donors, even if matched for one or two antigens, there may still be very substantial disparity.

Thus, in order to avoid rejection, the concept of tissue typing — trying to more accurately match donor and recipients — has gained wide acceptance. Serological methods allow class 1 HLA antigens to be defined using typed serum obtained from nulliparous women. Using a microcytotoxicity assay multiple antisera against HLA-A, B, C, and DR antigens are provided on Terasaki trays and then frozen until needed. When needed the trays are thawed and the donor lymphocyte cells are added to the wells containing complement and the antisera against specific HLA types. If the antibody causes the cells to lyse, acridine orange (a dye) enters the damaged cell and appears orange under fluorescence microscopy. Thus using microcytotoxicity tests it is possible to identify quite rapidly the HLA class 1 antigens present in a donor.

Class 2 antigen typing until recently required a mixed leucocyte reaction to determine individual constituents, but more recent techniques have avoided this laborious investigation.

From the clinical standpoint the practical importance of identification of the degree of compatibility between donor and recipient is clearly defined in many organ grafting systems. Cadaveric grafting can only achieve this level when beneficially matched donor and recipient pairs, in which all major class 1 and class 2 antigens are identical, are grafted. This so-called 'full house' HLA match can give one year cadaveric graft survival approaching 90%. However, this is only when combined with chemical non-specific immunosuppression.

When grafts are transferred between donor and recipient with a complete mismatch an additional 20–25% of grafts will be lost over the ensuing five years. Thus, in cadaveric grafting the degree of matching has an important role in determining the severity of the immune response and ultimate success or otherwise of the graft.

Nevertheless, no matter how good the matching is in cadaveric situations modulation of the immune response continues to be necessary to ensure graft survival.

## Reduction of immune response

Reduction in the immune response occurs frequently in clinical practice in such situations as uraemia, profound jaundice and in patients with advanced malignancy and AIDS. The controlled reduction of an immune response to foreign antigen on graft requires careful clinical judgement. Initial attempts using widespread radiation produced severe depletion of not just lymphocytes, but also a pancytopenia, and although skin grafts and other organs were readily accepted immunologically by the recipients the majority of patients quickly died from overwhelming infection.

A refinement of this technique in which partial lymphocyte irradiation was used has been successful experimentally and in clinical practice, for depleting the immune response so that grafts can be accepted.

### Chemical immunosuppression

Since the mid-1950s the primary mode of immunomodulation has been the administration of chemical agents. A demonstration by Hitchings & Elion (1959) over 40 years ago that 6-mercaptopurine had immunosuppressive potential allowed Schwartz & Dameschek (1959) to treat rabbits stimulated by foreign antigen. The treated animals did not produce antibodies to the antigen stimulation and work by Calne in 1960 showed that 6-mecaptopurine could also inhibit the immune response in dogs. A number of other agents were studied at that time and of clear benefit were steroids, reducing the cellular response, and eventually azothioprine showed improved results when compared to 6-mercaptopurine.

For more than 20 years chemical immuno-modulation with the combination of steroids (prednisolone) and azothioprine was to be the main non-specific immunosuppressant used. They inhibited the immune response largely by depressing circulating T-cells.

The production of antilymphocytic globulin by sensitization in animals was also demonstrated to inhibit the immune response, although variability and efficacy limited its clinical use.

## Cyclosporin

Clearly the ultimate goal of selectively inhibiting the recipient's immune response remains a long way off and in clinical practice non-specific agents continue to be used. In 1976 Borel working in Sandoz laboratories assessed the potent immunosuppressive properties of cyclosporin A, a cyclical peptide with 11 amino acids. The demonstration of both the in vitro and in vivo immunosuppressive activity was quickly followed by extended clinical studies. It was clearly demonstrated that cyclosporin could suppress both antibody production and cell-mediated immunity, exhibiting a selective inhibitory effect on T-cell-dependent responses. Of critical importance was the observation that the drug was neither profoundly lympho- nor myelotoxic and had no influence on the viability of the mature T-cells or the antibody-producing B-cells.

## CURRENT CLINICAL IMMUNOSUPPRESSIVE USE

For nearly 25 years the mainstay of clinical immunosuppression was the combined use of steroids and azothioprine. With increasing clinical experience it became possible to adjust the dosage of these agents so that in many individuals it was possible to maintain 'immunosuppression' and thus prevent rejection, while minimizing the risk to the recipient of over immunomodulation — a delicate balance, which requires considerable clinical skill.

Patients receiving steroids and azothioprine required careful, meticulous monitoring for signs of early infection and the presence of organ rejection. Progressive reduction in haemopoietic production leads to thrombocytopenia and leucopenia, with the attendant risk of infection, bacterial, fungal and viral. The major complications of long-term steroid and azothioprine immunosuppression are outlined in Table 15.2.

**Table 15.2**  Side-effects of steroids and azothioprine

| Side-effects of steroids | Side-effects of azothioprine |
| --- | --- |
| Avascular necrosis of bones | Bone marrow suppression |
| Diabetes | Polycythaemia |
| Obesity | Hepatotoxicity |
| Cushing's syndrome | |
| Pancreatitis | |
| Cataract | |
| Skin problems | |
| Psychosis | |

Thus, considerable clinical skill was needed to avoid the risks of infection, and in cadaveric grafting, when the degree of matching between donor and recipient was often less than optimal, death from infection was the commonest cause of patient loss in the first three months after grafting. In addition, the need to administer steroids continually became a major limiting factor, particularly in children, where the complications of steroids could be so crippling. (Table 15.3).

**Table 15.3**  Side-effects of steroids in children

| |
| --- |
| Growth retardation |
| Cushingoid appearance |
| Diabetes |
| Obesity |

The results of organ grafting using prednisolone and azothioprine left much to be desired and so the introduction of cyclosporin into clinical trials in the early 1980s was an important step forward in the more selective use of immunomodulation. Not only could steroids be minimized or avoided in some individuals, but pancytopenia was rarely encountered. Nevertheless cyclosporin was rapid-

**Table 15.4**   Side-effects of cyclosporin

Nephrotoxicity
Hepatotoxicity
Tremors, convulsions
Skin problems
Gingival hypertrophy
Haemolytic anemia
Hypertension
Malignant change

ly found to have its own attendant problems and difficulties and nephrotoxicity remains a persistent problem. (Table 15.4).

With increasing clinical experience, however, many of these toxic effects can now be minimized such that excellent rehabilitation can be achieved and organs can now be grafted which previously would have been unsuccessful in the prednisolone and azotioprine era. The overall results of cyclosporin will be outlined in the individual sections, but there have been no clinical series in which the results of cyclosporin have been inferior to the treatment with azothioprine and prednisolone and for the most part an improved benefit of between 15% and 20% of graft survival at one year has been reported.

Postoperative monitoring of all patients with transplanted organs involves regulation of the immunosuppressive regime, detection of the development of organ rejection and constant vigilance for signs of infection.

## CADAVERIC ORGAN DONATION

The concept of the diagnosis of brain death and increased awareness by both the public and doctors alike of the need for organ donation have improved the supply of cadaveric organs for grafting. In the UK about a third of patients who become organ donors have died from spontaneous intracranial haemorrhage, although head injuries and road traffic accidents also provide a significant number.

## SPECIFIC ORGAN TRANSPLANTATION

### KIDNEY

Kidney transplantation is now well established as the most effective way of helping patients with end-stage renal failure. Despite a significant expansion in the number of kidney transplants, long waiting lists exist for those on dialysis awaiting treatment. In the UK an integrated approach has shown a steady increase in the proportion of patients treated by transplantation, such that nearly 50% of patients now have a functioning transplant.

### Patient selection

With kidney transplantation affording the optimal quality of rehabilitation few patients will be denied the prospect, although the patient's age and underlying renal condition may need to be taken into account.

### Age

In general children do very well after transplantation, although infants below the age of 5 years present a more controversial issue because of the difficulty of management of immunosuppressive agents. The newer immunosuppressive regimes, however, allow adequate growth and physical development. The goal for children must be the establishment of normal renal function before maturity and to take full advantage of the growth spurt that occurs at puberty.

While in the early days patients over the age of 55 were frequently denied transplantation, many centres now offer renal transplantation to patients over 65 or 70 years. Patient and graft survival has been very satisfactory in this group but immunosuppressive schedules frequently need to be reduced in the elderly to ensure overwhelming infection does not occur.

### Renal disease

Renal transplantation is now offered for many primary and secondary renal conditions resulting in chronic renal failure, including glomerulonephritis, pyelonephritis and polycystic disease. Some types of autoimmune glomerulonephritis antibodies have been demonstrated to cause damage to the transplanted kidney but this is not a contraindication to transplantation since probably less than 10% of grafts will be seriously injured.

## Assessment of potential recipient

Careful review of both the physical and psychological status of the patient is needed prior to transplantation and factors which may increase the hazards of surgery or immunosuppressive management require evaluation. Patients in renal failure frequently suffer from cardiovascular problems — hypertension with left ventricular hypertrophy, coronary artery disease — and the symptoms are increased by anaemia. There is a high incidence of peptic ulceration in uraemic patients and of metabolic bone disease, causing renal osteodystrophy. All these associated conditions must be optimally treated or controlled prior to transplantation surgery. Sources of underlying or potential infection such as an infected urinary tract or peritoneal cavity from peritoneal dialysis must be irradicated or treated and the patient's status for viruses such as hepatitis B, HIV and cytomegalovirus must be known to minimize activation following immunosuppression. Careful surgical review related to previous abdominal operations, peripheral vascular ischaemia, or the presence of ileal conduits following previous urogenital surgery needs also to be carefully taken into account and a surgical plan initiated.

Careful counselling and support are also needed to ensure that the patient understands and is prepared for transplantation.

## Surgical technique

The technique of renal implantation has remained unchanged now for nearly 40 years, with the donor kidney being implanted extraperitoneally in one of the iliac fossae. The renal artery is anastomosed to either the internal or external iliac artery and the renal vein to the recipient's external iliac vein. The donor ureter is then implanted into the recipient's bladder. Over 100 000 kidney grafts have been performed around the world but total transplantation rates vary significantly from one country to another.

## Postoperative problems

Monitoring of the kidney allograft is required to detect signs of rejection, suggested by a reduction in urinary output and an elevation in serum creatinine, then confirmed by biopsy or aspiration cytology. This allows the prompt recognition of acute rejection crisis and its treatment by steroids.

With increased clinical experience the hurdles of acute rejection and infectious complications can usually be overcome and patient survival at one year is in excess of 95% in many programmes, with over 85% of kidney grafts functioning well. However, a steady attrition of renal grafts will occur over the next ten years, so that only just half of all renal transplants will be functioning well at ten years, with many having been lost from the slow process of chronic rejection.

Rehabilitation can be spectacular, allowing patients the freedom to eat without restriction of salt, protein or potassium, the resolution of anaemia and infertility and an improvement in overall sense of well-being.

Renal transplantation in the diabetic patient can be combined with pancreas transplantation, with implantation of the whole organ and drainage of the pancreatic duct into the gastrointestinal tract or the urinary bladder. Transplantation of isolated pancreatic islets is in its infancy.

## HEART

While the patient afflicted by renal disease has the benefit of chronic haemodialysis, the individual with progressive cardiac problems has no life support system and death invariably ensues unless cardiac transplantation is undertaken. Initial efforts in the late 1960s by Barnard (1967) have led to a progressive expansion of increasingly successful programmes. The majority of patients will suffer from cardiomyopathy, terminal ischaemic cardiac disease or more rarely some congenital form of cardiac disease. Donor selection must be rigorous because immediate life-sustaining function is required of the graft.

Orthotopic replacement of the diseased heart has been the most frequently undertaken procedure, although the heterotopic placement of auxiliary cardiac implants has been undertaken. The donor atria are anastomosed to the posterior walls of the corresponding chambers of the recipient prior to joining the pulmonary artery and the aorta.

Postoperative cardiac function is monitored and endomyocardial biopsy allows histological examination of heart muscle for ventricular cellular infiltration indicative of acute rejection.

While the early attempts at cardiac grafting resulted in poor overall survival, the situation has improved remarkably. One-year survival of over 85% and a five-year survival of 60% of patients with excellent quality of rehabilitation is most encouraging.

This solid foundation of cardiac grafting inevitably led to an extension to combined heart and lung transplantation, primarily for those suffering from pulmonary hypertension, or for some terminal lung diseases, such as cystic fibrosis or emphysema. If the recipient has lung disease but a good functioning heart on recipient of a combined heart–lung graft the heart from the first recipient can be implanted into a second cardiac patient — the 'domino' procedure. As a result of technical advances transplantation of single lung is now possible. Because of the risk of infection in the implanted lungs immunosuppressive management is critical. Sputum cytology and even lung biopsy may be needed to differentiate infection from rejection. In spite of this, the Standard University Series now reports two-year survival of over 60% in heart–lung recipients.

## LIVER

Although first attempts at liver transplantation occurred in the early 1960s, the formidable technical, preservation, immunological and organ availability difficulties meant that it was only in the early 1980s that successful programmes were established. The majority of adult patients coming to liver grafting have extensive cirrhosis (primary biliary cirrhosis, chronic active hepatitis and hepatitis B) or less frequently primary liver cancer. In the paediatric group the most common indication for liver transplantation is biliary atresia.

The liver is particularly susceptible to ischaemic injury and the ability to harvest and store livers for only a few hours led to an extremely complex surgical procedure, under-

taken often in the most difficult emergency situations.

The liver is placed orthotopically after removal of the diseased organ, and to reduce the physiological changes during the anhepatic phase venovenous bypass is employed.

Improvements in organ preservation (principally the introduction of University of Wisconsin solution) mean that livers can now be stored from 12 to 14 hours and transferred from one country to another. The evidence that tissue matching is important in liver grafting has yet to be fully established, but as in other forms of transplantation may be important.

Patients coming to liver grafting are frequently critically ill with multisystem failure, and the complexity of the operation inevitably has meant that technical failures have been frequent. In spite of this, results have continued to improve and with nearly 7000 liver transplants performed in Europe alone and one-year survival of over 75%, liver transplantation is increasingly being established as one of the most effective modalities of treatment for liver disease. In some groups the results have shown even more impressive improvement. Infants and children with biliary atresia undergoing grafting stand a more than 90% chance of one-year survival, with the majority going on for many years. The longest survivor is now over 20 years after transplantation.

The major limiting factor in liver grafting now is donor availability and while in the UK some 380 grafts were performed in 1990, the need is probably double that. The most acute shortage is of paediatric organs and often a larger liver has to be divided and only part transplanted into a child.

## ETHICAL ISSUES

The development of transplantation in the 1950s and 1960s caught not just the imagination of the medical profession but the public as well, and led to the reappraisal of fundamental beliefs in many areas. The concept of death was challenged from the traditional one of the cessation of the heart beat to that of the concept of brain stem death, and wide public and professional debates ensued. Death, the great taboo of the twentieth century, was addressed in a new fundamental way. The majority of countries enacted legislation or medical guidelines identifying new criteria which would allow more effective recognition of an individual's incapacity to regain essential and vital functions. Some of these issues were challenged in courts of law and were often widely reported in the media.

Thus ethical and moral issues were raised from the very outset of organ grafting. With the increasing success of organ transplantation these pressures have grown. The rights of the individual to dispose of his or her own organs as wished has been a matter of debate and the profession has loudly condemned the commercialism which is in danger of entering clinical practice. The purchase or sale of organs is now condemned by almost all international transplantation organizations.

Should a living individual during his lifetime voluntarily donate an organ to another? The first successful grafts between identical twins from within a family were clearly perceived to be an act of great charity and compassion. Living kidney grafting in the USA accounts for more than a third of all grafts, but should such altruism be permitted between non-familiar members, or those in whom a loving and caring bond does not exist? These new issues continue to be addressed by society.

One other issue has particularly focused on cardiac and liver transplantation and this relates to the consumption of economic resources for an individual. In the UK the cost of renal transplantation in total is approximately £8000–£10 000, whereas the cost of dialysis per year per patient approaches £15 000. While renal transplantation is clearly the most cost-effective way of dealing with renal failure compared with some other forms of medical and surgical treatment and perhaps health care initiative, it is seen as being 'expensive'. Cardiac and liver transplantation can equally be seen to consume an inappropriate amount of the health resources available in some areas, and indeed the State of Oregon has now withdrawn financial support from liver transplantation programmes, giving them a very low priority compared with their other health schedules.

Each new development in science and clinical medicine raises its own issues which need to be addressed, and as these modalities of treatment spread to other countries different cultural approaches may be required. It will be for the individual community to decide whether such treatments are appropriate for its fellow human beings and what extent of resources can be made available.

Clinical organ transplantation has evolved rapidly over the last 25 years, affording treatment to many thousands of patients who would otherwise be dead or enduring an existence of chronic illness. Further advances are sought in the fight against the recipient immune response and to procure donor organs of the highest quality, thus enabling even more patients to experience the increasing benefits of transplantation.

REFERENCES

Barnard C N 1967 The operation. A human cardiac transplant: an interim report of a successful operation performed at Groote Schuur Hospital, Cape Town. South African Medical Journal 41: 1271–1274
Borel J F, Feurer C, Gubler H U, Stahelin A 1976 Biological effects of cyclosporin A: a new antilymphocytic agent. Agents and Actions 6: 468–475
Calne R Y 1960. The rejection of renal homografts: inhibition in dogs by 6-mercaptopurine. Lancet i: 417–418
Gibson T, Medawar P B 1943 The fate of skin homografts in man. Journal of Anatomy 77: 299–309
Hitchings G H, Elion G B 1959, Activity of heterocyclic derivatives of 6-mercaptopurine and 6-thioguanine in adenocarcinoma 755. Proceedings of the American Association for Cancer Research 3: 27
Medawar P B 1944 Behaviour and fate of skin autografts and skin homografts in rabbits. Journal of Anatomy 78: 176–99
Mitchison N A 1953 Passive transfer of transplantation immunity. Nature 171: 267–268
Murray J E, Merrill J P, Harrison J H 1955 Renal homotransplantation in identical twins. Surgery Forum 6: 423–426
Schwartz R, Dameschek W 1959 Drug induced immunological tolerance. Nature 183: 1682–1683

# 16. Fluid, electrolyte and acid–base balance

*W. Aveling*

## FLUID COMPARTMENTS

Every medical student knows that man is mostly water. For the surgeon, the key to fluid and electrolyte balance is a knowledge of the various fluid compartments. An adult male is 60% water, a female, having more fat, is 55% water, newborn infants are 75% water. The most important compartments are the intracellular fluid (ICF) — 55% of body water — and the extracellular fluid (ECF) – 45%. ECF is further subdivided into the plasma (part of the intravascular space), the interstitial fluid, the transcellular water (e.g. fluid in the gastrointestinal tract, the cerebrospinal fluid (CSF) and aqueous humour) and water associated with bone and dense connective tissue which is less readily exchangeable and of much less importance. The partitioning of the total body water (TBW) with average values for a 70 kg male, who would contain 42 litres of water, is shown in Figure 16.1 (Edelman & Leibman 1959).

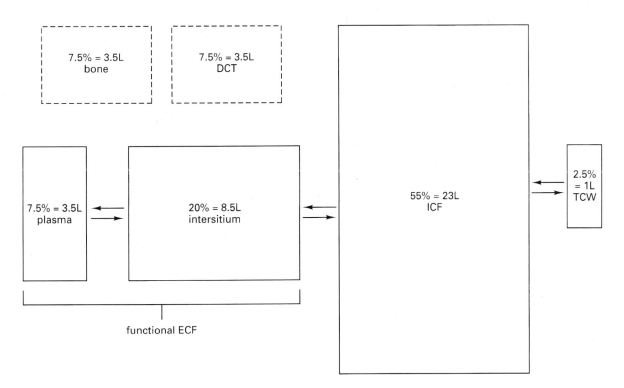

**Fig. 16.1** Distribution of total body water in a 70 kg man. ECF, extracellular fluid; ICF, intracellular fluid; DCT, dense connective tissue; TCW, transcellular water.

To understand fluid balance one needs to know from which compartment or compartments fluid is being lost in various situations, and in which compartments fluids will end up when administered to the patient. For practical purposes we need only consider the plasma, the interstitial space, the intracellular space and the barriers between them.

## The capillary membrane

The barrier between the plasma and interstitium is the capillary endothelium, which allows the free passage of water and electrolytes (small particles) but restricts the passage of larger molecules such as proteins (the colloids). Although no one has demonstrated holes in the membrane, capillaries behave as if they had pores of 40–50 Å in most tissues. Kidney and liver have larger pores and brain capillaries are relatively impermeable. The osmotic pressure generated by the presence of colloids on one side of a membrane which is impermeable to them is known as the colloid osmotic pressure (COP). Only a small quantity of albumin (mol. wt 69 000) crosses the membrane and it is mainly responsible for the difference in COP between the plasma and the interstitum. The COP is normally about 25 mmHg and tends to draw fluid into the capillary, while the hydrostatic pressure difference between capillary and interstitium tends to push fluid out. This balance was first described by Starling (1896).

Staverman (1952) introduced the concept that different molecules will be 'reflected' to a different extent by the membrane. This term, the reflection coefficient, varies between zero (all molecules passing through the membrane) and +1 (all molecules reflected). In disease states when the capillary membrane becomes leaky the reflection coefficient will fall. Flow across the membrane is represented in the equation:

$$V = K_f S [P_c - P_{IF}) - \sigma(\pi_p - \pi_{IF})]$$

where $V$ is the rate of movement of water; $K_f$ the capillary filtration coefficient; S the surface area; $P_c$, $P_{IF}$ the capillary and interstitial hydrostatic pressures; $\pi_p$, $\pi_{IF}$ the plasma and interstitial oncotic pressures; and $\sigma$ the reflection coefficient.

## The cell membrane

The barrier between the extracellular and intracellular space is the cell membrane. This is freely permeable to water but not to sodium ions, which are actively pumped out of cells. Sodium is therefore mainly an extracellular cation, while potassium is the main intracellular cation. Water will move across the cell membrane in either direction if there is any difference in osmolality between the two sides. Osmolality expresses the osmotic pressure across a selectively permeable membrane and depends on the number of particles in the solution, not their size. Normal osmolality of ECF is 280–295 mosmol kg$^{-1}$. Since each cation is balanced by an anion, an estimate of plasma or ECF osmolality can be obtained from the formula:

osmolality (mosmol kg$^{-1}$)
= 2 (Na$^+$ + K$^+$) + glucose + urea (mmol l$^{-1}$)[*]

Note that the colloids contribute very little to total osmolality as the number of particles is small, although as we saw above they play an important role in fluid movement across the capillaries.

## Movement of water between compartments

Consider what happens when a patient takes in water, either by drinking or in the form of a 5% glucose infusion, whose glucose is soon metabolized. It will rapidly distribute through the ECF with a resultant fall in ECF osmolality. Since osmolality must be the same inside and outside cells, water will move from ECF to ICF until the osmolalities are the same. Thus a litre of water or 5% glucose given to a patient will distribute itself throughout the body water. By a converse argument we can see that someone marooned on a life raft with no water will lose water from all compartments.

Normal saline (0.9%) contains Na$^+$ and Cl$^-$ 150 mmol l$^{-1}$ and has an osmolality of 300

---

[*] Osmolality is expressed per kilogram of solvent (usually water) whereas osmolarity is expressed per litre of solution. The presence of significant amounts of protein in the solution, as in plasma, means that the osmolality and osmolarity will not be the same.

mosmol $kg^{-1}$. If this is infused into a patient it will stay in the ECF and because the osmolality matches that inside the cells there is no movement of water into the cells. Conversely a patient losing electrolytes and water together, as in severe diarrhoea, loses the fluid from the ECF and not the ICF.

Finally, consider the infusion of human plasma protein fraction (4.5% albumin). The electrolyte and protein content are like that of plasma, so there is no change in colloid osmotic pressure and the solution stays in the plasma compartment (there are, of course, circumstances in which it can leak out). A burned patient losing plasma loses it from the vascular compartment and initially there is no shift of fluid from the interstitial space. As blood pressure falls, hydrostatic pressure in the capillary falls, and if colloid osmotic pressure is maintained the Starling forces will draw water and electrolytes into the vascular compartment from the interstitium. Because there are only 3.5 litres of plasma, losses from this compartment lead to hypoperfusion and reduced oxygen transport to tissues and are potentially life threatening.

Since the plasma is part of the ECF, any loss of ECF results in a corresponding decrease in circulating volume and is potentially much more serious than loss of an equivalent volume from the total body water. For example, compare a man losing 1 litre a day of water, because he is marooned on a life raft, with a man losing 1 litre a day of water and electrolytes, due to a bowel obstruction. The man on the life raft will lose 7 litres in a week from his total of 42 litres body water, i.e. a 17% loss. The plasma volume will fall by 17%, which is survivable. The man with a bowel obstruction, on the other hand, loses his 7 litres from the functional ECF of 12 litres, i.e. a 58% loss. Losing more than half of the plasma volume is not compatible with life.

## NORMAL WATER AND ELECTROLYTE BALANCE

We take in water as food and drink and also make about 350 ml per day as a result of the oxidization of carbohydrates to water and carbon dioxide, known as the metabolic water. This has to balance the output. Water is lost through the skin and from the lungs; these insensible losses amount to about 1 litre a day. Urine and faeces account for the rest. A typical balance is shown in Table 16.1

**Table 16.1** Average daily water balance for a sedentary adult in temperate conditions

| Input (ml) | | Output (ml) | |
|---|---|---|---|
| Drink | 1500 | Urine | 1500 |
| Food | 750 | Faeces | 100 |
| Metabolic | 350 | Lungs | 400 |
| | | Skin | 600 |
| Total | 2600 | Total | 2600 |

The precise water requirements of a particular patient depend on their size, age and temperature. Surface area (1.5 l water per $m^2$ daily) is the most accurate guide but it is more practical to use weight, giving adults 30–40 ml $kg^{-1}$ per day. Children require relatively more water than adults, as set out in Table 16.2.

**Table 16.2** Water requirements of children

| Weight (kg) | Water requirements |
|---|---|
| 0–10 | 100 ml $kg^{-1}$ |
| 10–20 | 1000 ml + 50 ml $kg^{-1}$ for each kg >10 |
| >20 | 1500 ml + 25 ml $kg^{-1}$ for each kg >20 |

The average requirements of sodium and potassium are 1 mmol $kg^{-1}$ daily of each. Humans are very efficient at conserving sodium and can tolerate much lower sodium intakes but they are less good at conserving potassium. There is an obligatory loss of potassium in urine and faeces and patients who are not given potassium will become hypokalaemic. As potassium is mainly an intracellular cation there may be a considerable fall in total body potassium before the plasma potassium falls.

## PRESCRIBING FLUID REGIMES

In prescribing fluid regimes for patients, we need to consider three things:

**Table 16.3**  Content of crystalloid solutions

| Name | Known as | Na+ | Cl- | K+ | HCO₃- | Ca²⁺ | Calculated |
| --- | --- | --- | --- | --- | --- | --- | --- |
| | | | | mmol l⁻¹ | | | (mosmol l⁻¹ |
| Sodium chloride 0.9% | Normal saline | 150 | 150 | | | | 300 |
| Sodium chloride 0.9%, potassium chloride 0.3% | Normal saline + KCl | 150 | 190 | 40 | | | 380 |
| Sodium chloride 0.9%, potassium chloride 0.15% | Normal saline + KCl | 150 | 170 | 20 | | | 340 |
| Ringer's lactate | Hartmann's | 131 | 111 | 5 | 29 (as 12 lactate) | | 280 |
| Glucose 5% | 5% dextrose | | | | | | 280 |
| Glucose 5%, potassium chloride 0.3% | 5% dextrose + KCl | | 40 | 40 | | | 360 |
| Glucose 5%, potassium chloride 0.15% | 5% dextrose + KCl | | 20 | 20 | | | 320 |
| Glucose 4%, sodium chloride 0.18% | Dextrose saline | 30 | 30 | | | | 286 |
| Glucose 4%, sodium chloride 0.18%, potassium chloride 0.3% | Dextrose saline + KCl | 30 | 70 | 40 | | | 366 |
| Glucose 4%, sodium chloride 0.18%, potassium chloride 0.15% | Dextrose saline + KCl | 30 | 50 | 20 | | | 326 |
| Sodium chloride 0.45% | Half normal saline | 75 | 75 | | | | 150 |
| Sodium chloride 1.8% | Twice normal saline | 300 | 300 | | | | 600 |
| Sodium bicarbonate 8.4% | – | 1000 | | | 1000 | | 2000 |
| Sodium bicarbonate 1.4% | – | 167 | | | 167 | | 334 |

1. basal requirements
2. continuing abnormal losses over and above basal requirements
3. pre-existing dehydration and electrolyte loss.

Intraoperative fluid balance needs special consideration as all three of the above apply. Normally nourished patients who are 'nil by mouth' for a few days during surgery do not need feeding intravenously. Only in special circumstances is intravenous feeding required and that is outside the scope of this chapter.

## Basal requirements

We have seen above the daily requirements of water and electrolytes. If we look now at the various crystalloid solutions that are available (Table 16.3), we can design fluid regimes for basal requirements. Normal saline, Hartmann's, 5% dextrose and dextrose saline are the most commonly used. Note that their osmolalities are similar to that of ECF, i.e. they are isotonic with plasma. The purpose of the glucose is to make the solution isotonic, not to provide calories, although a small amount of glucose does have a protein sparing effect during the catabolism that follows major surgery and trauma.

Our standard 70 kg patient can be provided with the 24-hour basal requirements of 30–40 ml kg⁻¹ water and 1 mmol kg⁻¹ of sodium in any of the ways shown in Table 16.4.

**Table 16.4.**  Basal water and sodium regimes for a 70 kg patient on intravenous fluids

| Solution | Volume (ml) | Na⁺ (mmol) | K⁺ (mmol) |
| --- | --- | --- | --- |
| 5% glucose | 2000 | – | |
| 0.9% saline | 500 | 75 | |
| 5% glucose | 2000 | – | – |
| Hartmann's | 500 | 65.5 | 2.5 |
| 4% glucose | 2500 | 75 | – |
| 0.18% saline | | | |

### Potassium

None of these regimes supply significant amounts of potassium. Potassium chloride can be added to the bags and is supplied as ampoules of 20 mmol in 10 ml or 1 g (= 13.5 mmol) in 5 ml. Bags of crystalloid are available with potassium already added and this is safer than adding ampoules. It cannot be stressed enough that potassium can be very dangerous because hyper-kalaemia causes cardiac arrhythmias and asystole. It should never be injected as a bolus. There have been a number of tragedies reported to the medical defence societies in which potassium chloride ampoules were mistaken for sodium chloride and used as 'flush', with fatal consequences. Hyper-kalaemia may also occur if potassium supplements are given to anuric patients. For this reason one usually waits until one is certain of reasonable urine output before adding potassium to the regime postoperatively. Safe rules for giving potassium are:

1. urine output at least 40 ml h$^{-1}$
2. not more than 40 mmol added to 1 litre
3. no faster than 40 mmol h$^{-1}$.

## Continuing loss

Patients with continuing losses above the basal requirements need extra fluid. The commonest example in anaesthetic and surgical practice is the patient with bowel obstruction. Fluid can be aspirated by a nasogastric tube to assess both volume and electrolyte content. Saline with added potassium should be given to replace it. Dextrose saline is not an appropriate fluid for this purpose because it only contains Na 30 mmol l$^{-1}$, and 5% glucose is even worse. Hyponatraemia will result if these solutions are used to replace bowel loss.

To keep track of the fluids, a fluid balance chart should be kept. This records all fluid in (oral and intravenous) and all fluid out (urine, drainage, vomit, etc.). Every 24 hours these are totalled, allowance made for insensible losses and the balance, positive or negative, recorded. Any patient on intravenous fluids should have a daily balance, daily electrolyte measurements and a new regime prescribed every day. The instruction 'and repeat' should never be used in fluid management and has led to disasters in the past.

## Correction of pre-existing dehydration

Patients who arrive in a dehydrated state clearly need to be resuscitated with fluid over and above their basal requirements. Usually this will be done intravenously. The problems are (1) to identify which compartment or compartments the fluid has been lost from and (2) to assess the extent of the dehydration. The fluid used to resuscitate the patient should be similar in composition and volume to that which has been lost.

From what we know about the movement of fluid between compartments (see above) and the patient's history, one can usually decide where the losses are coming from. As we have seen, bowel losses come from the ECF, while pure water losses are from the total body water. Protein-containing fluid is lost from the plasma and there may sometimes be a combination of all three types of loss.

### Assessment of deficit

To estimate the extent of the losses, history, clinical examination, measurement and laboratory tests all play a part. A dehydrated patient will be thirsty, have dry mucous membranes, sunken eyes and cheeks, loss of skin elasticity and weight loss. They will feel weak and in severe cases will be mentally confused. The cardiovascular system responds with tachycardia and peripheral vasoconstriction, so that the patient feels cold. Eventually, blood pressure and cardiac output fall, at which point the vital organs, brain, liver and kidneys, which up to now have been protected, are affected. Clouding of consciousness and oliguria are signs of severe dehydration. Weight, pulse, blood pressure and urine output are essential and simple measurements in the assessment and treatment of fluid loss.

***Venous pressure.*** Equally important is the measurement of central venous pressure (CVP). An intravenous catheter is inserted into a central vein. The tip should lie within the thorax, usually in the superior vena cava or right atrium. In this position, blood can be aspirated freely and there is a swing in pressure with respiration. The pressure is usually measured by an electronic transducer but can be done quite simply by connecting the patient to an open-ended column of fluid and measuring the height above zero with a ruler.

The zero point for measuring CVP is the fifth rib in the mid-axillary line with the patient supine (this corresponds to the position of the left atrium).

The normal range for CVP is 3–8 cmH$_2$O (1 mmHg = 1.36 cmH$_2$O). A low reading, particularly a negative value, confirms dehydration, but CVP measurements are more use as a guide to the adequacy of treatment. The response of the CVP to a fluid challenge of 200 ml 5% glucose tells you more about the state of the circulation than a single reading. A dehydrated patient's CVP will rise in response to the challenge but then fall as the circulation vasodilates to accommodate the fluid. If the CVP rises and does not fall again this indicates overfilling or a failing myocardium.

The CVP reflects the function of the right ventricle; usually this parallels left ventricular function. In cardiac disease there may be disparity between the function of the two ventricles. The left ventricular function can be assessed by the use of a balloon-tipped catheter (Swan Ganz) in a branch of the pulmonary artery. When the balloon is blown up to occlude the vessel the pressure measured distally gives a good guide to the left atrial pressure. This is called the pulmonary capillary wedge pressure (PCWP) and is normally 5–12 mmHg. For the assessment of volume replacement in patients who have normal cardiac function CVP is quite adequate and PCWP is unnecessary and expensive.

*Quantification of plasma and ECF loss*

If plasma is lost from the circulation, the plasma remaining still has the same albumin concentration although the volume is diminished. Since no

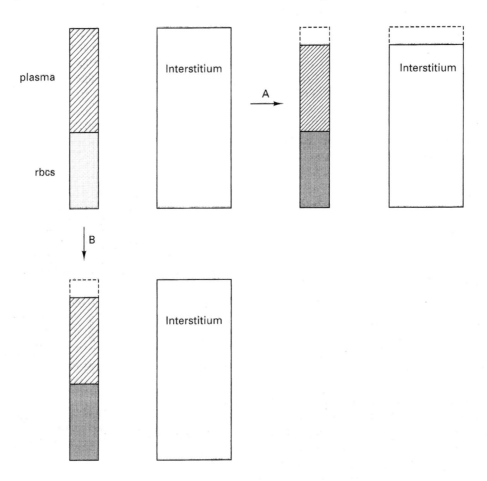

**Fig. 16.2** **A** Loss of ECF leading to a rise in albumin concentration and haematocrit. **B** Loss of plasma leading to a rise in haematocrit but no change in albumin concentration.

red cells are lost they become concentrated, resulting in a rise in haematocrit. Plasma is of course part of the ECF, so that losses of fluid and electrolytes without protein loss will cause a rise in haematocrit but also a rise in plasma protein concentration (Fig. 16.2). Changes in plasma albumin and haematocrit thus provide a good guide to ECF losses, while only haematocrit is of use in monitoring plasma loss (Robarts et al 1979).

In ECF depletion the total amount of albumin stays the same although its concentration goes up. If $Pr_1$ is the initial albumin concentration and $Pr_2$ is the concentration after dehydration it can be shown that:

$$\% \text{ fall in ECF volume} = (1 - \frac{Pr_1}{Pr_2}) \times 100$$

For example, if the albumin rises from 35 to 45 g l$^{-1}$

$$\text{fall in ECF volume} = (1 - \frac{35}{45}) \times 100 = 22\%$$

By a similar argument one can calculate the fall in plasma volume as follows:

$\%$ fall in plasma volume

$$= 100 \left[1 - \left(\frac{Hct_1}{100 - Hct_1} \times \frac{100 - Hct_2}{Hct_2}\right)\right]$$

For example, haematocrit (Hct) rises from 40% to 50%:

fall in plasma volume

$$= 100 \left[1 - \frac{40}{60} \times \frac{50}{50}\right] = 33\%$$

Haematocrit and plasma albumin are thus very useful in the assessment of ECF and plasma losses — much more so than the sodium which, though being lost, does not change in concentration.

A practical application of this from the paper by Robarts et al (1979) is shown in Figures 16.3. and 16.4. Figure 16.3 shows the results in a patient with acute pancreatitis. The plasma vol-

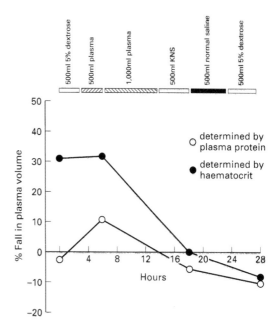

**Fig. 16.3**  Changes in plasma volume as determined by changes in plasma protein and haematocrit, during treatment of acute pancreatitis (see text).

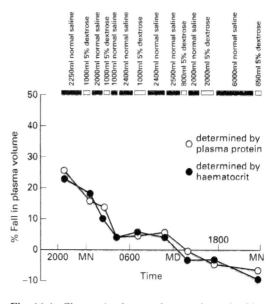

**Fig. 16.4**  Changes in plasma volume as determined by changes in plasma protein and haematocrit, during treatment of bowel obstruction (see text).

**Table 16.5**   Changes resulting from three kinds of expansion and contraction of body fluids

| Acute change | Example | Change in ECF vol | Change in ICF vol | Change in [Na] | Change in [Hct] | Change in [protein] |
|---|---|---|---|---|---|---|
| Loss H$_2$O + NaCl | Cholera | ↓ | → | → | ↑ | ↑ |
| Loss H$_2$O>Na | Excess sweating | ↓ | ↓ | ↑ | → | ↑ |
| Loss Na>H$_2$O | Addison's | ↓ | ↑ | ↓ | ↑ | ↑ |
| Isotonic expansion | Saline infusion | ↑ | → | → | ↓ | ↓ |
| Hypertonic expansion | 2 × normal saline | ↑ | ↓ | ↑ | ↓ | ↓ |
| Hypotonic expansion | 5% glucose infusion | ↑ | ↑ | ↓ | → | ↓ |

ume has fallen 30% (as determined by a rise in haematocrit), but the rest of the ECF volume is unchanged as there was no change in plasma protein concentration. After giving 1.5 litres of plasma, the plasma volume has been restored. By contrast, Figure 16.4 illustrates a patient who had lost ECF through the bowel and both haematocrit and plasma protein estimations show a 25% fall in plasma, hence ECF volume. As saline is administered, the values return to normal.

Table 16.5 summarizes the changes in volume and composition of various compartments in (1) isotonic fluid loss, (2) loss of water in excess of electrolytes, and (3) loss of sodium in excess of water. The corresponding expansion of compartments is also shown. It is a useful exercise to work through the various boxes predicting what change, if any, will occur. In the case of water loss (from both ECF and ICF) remember that the red cells are part of the ICF, so when water is lost from both compartments the haematocrit may not change. Similarly, when there is hypotonic expansion, red cells increase in volume as part of the ICF and with the simultaneous expansion of ECF there may again be no change in haematocrit.

*Water and electrolyte replacement*

Having assessed the amount of deficit, as discussed above, we come to the question of what to give to restore the situation. A look at the composition of various body fluids (Table 16.6) shows us that ECF losses of water and electrolytes should be replaced with either normal saline or ringer–lactate with added potassium (see above: Basal requirements).

The only hypotonic secretions are saliva and sweat. The sodium content of sweat varies and responds to aldosterone. Gastric secretion, though having a sodium content of only 50 mmol l$^{-1}$, is isotonic with ECF because of the hydrogen it contains. Where the losses are primarily of gastric secretion, e.g. pyloric stenosis, one might think it necessary to supply hydrogen ions. In fact, the kidney compensates by retaining hydrogen and

**Table 16.6**   Electrolyte content and daily volume of body secretions

| | Na | K (mmol l$^{-1}$) | Cl | Volume (litres daily) |
|---|---|---|---|---|
| Saliva | 15 | 19 | 40 | 1.5 |
| Stomach | 50 | 15 | 140 | 2.5 |
| Bile, pancreas, small bowel | 130–145 | 5–12 | 70–100 | 4.2 |
| Insensible sweat | 12 | 10 | 12 | 0.6 |
| Sensible sweat | 50 | 10 | 50 | Variable |

**Table 16.7** Characteristics of colloid solutions

| Name | Brand name | No. average* mol. wt | Mol. wt range | Na$^+$ K$^+$ Ca$^{2+}$ (mmol l$^{-1}$) | $t\frac{1}{2}$ in plasma | Adverse reactions Mild (%) | Severe (%) | Effect on coagulation | Cost (UK 1991) |
|---|---|---|---|---|---|---|---|---|---|
| Human plasma protein fraction | HPPF | 69 000 | 69 000 | 150  5  2 | 20 days | 0.02 | 0.004 | None | £40 |
| Dextran 70 in saline 0.9% or glucose 5% | Macrodex Lomodex 70 Gentran 70 | 38 000 | <10 000 –>250 000 | 150  –  – | 12 h | 0.7 | 0.02 | Inhibit platelet aggregation Factor VIII↓ Interfere with cross-match | £3.66 £4.11 |
| Polygeline (degraded gelatin) | Haemaccel | 24 500 | <5 000 –>50 000 | 145  5  6.25 | 2.5 h | 0.12 | 0.04 | None | £3.81 |
| Succinylated gelatin | Gelofusin | 22 600 | <10 000 –>140 000 | 154  0.4 0.4 | 4 h | 0.12 | 0.04 | None | £3.16 |
| Hydroxyethyl starch 6% in saline (Hetastarch) | Hespan | 70 000 | <10 000 –>10$^6$ | 154  –  – | 25 h | 0.09 | 0.006 | >1.5 g kg$^{-1}$ d$^{-1}$ can cause coagulopathy | £15.39 |

* Number average molecular weight should not be confused with weight average molecular weight, which is usually quoted by the manufacturers. No average molecular weight is more appropriate.

excreting sodium and bicarbonate, so that the net effect is a loss of sodium and chloride. Normal saline with potassium should therefore be used in rehydration.

### Plasma replacement and plasma substitutes

When we need to replace lost plasma there is a choice between giving plasma prepared from donated blood or one of the synthetic plasma substitutes. Human plasma protein fraction (HPPF) is prepared by separating red cells from donated blood. A bottle contains plasma from several donors and has been pasteurized to prevent the transmission of disease (e.g. hepatitis or HIV). It contains 4.5% albumin, has no clotting factors and is stable at room temperature. The main disadvantage is its cost (£40 in the UK, 1991), which reflects its limited availability.

A number of solutions containing molecules large enough to stay within the capillaries and generate colloid osmotic pressure are available as plasma substitutes (Table 16.7).

**Dextrans.** The dextans are glucose polymers available in preparations of different molecular weights. There is a large range of molecular weights in the solution. Dextran 70 is so called because the average molecular weight is supposed to be 70 000. In fact, the number average molecular weight which is much more relevant to the colloid osmotic pressure is 38 000 (see footnote to Table 16.7) (Webb et al 1989). Dextran 40 has smaller molecules and can be nephrotoxic. Dextran 110 has larger molecules. Neither of these will be considered further. Dextran 70 is quite a good plasma substitute but has declined in popularity because of its adverse effects on coagulation and cross-matching and the relatively high incidence of allergic reactions.

**Gelatins.** Gelatin solutions are prepared by the hydrolysis of bovine collagen. They have the advantage over dextrans of not affecting coagulation and having a low incidence of allergic reactions. Being of smaller average particle size they stay in the intravascular space a shorter time. Haemaccel contains potassium and calcium ions, which can cause coagulation if mixed with citrated blood in a giving set. Haemaccel stays a shorter time in the circulation, 30% of the molecules being dispersed to the interstitial tissues in 30 minutes. Gelofusin is probably preferable from this point of view.

**Hetastarch.** Six per cent hetastarch in saline has become available in the last few years. It has the largest average molecular weight of any of the plasma substitutes and therefore stays in the circulation longer. The dose should be limited to 1500 ml 70 kg$^{-1}$; more can cause coagulation problems. About 30% of a dose is taken up by the reticuloendothelial system without apparent detriment to its function. Smaller molecules (<50 000 mol wt) are filtered by the kidneys. Larger ones are broken down by plasma amylase until small enough for renal excretion.

***Choice of solution for plasma expansion.*** The intravascular space can be expanded by the use of crystalloid solutions, e.g. saline, but because the fluid spreads throughout the ECF 4 litres of crystalloid are needed to expand the plasma by 1 litre. In an emergency crystalloid is useful. All the battle casualties in the Falklands War were resuscitated in the field with Hartmann's solution.

For most patients with acute hypovolaemia the best combination of advantages at low cost is offered by succinylated gelatin (Gelofusin). Being relatively short acting it is particularly useful as a holding measure until blood becomes available.

In continuing hypovolaemia hetastarch gives more prolonged expansion and its larger molecules are better retained in the circulation when the capillaries are leaky, e.g. in septicaemic shock.

**Table 16.8**  Hazards of blood transfusion

| | |
|---|---|
| A. | *Any transfusion*<br>Transmission of disease, e.g. AIDS, malaria<br>(donor blood screened for HIV, hepatitis, syphilis)<br>Bacterial contamination<br>Pyrogenic reactions (antibodies to white cells)<br>Incompatibility reactions<br>± Haemolysis (clerical error commonest cause) |
| B. | *Massive transfusion*<br>Hypothermia<br>Hyperkalaemia<br>Citrate toxicity<br>Acidosis<br>Microaggregate embolism, 'shock lung'<br>Dilution and consumption of clotting factors |

*Blood loss and blood transfusion*

So far we have talked about plasma loss and plasma expansion. Most of what has been said about the assessment and replacement of plasma volume applies to blood loss. Transfusion of donated blood is possible in most circumstances but has several disadvantages to be weighed against the fact that only haemoglobin carries oxygen. With a haemoglobin of 14 g dl$^{-1}$ evolution has equipped us with spare capacity as far as oxygen-carrying capacity is concerned. Indeed, as haematocrit falls, the decrease in oxygen carrying is compensated by better tissue perfusion due to reduced blood viscosity. It has been shown that the best balance between oxygen carrying and viscosity occurs around a haematocrit of 30%. It is also suspected that blood transfusion at the time of surgery for certain cancers leads to immunological suppression and poorer long-term survival. Since the AIDS scare there is greater reluctance on the part of the public to accept blood transfusion. For all these reasons, as well as the hazards of blood transfusion listed in Table 16.8, the expense of blood and rarity of some blood groups, one is reluctant to transfuse blood. In practical terms operative blood loss up to 500 ml can be replaced with crystalloid, remembering that four times as much will be needed (see above) or plasma substitutes. Only if more than 1 litre of blood has been lost should one consider giving blood.

Rather than supply whole blood, it is more efficient for the transfusion service to separate it into components as listed in Table 16.9. Blood cross-matched for patients undergoing surgery usually comes as plasma-reduced blood ('packed cells'). This is more viscous than whole blood and needs to be given with appropriate amounts of crystalloid or colloid solution to restore the volume.

The quantity of blood lost is assessed clinically as outlined above, and at operation by watching the suction bottle and weighing swabs, but this generally underestimates the loss. In operations like transurethral resection of prostate, measurement of haemoglobin in the irrigating fluid gives an accurate measure of blood loss. In acute blood loss haematocrit and haemoglobin concentrations do not change until the blood remaining in the patient has been diluted by shift of fluid from the interstitial space or intravenous infusion. Plasma-reduced blood and whole blood more than a day old (which it almost always is) contain no viable platelets and few clotting factors. The same applies to plasma protein fraction. In massive transfusion both dilution and consumption of clotting factors make it necessary to send blood for a clotting screen and give platelets and fresh frozen plasma (FFP) according to the results. As a rule one gives a unit of FFP for every 4–6 units of stored blood transfused.

**Table 16.9** Blood products

| |
| --- |
| Plasma-reduced blood (packed cells) |
| Washed red cells: if transfusion reaction a problem |
| Plasma protein fraction (HPPF) |
| Fresh frozen plasma (FFP): contains clotting factors more dilute than the concentrates below |
| Cryoprecipitate: rich in factor VIII |
| Factor VIII concentrate: even richer in VIII |
| Factor II VII IX X concentrate |
| Factor XI concentrate |
| Fibrinogen |
| Platelet concentrate |

## Intraoperative fluid balance

During an operation everything we have discussed so far may be going on at the same time. The patient is starved for 6–12 hours, there may be blood loss, plasma loss, ECF loss and evaporation of water from exposed bowel. As part of the stress response to surgery the patient retains water and sodium. The importance of careful monitoring in major surgery will be obvious; this includes accurate assessment of blood loss, haemodynamic variables and urine output.

As a rule of thumb, in intra-abdominal surgery Hartmann's solution 5 ml kg$^{-1}$ h$^{-1}$ may be given up to 2 litres. This will compensate for starvation, ECF loss, evaporation and some blood loss. Blood or colloids may have to be given in addition.

For the first 36 hours postoperatively there is water retention and there is sodium retention lasting three to five days. Obligatory potassium loss of 50–100 mmol per day continues. If additional sodium is given it is simply retained, although the urine may show an increase in sodium output. Provided that intraoperative losses have been replaced by the end of the operation one should give the basal requirements (30–40 ml kg$^{-1}$ H$_2$O + 1 mmol kg$^{-1}$ Na$^+$ and K$^+$) plus additional blood or colloid if there is significant wound drainage. Remember not to start potassium until urine output is established; the operation of inadvertent bilateral ureteric ligation is not unknown.

## ACID–BASE BALANCE

Claude Bernard was the first to recognize that to function effectively the body needs a stable 'milieu interieur'. The hydrogen ion concentration is a most important part of this. An acid is a hydrogen ion (proton) donor and a base accepts hydrogen ions. Throughout life the body produces hydrogen ions and they must be excreted or buffered to keep the internal environment constant.

### Terminology and definitions

#### Hydrogen ion activity

Hydrogen ion activity is traditionally expressed in pH units, pH being the negative log$_{10}$ of the hydrogen ion concentration:

$$pH = -\log[H^+] = \log \frac{1}{[H^+]}$$

Hydrogen ion concentration can also be expressed directly in nanomoles per litre (see Table 16.10).

**Table 16.10**    Conversion table for pH units and hydrogen ion concentration

| pH unit | H$^+$ (nmol l$^{-1}$) |
|---------|------------------------|
| 8.00    | 10                     |
| 7.70    | 20                     |
| 7.44    | 36                     |
| 7.40    | 40                     |
| 7.36    | 44                     |
| 7.10    | 80                     |
| 7.00    | 100                    |

Note that the pH is a log scale, so that each 0.3 unit fall in pH represents a doubling of hydrogen ion concentration.

#### Acidosis and alkalosis

The normal ECF pH is 7.36–7.44 (44–36 nmol l$^{-1}$). Acidaemia is a blood pH below this range and alkalaemia above it. Acidosis is a condition that leads to acidaemia or would do if no compensation occurred, but the terms acidosis and acidaemia are often used loosely to mean the same thing, which is not strictly correct. Alkalosis and alkalaemia are defined in a similar way.

**Respiratory acidosis.** A fall in pH resulting from a rise in the PCO$_2$ is a respiratory acidosis, e.g. opiate overdose leading to hypoventilation causes a rise in PCO$_2$.

**Respiratory alkalosis.** This is a rise in pH due to a lowering of the PCO$_2$, such as occurs in hyperventilation.

**Metabolic acidosis.** This is a fall in pH due to anything other than carbon dioxide (sometimes referred to as non-respiratory acidosis). There is a primary gain of acid or loss of bicarbonate from ECF.

**Metabolic alkalosis.** This is a rise in pH from non-respiratory causes. There is either a gain in bicarbonate or a loss of acid from the ECF.

**Compensatory changes.** If the initial problem is respiratory, the result is called a *primary* respiratory acidosis or alkalosis. If the respiratory problem persists for more than a few hours the kidney will excrete or retain bicarbonate to try and compensate for the respiratory disturbance. This is referred to as *secondary* or *compensatory* metabolic acidosis or alkalosis.

Thus a *primary* respiratory acidosis may be accompanied by a *secondary* metabolic alkalosis. For example, chronic obstructive airways disease leads to a rise in the PCO$_2$: *primary respiratory acidosis*. To compensate for this the kidney retains bicarbonate, leading to a rise in ECF bicarbonate: *secondary or compensatory metabolic alkalosis*.

In the same way primary respiratory alkalosis (e.g. the hyperventilation that occurs at high altitude) will be compensated by a secondary metabolic acidosis.

Where the first disturbance is metabolic, e.g. the build-up of acid in diabetic ketoacidosis, the primary metabolic acidosis will cause hyperventilation (secondary respiratory alkalosis), which will tend to restore the pH to normal. This respiratory compensation for a metabolic change happens much more rapidly than the metabolic compensation for a respiratory problem.

The fourth possible combination of changes is to have a metabolic alkalosis (e.g. loss of H⁺ in pyloric stenosis) compensated by a respiratory acidosis. However, hypoventilation (respiratory acidosis) leads to a fall in $PO_2$, which stimulates ventilation so that in practice compensatory respiratory acidosis is not usually seen.

In deciding which is the primary and which is the secondary change it is important to realize that the compensatory changes do not bring the pH back to normal — they bring it back *towards* the normal range. In other words, even after compensation the measured pH is altered in the direction of the primary problem (acidosis or alkalosis). Compensatory mechanisms merely make the disturbance in pH less than it otherwise would have been. It is also important to consider the history. Examiners may give candidates blood gas results to interpret but in real life blood gases come from patients. Knowing that a patient is an unconscious diabetic breathing spontaneously, rather than an anaesthetized patient on a ventilator, certainly helps one's interpretation.

*Buffers*

Buffers are substances which by their presence in solution minimize the change in pH for a given addition of acid or alkali. Three-quarters of the buffering power of the body is within the cells; the rest is in the ECF. Proteins, haemoglobin, phosphates and the bicarbonate system are all important buffers. The particular importance of the bicarbonate system is that carbon dioxide is excreted in the lungs and can be regulated by changes in ventilation. Bicarbonate excretion in the kidney can also be regulated. The lungs are responsible for the excretion of 16 000 mmol per day of acid and the kidneys for only 40–80 mmol per day. The formation of carbonic acid from carbon dioxide and water is catalysed by carbonic anhydrase (present in red cells). The reaction may go in either direction:

$$H^+ + HCO_3^- \rightleftharpoons H_2CO_3 \rightleftharpoons H_2O + CO_2$$

The Henderson–Hasselbalch equation is derived from this and expresses the relationship between the bicarbonate concentration, the carbon dioxide and the pH:

$$pH = pK + \log \frac{[HCO_3^-]}{[H_2CO_3]}$$

The carbonic acid can be expressed in terms of carbon dioxide, so that a more useful form of the equation is:

$$pH = pK + \log \frac{[HCO_3^-]}{0.03\ PCO_2}$$

As this is a buffer system which minimizes changes in pH, we can see that if the carbon dioxide rises so will the bicarbonate, to keep $[HCO_3^-]/PCO_2$ constant. Similarly a fall in bicarbonate will be accompanied by a fall in $PCO_2$ to prevent a change in pH.

**Interpretation of acid–base changes**

As the patient's acid–base status varies, three things are changing at once: pH, $[HCO_3^-]$ and $PCO_2$. Blood gas machines measure directly $PO_2$, pH and $PCO_2$. The actual bicarbonate $[HCO_3^-]$ is calculated from the Henderson–Hasselbalch equation. They also derive other variables which help in the interpretation of the acid–base status. These are as follows.

*Standard bicarbonate (SBC)*

This is the concentration of bicarbonate in the plasma of fully oxygenated blood at 37°C at a $PCO_2$ of 5.3 kPa (40 mmHg). In other words, it tells you what the bicarbonate would be if there was no respiratory disturbance. Looking at the standard bicarbonate therefore tells you what is going on on the metabolic side. Normal standard bicarbonate is 22–26 mmol l⁻¹. Values above this indicate metabolic alkalosis and those below, metabolic acidosis.

*Base excess (BE)*

This is the amount of strong base or acid that would need to be added to whole blood to titrate the pH back to 7.4 *at a $PCO_2$ of 5.3 kPa and*

$37°C$. It tells you the same thing as standard bicarbonate, namely the metabolic status of the patient. Normal base excess is obviously 0 (±2 mmol $1^{-1}$). Positive base excess occurs in metabolic alkalosis, and negative base excess (sometimes called base deficit) indicates metabolic acidosis. The base excess is an in vitro determination in whole blood. It is also known as the actual base excess (ABE) or the base excess (blood) (BE b).

### Standard base excess (SBE)

This is an estimate of the in vivo base excess and takes into account the difference in buffering capacity between the patient's ECF and the blood that was put in the blood gas machine. Interstitial fluid, having less protein and no haemoglobin, has a lower buffering capacity than blood. SBE is therefore ±1–2 mmol $1^{-1}$ greater than BE but this makes very little difference in practice. SBE is sometimes called base excess (e.c.f.).

### Total carbon dioxide (TCO₂)

This is the total concentration of carbon dioxide in the plasma as bicarbonate and dissolved carbon dioxide.

$$TCO_2 = [HCO_3^-] + (PCO_2 \times solubility)$$

### Oxygen saturation (O₂ sat.)

The percentage saturation of haemoglobin by oxygen is derived from the haemoglobin oxygen dissociation curve and the measured $PO_2$. Normal value is >95%.

### PO₂ and inspired oxygen (F₁O₂)

To interpret the $PO_2$ one needs to know the age of the patient and the $F_1O_2$. Normal arterial $PO_2$ declines with age. Roughly speaking $PO_2$ = 100–age in years/3 mmHg or 13.3–0.044 × age kPa.

The expected alveolar $PO_2$ ($PAO_2$) can be predicted from the inspired oxygen by the simplified alveolar gas equation: $PAO_2 = P_1O_2 - PACO_2/R$, where R is the respiratory exchange

ratio (normally 0.8). In dry gas $P_1O_2$ in kPa = fractional inspired oxygen $(F_1O_2)$%. Alveolar gas is saturated with water vapour (6.3 kPa), for which allowance must be made. If the $F_1O_2$ was 40% and the $PCO_2$ 5.3:

$$PAO_2 = \frac{(40 - 40 \times 6.3)}{100} - \frac{5.3}{0.8} = 30.85 \text{ kPa}$$

As an approximate rule of thumb one can deduct 10 from the $F_1O_2$% to give the expected $PAO_2$ in kPa, e.g. $F_1O_2$ 50% — approx. $PAO_2$ = 40 kPa. The difference between the estimated $PAO_2$ and the measured arterial $PO_2$ is called the (A–a) $PO_2$ gradient. It is normally 0.5–3 kPa.

Without considering the inspired oxygen it is not possible to comment sensibly on the observed $PAO_2$. A rough calculation of the (A–a) $PO_2$ gradient should be made when commenting on blood gas results. Some machines even calculate this for you as well!

A blood gas machine usually prints out the variables shown in Table 16.11. There is often a haemoglobin measurement and the temperature of measurement (37°C) is quoted.

**Table 16.11** Printout from a blood gas machine with normal values

| Temp. | 37° |
|---|---|
| pH | 7.36–7.44 (44–36 nmol $1^{-1}$) |
| $PCO_2$ | 4.6–5.6 kPa (35–42 mmHg) |
| $PO_2$ | 10.0–13.3 kPa (75–100 mmHg) |
| $HCO_3^-$ | 22–26 mmol $1^{-1}$ |
| $TCO_2$ | 24–28 mmol $1^{-1}$ |
| SBC | 22–26 mmol $1^{-1}$ |
| BE | –2 to +2 mmol $1^{-1}$ |
| SBE | –3 to +3 mmol $1^{-1}$ |
| $O_2$ sat. | >95% |
| Hb | 11.5–16.5 g d$1^{-1}$ |

### Temperature correction

The blood gas machine operates at 37°C. Because gases are more soluble in liquid at lower temperatures (as drinkers of cold lager will know) the blood gases would be different if measured at another temperature. Blood gas machines are programmed to correct the gases if you tell the machine the patient's actual temperatures.

However, there has been much debate as to whether it is appropriate to correct for temperature. Suffice it to say that the protagonists of not correcting for temperature (the alpha stat theory) hold sway and one should probably act on the blood gases as measured at 37°C and not the temperature-corrected values.

### The anion gap

For electrochemical neutrality of the ECF the number of anions must equal the number of cations. The main cations are sodium and potassium and the main anions are chloride, bicarbonate, proteins, phosphates, sulphates and organic acids.

Normally only $Na^+$, $K^+$, $HCO_3^-$ and $Cl^-$ are measured in the laboratory. Thus when we add the normal values for these they do not balance:

| Cations | | Anions | |
|---|---|---|---|
| $Na^+$ | 140 | $Cl^-$ | 105 |
| $K^+$ | 5 | $HCO_3^-$ | 25 |
| Total | 145 | Total | 130 |

The difference is known as the anion gap and represents the other anions not usually measured. Anion gap $= (Na^+ + K^+) - (HCO_3^- + Cl^-) = 11-19$ mmol $l^{-1}$. Its significance is that in certain metabolic acidoses, e.g. ketoacidosis or lactic acidosis, the anion gap will be increased by the presence of organic anions. However, in metabolic acidosis in which chloride replaces bicarbonate, e.g. bicarbonate loss due to diarrhoea, the anion gap will be normal.

### Plan for interpreting blood gases

1. Check for internal consistency. Remember that the machine only measures pH, $PCO_2$ and $PO_2$. If it measures any of these wrongly, which is not infrequent, the derived variables will be wildly abnormal too. If the results do not fit with the clinical picture, suspect the machine. Example: a patient on a ventilator in theatre with an end-tidal carbon dioxide of 5% has the following gases:

| | |
|---|---|
| $PO_2$ | 13.0 |
| pH | 7.64 |

| | |
|---|---|
| $PCO_2$ | 5.1 |
| $HCO_3^-$ | 37.5 |
| $TCO_2$ | 38.5 |
| SBC | 39.0 |
| BE | +15 |
| SBE | +16 |
| $O_2$ sat. | 99% |

It is much more likely that the pH has been measured wrongly than that the patient has a gross metabolic alkalosis.

2. Look at the pH. Remember the pH change is always in the direction of the primary problem acidosis or alkalosis.

3. Look at the $PCO_2$. Abnormality of the $PCO_2$ indicates the respiratory component.

4. Look at the base excess or standard bicarbonate. Both give the same information, i.e. the metabolic acid-base status after correcting for the $PCO_2$.

5. Calculate the anion gap.

6. Look at the $PO_2$ and calculate the A-a gradient.

### Examples of abnormal blood gases

| | | |
|---|---|---|
| pH | 7.51 | The alkalaemia is due to |
| $PCO_2$ | 3.7 | primary respiratory alkalosis |
| $PO_2$ | 29 | (low $PCO_2$). There is no |
| $HCO_3^-$ | 22.1 | metabolic compensation |
| $TCO_2$ | 23.6 | (normal base excess). The $PO_2$ |
| SBC | 25 | would be expected if breathing |
| BE | +1.1 | 40% oxygen $P_1O_2-10$ |
| SBE | +2 | $= (40-10) = 30$. The patient is |
| $O_2$ sat. | 100% | hyperventilating. |
| ($F_1O_2$ 40%) | | |

| | | |
|---|---|---|
| pH | 7.28 | A respiratory acidosis with |
| $PCO_2$ | 7.33 | high $PCO_2$ due to hypo- |
| $PO_2$ | 9.21 | ventilation. Again no |
| $HCO_3^-$ | 25.2 | metabolic compensation |
| $TCO_2$ | 28.4 | (normal SBC and BE). Low |
| SBC | 22.3 | $PO_2$ due to hypoventilation. |
| BE | -1.9 | |
| SBE | -2.5 | |
| $O_2$ sat. | 91% | |
| ($F_1O_2$ air) | | |

| | | |
|---|---|---|
| pH | 7.35 | Again a respiratory acidosis |
| $PCO_2$ | 9.33 | (high $PCO_2$) but this time |
| $PO_2$ | 7.11 | compensated by metabolic |
| $HCO_3^-$ | 39.1 | alkalosis (high SBC and |
| $TCO_2$ | 41.2 | positive base excess). This is |
| SBC | 32.4 | typical of chronic obstructive |
| BE | +8.2 | airways disease with renal |
| SBE | +9.1 | compensation. |
| $O_2$ sat. | 85% | |
| ($F_1O_2$ air) | | |

| | | |
|---|---|---|
| pH | 7.21 | The acidaemia (low pH) is |
| $PCO_2$ | 4.0 | primarily due a metabolic |
| $PO_2$ | 13.3 | acidosis (low SBC, base excess |
| $HCO_3^-$ | 11.5 | −15). Compensatory |
| $TCO_2$ | 12.8 | respiratory alkalosis (low |
| SBC | 9.3 | $PCO_2$) does not return the pH |
| BE | −15.2 | to normal. $PO_2$ normal. |
| SBE | −16.4 | |
| $O_2$ sat. | 99% | |
| ($F_IO_2$ air) | | |

| | | |
|---|---|---|
| pH | 7.36 | The pH is in the normal range |
| $PCO_2$ | 4.21 | despite low $PCO_2$ (respiratory |
| $PO_2$ | 10.49 | alkalosis) and low standard |
| $HCO_3^-$ | 17.6 | bicarbonate (metabolic |
| $TCO_2$ | 18.5 | acidosis). The important thing |
| SBC | 17.8 | here is the $PO_2$. It is apparently |
| BE | −6.2 | in the normal range but not |
| SBE | −6.9 | when breathing 60% oxygen. |
| $O_2$ sat. | 96% | The (A–a) $PO_2$ gradient is |
| ($F_IO_2$ 60%) | | roughly 40 kPa. These gases |
| | | are typical of a patient with |
| | | adult respiratory distress |
| | | syndrome. |

## Treatment of acid–base disturbances

As in any other field of medicine treatment should be directed at the underlying cause. Correcting the $PCO_2$ is usually possible by taking over the patient's ventilation and adjusting the minute volume to give the desired $PCO_2$.

Treatment of a metabolic acidosis is more controversial. It was traditional to treat a metabolic acidosis by giving sodium bicarbonate according to the formula (base excess × body weight in kg ÷ 3) mmol starting by giving half the dose; 8.4% sodium bicarbonate contains 1 mmol ml$^{-1}$.

It is now argued that, particularly in a hypoxic state such as exists at cardiac arrests, bicarbonate administration may do more harm than good. (Graf & Arieff 1986). The bicarbonate generates carbon dioxide which crosses easily into cells, making the intracellular acidosis worse. If ventilation is impaired the carbon dioxide generated is unable to escape via the lungs. The traditional practice of giving 50–100 mmol of bicarbonate at a cardiac arrest is probably unjustified.

There is still a place for bicarbonate therapy in acidosis due to diarrhoea, renal tubular acidosis and uraemic acidosis. As outlined above the base excess is used to calculate the dose; 8.4% sodium bicarbonate is hyperosmolar and must be given into a large central vein. Accidental subcutaneous administration can cause tissue necrosis. One must also bear in mind that each mmol of $HCO_3^-$ is accompanied by $Na^+$ and it is easy to overload the patient with sodium. Frequent blood gas and electrolyte analyses must be made during treatment with bicarbonate.

REFERENCES

Edelman I S, Leibman J 1959 Anatomy of body water and electrolytes. American Journal of Medicine 27: 256
Graf H, Arieff A I 1986 Use of sodium bicarbonate in the therapy of organic acidosis. Intensive Care Medicine 12: 285–288
Robarts W M, Parkin J V, Hobsley M 1979 A simple clinical approach to quantifying losses from the extracellular and plasma compartments. Annals of the Royal College of Surgery 61: 142–145
Starling E H 1896 On the absorption of fluids from the connective spaces. Journal of Physiology 19: 312–326
Staverman A 1952 Apparent osmotic pressure of solutions of heterodisperse polymers. Rec Trav Chim 71: 623–633
Webb A R, Barclay S A, Bennett E D 1989 In vitro colloid pressure of commonly used plasma expanders and substitutes. Intensive Care Medicine 15: 116–120

# 17. Correction of preoperative, perioperative and postoperative anaemia: use of blood and blood products

## B. Brozović

The administration of blood and blood products represents substitution therapy and can correct almost immediately and invariably the existing anaemia, thrombocytopenia, coagulopathy or hypoproteinaemia in the patient. However, the administration of blood and blood products is not without risk and should be carried out where the indications are clearly established, i.e. where the benefits to the patient outweigh the risks of transfusion. In this chapter indications for preoperative, perioperative and postoperative transfusion of blood and blood products will be presented, available products described, measures for monitoring the therapeutic effect discussed and adverse reactions to transfusion summarized. Note that in this chapter the term blood products is used for all therapeutic materials prepared from blood and includes both blood components and plasma products. The term blood components refers to red cell preparations, platelet concentrates, fresh frozen plasma and cryoprecipitate. Whole blood and blood components are administered to the patient as 'units', a unit having a quantity obtained from one blood donation. The term plasma products refers to all plasma protein preparations manufactured from large pools of donor plasma. The therapeutic potency of a plasma product is given in weight of protein (for example, a bottle of 20 g of albumin in 100 ml), or in units of activity (for example, a vial of 250 iu of factor VIII:C).

## INDICATIONS FOR TRANSFUSION

Indications for transfusion of blood and blood products are based on the assessment of the impaired haematological status of the patient.

Each of the main functions of blood — maintenance of intravascular volume, oxygen-carrying capacity, haemostasis and maintenance of oncotic pressure — may be impaired to a different degree in the patient with acute blood loss or chronic anaemia. Furthermore, each of the functions has a different 'critical level' which requires immediate corrective action if serious consequences or even death are to be prevented (Table 17.1). When critical levels for any of the blood functions are reached, and that may happen at any time before, during or after an operation, corrective action has to be taken by transfusion of blood, blood components or blood substitutes.

**Table 17.1** Main functions of blood and their critical levels

| Function | Blood constituents | Critical level (%)* |
|---|---|---|
| Maintenance of intravascular volume | Blood volume | 60 |
| Oxygen-carrying capacity† | Haemoglobin concentration | 50 |
| Haemostasis‡ | Platelet count | 10 |
| | Concentration of coagulation factors | 10 |
| Maintenance of oncotic pressure | Concentration of plasma proteins (mainly albumin) | 50 |

*Expressed as a percentage of normal function. Critical levels vary considerably in each patient and they should always be individually assessed.
†Several factors may affect oxygen-carrying capacity of haemoglobin; see also Table 17.2.
‡The third component of the haemostatic mechanism, the fibrinolytic system, has been excluded.

The main objective in the management of anaemia encountered in surgical practice is to ensure adequate oxygenation of tissues and particularly of the heart and the brain. Experience accumulated over the last few years has shown that that objective is achieved when the haemoglobin concentration is above 8.0 g dl$^{-1}$. That level of haemoglobin, at which a decision to transfuse the patient is usually made, is generally known as the 'transfusion trigger'. While the transfusion trigger can be useful as a pointer for action, it should never be used as an immutable value, as for example, a young patient with haemoglobin concentration substantially lower than 8.0 g dl$^{-1}$ may tolerate the operation much better than an old patient with a higher haemoglobin level but with a failing heart or compromised cerebral circulation. It has to be appreciated that oxygen delivery to the tissues is a function of partial pressure of oxygen in the air, which is raised during anaesthesia and haemoglobin oxygenation; it is also dependent on the function of the lungs and cardiovascular system (Table 17.2). Although it is well documented that the level of haemoglobin and postoperative survival are inversely correlated, neither clinical observations nor laboratory experiments have been able to define the lowest 'safe' haemoglobin concentration. Therefore, it is mandatory to assess each patient individually and to consider the type and probable duration of anaesthesia and of operation before a decision to administer blood is made. In a proportion of patients anaemia may be associated with thrombocytopenia and/or defective coagulation. These patients will require, in addition to red cells, transfusion support with platelet concentrates and fresh frozen plasma.

Table 17.2 Factors which may affect delivery of oxygen to the tissues.

Haemoglobin oxygenation
  Partial pressure of oxygen in air
  Haemoglobin concentration
  Haemoglobin oxygen saturation
  Haemoglobin affinity for oxygen
    Effects of pH, 2,3-DPG and haemoglobins with high
      affinity for oxygen
Blood volume
Cardiac output
Peripheral vascular resistance
Lung function
Type and duration of anaesthesia
Type and duration of surgery

The use of albumin solutions is rather limited to specific indications, which will be discussed later.

## PREOPERATIVE ANAEMIA

The determination of haemoglobin concentration — part of the preoperative assessment of the patient (see chapter 2) — will reveal the presence of anaemia (haemoglobin concentration less than 13.0 g dl$^{-1}$ in men and 11.5 g dl$^{-1}$ in women). Faced with the anaemic patient awaiting surgery, the surgeon should first ensure that the correct diagnosis of anaemia is made or at least that the samples required for the diagnosis have been collected. Second, he should decide whether to proceed with or defer the operation. Finally, he should decide whether the patient requires transfusion of blood. The decision to transfuse the patient should be based on the type and degree of anaemia and the urgency for surgery. Elective surgery should be delayed until haemoglobin concentration is raised to the level considered safe for the patient.

Anaemia is caused by the decreased production of red cells in the bone marrow, increased destruction of red cells in the circulation, or blood loss. Anaemia may be chronic or of sudden onset. In chronic anaemia compensatory mechanisms which increase oxygen delivery to the tissues are well developed; they are absent in acute anaemia. The current diagnosis of anaemia will most often make it possible to predict its progress and response to treatment. In the patient with functioning bone marrow an appropriate treatment will raise the haemoglobin concentration on average 1.0 g dl$^{-1}$ per week.

Types of anaemia and their management are presented in Table 17.3. Anaemias of interest to the surgeon are described below.

*Iron deficiency anaemia* due to chronic blood loss is the most frequently seen type of anaemia. It is usually caused by blood loss from the gastrointestinal tract or kidneys and in women by menorrhagia. Once the measures to prevent further blood loss are taken, anaemia will respond well and quickly to treatment with oral iron.

*Anaemia of chronic disease* is often found in association with a number of chronic diseases. It is usually mild and unresponsive to treatment. A

**Table 17.3** Main types of anaemia found by preoperative assessment and their management

| Type | Management |
| --- | --- |
| Anaemia due to decreased production of red cells<br>   Iron deficiency anaemia<br>Nutritional or due to malabsorption<br>Chronic blood loss | Establish diagnosis, deal with the cause and prescribe oral iron preparations. Usually good response |
| Vitamin $B_{12}$ deficiency<br>   Nutritional or due to malabsorption<br>   Pernicious anaemia | Establish diagnosis, deal with the cause and treat with parenteral vitamin $B_{12}$. Usually good response |
| Folic acid deficiency<br>   Nutritional or due to malabsorption | Establish diagnosis, deal with the cause and prescribe folic acid. Usually good response |
| Anaemia of chronic disease | Establish diagnosis and treat the primary disease. Usually poor response. Patients with renal disease respond to rhEPO* |
| Anaemia due to bone marrow failure<br>Aplastic anaemia, leukaemia, bone marrow infiltration with malignant cells | Establish diagnosis and treat the primary disease. Variable response. Transfuse as required. Sometimes transfusion of platelets is also needed |
| Anaemia due to increased destruction of red cells<br>   Inherited<br>      Haemoglobinopathies<br>      Thalassaemias<br>      Sickle cell disease | Establish diagnosis. Transfuse as and when required |
|    Acquired<br>Immune-mediated<br>Non-immune haemolytic anaemias | Establish diagnosis and treat primary disease. Avoid transfusion where possible |
| Anaemia due to blood loss<br>   Acute | Remove the cause of bleeding where possible, transfuse where required |
|    Chronic | Manage as iron deficiency anaemia |

*rhEPO, recombinant human erythropoietin.

severe degree of anaemia may occur in patients with renal failure and in these patients administration of recombinant human erythropoietin may raise the haemoglobin concentration to near normal values.

*Haemoglobinopathies.* Patients with sickle cell disease (HbSS, HbSC or HbS/thalassaemia) in general require exchange transfusion before major surgery, whereas intermediate and minor surgical procedures can be carried out safely without transfusion in the majority of patients. Particular attention should be paid to the hydration of the patient and to oxygenation during anaesthesia. Patients with sickle cell disease may develop painful crisis due to infarcts in tissues and organs, before, during or after an operation, which is best managed by symptomatic treatment, but occasionally may require blood transfusion.

*Haemolytic anaemia.* Patients with hereditary or long-standing acquired haemolytic anaemia are sometimes referred for splenectomy as the spleen is the major site of red cell destruction. Patients with long-standing haemolysis are prone to cholelithiasis and may be referred for cholecystectomy.

Patients with acquired autoimmune haemolytic anaemia may present a challenge to the blood bank to provide compatible blood for transfusion. When ordering blood sufficient time should be allowed for compatibility testing. Often blood issued for transfusion carries the warning that it is as compatible (or incompatible) as the donor's own red cells.

*Anaemia due to acute blood loss*, when severe, requires immediate restoration of circulatory volume with crystalloid solutions in the first instance and then colloid solutions afterwards. The decision to administer blood should be made after careful assessment of the patient's condition. Administration of albumin solutions as volume expanders is not recommended.

## PERIOPERATIVE LOSS OF BLOOD

In a number of operations blood loss of varying magnitude may occur. Programmes to minimize the blood loss are based on meticulous surgical haemostasis and the use of pharmacological agents (ε-aminocaproic acid, tranexamic acid, desmopressin, aprotinin) to decrease the blood loss. However, supportive treatment with blood may be needed when excessive bleeding due to inadequate surgical haemostasis and/or breakdown of haemostatic mechanisms are encountered. With that in view it is customary to order in advance compatible blood according to the locally agreed maximum surgical blood order schedule (MSBOS). In addition, surgeons wishing to eliminate or decrease the use of homologous blood transfusion in the surgical patient should consider using one or several forms of autologous transfusion: preoperative blood donation, intraoperative and postoperative blood salvage and acute normovolaemic haemodilution (see below).

It is well recognized that it is difficult to estimate blood loss during surgery. Although there are a number of methods available for monitoring the patient's homeostatic and haemostatic states, none of these is wholly satisfactory (Table 17.4). In addition, the decision to transfuse blood may be influenced by the local policy and personal preferences of the surgeon or anaesthetist in relation to the type of operation, test used for monitoring blood loss and availability of blood and blood components. The management of blood loss and associated adverse reactions is best illustrated by descriptions of massive blood transfusion and cardiopulmonary bypass.

### Massive blood transfusion

Massive blood transfusion is by definition transfusion of a volume of blood, greater than the recipient's blood volume, in less than 24 hours. It is used to combat hypovolaemic shock caused by profuse bleeding due to disease, trauma or surgical intervention.

Blood group-specific, compatible whole blood or red cell preparations can be transfused, usually using an in-line microaggregate filter. When a fast rate of transfusion is required a pressure infusor or a pump and blood warmer should be used. In massive blood transfusion, administration of fresh frozen plasma and platelet concentrates may also be required. These should be from the same blood group as the red cells. The following complications of massive blood transfusion can occur.

*Cardiac abnormalities* are usually ventricular extrasystoles, and rarely ventricular fibrillation progressing to cardiac arrest. They are due to the combined effect of low temperature, high potassium concentration and excess citrate with low calcium concentration. They can be prevented by using a blood warmer and a slower rate of transfusion, particularly in patients with hepatic or renal failure. Routine administration of calcium gluconate in massive transfusion has not been shown to be beneficial and may even be danger-

**Table 17.4**   Tests available for monitoring blood loss and substitution therapy with blood and blood products

Oxygen-carrying capacity of blood
   Haemoglobin concentration
   Packed cell volume (PCV)
   Pulse oxymetry
Haemostatic functions
   Whole blood coagulation time
   Coagulation screen[*]
      Prothrombin time (PT)
      Partial thromboplastin time (PTT)
      Thrombin time (TT)
      Platelet count
   Thromboelastography
Oncotic pressure of plasma
   Serum total protein concentration[*]

[*] Samples for testing usually have to be sent to a main laboratory.

ous unless calcium concentration in plasma can be monitored.

*Acidosis* in the patient with severe renal or liver disease may be aggravated by the low pH of stored blood. In practice, acidosis is rarely a problem and administration of sodium bicarbonate after determining the 'base deficit' from measurements of blood pH and $PCO_2$ is rarely justified.

*Failure of haemostasis.* The usual clinical manifestations are failure of local haemostasis and, infrequently, a generalized bleeding tendency due to the lack of factors VIII:C, V and XI, as well as platelets in the stored blood. The diagnosis of bleeding due to massive transfusion must be confirmed by the laboratory, as other haemostatic defects have an identical clinical presentation but require different management (Table 17.5). Fresh frozen plasma, 1–2 units, corrects the abnormalities of coagulation and should be given prophylactically after every 10 units of blood. Platelet transfusion may be required when the platelet count is lower than $30 \times 109$ $l^{-1}$, particularly if the patient is undergoing a neurosurgical procedure.

*Adult respiratory distress syndrome (ARDS)*, also called non-cardiogenic pulmonary oedema (NPE), occurs in severely ill patients after major trauma and/or surgery. A tetrad of clinical features characterizes ARDS: progressive respiratory distress, decreased lung compliance, acute hypoxaemia and diffuse radiographic opacification of the lungs. The mortality is high; post-mortem studies show widespread macroscopic and microscopic thrombosis in the pulmonary arteries. The pathogenesis of ARDS is unclear, but agglutination of donor leucocytes, recipient leucocytes or both may be responsible for direct damage to alveolar lining cells; local disseminated intravascular coagulation, microvascular fluid leakage and embolization by leucocyte aggregates and microaggregates from stored blood all contribute. Management consists of stopping the transfusion, administering corticosteroids and providing supportive treatment to combat pulmonary oedema and hypoxia by using oxygen and positive pressure ventilation.

*Jaundice* almost invariably follows massive blood transfusion. However, serum total bilirubin rarely exceeds 40 µmol $l^{-1}$ and haemoglobinaemia is slight. Investigation for a delayed haemolytic transfusion reaction is not indicated.

## Transfusion in open heart surgery

Patients undergoing open heart surgery require cardiopulmonary bypass (CPB) for maintaining the circulation with oxygenated blood. CPB as a

**Table 17.5** Differential diagnosis of haemostatic failure in massive blood transfusion

| Condition or platelet disease | Laboratory tests | | | |
|---|---|---|---|---|
| | Prothrombin time | Partial thromboplastin time | Thrombin time | Platelet Count* |
| Massive blood transfusion | ↑ | ↑ | N | ↓ |
| DIC[†] | ↑↑ | ↑↑ | ↑↑ | ↓↓ |
| Vit. K deficiency | ↑↑ | ↑ | N | N |
| Haemophilias | N | ↑↑ | N | N |
| ITP[‡] | N | N | N | ↓↓ |

*Platelet count rarely falls below $50 \times 10^9$ $l^{-1}$.
[†]DIC, disseminated intravascular coagulation.
[‡]ITP, idiopathic thrombocytopenic purpura.
N, normal; ↑, moderately prolonged; ↑↑, markedly prolonged;
↓, moderately decreased; ↓↓, markedly decreased.

part of open heart surgery is a complex procedure and the demand for blood and blood products is variable in individual patients.

The blood required should be of the same blood group as the patient. In adults blood is not required for priming of the heart–lung machine but it is needed in neonates and small children. For post operative transfusion, any of the red cell preparations are equally satisfactory. Blood less than five days old is preferred to stored blood, but the latter can be used safely.

In most cases of open heart procedures 4 units of blood are initially cross-matched. An additional 2–4 units are required in repeated procedures. Blood components may be required for the correction of the haemostatic defect (see below). The use of albumin solutions either for priming the heart–lung machine or postoperatively has not been proved to be advantageous.

*Bleeding associated with CPB* is rare in the patient operated on for the first time. It is due to activation and loss of platelets and coagulation factors in the extracorporeal circulation, failure of heparin neutralization by the first dose of protamine, activation of fibrinolysis in the oxygenator and pump, and/or disseminated intravascular coagulation in patients with poor cardiac output and long perfusion times. The differential diagnosis

of bleeding associated with CPB is presented in Table 17.6.

*Management of bleeding* associated with CPB requires: administration of 4–8 units of platelet concentrates when the platelet count is less than $30 \times 10^9 1^{-1}$; transfusion of 2–4 units of fresh frozen plasma to correct the loss of coagulation factors; neutralization of excess heparin by protamine (1 mg of protamine neutralizes approximately 100 iu of heparin); administration of tranexamic acid (or a similar antifibrinolytic agent) when hyperfibrinolysis is confirmed by laboratory testing; treatment of disseminated intravascular coagulation, in the first instance by correcting the underlying cause (e.g. poor perfusion, oligaemic shock, acidosis, infection, etc.), and then by transfusion of fresh frozen plasma and platelet concentrates as required.

## Autologous transfusion

Autologous transfusion is the administration of the patient's own blood collected prior to, during or after an operation. Indications for autologous transfusion are, first, provision of blood for the patient with antibodies to one of the high-frequency antigens (public antigens) who is awaiting elective surgery and for whom it is not possible to

**Table 17.6**  Differential diagnosis of bleeding associated with cardiopulmonary bypass

| Cause of bleeding | Prothrombin time | Partial thromboplastin time | Thrombin time Without protamine | Thrombin time With protamine | Platelet count |
|---|---|---|---|---|---|
| Loss of platelets | N | N | N | N | ↓↓ |
| Depletion of coagulation factors | ↑↑ | ↑↑ | N | N | N or ↓ |
| Excess of heparin | ↑ | ↑↑ | ↑ | N | N or ↓ |
| Hyperfibrinolysis | ↑ | ↑ | ↑↑ | ↑↑ | N or ↓ |
| DIC* | ↑↑ | ↑↑ | ↑↑ | ↑↑ | ↓↓ |

*DIC, disseminated intravascular coagulation.
N, normal; ↑, moderately prolonged; ↑↑, markedly prolonged; ↓, moderately decreased; ↓↓, markedly reduced.

obtain compatible homologous blood; second, rational utilization of shed blood during an operation and preservation of scarce resources — blood and blood products; finally, provision of blood for recipients who wish to avoid the risks of random donor blood (alloimmunization, transmission of infection). Procedures employed for autologous transfusion are as follows:

*Preoperative deposit* of blood from the patient awaiting surgery should take into account the volume required and the time available. It is possible to collect 1 unit of blood a week from a patient with normal erythropoiesis and on iron supplements; up to 5 units can be collected and stored during a five-week period (shelf-life of blood collected into CPDA-1 anticoagulant). When more than 5 units are required or when the patient cannot tolerate frequent donations, either freezing of red cells or administration of recombinant human erythropoietin may be used.

*Normovolaemic haemodilution* is performed by withdrawing 1 or 2 units of blood from the patient within 24 hours or up to 5 units immediately before an operation and simultaneous replacement with an equivalent volume of crystalloid or colloid solution; the blood is returned after the operation. Haemodilution is almost always used in open heart surgery and less commonly in other surgical procedures.

*Salvage of blood* lost during an operation is accomplished using a simple device (e.g. Solcotrans) or a cell saver (Haemonetics Cell Saver IV). Blood shed into the thoracic or abdominal cavity is aspirated and mixed with anticoagulant. It can then be returned to the patient (Solcotrans) or the red cells can be washed, suspended in saline and transfused to the patient (Haemonetics Cell Saver IV). The use of a cell saver may considerably reduce the number of units required for transfusion. Contraindications for use of the blood salvage procedure is exposure of blood to a site of infection or the possibility of contamination with malignant cells.

## POSTOPERATIVE ANAEMIA

Anaemia in the postoperative period is most often the consequence of blood loss during operation. In the absence of protracted bleeding the haemoglobin concentration will gradually rise by approximately 1 g $dl^{-1}$ in a week. Anaemia worsening in the postoperative period requires thorough investigation to exclude a bleeding point within the operative field or failing haemostatic processes.

Appearance of anaemia, sometimes associated with mild jaundice, a week or two after operation during which the patient received blood indicates the presence of delayed haemolytic transfusion reaction (see below).

The concern that anaemia in the postoperative period may impair wound healing or prolong convalescence is not shared by all surgeons. In view that there has not been a conclusive study to prove the deleterious effect of subnormal haemoglobin it would be prudent to avoid blood transfusions used solely for the purpose of improving wound healing in the postoperative period.

## BLOOD AND BLOOD PRODUCTS

Rational use of blood and blood products is based on a knowledge of the properties and indications for use (Table 17.7).

*Whole blood and red cell preparations.* A unit contains 450 ml of blood collected in 63 ml of a citrate anticoagulant (usually CPDA-1). Red cells are prepared by removing most of the plasma after centrifugation. Red cells can also be suspended in 100 ml of an optimal additive solution. Units of blood and red cells contain about 200 ml of red cells. Blood and red cells are primarily used to correct haemoglobin deficit and each unit administered is expected to raise haemoglobin concentration by 1.0 g $dl^{-1}$ in an adult patient with stable homeostasis.

The preparations of red cells have a shelf-life of 35 days stored at 4°C. During storage, concentration of 2,3-diphosphoglycerate (2,3-DPG) in the red cells gradually decreases, granulocytes and platelets rapidly lose function, coagulation factors V and VIII and to a lesser extent XI rapidly lose their coagulant activity, and aggregates of aged platelets, leucocytes, fibrin strands, cold-insoluble globulin and cellular debris are formed.

*Platelet concentrates* are available as single units (prepared from 1 unit of blood), pooled platelets (usually equivalent to 6 single units) or as platelets collected using a cell separator (also equivalent to 6 single units). Single units contain on average $75 \times 10^9$ platelets. Platelet concentrates are administered to thrombocytopenic patients who are bleeding or receiving prophylactic treatment. In surgical practice platelet concentrates are used for treating severe bleeding after cardiopulmonary bypass and massive transfusion as well as in preparation for surgery of patients with qualitative disorders of platelets — Glanzmann's thrombasthenia, Bernard–Soulier syndrome, etc..

Platelet concentrates have a shelf-life of five days when kept in packs for extended storage, at temperatures between 20 and 24°C, preferably in an incubator and continuously agitated on an agitator. Usually 6 units of platelet concentrate are administered as one dose for an adult patient, and using a rule of thumb 1 unit of platelet concentrate, with at least $50 \times 10^9$ platelets, will increase the platelet count 1 hour after transfusion by $10^{10}\,l^{-1}\,m^{-2}$ body surface.

*Fresh frozen plasma* (FFP) for clinical use is separated from single units of blood and rapidly frozen within 6 hours after collection. It contains all the constituents of fresh plasma (except platelets). FFP is used for supporting failing coagulation in disseminated intravascular coagulation, deficiency of vitamin K-dependent coagulation factors, overdose of oral anticoagulants, liver disease, massive blood transfusion, cardiopulmonary bypass and treatment of congenital deficiencies of factors V and XI. Although 2–4 units are usually administered to the patient, the volume and frequency of administration should be assessed for each patient separately. FFP, kept in a deep-freeze at a temperature below –30°C, has a shelf-life of one year.

*Cryoprecipitate and single coagulation factor concentrates* are rarely used in surgical practice. The properties, indications for use and monitoring of

**Table 17.7** Blood and blood components and indication for use

| Component | Volume/unit (ml) | Main indications for use | Special precautions |
|---|---|---|---|
| Whole blood (PCV* 0.35–0.45) | 510 | Acute massive blood loss | Possible abnormalities of haemostasis if loss and replacement exceed twice the blood volume |
| Red cells (PCV 0.55–0.75) | 280 | Anaemia | None |
| Red cells in OAS† (PCV 0.50–0.70) | 350 | Anaemia | Not to be used for neonates and exchange blood transfusion |
| Filtered red cells (PCV variable) | Variable | Non-haemolytic febrile transfusion reaction Prevention of HLA immunization | None |
| Platelet concentrates from random donors | 50 | Thrombocytopenia Qualitative disorders of platelets | None |
| obtained by plateletpheresis | 250 | As above | For patients with platelet refractoriness should be HLA matched |
| Fresh frozen plasma | 200 | Replacement of all coagulation factors Reversal of warfarin effect Thrombotic thrombocytopenic purpura | Allergic reactions; circulatory overload |
| Cryoprecipitate | 20 | von Willebrand's disease Hypofibrinogenaemia Factor XIII deficiency | Allergic reactions |

*PCV, packed cell volume.

†OAS, optimal additive solution.

therapeutic effect of these preparations are described in textbooks of haematology and blood transfusion.

*Albumin* is available as 5% and 20% solutions in a variety of dose units. The indication for administration of 5% albumin is the replacement of plasma proteins and expansion of plasma volume, as in hypoproteinaemia following burns (after the first 24 hours) and as a part of the replacement fluid in large-volume plasma exchange. Opinions are divided whether albumin solutions play a role in restoration of circulatory volume in haemorrhage shock, but the view that administration of colloid and crystalloid solutions is better for that purpose (and it is certainly cheaper) is gaining popularity. The indication for use of 20% albumin is solely the replacement of plasma proteins in severe hypoproteinaemia in renal or liver disease, after large-volume paracentesis, following massive liver resection and in some cases of Gram-negative septicaemia.

*Plasma substitutes* are colloid and crystalloid solutions which are used for maintaining the circulatory volume following acute haemorrhage, shock, burns and septicaemia. Plasma substitutes have no oxygen-carrying capacity and lack haemostatic properties. Crystalloid solutions have no plasma oncotic activity and colloid solutions possess it only temporarily as their half-life in circulation is rather short (Table 17.8). The use of plasma substitutes in an emergency 'buys time' necessary for provision of compatible blood and appropriate blood products.

## ADVERSE CONSEQUENCES OF BLOOD TRANSFUSION

In general, transfusion of blood and blood products is a safe and effective mode of treatment. However, a small proportion of patients will suffer from transfusion side effects and a few may be in danger from having potentially catastrophic reactions of transfusion. The main undesirable consequences of transfusion are transfusion reactions due to antigen/antibody binding and subsequent destruction of the target cell, modulation of the immune system of the recipient, graft-versus-host disease and transmission of diseases (Table 17.9).

*Immediate haemolytic transfusion reaction (HTR)* is almost always due to ABO incompatibility between the transfused red cells and the recipient. Over 90% of HTR is due to clerical error in the identification of the patient or the unit of blood.

Severe HTR is characterized by anxiety, chest pain, back pain, headache, dyspnea, rigors, vomiting, diarrhoea, restlessness, tachycardia, hypotension, shock, unexplained bleeding and renal shutdown, which occur in quick succession. In the anaesthetized patient persistent hypotension and unexplained oozing from the wound may be the only signs. Haemoglobinaemia and haemoglobinuria are present. Diagnosis is based on finding the clerical error, visual inspection of serum and urine and laboratory testing. Management consists of stopping the transfusion, administration of hydrocortisone 100 mg and an intravenous antihistamine (i.e. chlorpheniramine 10 mg), maintenance of blood volume and urinary flow with intravenous fluids, and in the presence of disseminated intravascular coagulation intravenous administration of heparin.

Moderate HTR presents less dramatically than severe HTR, while mild HTR presents with a mild degree of fever only and often passes unnoticed.

*Delayed haemolytic transfusion reaction.* Haemolysis of the transfused red cells in the recipient's circulation which occurs one to three weeks after transfusion is due to an anamnestic antibody re-

**Table 17.8** Plasma substitutes: colloid volume expanders (given in percentages)

| Product | Mol. w | Concentration | Half-life in circulation (h) |
| --- | --- | --- | --- |
| Modified gelatin | 35 000 | 3–4 | 5 |
| Hydroxyethyl starch | 450 000 | 6 | 24 |
| Dextran 70 | 70 000 | 6 | 24 |

**Table 17.9**  Adverse consequences of blood transfusion

Immune response to cellular and plasmatic alloantigens:
  Clinical syndromes following repeated transfusions
  Red cell antibodies              —  haemolytic transfusion reaction
  HLA antibodies                   —  non-haemolytic febrile transfusion reaction
                                   —  platelet refractoriness
  Platelet-specific antibodies     —  platelet refractoriness
                                   —  post-transfusion thrombocytopenia
                                   —  neonatal immune thrombocytopenia
  Anti-IgA*                        —  anaphylactic shock

Immunomodulation (e.g. reduced disease-free interval after resection of carcinoma of the colon)

Graft-versus-host disease (caused by transfusion of live lymphocytes)
  In immunosuppressed patients (e.g. patients receiving tissue or organ transplants
  In immunocompetent patients (transfused with blood donated by first-degree relatives)

Transfusion of viruses†
  Hepatitis B virus
  Non-A, non-B hepatitis (including hepatitis C virus)
  Cytomegalovirus
  Epstein–Barr virus
  HIV 1 and 2
  HTLV I and II

---

*Only seen in some individuals with IgA deficiency.
†Transfusion of *Treponema pallidum* (syphilis) is exceedingly rare in the UK. In tropical areas the transmission of
  *Plasmodium* species (malaria) and in South America transmission of *Trypanosoma cruzi* (Chagas' disease) presents
  a serious problem.

sponse, most often against antigens in the Rh system. Jaundice, progressive anaemia, fever, arthralgia and myalgia are commonly encountered. Diagnosis is easily established by a positive direct antiglobulin test (DAT) and a positive antibody screen.

Usually no treatment is required, but when hypotension and renal failure are present the patient should be treated symptomatically. Blood transfusions should be avoided but when necessary compatible red cells should be administered. Patients with delayed haemolytic transfusion reaction have an increased risk of thrombosis and should be considered for administration of prophylactic subcutaneous heparin.

*Non-haemolytic febrile transfusion reaction (NHFTR)* usually occurs within hours after the onset of transfusion. NHFTR occurs in multi-transfused patients with antibodies against HLA antigens or granulocyte-specific antibodies. The reaction is due to pyrogens, released from granulocytes damaged by complement in an antigen/antibody reaction. It presents with a rise of temperature with flushing palpitations and tachycardia, followed by headache and rigors. In severe forms of NHFTR, cough, breathlessness and respiratory distress may ensue. Diagnosis is made clinically and confirmed by laboratory tests showing absence of haemolysis. Management of NHFTR consists of administration of antipyretics (aspirin or paracetamol) and in patients with severe symptoms 100 mg of hydrocortisone i.v. can also be given. Prevention in patients who repeatedly suffer from NHFTR is achieved by administration of blood filtered using one of the specific leucocyte depletion filters (Sepacell R-500, Pall RC-100).

*Platelet refractoriness* is the term used to describe the failure of platelet transfusion to raise the platelet count in the recipient. It represents one of the serious manifestations of alloimmunization to HLA and platelet-specific antigens. Diagnosis of platelet refractoriness and management of the patient are usually in the province of the haematologist.

*Transfusion reactions associated with plasma proteins* are urticaria and anaphylactoid reactions. Urticaria is one of the most common transfusion reactions and consists of circumscribed areas of cutaneous oedema. It is caused by the degranulation of mast cells in the skin and subsequent release of histamine. Urticaria is easily recognizable clinically and it is treated by administration of an antihistamine drug. Severe urticaria recurring with each transfusion can be prevented by administration of chlorpheniramine or transfusion of washed red cells or frozen and thawed red cells, free of plasma proteins.

Anaphylactoid reaction is a term used to describe an immediate hypersensitivity reaction. It is a rare reaction which occurs in individuals with IgA deficiency who have anti-IgA due to previous immunization. The clinical manifestations vary from mild erythema, pruritus, urticaria and angiooedema of lips to severe oedema of the larynx or epiglottis, and bronchospasm, hypotension and shock. The mainstay of treatment is administration of adrenaline, as well as maintenance of unimpeded breathing and treatment of hypotension.

*Immunomodulation.* There is now little doubt that transfusions of blood can cause immunosuppression in the recipient. This effect of transfusion was used for the benefit of recipients of kidney transplants before the introduction of cyclosporin into the treatment schedules. However, adverse effects of blood transfusion have been reported in patients after surgical removal of malignant tumours (shortened disease-free interval). Furthermore, several reports have highlight-

ed increased incidence of postoperative infections in patients transfused before or during operation. Detailed discussion on immunomodulation is beyond the scope of this chapter.

*Graft-versus-host disease (GVHD)* is caused by engraftment of donor lymphocytes in severely immunosuppressed or immunodeficient recipients as well as in premature babies. It can also occur in immunocompetent recipients who are transfused with blood donated by first-degree relatives (directed donations). In most instances manifestations of GVHD are mild but in immunocompetent patients the disease is often fatal. To abolish the capacity for engraftment of donor lymphocytes it is recommended that blood, platelet and granulocyte concentrates are irradiated with 15–30 Gy before administration to patients likely to develop GVHD.

*Transmission of infectious diseases.* While the transmission of bacterial and parasitic infections by transfusion is exceptionally rare in the UK, the transmission of viruses is the focus of interest of the public and medical profession alike. Transfusion services maintain a safe blood supply by a rigorous process of selection of prospective blood donors and by the use of specific microbiological screening tests for markers of the disease. In addition, safety of the fractionated plasma products is enhanced by the use of viral inactivation procedures. A description of the manifestation

**Table 17.10**  Estimates of virus transmission rates by transfusion of blood and blood components[*]

| Virus | Incidence of carriers[†] | Tests Available | Used | Estimate of units required for transfusion |
|---|---|---|---|---|
| Hepatitis B virus | 1 : 1000 | Yes[‡] | Yes | 20 000 |
| Non-A, non-B viruses[§] | 1 : 1700 | Yes | Yes | 20 000 |
| Cytomegalovirus | 1 : 2 | Yes | No[‖] | 10[•] |
| Epstein–Barr virus | 9 : 10 | Yes | No | Most recipients are immune |
| HIV 1 and 2 | 1 : 25 000 | Yes | Yes | 1 000 000 |
| HTLV I and II | 1 : 20 000 | Yes | No | 1 000 000[•] |

[*]Transmission of viruses by plasma products is excluded; all plasma products undergo viral inactivation in production.
[†]Seen in first-time blood donors following self-exclusion of those in risk categories, donating blood in London, February 1992.
[‡]Test for HB$_S$ antigen.
[§]Includes hepatitis C virus; test for anti-HCV is reactive in about 80% of carriers capable of trasmitting non-A, non-B hepatitis.
[‖]Test is used to provide anti-CMV negative blood for patients in 'at risk' groups: recipients of kidney transplants, recipients of bone marrow transplants, preterm babies of less than 1500 g weight and pregnant women. Patients with AIDS who are anti-CMV negative can be also considered as at increased risk from acquiring CMV infection.
[•]Only about 1 in 5 recipients negative on testing will seroconvert following transfusion of a unit of blood found positive on testing.

and management of the viral diseases which can be transmitted by transfusion can be found elsewhere and only the estimates of risk of transmission are discussed below.

The risk of transmission of a viral disease depends, in addition to a vigorous selection procedure, on the incidence of carriers (individuals who are healthy but harbour the virus), availability of a screening test and its sensitivity and specificity, the use of the test for screening purposes, and the susceptibility to infection of the recipient (Table 17.10). It is mandatory in the UK to test for markers of hepatitis B virus (HBV), hepatitic C virus (HCV), human immunodeficiency virus types 1 and 2 (HIV 1 and 2) and for *Treponema pallidum*.

It can be seen from Table 17.10 that the incidence of most of the viral infections in the general population is low; donor selection procedures are effective and the screening for disease markers is highly successful. The absolute number of infections transmitted by blood transfusion is exceedingly small. However, the risk of transmitting a disease still remains and has to be taken into account when the decision to transfuse the patient is made.

FURTHER READING

British Committee for Standards in Haematology 1990 Guidelines for implementation of a maximum surgical blood order schedule. Clinical and Laboratory Haematology 12: 321–327

British Society for Haematology and the British Blood Transfusion Society 1988 Guidelines for autologous transfusion. Clinical and Laboratory Haematology 10: 193–201

Consensus conference 1985 Fresh-frozen plasma: indications and risks. Journal of the American Medical Association 253: 551–553

Consensus conference 1987: Platelet transfusion therapy. Journal of the American Medical Association 257: 1777–1780

Consensus conference 1988 Perioperative red cell transfusion. Journal of the American Medical Association 260: 2700–2703

Contreras M (ed) 1990 ABC of transfusion. British Medical Journal, London

Goodnough L T, Johnston M F M, Ramsey G et al 1990 Guidelines for transfusion support in patients undergoing coronary artery bypass surgery. Annals of Thoracic Surgery 50: 675–683

Hunt B J 1991 Modifying perioperative blood loss. Blood Reviews 5: 168–176

Kruskall M S, Mintz P D, Bergin J J et al 1988 Transfusion therapy in emergency medicine. Annals of Emergency Medicine 17: 327–335

McClelland D B L (ed) 1989 Handbook of transfusion medicine. Her Majesty's Stationery Office, London

# 18. Nutritional support

*J. J. Payne-James*

Nutritional support is administered to patients because a number of studies have demonstrated poorer outcomes of treatment in patients who are suffering from protein calorie (energy) malnutrition (PCM). Patients may be at increased risk of infection (e.g. chest, urinary, wound), slow healing, wound breakdown and dehiscence, and death. Defining 'the nutritionally compromised patient' is a problem. It is possible to consider a variety of parameters including biochemical (e.g. serum albumin, transferrin, retinol-binding protein), anthropometric (e.g. triceps skin-fold thickness (TSF), mid-arm muscle circumference (MAMC)), immunological (e.g. lymphocyte count, delayed hypersensitivity skin-testing) and dynamometric (e.g. hand-grip strength) measurements. Different studies examining each type of parameter in turn have shown that each may (if values are low or impaired) reflect an increased likelihood of increased morbidity and mortality. Unfortunately it has been less easy to demonstrate that improving the nutritional state improves patient outcome, and often this has been due to poor or flawed study design. It is often considered surprising that malnutrition can be considered a problem in hospitals. Hill et al 1977 and Bistrian et al 1976 in two widely quoted studies showed incidences of malnutrition (using parameters such as serum albumin, TSF, MAMC) for up to 60% of hospital patients over ten years ago. Despite advances in the practice of clinical nutrition, recent studies confirm that malnutrition is still a significant problem. The aim of nutritional support should therefore be to identify the malnourished (or potentially malnourished) patient, to correct or improve the nutritional status such that morbidity and mortality related to poor nutritional status are reduced. This in turn will shorten in-patient stay and lessen the financial burden on hospitals.

## INDICATIONS FOR NUTRITIONAL SUPPORT

In the absence of a single specific measure of nutritional state it is necessary for the practising clinician to define groups of patients who should receive nutritional support. All patients admitted to hospital, even for elective procedures, should have a nutritional assessment. The routine history and clinical examination of a patient should enable patients who may require nutritional support to be identified and placed in one of the following three groups:

1. Obvious severe malnutrition (recent or long term) ( >10% recent weight loss; serum albumin <30gl⁻¹; gross muscle wasting ± peripheral oedema)
2. Moderate malnutrition (some nutritional parameters suggestive; dietary history shows impaired nutrient intake for preceding two to four weeks or more; there may be no obvious physical evidence of malnutrition)
3. Normal or near-normal nutritional status (but underlying pathology is likely to result in malnutrition if nutritional support withheld — e.g. trauma patients, ventilated patients).

Once it has been decided that a patient needs nutritional support, a decision about whether to use parenteral (intravenous) or enteral (via the gastrointestinal tract) feeding must be made. The main consideration when choosing the optimal route of access is that: *the enteral route should be used as the technique of choice in all patients with a normal or near-normal functioning, accessible gastrointestinal tract.*

The main contraindications to enteral nutrition are intestinal obstruction, paralytic ileus, major abdominal sepsis and multi-organ failure with or without complex fluid-balance problems. In those patients with complex fluid-balance abnormalities, enteral nutrition may cause problems as it is difficult to assess the time course over which enteral substrates and their fluid load may be absorbed. The main contraindication to parenteral nutrition is a functioning gastrointestinal tract. Access to the gastrointestinal tract may be achieved in a number

**Table 18.1**    Routes of administration

| Enteral | |
| --- | --- |
| Oral feeding | |
| Tube feeding | |
| Nasoenteral | — gastric |
| | — duodenal |
| | — jejunal |
| Cervical pharyngostomy | |
| Cervical oesophagostomy | |
| Gastrostomy | — surgical |
| | — percutaneous endoscopic gastrostomy (PEG) |
| Jejunostomy | — surgical |
| | — needle catheter jejunostomy (NCJ) |

(Payne-James 1992)

**Table 18.2**    Categories of patients suitable for enteral nutrition

| Patient group | Disease state |
| --- | --- |
| Medical | Inflammatory bowel disease |
| | Hepatic failure |
| | Renal failure |
| | Respiratory failure |
| Neurological | Cerebrovascular accident |
| | Motor neurone disease |
| | Multiple sclerosis |
| Geriatric | |
| Surgical | Preoperative |
| | Postoperative |
| | Fistula |
| | Burns |
| | Sepsis |
| Orthopaedic | Trauma |
| Psychiatric | Anorexia nervosa |
| Paediatric | Cystic fibrosis |
| Miscellaneous | ITU |
| | Cancer |
| | Short bowel |
| | AIDS/HIV |

**Table 18.3**    Categories of patients suitable for total parenteral nutrition

| Patient group | Disease state |
| --- | --- |
| Medical | Inflammatory bowel disease |
| | Hepatic failure |
| | Renal failure |
| | Respiratory failure |
| Surgical | Preoperative |
| | Postoperative |
| | Fistula |
| | Burns |
| | Sepsis |
| | Pancreatitis |
| Orthopaedic | Trauma |
| Miscellaneous | ITU |
| | Cancer |
| | Short bowel |
| | AIDS/HIV |

of ways (see Table 18.1). Examples of disease states that may be appropriate for either enteral or parenteral nutrition are listed in Tables 18.2 and 18.3.

It will be noted that there is a great deal of overlap, emphasizing that these therapies are *complementary*, not *competing*. It is because of this that clinical nutrition within a hospital setting should be monitored and managed by practitioners experienced with both techniques. It is very important to emphasize that the best way of providing nutritional support for a patient is by mouth. If there is uncertainty about a patient's required versus achieved food intakes then techniques of nutritional support highlighted in this chapter should be used only after formal dietary assessment has established that the patient cannot (even with sip feeds and diet supplements) achieve the required goals. In general this assessment is best done by a dietitian.

## PERIOPERATIVE NUTRITION

A considerable number of patients undergoing surgical procedures may be malnourished and be at risk for postoperative complications such as infection or wound breakdown. There are few randomized controlled studies showing a benefit of improving nutritional status on patient outcome (Buzby et al 1987) but the consensus of opinion is that there is no evidence of benefit in administering routine preoperative nutritional support to any patient with normal or near-normal status whatever the procedure they are to undergo. The patient who *is* severely malnourished, however, may benefit from receiving preoperative nutritional support (von Meyenfeldt et al 1992). Clearly the reason for operation, the degree of malnutrition and expected postoperative course are important in making this decision. A severely malnourished elderly patient who is a smoker, requiring oesophagectomy, would be a candidate for preoperative nutritional support. A patient with a prolonged exacerbation of inflammatory bowel disease unresponsive to medical management who presents with a perforated viscus requires surgery first and nutritional support later.

The length of preoperative nutritional support should not be such that the patient's condition can deteriorate as a result of progression of the disease. However, neither should it be so short as to have no effect on any nutritional parameters. In practice this means a minimum period of nutritional support 7–14 days.

Postoperative nutrition should be considered for any patient who fails to have an adequate oral intake (as assessed by a dietitian) after five days of surgery. For some patients it may be clear at the time of operation that adequate oral intake will not be possible (because of major oropharyngeal/maxillofacial surgery) for some time postoperatively, or that normal gut function will take more than a few days to recover (major upper gastrointestinal resection). In cases such as these it may be advisable to insert routes of access (e.g. gastrostomy, jejunostomy, central lines) while the patient is still in the operating theatre anaesthestized. If unexpected rapid recovery ensues, these may be removed. If they *are* required the patient is not subject to, and the surgeon does not have to arrange, placement at a later date.

## ENERGY AND NITROGEN REQUIREMENTS

Most surgical patients in need of nutritional support are stressed, septic or have been subject to trauma (accident or operation). These patients (particularly those with burns or head injuries) are likely to be hypermetabolic as a result of the normal neuroendocrinological response to injury. Specific energy requirements may be determined from indirect calorimetry but this is not practical for most clinicians. In general, energy requirements are rarely more that 2200–2400 kcal per 24 hours for surgical patients to achieve positive energy balance. Thus 35–40 kcal kg$^{-1}$ per 24 hours energy will be appropriate for most patients, and this will be supplied as a mixture of carbohydrate and fat. Nitrogen (protein) requirements are often considerably greater than normal, and in hypermetabolic, stressed and injured patients nitrogen balance may be impossible to achieve until the primary pathology has been treated. The amount of nitrogen administered should ideally minimize net losses without wasting administered nitrogen; permit maintenance of the patient's lean body mass, allowing an adequate supply of nitrogen for repair; and allow active repletion of lean body mass in the previously compromised patient. For most adult patients 14–16g nitrogen will be appropriate. Those patients with increased energy needs will require increased nitrogen and amounts up to 0.4 g nitrogen kg$^{-1}$ per 24 hours have been suggested.

## Monitoring

The main parameters that should be considered when monitoring a patient receiving nutritional support are listed in Table 18.4.

**Table 18.4** Patient monitoring

Diet charts
Weight
Haematology
Biochemistry
Anthropometry
Dynamometry

Diet charts (for patients on enteral nutrition) enable an accurate record of the patient's actual versus prescribed intake to be kept, and the charts will allow correction of intake problems to be undertaken. These charts are also of importance during the changeover from enteral feeding to per os nutrition. Weighing is probably the simplest but most valuable way to ensure that the nutrition regimen prescribed for a particular patient is satisfactory. A steady increase in weight of 1–2 kg per week suggests adequate nutrition in those requiring body mass repletion. Basic haematological and biochemical parameters should be measured at the commencement of nutrition. Initially close monitoring of the plasma potassium, phosphate and glucose are important, particularly in the severely malnourished patient. In patients on long-term feeding, vitamin levels or trace element levels may be required if clinically indicated. The plasma proteins albumin, transferrin and thyroid binding pre-albumin can all be useful markers for indicating a response to nutritional support over a period of time. Anthropometric and dynamometric measurements are often considered as research tools, but they can offer sensitive and effective measurement of the efficacy of nutritional support over a period of time.

## Nitrogen balance

Nitrogen balance is frequently used as an assessment technique for monitoring day-to-day progress of nutritional support. One of the aims of nutritional support should be to place the patient in positive nitrogen balance. This is often difficult or impossible to achieve in the very stressed or catabolic patient. The components of nitrogen balance are those of whole-body protein turnover — it represents the difference between whole-body protein synthesis and breakdown. Thus it is a measure of metabolic state rather than nutritional status. In most patients nitrogen balance can be calculated from urinary and faecal nitrogen losses and whenever possible 24-hour collections of urine should be undertaken on all patients receiving nutritional support. Often faecal output is negligible. Lee & Hartley (1975) showed that there is a reasonable correlation between urinary urea excretion and total urinary nitrogen, with urea accounting for about 80%. Allowances must be made for plasma urea levels and a figure of 2–3 g allowed for other routes of loss, including faeces. These figures are not appropriate for the severely ill patient, where the urinary urea may represent considerably less than 80% of the total nitrogen because of excessive excretion of ammonium and other non-urea nitrogenous compounds. In recent years it has become possible to measure total urinary nitrogen by chemiluminescence routinely, thereby obviating the need to estimate output from urea values.

## ENTERAL NUTRITION

### Types of enteral diets

There are three main types of nutritionally complete enteral diets appropriate for the surgical patient: polymeric, predigested (or elemental), and disease-specific.

*Polymeric* diets are indicated for the vast majority of patients with normal or near-normal gastrointestinal function (Payne-James & Silk 1988). They contain whole protein as a nitrogen source, energy is derived from triglycerides and glucose polymers, while electrolytes, trace elements and vitamins are included in standardized amounts. Generally one of two polymeric diets, a 'standard' or an 'energy', nitrogen-dense' diet, is prescribed. The standard polymeric diets contain approximately 6 g nitrogen per litre with an energy density of 1 kcal ml$^{-1}$. The energy, nitrogen-dense diets contain between 8 and 10 g nitrogen per litre and an energy density of 1–1.5 kcal ml$^{-1}$. Polymeric diets are suitable for over 90% of patients with normal or near-normal gastrointestinal function. In a few patients with very severe exocrine pancreatic insufficiency or with intestinal failure because of short bowel syndrome, intraluminal hydrolysis may be severely impaired, thereby limiting diet assimilation. In such cases a *predigested or elemental* diet may be indicated. These diets have a nitrogen source derived from free amino acids or oligopeptides. Energy is derived from glucose polymer mixture predominating with polymers of chain length >10 glucose molecules. The fat source consists of a combination of long and medium-chain triglycerides. Specially formulated *'disease-specific'* diets have been developed for patients with specific diseases such as encephalopathy associated with chronic liver disease, and respiratory failure. Malnourished patients with cirrhosis who present with encephalopathy, or who have a previous history of episodes of encephalopathy, present a difficult problem of nutritional management. Branched-chain amino acid-enriched diets have been advocated to normalize plasma amino acid profiles with the aim of improving nutritional state and preventing worsening of encephalopathy. At present the results of controlled clinical trials are conflicting, and more research is required before recommendations for usage can be made. The same factors apply to the use of 'renal formulas' containing essential amino acids for treatment of patients with renal failure. Patients with respiratory failure on ventilators have been shown to be adversely affected by diets with high carbohydrate loads which increase carbon dioxide production. The administration of a diet with a higher fat energy component is beneficial in allowing earlier weaning off the ventilator as a result of decreased carbon dioxide production and reduced respiratory quotient.

## Route of administration

Most patients will require nutritional support for less than a month. For these patients the best method of enteral delivery is via a fine-bore nasogastric feeding tube. The most frequent complication (less than 5% of patients) is tube malposition at insertion, generally into the trachea and bronchi. If the presence within the bronchus has not been recognized then accidental intrapulmonary aspiration of feed may occur. This complication occurs most commonly in patients with altered swallowing, diminished gag reflex or who have had upper airway or pharyngeal surgery. In patients who are alert and orientated tube positioning may be confirmed by aspiration of gastric contents and auscultation of the epigastrium. If aspiration or auscultation is unsuccessful, *X-ray confirmation of the position of the tube is essential, and must be undertaken routinely in all patients with altered consciousness, altered cough or gag reflex, who are mechanically ventilated or who have had upper airway surgery.* In some patients nasogastric delivery of nutrients may not be appropriate because of an increased risk of regurgitation and/or pulmonary aspiration of feed (see Table 18.5).

All patients in the groups indicated in Table 18.5 and those with gastric atony or paresis for any reason should at least be considered for postpyloric nasoduodenal or nasojejunal feeding to

**Table 18.5** Examples of diseases with an increased risk of regurgitation and aspiration

Diabetes with neuropathy
Hypothyroidism
ITU patients on ventilators
Neuromotor deglutition disorders
Neurosurgical patients
Postabdominal surgery

reduce the risk of regurgitation or aspiration. Placement of fine-bore tubes beyond the pylorus remains a problem. Controlled trials have clearly demonstrated that tube design will not affect the incidence of spontaneous transpyloric passage of lengthened fine-bore tubes. Other techniques using metoclopramide, manipulation of the tube at the bedside or under fluoroscopic control have all been tried, with varying success. For the surgical patient in whom postoperative feeding is anticipated, placement at laparotomy is advised. In other cases a fine-bore tube of appropriate length may be introduced pernasally, and if spontaneous passage has not occurred after 12–24 hours endoscopic positioning is undertaken. For some patients other routes of administration may be more appropriate or preferable than the nasoenteral route. Pharyngostomy and oesophagostomy have not found widespread acceptance although are used by a few enthusiasts. Surgically placed gastrostomies are still used for long-term administration of feed for patients with incurable deglutition disorders (motor neurone disease, multiple sclerosis) but the percutaneous endoscopic gastrostomy (PEG) is becoming increasingly recognized as the technique of choice for indefinite administration of enteral nutrition. This technique enables a gastrostomy tube to be inserted under endoscopic control using local anaesthesia. This technique has proved to be effective, with a satisfactorily low morbidity and mortality, when compared with the conventional surgical placement. The technique of needle catheter jejunostomy (NCJ) described by Delaney in 1973 has gained some acceptance. The catheter is inserted either as a separate surgical procedure or concurrently at the time of abdominal surgery. It has been suggested that an NCJ could be recommended for patients (a) malnourished at the time of surgery, (b) undergoing major upper gastrointestinal surgery,

(c) who may receive adjuvant radio- or chemo-therapy after surgery and (d) for patients under-going laparotomy after major trauma. The avail-ability of this route means that total parenteral nutrition (TPN) with its attendant risks may be avoided.

## Reservoirs and giving sets

Enteral diets may be dispensed from different-sized containers ranging from 500 ml to 2 litres in vol-ume. The policy of using larger reservoirs improves the ratio of administered diet/prescribed diet and reduces the amount of handling time needed. Giving sets should be changed every 24 hours as there is a risk of contamination of the diet con-tainer with bacteria spreading retrogradely up the giving set from the patient.

## Infusion versus bolus administration

Bolus feeding of enteral diets, whereby a volume of 200–400 ml of feed was instilled into the stom-ach via a nasogastric tube over a period of time ranging from 15 minutes to 1 hour, was the stan-dard method of administration for many years. There is now substantial evidence to show that this is a poor method of administering enteral diet, because it has greater incidence of side-effects such as bloating and diarrhoea, in addition to which a considerable amount of nursing time is required and feeds may often be accidentally omitted. A continuous infusion either by gravity feed or by using a peristaltic pump is therefore the method of choice. A continuous overnight infusion followed by disconnection during the day may be the optimal technique, as nutritional parameters may be addi-tionally improved in this way.

## Starter regimens

Controlled clinical trials have convincingly demon-strated that the use of starter regimens (either by diluting the feed or reducing the volume) only results in limiting the intake of diet in the first few days of feeding, thereby prolonging the length of negative nitrogen balance. The incidence of gastrointestinal side effects is unchanged in patients with normal bowel, or those with inflammatory bowel disease, when a full-strength full-volume diet is used to commence enteral nutrition. Starter regimens should not therefore in general be used.

## Commencing enteral feeding

For those patients who are immobile or confined to bed, or with altered consciousness, our practice is to elevate the head of the patient's bed by 20 or 30° to help reduce the risk of regurgitation and aspiration. In most adult patients with no other metabolic or fluid balance problems, between 2 and 2.5 litres of diet are prescribed on a daily basis. This volume is infused from day one.

## Complications

The potential complications of enteral nutrition are summarized in Table 18.6.

Tube blockage most commonly occurs after dis-connection of the giving set from the feeding tube, and the residual diet solidifies. This complication may be prevented by flushing the tube with water after disconnection. An obstructed tube may occa-sionally be unblocked by instilling pancreatic en-zyme or cola. Diarrhoea occurs in about 10% of patients (Payne-James et al 1992), although definitions of the term diarrhoea are unreliable. The definition of diarrhoea as 'passage of too loose or too frequent stools, or both, sufficient to have been observed by patient and nursing staff' is use-ful in clinical practice. Its aetiology remains

Table18.6   Complications of enteral nutrition

| Feeding tube related | Malposition |
| --- | --- |
| | Unwanted removal |
| | Blockage |
| Diet and diet administration related | Diarrhoea |
| | Bloating |
| | Nausea |
| | Cramps |
| | Regurgitation |
| | Pulmonary aspiration |
| | Vitamin, mineral, trace element deficiencies |
| | Drug interactions |
| Metabolic/biochemical | |
| Infective | Diets |
| | Reservoirs |
| | Giving sets |

unclear. There is a definite association with concomitant antibiotic therapy, and there seems to be increasing evidence that hypoalbuminaemia may play a role. For the present, until the aetiology is clearly established symptomatic treatment (with antidiarrhoeals such as codeine phosphate or loperamide) is appropriate and only rarely does enteral feeding have to be discontinued. Antibiotics that are no longer clinically indicated (not an uncommon occurrence) should be stopped. Nausea and vomiting rarely occur and may result from slowed gastric emptying. Antiemetics may be of benefit. The symptoms of bloating, abdominal distension and cramps most commonly occur following inadvertent too rapid administration of feed, and are very similar to the symptoms described in association with bolus-type feeding. Enteral diets will interact with enterally administered drugs. Specifically problems have been reported with theophylline, warfarin, methyldopa and digoxin. Failure of drug therapy in previously stable patients receiving enteral nutritional support must be assumed to be feed related until proved otherwise.

## TOTAL PARENTERAL NUTRITION

The successful use of intravenous nutrition (total parenteral nutrition) in maintaining body weight and allowing growth to progress normally was first demonstrated by Stanley Dudrick and coworkers over 20 years ago (Dudrick el at 1968). TPN plays an essential role in the management of some acutely ill patients. Up to 25% of patients in hospital requiring nutritional support need it administered via the parenteral route. *TPN can be considered for all malnourished or potentially malnourished patients with non-functioning and/or non-accessible gastrointestinal tract.* Four main areas need to be considered when providing TPN for a patient (see Table 18.7).

### Access

**Table 18.7** Considerations for TPN

| Access | — techniques |
| | — complications |
| Nutrients | — delivery |
| Monitoring | |
| Metabolic complication | |

TPN solutions have high osmolalities. As a result administration of TPN solutions into peripheral veins can result in rapid development of thrombophlebitis and line failure. This problem is overcome by using central venous catheters to deliver TPN solutions into large veins such as the superior vena cava (SVC), most commonly via the subclavian or internal jugular veins. Getting access to, and the presence of central venous catheters within these veins, give rise to certain complications, the most well recognized of which are listed in Table 18.8. These catheter-insertion complications represent most of the serious complications associated with TPN.

**Table 18.8** Complications of central venous catheter

*Insertion-related*

| Air embolism | Haematoma |
| Arterial puncture | Haemothorax |
| Arrhythmias | Hydro-TPN-othorax |
| Catheter embolus | Malposition |
| Chylothorax | Neurological injury |
| Haemo/hydropericardium | Pneumothorax |

*Late complications*
Catheter infection/sepsis
Luminal occlusion
Catheter displacement
Central venous thrombosis

A variety of routes, catheters and techniques of insertion are available. The two main methods of insertion are by blind percutaneous puncture of a vein or by open surgical exposure. The advantages of the percutaneous technique in experienced hands are that insertion is quick and may be done under local anaesthesia at the patient's bedside as long as sterile procedure is observed. A catheter should be used that is inserted by the Seldinger technique so that guidewire exchange of catheters is possible. Complications should occur in less than 5% of patients and are dependent on operator experience. Open surgical exposure generally requires an operating theatre and occasionally general anaesthesia. However, there are three groups of patients where catheter insertion should always be undertaken by using the surgical 'open' technique if possible because the risks associated with development of complications are more likely to be fatal. These are patients with chronic respiratory disease, those on a ventilator, and those with severe clotting disorders. The majority of catheters used for TPN in the UK are still single-lumen central venous catheters. Most of these are inserted with a short subcutaneous tunnel fashioned to allow the catheter to exit away from the point of vein penetration. Originally the 'tunnel' was fashioned in an attempt to reduce the incidence of catheter infection but it is now clear that catheter contamination originates not only locally from the insertion site but also from catheter manipulation at the junctions between catheter and giving set. There is probably little difference in infection rates between tunnelled and non-tunnelled catheters if strict catheter care protocols are followed and monitored by an infection control or nutrition nurse. The most serious complication unrelated to catheter insertion is catheter-related infection or sepsis. If a patient on TPN develops a pyrexia and leucocytosis in the absence of any other focus of infection, then the CV catheter should be considered the source of infection. Therefore in addition to culture of sputum, urine and other possible sites of origin of sepsis the treatment plan in Table 18.9 should be pursued. Increasingly multiple-lumen central venous catheters are used for administration of TPN. Other functions such as central venous pressure measurement, blood product administration, drug administration and blood sampling may be undertaken concurrently. Early fears that the increase in handling of such catheters would result in worse catheter infection rates have not been confirmed, as long as the strict catheter care protocol is observed.

In recent years great interest has been expressed by a number of groups about the feasibility of administering TPN by the peripheral route (peripheral parenteral nutrition—PPN) (MacFie 1992). Historically the central venous route was used

because of the high incidence of thrombophlebitis using parenteral nutrition infusion mixtures. It is now clear that peripheral cannula-associated thrombophlebitis is multifactorial and not related solely to the osmotic load of the infusion mixture. Amongst other factors microparticulates from small-volume parenterals and cannula material may have an effect on the development of thrombophlebitis. A number of methods have been investigated to reduce the incidence of peripheral vein thrombophlebitis, including heparin, in-line filtration, cortisol, buffering, glyceryl trinitrate and using fine-bore cannulas. Reducing the osmolality by altering the formulation of carbohydrate energy components and nitrogen source may also have a role, and specially formulated commercial mixtures have been shown in clinical studies to be suitable for PPN. Thrombophlebitis cannot be totally abolished, however, but it should be borne in mind that most courses of TPN rarely last more than 10–14 days. Thus if a peripheral line can be safely maintained for five days, just two peripheral cannula changes will be required to administer parenteral nutrition, while at the same time avoiding the main current risk of central venous administration of TPN, the central venous catheterization itself.

## TPN nutrients

Macronutrients consist of energy sources, nowadays consisting of carbohydrate (glucose)and lipid emulsions. Most regimens consist of a combination in proportions up to 50% : 50%. The nitrogen sources at present are *l*-amino acids, although much work is being undertaken in developing peptides and protein hydrolysate solutions which may have considerable potential benefits. Micronutrients are electrolytes, trace elements and vitamins, deficiencies of which may present interesting clinical problems.

Commercial sterile solutions of the parenteral nutrition requirements may be mixed together safely in a single container (generally made of ethyl vinyl acetate), the contents of which can be infused safely over a given period. Mixing of these solution is undertaken in a sterile laminar flow room. This method of administration has been used in the UK for almost ten years and has proven safe

**Table 18.9**   Treatment plan in the presence of pyrexia and leucocytosis

---

Take sample for peripheral blood culture
Take sample for central line drawback culture
If either positive — GUIDEWIRE EXCHANGE
Culture catheter tip
If catheter tip positive — resite catheter
If catheter tip negative — leave in place

---

**Table 18.10**  TPN regimens

| Nutrient | | Moderate injury | (ml) | Severe injury | (ml) |
|---|---|---|---|---|---|
| Nitrogen* | | 14g | 1000 | 17 g | 1000 |
| Energy | | | | | |
| Glucose* | Dextrose 50% | 1000 kcal | 500 | 1000 kcal | 500 |
| | Dextrose 20% | 400 kcal | 500 | 800 kcal | 1000 |
| Lipid | (20% emulsion) | 1000 kcal | 500 | 1000 kcal | 500 |
| Total volume | | | 2500 | | 3000 |
| As required: | Potassium, phosphate, sodium | | | | |
| | Trace elements | | | | |
| | Vitamins (water soluble) | | | | |
| | Vitamins (fat soluble) | | | | |
| | (Insulin) | | | | |

*Differences in nitrogen densities, glucose and lipid concentrations allow manipulation of total volume.

and reliable. The benefits of using such a system include reduced handling for bottle changes, thereby decreasing infection risks and nursing time. Three-litre solutions may be used effectively in clinical practice and solutions can be compounded and stored for several weeks without deleterious effect. Compatibilities of solutions vary and if in doubt manufacturers should be consulted for advice. Example of regimens are shown in Table 18.10.

## Monitoring

It is important that an accurate record of the administration of TPN is maintained. Thus wherever possible TPN should be administered using infusion pumps or flow-control devices. In the first week of TPN glucose should be measured 6-hourly, as many patients will develop some degree of insulin resistance because of their underlying pathology and may require exogenous insulin administered by injection/infusion, or occasionally incorporated in the TPN regimen. Electrolytes should be measured daily to allow correction of initial electrolyte imbalance and fluctuations, and to detect changes before severe metabolic/biochemical changes can affect the patient's clinical status. Liver function tests should be monitored to observe changes in serum albumin, and to detect TPN-related hepatobiliary dysfunction (see below).

## Metabolic complications

A wide variety of metabolic complication can occur with TPN, and the results of a study documenting complications in order of frequency are listed in Table 18.11.

**Table 18.11**  Metabolic complications of TPN

Hyperglycaemia
Hypoglycaemia
Hypophosphataemia
Hypercalcaemia
Hyperkalaemia
Hypokalaemia
Hypernatraemia
Hyponatraemia
Hyperosmolar diuresis
Other: deficiencies of folate, zinc, magnesium, other trace elements, vitamins and essential fatty acids

Although wide ranging these complications only occurred in under 5% of patients, the majority of whom were in intensive care. A specific complication of TPN of as yet unknown aetiology is the development of hepatic dysfunction. This is characterized by elevated hepatic enzymes, intrahepatic cholestasis and fatty infiltration of the liver. This is generally self-limiting and hepatic function returns to normal after cessation of TPN. The causes are multifactorial but certain ways of reducing the incidence and degree of dysfunction have been proposed (see Table 18.12 a & b).

## NUTRITION SUPPORT TEAM

It must be emphasized that the key to correct application of nutritional support techniques is the use of a multidisciplinary nutrition support

**Table 18.12**    (a) Associated factors in the development of hepatobiliary dysfunction

Pre-existing nutritional depletion
Underlying disease
Sepsis
Pre-existing liver disease
Duration of TPN
Excess non-protein calories
Excess glucose calories
Essential fatty acid deficiency
Hypophosphataemia
Lithocholic acid production
Toxicity of specific amino acids
Tryptophan
Carnitine deficiency

(b) Methods (practical and theoretical) by which the incidence and degree of hepatobiliary dysfunction may be reduced

Oral feeding
Stopping TPN
Cyclic administration of TPN
Avoid sepsis
Avoid unnecessary surgical procedures
Reduce non-protein calories
Reduce glucose calories
Review amino acid profile of TPN solution
Use of lipid (as calories and supplier of essential fatty acids)
Glucagon
Metronidazole
Gentamicin
Phenobarbitone
Carnitine supplementation
Taurine supplementation

team. The different members of the team can provide expert advice within their own field, but this advice can be tempered or modified by other team members. In this way the patient is most likely to be given the most appropriate nutritional support for his or her particular circumstance with the minimum of nutrition support-related complications (Payne-James 1991b).

## FURTHER READING

Bistrian B R, Blackburn G L, Vitale J, Cochran D, Naylor J 1976 Prevalence of malnutrition in general medical patients. Journal of the American Medical Association 235: 1567–1570

Buzby G P, Williford W O, Peterson O L et al 1988 Veterans Administration cooperative trial of perioperative total parenteral nutrition in malnourished surgical patients. American Journal of Clinical Nutrition 47 Suppl: 351–391

Chang R W S, Hatton I, Henley J, Richardson R, Egail S 1986 Total parenteral nutrition: a four year audit. British Journal of Surgery 73: 656–658

Dudrick S J, Wilmore D W, Vars H M, Rhoads J E 1968 Long-term total parenteral nutrition with growth, development and positive nitrogen balance. Surgery 64: 134–142

Grimble G K, Payne-James J J, Rees R G, Silk D B A 1989 a TPN: novel energy substrates. Intensive Therapy and Clinical Monitoring 10: 8–13

Grimble G K, Payne-James J J, Rees R G, Silk D B A 1989b Total parenteral nutrition: novel nitrogen substrates. Intensive Therapy and Clinical Monitoring 10: 92–8

Hansell D T 1989 Intravenous nutrition: the central or peripheral route. Intensive Therapy and Clinical Monitoring 10: 184–190

Hill G L, Blackett R L, Pickford I et al 1977 Malnutrition in surgical patients. Lancet i 689–692

Lee H A, Hartley T F 1975 A method of determining daily nitrogen requirements. Postgraduate Medical Journal 51: 441–445

MacFie J, Nordenstrom J 1992 Full circle in parenteral nutrition. Clinical Nutrition II: 237–239

MayenFeldt M F, Meijerine W J H J, Rouflat M M J et al 1992 Perioperative nutrition support: a randonised clinical trial. Clinical Nutrition II: 180–186

Payne-James J J, Silk D B A 1988 Enteral nutrition: background, indications and management. Baillière's Clinical Gastroenterology 2: 815–847

Payne-James J J, Silk D B A: 1990 Clinical nutrition support: better control and assessment needed. British Medical Journal 301: 1–2

Payne-James J J, Silk D B A 1991 Hepatobiliary dysfunction associated with total parenteral nutrition. Digestive Diseases 9: 106–124

Payne-James J J 1991 b Are nutritional support teams justified? Current Medical Literature – Gastroentrology 2: 4–7

Payne-James J J, Grimble G K, Rees R G, Silk D B A 1989 Total parenteral nutrition: clinical applications. Intensive Therapy and Clinical Monitoring 10: 19–26

Payne-James J J 1992 Enteral nutrition: accessing patients. Nutrition 8: 223–231

Payne-James J J, de Gara C J, Grimble G K et al 1992 Artificial nutrition support in hospitals in the United Kingdom 1991. Second National Survey. Clinical Nutrition 11: 182–192

Shanbhogue L K R, Chwals W J, Weintraub M, Blackburn G L, Bistrian B R 1987, Parenteral nutrition in the surgical patient. British Journal of Surgery 74: 172–80

Shenkin A 1988 Clinical aspects of vitamin and trace element metabolism. Baillière's Clinical Gastroenterology 2: 765–798

Wilmore D W 1989 The Practice of clinical nutrition: how to prepare for the future. Journal of Parenteral and Enteral Nutrition 13: 337–343

Woolfson A M J 1986 Energy and nitrogen requirements. In: Woolfson A M J (ed) Biochemistry of hospital nutrition. Churchill Livingstone, Edinburgh, pp 140–158

# 19. Postoperative care

*J. J. T. Tate*

## POSTOPERATIVE MONITORING

Postoperative care of the surgical patient has three phases:

1. immediate postoperative care (the recovery phase)
2. care on the ward until discharge from hospital
3. continuing care after discharge (e.g. district nurse visits for wound care).

The intensity of postoperative monitoring depends upon the type of surgery performed and the severity of the patient's condition.

## MONITORING OF THE RECOVERY PHASE

### Basic management

Immediately after surgery patients should go to a recovery ward adjacent to the theatre where they can be closely monitored, usually by one nurse to each patient. Monitoring of airway, breathing and circulation is the main priority but a smooth recovery can only be achieved if pain and anxiety are relieved; thus monitoring the patient's overall comfort is essential also. Particular attention must be paid to children, the elderly, patients with other medical problems such as cardiac disease and patients who have had major surgery. Patients may be discharged from the recovery area when they are able to maintain their vital functions independently (i.e. full consciousness and stable respiratory and cardiovascular observations). Thus some patients may need to be recovered for a few minutes only, while those having had major surgery may need to stay an hour or more.

Monitoring of the general comfort of the patient includes:

- relief of pain and anxiety

- administering mouthwashes (a dry mouth is common after general anaesthesia)
- the patient's position, including care of pressure points
- prophylactic measures against:
  a. atelectasis by encouraging deep breathing
  b. venous stasis by passive leg exercises.

These steps, including the prophylactic measures, all start in recovery and will continue on the main ward.

### Airway and breathing

Patients may have an oral airway, a naso-pharyngeal airway or, rarely, may still be intubated on arrival in recovery; all secretions must be cleared by suction and the artificial airway left until the patient can maintain their own. Breathing may be depressed and a patient hypoxic due to three factors:

1. airway obstruction
2. residual anaesthetic gases
3. the depressant effects of opioids.

Oxygen is given, ideally by mask, and the oxygen saturation monitored by a pulse oximeter. Expired carbon dioxide can also be monitored if a patient is being ventilated. Special care is needed for patients with a new tracheostomy (see Ch. 6).

If there is concern about vomiting and the risk of aspiration, patients may be sat up or nursed head up rather than in the supine position.

### Circulation

Blood pressure is recorded quarter-hourly or, after very major surgery, continuously via a cannula placed in the radial artery. The pulse is also recorded regularly but continuous monitoring of pulse rate is provided by a pulse oximeter (which is rapidly becoming an essential monitoring tool for all patients after general anaesthesia). The wound and any drains are monitored for signs of reactionary bleeding.

Before patients are returned to the ward their calculated fluid losses should be replaced with blood, blood products or crystalloids, and, ideally, fluid balance achieved. Monitoring of central venous pressure (CVP) can assist fluid balance management in severely ill patients or after major surgery; similarly urine output measurement may provide useful information about circulating volume and perfusion.

The patients' temperatures are monitored as there may be a significant drop during surgery which should be corrected before they leave the recovery room (e.g. space blanket). As the temperature rises there may be peripheral vasodilation and this can lead to hypotension if not anticipated.

## Miscellaneous

Specific medical conditions and certain types of surgery will require special additional monitoring:

- diabetes mellitus — blood sugar monitoring
- cardiac disease — ECG monitor
- orthopaedic and vascular surgery — monitoring of distal perfusion in a treated limb
- neurosurgery — quarter-hourly neurological observations (in some cases continuous intracranial pressure monitoring by an intraventricular catheter or a transducer in the subarachnoid space is indicated)
- urology — after transurethral prostatectomy bladder irrigation is usually implemented and pulmonary oedema can develop if glycine has been absorbed into the circulation; fluid balance is particularly important in these cases.

## WARD MONITORING

Patients return to the main ward when their general condition is stable; thus, the aim of further monitoring is early detection of complications. Clearly, closer and more frequent observation is necessary in the first few hours and the priorities are the same as in the recovery room. Nursing staff perform routine observations; medical staff must undertake additional, clinical monitoring dictated by the nature of the case, including daily review of drug prescriptions. General care includes those measures described previously and early ambulation is an aim to reduce the risk of thrombotic complications. Appropriate explanation of the results of the operation and the expected postoperative course should be given to the patient and relatives.

## Postoperative infection

The patient's temperature is recorded 4–6-hourly initially as a basic, but crude, observation for infection. Clinical monitoring includes examination of the chest and inspection of the wound. The upper limit of normal temperature is 37°C but there is considerable variation and occasionally a patient may be pyrexial despite a temperature below this 'magic' figure. The timing of postoperative pyrexia may suggest a cause; after a large bowel resection, for example, the development of pyrexia within the first 48 hours is usually due to chest infection, whereas a pyrexia on the fifth or sixth day may indicate anastomotic leakage or wound infection, and fever associated with venous thrombosis typically occurs on the tenth day.

If a patient develops a pyrexia, a routine 'infection screen' is carried out;

- examine the chest — chest X-ray; sputum for culture; ECG (if ? pulmonary embolus)
- examine the wound — wound swab for culture
- enquire about urinary symptoms — urine sample for culture
- examine for signs of deep vein thrombosis
- examine intravenous sites (phlebitis)
- examine pressure areas
- if a child — look in the ears and mouth
- if cause uncertain — send blood cultures; measure white cell count; consider the underlying disease (e.g. pyrexia of malignancy); consider hidden infection (e.g. subphrenic abscess).

## Monitoring fluid balance

After major surgery regular monitoring of fluid balance is important and many such patients have a urinary catheter to allow accurate charting of urine output. Visible fluid losses will be recorded on a fluid balance chart at regular intervals (e.g. hourly for urine output, 4-hourly for nasogastric aspirations, 12 or 24-hourly for output into drains) and totalled every 24 hours. Unrecorded fluid losses (e.g. evaporation from skin, losses into hidden spaces such as the intestine, diarrhoea) must be estimated and added to the recorded losses to calculate the patient's subsequent fluid requirements.

For most patients requiring intravenous fluids after operation a standard regimen would be 2.5 litres per day, of which 1 litre is normal saline and the remainder 5% dextrose; potassium being added after the first 24 hours once 1.5 litres of urine have been passed. Typically, sodium requirement is 2 mmol kg$^{-1}$ (normal saline contains 140 mmol l$^{-1}$ of sodium) and potassium 1 mmol kg$^{-1}$. If the dissection area at operation has been large there will be a greater loss of plasma into the operation site and this may need to be replaced with colloid (e.g. Haemaccel) in the early postoperative period. In addition to these basic requirements gastrointestinal losses are replaced volume-for-volume with normal saline. Daily plasma urea and electrolyte measurement are advisable while the patient is dependent on intravenous fluids.

Clinical monitoring should include asking the patient about thirst, assessing central and peripheral perfusion, examination of dependent areas for oedema and auscultation of the chest. Tachycardia is an important sign that can indicate fluid overload or dehydration but is also caused by inadequate analgesia.

Oliguria (defined as a urine output of less than 20 ml h$^{-1}$ in each of two consecutive hours) in postoperative patients is caused by hypovolaemia in the majority of cases; occasionally causes such as cardiac failure or simply a blocked catheter must be considered. Hypovolaemia may be due to unreplaced blood loss, loss of fluid into the gastrointestinal tract, loss of plasma into the wound or abdomen or sequestration of extracellular fluid into the 'third' space. Patients in whom fluid balance is difficult to manage, or where there is a particular risk of cardiac failure, may require central venous pressure monitoring or even left atrial pressure recording.

## Blood transfusion

Haemoglobin measurement will be a guide to the need for blood transfusion unless plasma or extracellular fluid loss causes an artificially high measurement; this is most likely in the first 24 hours after surgery and it is generally not necessary to monitor haemoglobin levels more than 72 hours postoperatively. Transfusion is usually considered if the haemoglobin concentration falls below 10 g%.

If blood transfusion is given, frequent, regular monitoring of pulse, blood pressure and temperature are routine to detect a transfusion reaction. A major ABO incompatibility can result in anaphylactic hypersensitivity reaction. Incompatibility of minor factors is usually less severe and is indicated by tachycardia, pyrexia and possible rash and pruritus. The transfusion should be stopped, some blood sent for culture and the remainder of the unit returned to the blood bank for further cross-matching against the patient's serum. However, if the reaction is mild it may be appropriate to give steroids or an antihistamine and continue the transfusion.

## Nutrition

Patients who are poorly nourished do not heal well, hence nutrition is important in surgical patients. Dietary intake should be monitored in all patients but usually only requires specific management in patients undergoing major abdominal surgery or in whom eating or swallowing is impossible. Serum protein is a crude but easily measured index of nutrition, and measurement of weight is useful over a period of time; more specific tests such as skinfold thickness or estimation of nitrogen balance are used infrequently.

Abdominal surgery is frequently associated with delayed gastric emptying and impaired colonic motility even though small bowel activity, and hence bowel sounds, may return relatively early.

If there is intra-abdominal sepsis, metabolic disturbances or retroperitoneal haematoma or inflammation there may be prolonged inactivity of the small bowel also (paralytic ileus). Too early reintroduction of diet can lead to gastric dilation with vomiting and the risk of aspiration. Monitoring nasogastric aspirates, abdominal distension and the passage of flatus determines the timing of reintroduction of normal diet. However, a restricted intake of oral fluids (30 ml h$^{-1}$) is permissible almost without exception and increases patient comfort.

If nutritional support is required, enteral feeding is preferable, if possible, because it has a lower complication rate than parenteral nutrition (see Ch. 18). Fluid balance and electrolyte monitoring are required and treatment should be given to reduce diarrhoea, which may be precipitated by high-calorie regimes. Parenteral feeding requires monitoring of the venous access point for sepsis, plasma and urinary electrolytes, blood sugar, plasma trace elements (e.g. magnesium) and liver function. The patient's fluid balance must be carefully managed.

## Surgical drains

Nasogastric tubes drain the stomach of fluid and swallowed air. They should be left on free drainage at all times with intermittent aspiration (4-hourly). There is rarely a need to leave a nasogastric tube spigoted; once drainage has fallen below 100–200 ml per day it can be removed.

Chest drains are attached to an underwater seal because the pleural space is at subatmospheric pressure. If the lung does not expand fully, then low-pressure, high-volume suction may be added. When a drain is bubbling it should not be clamped because there is a danger of tension pneumothorax if the clamp is forgotten or left too long; however, it is essential that the bottle is never raised above the level of the patient's chest or else there is a risk that fluid will syphon back into the pleural cavity. The drain is removed when:

- bubbling has stopped for 24 hours
- there is no bubbling when the patient coughs
- the daily chest X-ray shows that the lung is fully expanded.

Check X-rays should be taken at 24 and 48 hours after removal of the drain.

Drains at the operative site are used for the removal of anticipated fluid collections, not as an alternative to adequate haemostasis, and are usually simple tube drains or suction drains (it is important to check that the vacuum is maintained). Such drains should be removed early; if left in place they will not reduce the risk of a subsequent abscess and may introduce infection. If there is a chronic collection of fluid (such as an abscess or empyema) the drain may be left for several days to create a track. This type of drain is often removed a few centimetres at a time over several days (shortening) in an attempt to prevent the track closing too quickly; a sinogram may be used to confirm that the abscess cavity is shrinking.

All drains have similar potential complications:

- trauma during insetion
- failure to drain adequately due to:
  a) incorrect placement
  b) too small size
  c) blocked lumen
- complications due to disconnection
- introduction of infection from outside via the drain track
- erosion by the drain of adjacent tissues
- fracture of drain during removal (retained foreign body).

## Day-case surgery

After a general anaesthetic day-case operation the postoperative monitoring period is inevitably short but should follow the same basic principles outlined above.

For local anaesthesia the likely problems are systemic toxicity of the anaesthetic agent and reactionary haemorrhage. All the commonly used local anaesthetics (lignocaine, bupivicaine and prilocaine) are cardiotoxic. Initial symptoms are paraesthesiae around the lips, followed by dizziness which may progress to convulsions and cardiac arrhythmia and collapse. Such complications are prevented by strict adherence to maximum dosage schedules (Table 19.1) rather than by additional monitoring.

**Table 19.1** Maximum doses of local anaesthetic agents

|  | Plain solution | With adrenalin |
|---|---|---|
| Lignocaine | 200 mg | 500 mg |
|  | (20ml of 1%) | (50 ml of 1%) |
| Bupivicaine | 150 mg | 200 mg |
|  | (30 ml of 0.5%) | (40 ml of 0.5%) |
| Prilocaine | 400 mg | 600 mg |
|  | (80 ml of 0.5%) | (120 ml of 0.5%) |

For sedoanalgesia or sedation alone (e.g. endoscopy patients) particular attention is paid to monitoring respiration. Ideally, all patients should have a pulse oximeter attached until they are fully awake. The use of a specific antagonist to reverse the sedative effects of benzodiazepines can be associated with delayed respiratory depression as the reversal agent, which has a shorter half-life than the sedative itself, wears off. All patients given sedation should be observed for at least 2 hours before being sent home.

Patients who have had a general anaesthetic or sedation must be accompanied home and should not be allowed to drive for at least 24 hours. Written advice and instructions should be given both to the patient and their accompanying relative or friend.

## CARE AFTER HOSPITAL DISCHARGE

Good communication is crucial to the patient's full recovery after discharge from hospital. The patient should understand what treatment they have had, its effect, the likely time period to complete their recovery and special restrictions on normal activity. Whenever appropriate the relatives should also have this information. As many complications (e.g wound infection) occur in the first week or two after hospital discharge it is essential that the patient's general practitioner is told the diagnosis and treatment given and also what information the patient has received.

## MONITORING TECHNIQUES/EQUIPMENT

### Measurement of blood pressure

The sphygmomanometer is the standard method of blood pressure measurement. When continuous monitoring is required, automated machines can measure blood pressure at intervals as short as every 2 minutes. If greater accuracy is needed, invasive monitoring with a transducer attached to an arterial line, usually placed in the radial artery, is performed. This method also provides a display of the pulse waveform.

### ECG monitoring

Continuous ECG monitoring employs three chest leads to provide accurate information of cardiac rhythm. Careful placement of the leads also allows early detection of myocardial ischaemia by showing ST depression. A full 12-lead ECG is needed for accurate diagnosis.

### Pulse oximeter/blood gases

A pulse oximeter monitors three parameters: pulse rate, pulse volume and oxygen saturation. A sensor placed on the patient's finger tip contains two light-emitting diodes (LEDs); one is red and measures the amount of oxygenated haemoglobin, the other is infrared and measures the total amount of haemoglobin. The actual amount of oxygen carried in the blood relative to the maximum possible amount is computed — this is the oxygen saturation, $SaO_2$; the realtionship between oxygen in the blood and $SaO_2$ is linear. The delivery of oxygen to the tissues depends on:

- cardiac output
- haemoglobin concentration
- oxygen saturation ($SaO_2$).

Thus, a fall in oxygen reaching the tissues can be detected far more rapidly with $SaO_2$ monitoring than by clinical observation of the lips, nailbeds or mucous membranes for cyanosis (which may only be apparent when the $SaO_2$ is 60–70%) or by measuring arterial blood gases. However, pulse oximetry does not indicate adequate ventilation; the $SaO_2$ can be normal due to a high inspired oxygen level.

Arterial blood gases measure pH, arterial oxygen and carbon dioxide tensions ($PaO_2$, $PaCO_2$), bicarbonate and base excess. These measurements are affected by many variables and can be difficult to interpret. The $PaO_2$ has a non-linear relationship to oxygen content of the blood (the oxygen dissociation curve), hence oxygen saturation is easier to use in practice. $PaCO_2$ reflects the rate of excretion of carbon dioxide by the lungs and is thus inversely proportional to the ventilation (assuming constant production of carbon dioxide by the body). The base excess and bicarbonate reflect acid/base disturbances and may be used in conjunction with the $PaCO_2$ to distinguish respiratory from metabolic problems.

## Central venous pressure

A catheter placed in the superior vena cava, either via the internal jugular or subclavian vein, allows monitoring of the venous filling pressure of the heart. Measurements are made with a simple manometer against a zero reference point (usually 4th intercostal space, mid-axillary line) which must be kept constant for consecutive recordings. Changes in pressure reflect the physiological response to fluid therapy; it is the trend rather than the absolute value which is of most importance. Other factors which affect CVP values are:

- intrathoracic pressure (e.g. positive pressure ventilation increases the CVP)
- position and posture of the patient
- right ventricular function
- right-sided heart valve disease
- raised pulmonary artery resistance.

CVP monitoring is useful in patients with severe fluid imbalance, shock or with cardiac or renal impairment, and can demonstrate hypovolaemia before changes in pulse and blood pressure. The main complications are trauma at the time of insertion of the line, air embolism and sepsis in a line used for several days.

## Pulmonary artery wedge pressure

A pulmonary artery balloon catheter (Swan–Ganz) is inserted via a similar route to a CVP line and the catheter tip advanced through the right side of the heart into the pulmonary arterial tree. When the balloon is inflated, the arterial lumen is occluded and the pressure at the catheter tip then approximates the left atrial pressure. This device allows measurement of the filling pressure of the left side of the heart and is usually indicated in patients with severe cardiac insufficiency (e.g. left heart failure). In addition, some catheters incorporate a thermistor so that cardiac output may be measured by a dilutional technique. Pulmonary artery pressure monitoring is associated with significant morbidity (e.g. persistent arrhythmias, pulmonary infarction) and should only be used in experienced units.

# 20. The management of postoperative pain

*D. L. Crosby*

Unfortunately, pain is still recognized as a common consequence of surgery and doubtless deters some patients from seeking surgical advice. However, in recent years there has been an increasing awareness that postoperative pain is essentially avoidable, and that special efforts must be made if this is to be achieved. It is instructive to identify the previous causes of failure:

1. Failure of perception of patients' pain by doctors and nurses. This is made more difficult by the fact that many patients believe that pain is an inevitable consequence of surgery and, there-fore, do not complain about it. Also, some patients conceal their pain because of fear of appearing cowardly.

2. Variability in patients' perception of pain, and pharmacokinetic variation between patients in their handling of various drugs. Thus, for example, some patients may be more sensitive to opioids, and others more likely to have unwanted side-effects.

3. Legitimate but exaggerated fears of untoward side-effects such as respiratory depression and drug addiction.

4. Delays in the administration of post-operative analgesics engendered by the necessity of detailed checking arrangements.

5. Traditional methods of postoperative pain relief have depended mainly upon injections of morphine-like drugs. Newer methods of pain relief such as epidural and patient-controlled analgesia require expertise and resources which are not always available.

A considerable bar to progress in the past has been the absence of any generally acceptable criteria for the objective measurement of pain.

Currently, the simplest measurement techniques are single-dimensional methods whereby patients are simply asked to match pain severity to a scale provided by the observer. Such subjective visual analogue scales have been widely used. The simplest version is the verbal scale which asks the patient to rate pain as 'none', 'mild', 'moderate' or 'severe'. The inclusion of such measurements (i.e. pain charts) with other routine postoperative observations and linked to an analgesic regime is a simple and effective way to improve post-operative pain relief.

## CURRENTLY AVAILABLE METHODS FOR THE MANAGEMENT OF POSTOPERATIVE PAIN

### Counselling and psychological methods

The provision of adequate information concerning the nature, aims and consequences of a particular operation, together with reassurance about the availability of postoperative pain relief, undoubt-edly improves the quality of postoperative care. Instruction in coping techniques, relaxation and behavioural instruction have also been shown to reduce requirements for post operative analgesia.

### Oral

Mild postoperative pain can often be controlled by regular doses of analgesics such as codeine (30–60 mg every 6 hours q.d.s.), paracetamol (0.5–1.0 g every 6 hours q.d.s.) and dextro-propoxyphene (60 mg every 6 hours q.d.s.). For more severe pain, most opioids can be given orally. However, vomiting and delayed gastric emptying following anaesthesia and surgery may make this route impractical.

## Intramuscular

Repeated doses of opioids given by this route remains the standard and traditional method of postoperative pain relief e.g. morphine 10 mg 1.m 4 hourly p.r.n. To be effective and to avoid untoward side-effects the dosage and frequency need to be closely monitored.

## Intravenous

Intravenous infusions of opioids at a constant rate eventually reach a steady tissue concentration which can be titrated to achieve continuous pain relief without serious side-effects initial loading dose of morphine (5–10 mg) followed by 2–3 mg/h with appropriate individualisation as required. However, there may be a significant delay before this effect is achieved and it is essential that signs of hypoxia and respiratory depression are monitored. Consequently, such patients should be cared for either in high dependency units or areas where the required monitoring (including pulse oximetry) and an appropriate level of nursing care are constantly available.

## Patient-controlled analgesia (PCA)

PCA systems deliver intravenous opioids at a rate which is controlled by the patient. The theoretical basis is that the patient will titrate the delivery of drug to achieve good analgesia with minimal side-effects. The opioid is contained within an electronic delivery system which will administer a preset dose when a button is pressed by the patient. The regimen requires consideration of the bolus dose, maximum dose and background infusion rate. Also, there must be a 'lock out interval' during which time further doses cannot be given the usual dose of morphine is 1mg bolus with a 'lock out' interval of 5 minutes amended as required. Small and portable devices are now available. Regular concomitant monitoring of respiratory function and sedation are essential.

## Local anaesthesia

The local anaesthetic drugs used most commonly are Lignocaine, Prilocaine and Bupivacaine and they act by blocking the conduction of impulses along nerves. However, they have potentially dangerous side-effects when given in large doses including myocardial depression and disturbances of the central nervous system. Consequently, the volume of solution required to block all nerves at an operation site may be greater than the safe dose.

## Local infiltration

This is a simple technique which can be used in some wounds such as hernia repairs, resulting in analgesia lasting for 6 hours or so (10–20 ml of 0.25% at 0.5% bupivacaine). Prolongation can be achieved by the use of wound catheters, though these may increase the risk of wound infection. Pleural catheters can be used to maintain pain relief after thoracotomy and upper abdominal surgery and this technique is presently being evaluated.

### Nerve blocks

Individual or groups of peripheral nerves may be blocked to provide analgesia after many operations. This is usually performed by the anaesthetist while the patient is under general anaesthesia. Excellent pain relief can be provided in situations such as hernia repair and after operations on the limbs or chest.

### Epidural analgesia

Local anaesthetic agents introduced into the epidural space will block spinal nerves as they leave the spinal canal and will consequently result in analgesia in the deep as well as superficial tissues e.g. epidural infusion of 1 mg bupivacaine and 10 μg ml fentanyl at 2–5 ml/h. Opioids can also be used by this route. It is a useful technique in major abdominal and pelvic surgery since it usually avoids the respiratory depression inherent in other techniques. When used as a 'caudal block', excellent analgesia using small volumes of local anaesthetic can be achieved after procedures such as haemorrhoidectomy and circumcision. However, careful monitoring and good technique are again essential. Hypotension may sometimes occur and other complications may include infection, haematoma, muscle weakness and respiratory depression if the cerebrospinal space is entered.

## Other methods

Acupuncture, transcutaneous nerve stimulation, cryoanalgesia, inhalational analgesia, rectal opioids and hypnosis have all been used in the relief of pain but have not found a regular place for postoperative patients.

All these techniques can be used with the same precautions in children, though experience with PCA in this context is limited.

The immediate future for more effective pain relief depends mainly on the education and application of existing knowledge. Any busy surgical unit should designate a multidisciplinary team comprising a surgeon, nurse, anaesthetist and pharmacist, who have a particular interest in this field, i.e. a 'pain team'. The continuing increase in short-stay and day-case surgery will provide new challenges, while the concomitant development of ambulatory therapeutic techniques will hopefully provide new solutions. The more distant future will depend on the development of better analgesics with fewer unwanted side-effects and thereby improved safety. The continuing need to audit the risks and benefits of existing and new methods is self-evident.

## FURTHER READING

Report of the Working Party on Pain after Surgery September 1990 Royal College of Surgeons of England and the College of Anaesthetists

# 21. Complications — prevention and management

*J. A. R. Smith*

It is often assumed that complications are the domain of 'someone else'. It is also a truism that the surgeon who denies complications is either a stranger to the truth or does no surgery! Accepting the fact of complications in the postoperative period allows recognition of the risk factors involved, institution of selective appropriate prophylaxis, and early diagnosis and treatment of the established problem.

## RISK FACTORS

Every anaesthetic and surgical procedure carries a risk to the patient of mortality and morbidity, the risks varying according to the patient's condition and the severity of the operation. Every decision to operate must involve a balance between the danger to the patient and the potential benefit.

There are certain risk factors which are specific to a complication and others which are more general. The latter will be considered first.

### Age

Any procedure at the extremes of age is more likely to be hazardous. In older age this relates more to those condition which are found more commonly in the elderly, such as neoplastic, peripheral vascular and respiratory diseases, rather than to older age per se. In the fifth decade the incidence of cerebrovascular disease is 6% but in the seventh decade it rises to 41% and by the eighth to 100%. The risk of postoperative myocardial infarction over the age of 50 is 6%, with a 70% mortality. Furthermore, in the elderly the risk of heart block, atrial fibrillation and hypertension are all higher with consequent risk of serious dysrhythmias and death. Capillary fragility is increased, so that bruising and haematoma formation are more common.

With increasing age there is a reduction in arterial oxygen tension, especially over 80 years. This is compounded by the increase in physiological dead space and by the decrease of lung capacity, vital capacity, maximal breathing capacity, forced expiratory volume and peak expiratory flow rate.

Renal function deteriorates with age, partly because of vascular disease, partly because of loss of nephrons and partly secondary to impaired cell function. Therefore fluid overload, acid–base and electrolyte disturbance are more common in the elderly.

The older patient is more likely to be on medication for various disorders, so that the risk of drug interaction is higher.

At the other end of the spectrum, surgery in the neonatal period is also hazardous. The margins of safety in tolerance of fluid infusion are much less, but diarrhoea is common and accurate replacement of fluid and electrolytes is difficult. There is an increased susceptibility to acid–base disturbance.

Thermoregulation is poor, so that the risk of hypothermia is considerable. Congenital abnormalities are often multiple and major. Enzyme systems are immature, so that jaundice may occur and general and drug metabolism may be affected adversely.

The physical size of the child and the delicacy of the tissues make surgery more difficult.

## Obesity

Operating on a fat patient is always difficult. Exposure can be limited, and the view obscured by adipose tissue. This makes accidental trauma a greater risk. Vessels are less well supported and therefore more likely to bleed and to retract, making wound haematoma more common.

Fat patients are less mobile and, by sheer weight, exert direct pressure on a calf vein while lying on the operating table, increasing the risk of venous thromboembolism. Respiratory movements may also be limited, increasing the risk of atelectasis and infection.

There is an association in some obese patients with atherosclerosis and the consequences of peripheral vascular disease.

## Cardiovascular disease

The presence of any cardiovascular disorder increases the risk of serious morbidity and mortality in the postoperative period.

### Myocardial infarction

Recent myocardial infarct is the most serious predisposing factor (Table 21.1). The risk is highest if surgery is performed in the first six months after infarction, but even after three years the risk is higher than in a patient of similar age without history of infarct. Furthermore, the risk of mortality from infarction is high (25–70%).

**Table 21.1**   Risk of myocardial infarction with time

| Time since infarct | Incidence of further infarction after surgery (%) |
|---|---|
| 0–6 months | 55 |
| 1–2 years | 22 |
| 2–3 years | 6 |
| Over 3 years | 1 |
| No infarct | 0.66 |

### Angina

The more severe the symptoms of angina the higher the risk of cardiovascular complications in general, and infarction in particular.

### Dysrhythmias

Atrial fibrillation and heart block carry the worst prognosis. The risk is reduced but not abolished, when medical control of the dysrhythmia is achieved.

### Cardiac valve disease

Any valve disease or artificial valve is at risk of colonization with bacteria after surgery, so that even for clean surgery prophylactic antibiotics are indicated. In addition to the risk of fibrillation or atrial thrombosis, the presence of valvular disease impairs cardiovascular responses to surgery and to infused fluids.

### Cardiac pacemaker

The patient with a fixed-rate pacemaker cannot produce a tachycardia and is therefore particularly vulnerable to hypovolaemia. Care is required if diathermy is used.

### Arteriosclerosis

The incidence of atheroma increases with age and is associated with a similar increase in cardiovascular complications. The patient aged 50 years has a 23% incidence of atheroma and a 0.66% incidence of infarction. Over age 70 the incidence of atheroma approaches 100%.

### Hypertension

There is no clear relationship between hypertension and cardiovascular complication after abdominal surgery. In cardiac surgery there is an increased risk of myocardial infarction in the hypertensive patient. It is important to remember that in removing a phaeochromoctyomae blood pressure can fluctuate widely, with consequent risk of a cerebrovascular accident.

### Other factors

The combination of respiratory and cardiovascular disease is very serious because of the resulting arterial hypoxia.

If renal function is impaired the risk of fluid overload is increased greatly.

Down to a haemoglobin of 10 dl⁻¹ a normal myocardium can compensate well. Below this level, or in the presence of myocardial disease, peripheral hypoxia is more likely. Subendocardial ischaemia and fibrosis may also result.

## Respiratory disease

Smokers and patients with bronchiectasis and emphysema are at increased risk of respiratory complications. More common problems such as tonsilitis, bronchitis and even coryza make respiratory infection more common in the postoperative period and indicate the need to postpone elective surgery.

With advancing years there is a greater reduction in arterial oxygen tension, the decrease being greater over age 80. Age also produces reductions in total lung and vital capacities, and in peak expiratory flow rate and forced expiratory volume. The physiological dead space is increased and the alveolar–arterial oxygen difference is greater. Thus any respiratory complication produces more severe hypoxaemia. In addition it is estimated that the combination of cor pulmonale and ischamemic heart disease produces a mortality of about 50%.

## Diabetes mellitus

Insulin-dependent diabetics are high-risk patients for a number of different reasons.

### Metabolic

Maintenance of blood sugar can be difficult in the perioperative period, and even non-insulin-dependent diabetics may require insulin for a short time. The metabolic response to surgery results in hyperglycaemia, and if complications such as infection arise both hyperinsulinaemia and hyperglycaemia may coexist — so-called insulin 'resistance'.

The major danger is the development of severe ketoacidosis, most commonly seen in undiagnosed or poorly controlled diabetic patients.

### Infection

In diabetes, polymorphonuclear phagocyte function is impaired. The incidence of peripheral vascular disease affecting both medium and small vessels is increased. Diabetic neuropathy reduces sensation to touch and pain, so that skin ulceration is more common. It is also suggested that a higher sugar level in blood and tissues encourages bacterial growth.

For all these reasons, infective complications are more common and more likely to give rise to serious morbidity.

### Wound healing

The reduced blood supply and impaired polymorph function, combined with the increased risk of infection, all contribute to impaired wound healing.

### Peripheral vascular disease

There is an increased risk of atheroma affecting both medium and small arteries. If gangrene does result, infection is more common for the reasons given above, and because of the ulceration. Thus wet gangrene is more common in diabetic patients.

### Renal disease

In diabetes mellitus of 20 year's duration there is a 15% incidence of glomerulosclerosis. Impaired renal function makes fluid and electrolyte balance more complex. Furthermore, diabetic patients are more sensitive to protein depletion, and are at risk of severe ketoacidosis during a surgical illness.

## DRUG THERAPY

In general terms, details of medicaments taken are important to minimize the risk of allergic reaction and drug interactions. Certain drugs carry specific risks of surgical interest.

## Corticosteroids

The longer the patient is on steroid therapy and

the higher the dose, the greater the risk of complications.

Glucocorticoids interfere with the mobility and phagocytic activity of polymorphonuclear leucocytes, so that acute inflammation and the handling of bacteria are impaired. Thus deficient wound healing and wound infection are more common.

Ground substance is reduced and capillary fragility greater, so that wound haematoma is more common, contributing both to impaired wound healing and to infection. However, experimentally, the short-term use of methylprednisolone has not been associated with impaired healing of colonic anastomoses.

Intake of steroids in the six months before surgery may be associated with impaired stress response. The output of endogenous glucocorticoid is an essential part of the response to surgery and anaesthesia, and is depressed by exogenous steroid therapy. In order to avoid this complication the patient should have 100 mg hydrocortisone intravenously at induction of anaesthesia, continued 6-hourly for 48 hours, and then reduced gradually either to zero or to the preoperative intake over the next five to seven days.

Remember that steroid therapy may delay the diagnosis of postoperative complications or make them more likely to occur. Exacerbation of peptic ulcer disease is one example — and ulcer perforation may be masked by the anti-inflammatory effect of glucocorticoids. More contentious is the role of immunosuppressive dosage of steroids in the pathogenesis of neoplasia. There is some evidence that the incidence of head and neck tumors and the virally induced tumours may be increased in transplant patients but this does not apply to the more common tumours of lung, breast or gastrointestinal tract.

## Antibiotic therapy

The most serious complication of antibiotic therapy is anaphylaxis, closely followed by hypersensitivity. There remains a significant problem of development of resistant strain, such as methicillin-resistant *Staphylococcus aureus* (MRSA). Therefore, use antibiotics for specific indications and for a clearly defined duration.

From the surgical point of view, pseudomembranous colitis, caused by *Clostridium difficile*, is a more urgent problem. It seems likely that exposure to antibiotics, combined with hypovolaemia or hypotension, is required for colitis to develop. Treatment with vancomycin or metronidazole intravenously is usually effective. Occasionally, total colectomy is required for resistant cases.

The aminoglycosides have potential for ototoxicity and nephrotoxicity, such that peak and trough blood levels must be monitored. Gentamicin causes ototoxicity in 3% of patients, more commonly in the elderly and in those with impaired renal function. Nephrotoxicity occurs in 2% of patients.

## Cytotoxic agents

In addition to general problems such as gastrointestinal upset and hair loss, patients on cytotoxic chemotherapy who undergo surgery risk several complications.

Depression of the white cell count and function interfere with acute inflammation, increasing the incidence of wound infection and of impaired wound healing.

Reduction in cell-mediated immunity increases the risk of development of a second neoplasm, as exemplified by a 3% incidence in patients successfully treated for primary lymphoma.

Bone marrow depression is common, and in addition to the problems of infection, especially with opportunistic organisms, there is a risk of purpuric eruption and frank bleeding.

## Cyclosporin

Cyclosporin A carries the risk of depressing immune responses, but more specifically it can result in depression of renal function. Often this is a barrier to continued therapy with this agent.

## BLOOD TRANSFUSION

### Incompatibility

Major incompatibility reactions are now rare, even with emergency cross-matching. In patients who have had repeated transfusions, minor group incompatibility is more common. This involves Kell Duffy or Kidd systems in order of importance. Do not attribute all febrile reactions to incompatibility. Transfusion of pyrogens, or antibodies to white cells, are alternative explanations for a febrile reaction.

## Consequences of storage

Because of the finite lifespan of red cells, lysis is an inevitable consequence of storage. Transient jaundice after massive transfusion is not of dire consequence but the potential for hyperkalaemia is significant.

Acid citrate dextrose is the most commonly used anticoagulant. Transfused citrate may bind free calcium and result in hypocalcaemia. On storage, both platelets and clotting factors are consumed within some hours. Thus transfused stored blood cannot be relied upon to correct hemorrhagic tendencies.

The level of 2, 3-diphosphoglycerate falls in stored red cells. The resulting shift of the oxy-haemoglobin dissociation curve to the left increases the affinity of haemoglobin for oxygen. Delivery of oxygen at tissue level is thereby reduced.

Stored red cells become more rigid, thus impairing capillary circulation and encouraging sludging.

## Transmission of disease

In the past both syphilis and hepatitis B were transmitted by transfusion, but this has been virtually abolished by more stringent screening. More recently, HIV virus has been transfused, mainly to haemophilic patients, with disastrous consequences.

## Alteration in immunity

There is clear evidence that transplantation of a kidney is less likely to result in rejection after blood transfusion. The reduction in efficacy of cell-mediated immunity has deleterious effects in the surgical management of cancer patients. It is suggested that in colon cancer perioperative transfusion results in a poorer prognosis even when groups are matched for stage of disease, degree of operative trauma, age, sex, and other factors.

Other neoplastic processes, and the relevance of blood transfusion to prognosis, are under investigation.

## TYPE OF PATHOLOGY

### Obstructive jaundice

*Effect on coagulation*

The coagulation factors are manufactured in the liver. Interference with liver function by back-pressure and hepatocellular damage limits the production process. In addition, fat soluble vitamin K is not absorbed in the absence of bile salts, further interfering with the production of prothrombin.

All patients with obstructive jaundice have an increased risk of haemorrhage, which can be corrected by the systemic administration of Vitamin $K_1$ and by the infusion of fresh frozen plasma, depending on the results of the clotting screen. The intravenous route for vitamin $K_1$ reduces the risk of intramuscular haematoma.

*Effect on wound healing*

Disturbance of protein metabolism is also caused by the back-pressure causing hepatocellular disruption. Standard teaching has it that this results in impaired healing of wounds and anastomoses, with a consequent increase in the incidence of wound dehiscence and incisional herniae. More recent evidence suggests that only in obstructive jaundice due to a neoplastic cause is the problem of wound failure significant. However, sufficient doubt remains for all such patients to be considered at high risk.

*Effect on infective complications*

It is well established that opening the common bile duct produces a threefold increase in the incidence of wound infection relative to cholecystectomy alone. This effect is compounded by the presence of obstructive jaundice, especially when the obstruction is secondary to stones or postoperative stricture. The incidence of infected bile is at least 75%, and even with malignant obstructions ratios of 25% have been reported.

Wound infection and wound haematoma also contribute to the incidence of impaired wound healing. Infections play a significant role in the hepatorenal syndrome (see below). Because of reduced efficacy of the reticuloendothelial (Kupfer) cells in the liver, the incidence of septicaemia and endotoxinaemia is increased. Increased mortality and morbidity result from ascending cholangitis.

### Effects on renal function

Following surgery for obstructive jaundice, patients are at risk from acute renal failure — 'the hepatorenal syndrome'. There are a number of theories as to aetiology.

Acute renal failure is also a complication of Gram-negative septic shock, believed to be caused by the effects of endotoxin. These include activation of complement by the alternative pathway, and inappropriate disseminated intravascular coagulation. Microthrombi in the renal parenchyma interfere with renal function but it is likely that other toxic substances, released by the activation of complement, also interfere with renal function. It is said that at least some part of renal failure occurs because the tubules are blocked by excess bilirubin. Histological evidence of this is not invariable and at best it is only a contributing factor.

The hormones responsible for maintaining fluid and electrolyte balance are metabolized in the liver, so that disturbance of hepatic function may interfere with such hormonal activity.

Because of the difficulties with haemostasis, these patients are at greater risk of hypovolaemia. Protect them by ensuring that they receive adequate fluid infusion, and a good diuresis in the perioperative period.

### Effects in drug metabolism

It is generally assumed that drug metabolism is altered in the presence of obstructive jaundice. The evidence for this belief is not strong. A particular problem applies to drugs which are oxidized in the liver. In surgical practice great caution is recommended with analgesic and sedative therapy with, for example morphine-like agents.

## Neoplastic diseases

### Venous thromboembolism

The association between superficial thrombophlebitis migrans and pancreatic carcinoma is well established. The incidence of deep vein thrombosis (DVT) is also higher in patients with carcinomatous disease, probably because of factors released by tumours affecting the thrombotic cascade. Furthermore, oncological procedures tend to be prolonged, with greater operative trauma, often requiring blood transfusion.

### Wound healing

It is generally stated that patients with carcinoma are at higher risk of both primary wound failure (dehiscence) and later incisional herniation. This relationship has been most clearly confirmed in malignant obstructive jaundice, where malnutrition together with impaired protein metabolism in the liver combine to cause impaired healing. The whole concept of cancer cachexia is complex but the resulting protein malnutrition is of greatest significance as regards wound healing.

## TYPE OF SURGERY

### Orthopaedic

Operations on the hips and pelvis have an increased risk of DVT. Both with extensive elective procedures and after major trauma, DVT is also more common, especially if blood transfusion is required.

### Gynaecology

Trauma to the pelvic veins increases the risk of iliofemoral thrombosis. Extensive oncological eradication carries all the risks relevant to cancer surgery (see above).

## Thoracic/upper abdominal

Wound pain in these procedures increases the risk of respiratory complications, especially in the elderly (see above).

## Prolonged operations

It was always stated that long operations increased the risk of respiratory problems, fluid and electrolyte imbalance and DVT. However, prolonged 'keyhole' operations by the laparoscopic route have proved relatively free of complications and it seems likely that such factors as intraoperative trauma, blood transfusion, loss of fluid and heat from exposed cavities and tissues are more important than the duration per se.

## COMPLICATIONS AND THEIR MANAGEMENT

### Venous thromboembolism

*Risk factors*

- Obesity
- Age
- Malignant disease
- Length of operation
- Pelvic and hip surgery
- Past history of DVT or pulmonary embolism
- Varicose veins
- Pregnancy
- Oral contraceptive pill.

*Incidence*

The incidence varies with the type of operation and the risk factors mentioned. Overall it is estimated that for every 1000 operations there will be 100 DVTs, ten pulmonary emboli and one death. Pelvic and hip surgery, prolonged procedures and operations for neoplasia carry the highest risk of venous thrombosis.

*Diagnosis*

Early diagnosis is difficult and clinical diagnosis inaccurate. Experimentally $^{125}$I-fibrinogen scanning is sensitive in detecting developing thrombi but is of no value for established thrombosis.

Doppler ultrasound scans are increasingly valuable but only for peripheral sites. For iliofemoral thrombosis and more proximal lesions, venography is the definitive method of diagnosis. Two-criteria isotope venography shows great promise for the future.

*Prophylaxis*

Because of the difficulties of diagnosis, prophylaxis is the cornerstone of management. Such risk factors as obesity, contraceptive pill, etc., should be corrected if clinically possible.

The time of maximum risk of a thrombosis developing in surgical practice is during the operation when the three factors — stasis, endothelial trauma and increased coagulability — are most prevalent.

Mechanical and electrical methods of stimulating muscle function, thereby maintaining blood flow, are of value but have been superceded by pharmacological methods.

Subcutaneous calcium heparin (5000 units), injected 2 hours before surgery and continued postoperatively 12-hourly for five days or until the patient is fully mobile, is effective for all but high-risk patients. Up to now, orthopaedic surgeons have used full anticoagulation with warfarin to minimize the risk of DVT in major joint replacement. The new low-molecular-fragment heparin may well replace this method and reduce the risk of perioperative haemorrhage.

*Treatment*

If the thrombosis can be shown to be confined to the calf and is less than 5 cm long, no anticoagulation is indicated. Analgesics and support stockings may well be helpful.

Take care when actively treating patients with a dyspeptic history or with a history of cerebrovascular accident.

Most patients require:

1. Intravenous heparin, a loading dose of 10 000 units being followed by continuous intravenous infusion to prolong the activated partial thromboplastin time (APTT) by twice the control level

2. Anticoagulation with warfarin for at least three months.

### Complications

*Pulmonary embolism* may be fatal or multiple, producing pulmonary hypertension. Diagnosis is on the basis of a radio-isotope perfusion lung scan. If surgery is contemplated, as for a major embolism in a specialist centre, pulmonary angiography should be performed if time allows. Alternatively, thrombolyis with streptokinase or urokinase may be used. The alternative is full anticoagulation as described for DVT.

*Postphlebitic limb* is more likely to follow an occlusive iliofemoral thrombosis. Treatment is symptomatic with support stockings and analgesics or aimed at treating the venous ulcers which can complicate this condition, probably secondary to liposclerosis.

## Respiratory complications

Respiratory complications are the most common following surgery, but because of the various risk factors involved a true incidence is difficult to establish.

### Risk factors

Arterial oxygen tension falls gradually with age, especially over 80 years. Cardiovascular disease is more common. There is a reduction in vital capacity, lung capacity, peak expiratory flow rate and forced expiratory volume.

Smoking increases the risks, as obesity, excessive sedation, immobility, pre-existing lung disease and myocardial disease; the combination of heart and lung disease is particularly dangerous.

The type of operation is important. Cardiothoracic, upper abdominal and vertical wounds all reduce expiratory movement and increase the risk of respiratory complications.

### Pathology

The commonest problem after surgery is atelectasis. Small plugs of mucus block minor air passages and cause localized collapse. The plugs can usually be coughed clear by physiotherapy, but if not superinfection may result. Pulmonary embolus (see above) may also predispose to infection. Pleural effusion often complicates pulmonary pathology such as infection, infarct or metastatic disease, or may result from a subdiaphragmatic abscess or pancreatitis. It may also follow general causes such as congestive cardiac failure and hypoalbuminaemia. Pneumothorax can arise during ventilation, and may be caused by cannulation of central veins for monitoring central venous pressure or for parenteral nutrition.

Adult respiratory distress syndrome (ARDS) is the most serious pulmonary complication in surgical practice. It may complicate severe sepsis, fluid overload, chest trauma, fat emboli and inhalation pneumonitis. The cause is unclear but contributing factors are changes in types I and II alveolar cells, with loss of surfactant and alveolar collapse, impaired capillary to alveolar diffusion, arteriovenous shunts, the effects of endotoxin, resulting in complement activation by the alternate pathway and disseminated intravascular coagulation, and the effects of hyperoxide radicals.

### Management

Wherever possible correct risk factors such as weight and smoking habit before surgery. In all patients at risk ensure adequate analgesia without excessive sedation, regular physiotherapy administered not only by the therapist but also by the nursing and medical staff and indeed the patient.

Carefully monitor the pulse, respiratory rate and temperature, which all rise in patients with atelectasis and infection. Give appropriate antibiotics to patients who are pyrexial despite conservative measures, are ill, are at high risk as in combined myocardial and pulmonary disease, or who have features of ARDS. Administer supplementary oxygen by mask. Give ventilatory support if the PaO$_2$ falls below 75 mmHg.

## Infective complications

### Risk factors

Alimentary surgery not only has a higher incidence of infection but this is often associated with *endogenous* organisms. In 'clean' surgery, infection is usually secondary to *exogenous* agents.

The risk is increased in the presence of obesity, haematoma formation, diabetes mellitus, glucocorticoid therapy, immuno suppression, malnutrition and obstructive jaundice. Wounds may be classified as *clean*, such as thyroid or hernia surgery, *potentially contaminated*, as in elective gastrointestinal surgery, *contaminated*, as following bowel perforation, and *dirty*, where there is faecal contamination. The incidence of infection, morbidity and mortality increases from clean to dirty, and is greater in all categories if surgery is performed as an emergency.

## Prophylaxis

Identify the patients at risk. This refers both to those patients in whom the incidence of infection is higher and those for whom infection is particularly hazardous, such as those having joint or valve replacement, or those with cardiac valve disease. Reduce or control risk factors if possible. Ensure that your surgical technique is as perfect and as meticulous as possible. Select the appropriate antibiotic to give the greatest protection and tissue penetration, but take into account possible patient allergies and the cost involved. Give one dose intramuscularly with the premedication, or intravenously at the time of induction. Give more than one dose only if the operation is longer than 4 hours, or if there has been contamination. In this case, treatment rather than prophylaxis is indicated. Remember the value of mechanical bowel preparation.

Controversy persists about the need for and timing of shaving the operative area, the agent used for skin preparation, the value of intracavity antibiotics or antiseptics and the use of plastic drapes for wound protection. However, the use of 'danger' towels, separate knives for incising skin and deeper tissues and changing gloves after anastomoses are now of historical interest only.

It is difficult to overemphasize that antibiotics are no substitute for gentle handling of tissues, careful haemostasis, judicious use of diathermy, and avoiding strangling tissues with ligatures and sutures.

## Treatment

*Wound infection.* Open the wound to allow adequate drainage, obtain pus for culture, to establish the infecting organism(s) and antibiotic sensitivity. Irrigate the wound for adequate drainage and debridement. Formally reopen and surgically debride dirty wounds. If clean wounds became infected, consider cross-infections and investigate the likely sources.

Use antibiotics only if specifically indicated, for cellulitis, septicaemia, or if the consequences of infection would be disastrous — see above.

If the wound infection is chronic, consider the possibility of specific organisms such as Actinomyces, a foreign body in the wound such as a suture, an associated fistula as may occur in Crohn's disease, or associated factors such as irradiation and perineal wounds. Remember the danger of synergistic infections and dermal gangrene.

## Postoperative abscess

These are usually intraperitoneal but can be found deep in the wound. Localize the abscess and attempt drainage, if necessary under ultrasound or computed tomography (CT) control. Monitor resolution of the cavity radiologically if necessary. Exclude anastomotic leakage as a cause (see below).

If the patient remains toxic or the cavity fails to resolve, proceed to operative drainage and definitive treatment of any underlying cause.

## Septicaemia and septic shock

The septic complications mentioned above may progress to septicaemia and septic shock in patients who are debilitated by disease or drug therapy, such as steroids and cytotoxic chemotherapy. However, some organisms may be particularly virulent from the outset.

After surgery it is vital to remain alert for all septic problems. In terms of recognizing the more serious conditions remember the danger signs, which are:

- persistent, often swinging pyrexia with tachycardia

- signs of toxicity — flushed warm skin, glazed eyes, tachypnoea
- falling urinary output — less than 40 ml h$^{-1}$
- hypoxaemia.

Once the condition is suspected urgent effective therapy is essential to avoid low-output septic shock with its associated high mortality (>50%). The nature of death in such patients is multiple organ failure, and while a patient may survive failure of a single organ system such as the kidneys, the more organs which fail the higher the mortality.

Principles of treatment are:

- ensure adequate circulating blood volume using a mixture of crystalloid and colloid fluids, aiming for a central venous pressure 10–15 cm H$_2$O in a ventilated patient
- oxygen supplementation
- versatile intravenous antibiotic
- ventilatory support if the PaO$_2$ is less than 75 mmHg
- cardiac support with such drugs as dopamine, dobutamine, digitalis and catecholamines as indicated
- attention to renal function with dialysis for established renal failure.

More controversial are the methods used in some centres to ensure gastrointestinal decontamination. This involves a combination of enteral antibiotic and antiseptic agents, combined with a parenteral antibiotic, and this is gaining popularity. The value of enteral glutamine is considered vital in several intensive care units.

## Anastomotic leakage

Anastomotic leakage may complicate any anastomosis but is seen most commonly following oesophageal and colorectal surgery. In the latter group, leakage results in a threefold increase in operative mortality.

Anastomoses below the pelvic peritoneal reflection are associated with an increased risk of leakage, both clinical and radiological. The clinical rate always underestimates the true incidence of leakage detected by gastrografin or barium enema. (Table 21.2)

**Table 21.2**    Rates of clinically evident and radiologically detected leaks expressed as a percentage following colonic anastomoses performed above and below the pelvic peritoneal reflection.

| Pelvic peritoneum | Clinical | Radiological |
|---|---|---|
| Above | 1.2 | 18.3 |
| Below | 16 | 33 |

*Predisposing factors*

The general factors are similar to those which apply to wound healing in general, such as nutritional deficiencies, particularly protein, vitamin C and zinc, old age and impaired local blood flow from general conditions such as arteriosclerosis and cardiac disease.

Local factors include tension at the anastomosis and poor surgical technique as regards preparing the bowel ends, handling of tissues, excessive use of diathermy and the insertion and ligation of sutures. Contamination of the anastomosis with liquid faeces prejudices healing, as does an inadequate vascular supply to one or both sides of the anastomosis. Less important factors are the suture materials, the number of layers employed, and whether a stapling or suturing technique is used. However, there is preliminary evidence that tumour recurrence is lower in experimental studies when stainless wire is used for the anastomosis and, in clinical work if the anastomosis is stapled.

*Presentation*

Gastrointestinal contents may be identified in the wound or at a drain site. An intraabdominal abscess or more serious septic complication may develop. There may be prolonged ileus, unexplained pyrexia or tachycardia, sudden collapse postoperatively or development of an internal fistula.

Where there is any doubt, confirmation can often be obtained from a gently performed X-ray using a contrast medium.

*Management*

Management depends on the state of the patient and the volume draining. When the volume is small (i.e. less than 500 ml per 24 hours) and the patient is well, the initial treatment should be conservative:

- restricted oral intake
- intravenous fluids
- correct fluid, protein, electrolyte, acid–base and vitamin deficiencies
- treat associated sepsis
- institute nutritional support.

If such treatment fails to produce resolution, so that the output is high, or the patient is adversely affected by peritonitis, shock or infection, more interventional treatment is indicated.

- Adequate resuscitation
- Antibiotic cover
- Surgery.

The surgical procedure depends on the operative findings but the principles are:

- Thorough peritoneal lavage with tetracycline and warmed saline (1 gl$^{-1}$).
- Identification of the leak and any associated pathology such as Crohn's disease.
- Resection of the affected area — never try to insert a few extra sutures.
- Be prepared to establish a proximal stoma and a distal mucous fistula or carry out a Hartmann's type procedure, of closing the distal stump.
- *Very* occasionally, if contamination is slight, and conditions are satisfactory, an expert surgeon may elect to excise the margins and re-form the anastomosis.
- As a rule, after restoring the patients' health and nutritional status, the bowel ends are trimmed and re-joined.

## Problems with the wound

Failure of wound healing may result in wound dehiscence, incisional hernia or superficial wound disruption, in descending order of importance. Wound dehiscence should now be less than 0.1%. Incisional hernia is more common but should occur in less than 10% of abdominal wounds.

*Risk factors*

General risk factors include:

- respiratory disease
- smoking
- obesity
- obstructive jaundice, especially secondary to malignant disease
- nutritional deficiencies of protein: zinc and vitamin C
- Malignant disease
- Steroid therapy
- Emergency procedures.

Local risk factors include:

- wound infection
- impaired blood supply
- foreign body in the wound
- irradiation to the area
- type of wound — clean incised wounds heal better than ragged traumatic wounds
- site of wound — the anterior tibial area is motorious for wound breakdown and inappropriate length-to-width flap wounds heal less well
- poor surgical technique.

The best results are obtained by closing the abdominal wall en masse with a non-absorbable suture such as Nylon or an absorbable suture with prolonged tensile strength such as poly-dioxanone.

*Prevention*

As in all complications the cornerstone of success is to recognize risk factors, correct those which can be corrected and use appropriate surgical technique for all wounds.

*Management of superficial disruption*

- Evacuate haematoma and/or pus
- Excise and remove slough
- Remove any foreign body

● Irrigate with, for example, hydrogen peroxide and povidone iodine

● Pack *gently* to avoid too rapid healing over of the skin, but avoid trauma to granulation tissue

● Carefully monitor healing by secondary intention.

### Management of wound dehiscence

The mortality reported following abdominal wound rupture varies from 24% to 46%,

● Recognize the problem early.

● Do not overlook premonitory serious discharge from the wound, a prolonged ileus or low-grade pyrexia.

● Resuscitate the patient.

● Re-explore the abdomen and perform adequate peritoneal lavage.

● Proceed to re-suture the abdomen under general anaesthetic, using an adequate length of non-absorbable sutures without tension.

● Use 1 cm bites about 1 cm apart.

● Avoid pulling suture tightly in the tissues.

● It may be helpful to decompress the small bowel in retrograde fashion to reduce intra-abdominal tension.

Recurrence is uncommon but incisional herniation complicates approximately 25% cases.

### Management of incisional hernia

The indications for surgical intervention are obstruction, pain or increasing size. However, first spend time reducing such risk factors as obesity, smoking, constipation and prostatism and in assessing overall prognosis. Not all patients require or want surgical repair. In elderly and high-risk patients, an abdominal support controls symptoms in the majority of patients.

If you decide to proceed to herniorrhaphy, a number of options are available. The one selected depends on the site and size of the defect, the quality of the tissues, and your preferences.

Following repair the mortality should be less than 1% and the recurrence rate 5–10%. However, if a patient is greater than 50% over ideal body weight at the time of repair, a satisfactory result is less likely.

### Hypertrophic and keloid scarring

Hypertrophic scars are limited to the wound area and do not advance after six months. Keloids are more extensive, continue to expand beyond six months, and fortunately are much less common.

Predisposing factors are pigmented skin, burn trauma wounds on posterior aspects, younger age groups, and a past history of keloid scarring.

**Pathology.** There is excessive production and contraction of fibrous tissue. The synthesis of collagen is increased but the scar contains embryonic or fetal collagen. Only in hypertrophic scars is there an increased lysis of collagen.

The main complication is joint deformity, but the cosmetic problems can be considerable in exposed sites and with younger patients.

**Management.** Successful treatment is difficult, and should not be contemplated until six months from injury. There is no treatment for hypertrophic scars, and keloid scars should not be approached until they are mature.

Re-excision with and without pressure or plastic procedures is as disappointing as radiotherapy. Greater success has been claimed for injection of steroid into the wound. The mode of action appears to be increased collagen lysis, with depression of the proliferation of fibroblasts. Injection of triamcinolone can be repeated at intervals of one or two weeks depending on the result achieved.

## Haemorrhage

### Incidence

The incidence and severity of hemorrhagic complications are not easy to quantify. Re-exploration of a wound to evacuate haematoma and to secure haemostasis is uncommon. Wound haematoma and local bruising are sufficiently common to make it difficult to differentiate a complication from a normal sequel of surgery.

### Predisposing factors

● Obesity
● Long-term steroid therapy
● Jaundice
● Recent transfusions of stored blood

- Coagulation diseases
- Platelet deficiencies
- Anticoagulant therapy
- Older age
- Severe sepsis with disseminated intravascular coagulation.

## Pathology

It is conventional to consider *primary hemorrhage* within 24 hours of surgery, which is usually a technical problem of haemostasis, and *secondary hemorrhage*. This usually occurs five to ten days after operation and is due to local infection, sloughing of a clot or erosion of a ligature.

## Prevention

It is vital to recognize patients at risk and to reverse risk factors whenever possible. Even patients on long-term warfarin can be 'covered' by subcutaneous or intravenous heparin, on the basis that the latter agent can be reversed more rapidly than the warfarin.

Cooperation with a haematologist is essential in managing patients with coagulation disorders to infuse specific factors as required. Timing is vital e.g. fresh platelets after splenectomy. Vitamin K is used to reverse the problems associated with the obstructive element of jaundice.

Control of infection is essential. Above all, make sure your surgical technique is meticulous.

## Management

The need for intervention is dictated by the patient's symptoms and vital signs. Where haemorrhage is overt it is usually easier to decide whether exploration of the wound and cavity is indicated or not. When bleeding is internal reliance cannot be placed on any intra-cavity drain.

Check a clotting screen to assess any established, and identify any new problem. Correct any deficit appropriately with vitamin K by injection for problems with the clotting mechanism, expressed as international normalized ratio (INR). Use specific factors for deficiencies, fresh frozen plasma, and fresh platelets as indicated by the results of the coagulation study. Do not undertake surgical exploration until any deficit is corrected at least in part. It is unusual to identify a specific bleeding point.

The principles are:

1. Evacuate the blood and clot.
2. Identify any bleeding point or points, and control them appropriately.
3. If a troublesome ooze persists try the effect of a hemostatic agent such as Spongistan, or a collagen derivative.
4. If control remains difficult, pack the raw surface for 24–48 hours.
5. Consider leaving the superficial wound open, and give thought to the benefits of laparostomy (leaving the main wound open, packed with sterile packs), when a deeper source is suspected and recurrent bleeding is feared, as after pancreatic surgery. This facilitates re-exploration.

# 22. Screening for malignant disease

## T. Bates

At first sight, screening the population for the common forms of cancer seems a good idea since it should then be possible to cure the disease before it becomes symptomatic. Cancer of the lung, which is still the commonest malignancy (23 600 male: 10 200 female UK deaths per year) (Office of Population Censuses & Surveys 1990) has such a poor prognosis that prevention offers the only real hope of a significant impact on death rates, but screening programmes have been tried for carcinoma of the colon, stomach, breast and cervix. To be effective, early detection and treatment must lead to fewer deaths from the disease in the screened population but there are still remaining doubts that this has been achieved. An increased survival time from diagnosis to death could well be due to earlier and therefore more prolonged observation of the natural history of the disease, which might be unaffected by the treatment. This situation is known as lead time bias.

The acid test for a screening programme is to compare a screened population with an identical unscreened population, and this should ideally be set up as a randomized trial to avoid other biases (Shapiro 1981, Hardcastle et al 1989). If the disease carries a relatively good prognosis when adequately treated at an early stage, it may take many years of observation to show a difference in the number of deaths , and this will require enormous resources.

There are many questions which should be answered before very considerable amounts of time, money and effort are committed to a screening programme. These questions must be addressed by several disciplines: clinical scientists in the relevant specialty, epidemiologists with expertise in screening, social scientists and economists.

Is the screening test accurate in detecting cases in the population to be screened and is the subsequent treatment effective in curing the disease? In trying to answer these two critical questions the following specific issues must be considered.

## THE REQUIREMENTS FOR A SCREENING TEST

1. Is the screening test *sensitive:* i.e. does it detect most of the cases, with few false negatives?
2. Is the test *specific:* i.e. does it only detect cancer cases with few false positives?
3. The test must be safe, relatively inexpensive and capable of achieving adequate compliance in the population to be screened.

There are many examples of screening where these criteria have not been met. O- Toluidine-based dyes for detecting occult blood increased the risk of bladder cancer in laboratory staff, and the dose of irradiation used for the first breast screening mammograms is no longer regarded as safe.

## THE POPULATION TO BE SCREENED

To screen young people who rarely get cancer does not make sense but cancer of the cervix has become more common in younger women, which has led to a reduction in the age at which screening is offered. It is essential to have an accurate register of the population to be screened and in city areas it is vital that this is frequently updated if the client is to receive the invitation for screening. Screening the very elderly is likely to show poor compliance and the cost–benefit ratio is likely to be much less favourable. Screening high-risk groups, e.g. those with a strong family history, poses special problems and different criteria must be used.

## COLORECTAL CANCER (8100 male : 8600 female deaths per annum)

Colonoscopy is the gold-standard test for detecting colonic cancer or polyps, with both specificity and sensitivity nearing 100%, but high price and low compliance rule this out as a screening test unless a very high-risk population such as a family with familial adenomatous polyposis is being examined

Colorectal cancer should be an ideal candidate for screening since it seems that many cancers are preceded by benign adenomatous polyps and, furthermore, early cancer (Dukes' A) has a five-year survival of 90% with conventional operative treatment. However, the best available test is poor. The Haemoccult test is probably the best of several tests for faecal occult blood but it has a relatively low sensitivity (especially for right-sided and rectal tumours) and although the specificity is over 90%, this does give rise to false positive cases which require expensive and unnecessary investigation.

Hardcastle et al (1989) have set up a massive randomized controlled trial of Haemoccult screening which has shown a favourable downgrading of tumours in the screened group, but it is disappointing that survival benefit has not yet become apparent.

## CANCER OF THE BREAST (13 700 deaths per year)

There have been four randomly allocated trials of population screening for breast cancer by mammography, and of these only the Swedish Two-Counties study has shown a significant reduction in mortality (Tabar et al 1989). However, a recent overview of these trials and other non-randomized studies shows that all report fewer deaths in the screened versus the non-screened population (Wald et al 1991). There are unconfirmed reports of an initial increase in mortality in the screened group and our understanding of cause and effect is clearly incomplete.

Most authorities are confident that the UK National Breast Screening Programme (NBSP), in which women aged 50–64 are offered single-view mammography every three years, will reduce deaths from breast cancer, but some observers are still sceptical.

## CARCINOMA OF THE CERVIX (1900 deaths per year)

Unfortunately no randomized trial of cytological screening for carcinoma of the cervix has been carried out and, although death rates for this disease have fallen in many countries, this fall has often preceded the introduction of screening (Williams 1992).

Up to 60% of women who have developed cervical cancer in the UK have never been screened and the false-negative rate for examination of the smears is about 10%. Not all smears are adequate and cytoscreening is very labour intensive. Unlike the NBSP, there is not a prompt and efficient mechanism for the recall and treatment of patients with positive smears. This situation is unsatisfactory since the outcome of adequate treatment in cervical intraepithelial neoplasia (CIN) is highly successful. Considerable resources will be required to save the lives of a relatively small but increasingly young number of women.

## CARCINOMA OF THE STOMACH (5600 male : 3800 female deaths per year)

The incidence of cancer of the stomach seems to be falling as colon cancer rises, but these changes may be confounded by the vagaries of death certification.

Cancer of the stomach is much more common in Japan and there is considerable small-area variation in parts of the Middle East. Screening for early gastric cancer seems to be effective in Japan (Hisamichi & Sugawara 1984) but in the UK the search has been less successful and screening by gastroscopy should perhaps be confined to symptomatic patients over 55 (Hallissey et al 1990).

## WHAT COMPLIANCE IS TO BE EXPECTED?

Compliance varies with the social acceptability

and public awareness of the disease, the screening test and the perceived treatment. Screening for breast cancer by mammography will achieve 80% in areas with a stable population but this may be less than 50% in inner city areas. It is possible that compliance may be affected by fear of mastectomy, and discomfort at the initial screen may reduce attendance for re-screening. There is also some evidence that compliance may change due to media exposure in the short term.

In screening for colorectal cancer, enthusiasm in the population for faecal occult blood testing is very low, which leads to poor compliance unless considerable efforts are made to increase public awareness at the time that screening is offered. There are many reasons why people decline screening invitations, but failure to receive the letter is a common cause. The true refusers are an unusual group of people who have a poor outlook from both a health and a social standpoint. It seems that they neglect or abuse their health in many respects and it is therefore important not to use them as a control group for comparison with the accepters of screening, since whatever comparison is made the refusers will be disadvantaged. Compliance in screening for carcinoma of the cervix by cytology is worst in the socio-economic group most at risk from the disease.

## THE INTERVENTION TO BE USED

It has already been noted that an operation for early bowel cancer has a high cure rate, but we cannot be sure this is the case for breast cancer. In this latter disease the evidence so far fails to show survival benefit in screening women under 50 and it is therefore logical that screening on a national basis should be confined to older women until there is information to the contrary. Screen-detected breast cancer has many features known to indicate a good prognosis (Klemi et al 1992) but ductal carcinoma in situ is diagnosed in up to 20% of screened cases and the best treatment for this condition is still in doubt. It is possible that fear of over-treatment by mastectomy may lead to a sacrifice of survival advantage by inadequate surgery. Severe dysplasia of the cervix (CIN III)

has an extremely good outlook with local treatment and close surveillance. Node-positive carcnoma of the stomach has a five-year survival rate of less than 10% but in situ tumours carry a good prognosis if treated with adequate surgery. The Japanese have pioneered more radical surgery for gastric cancer than has been the norm in the West, and clinical trials are currently in hand to try and repeat their excellent results in the UK.

## WHAT SHOULD BE THE INTERVAL BETWEEN SCREENS?

In the NBSP the current intervals between screens is three years and in some trial centres this has been reduced to two. The most appropriate interval for cervical screening is still controversial and the case for screening in carcinoma of the colon or stomach is not sufficiently secure for the interval between screens to be a major issue. There will always be some tumours which are detected between screens and many of these 'interval cancers' will be rapidly growing tumours with a poor prognosis.

## WHAT IS THE COST?

The economist will want to know the cost per case detected, the cost per case treated and per life saved. The sociologist will want to know the psycho-social cost to those false-positive cases investigated unnecessarily (Ellman et al 1989) and the quality of life in those patients who have cancer detected sooner than it otherwise would have been.

## SUMMARY

A screening test for cancer must be able to detect the disease at a stage when earlier treatment will lead to fewer deaths. To achieve this the test must be sensitive, specific and acceptable: the treatment must be effective. The overall cost of a life saved may be difficult to quantify but this should be taken into account.

## REFERENCES

Ellman R, Angeli N, Christians A, Moss S, Chamberlain J, Maguire P 1989 Psychiatric morbidity associated with screening for breast cancer. British Journal of Cancer 60: 781–784

Hallissey M T, Allum W H, Jewkes A J, Ellis D J, Fielding J W L 1990 Early detection of gastric cancer. British Medical Journal 301: 513–515

Hardcastle J D, Chamberlain J, Sheffield J et al 1989 Randomised controlled trial of faecal occult blood screening for colorectal cancer: results from the first 107, 349 patients. Lancet i: 1160

Hisamichi S, Sugawara N 1984 Mass screening for gastric cancer by X-ray examination. Japanese Journal of Clinical Oncology 14: 211–223

Klemi P J, Joensuu H, Toikkanen S et al 1992 Aggressiveness of breast cancers found with and without screening. British Medical Journal 304: 467–469

Office of Population Censuses & Surveys 1990 Series DH2 No. 15. Mortality statistics for 1988. Cause. HMSO, London

Shapiro S 1981 Evidence on screening for breast cancer from a randomised trial. Cancer 39: 618–627

Tabar L, Fagerberg F, Duffy S W, Day N E 1989 The Swedish Two Counties Trial of mammographic screening for breast cancer: recent results and calculation of benefit. Journal of Epidemiology and Community Health 43: 107–114

Wald N, Frost C, Cuckle H 1991 Breast cancer screening: the current position. British Medical Journal 302: 845

Williams C 1992 Ovarian and cervical cancer. British Medical Journal 304: 1501–1504

# 23. Principles of surgery for malignant disease

*P. J. Guillou*

In 1989 malignant disease accounted for just under a quarter of all deaths in the UK, being second only to cardiovascular disease (45.9% of all deaths) in the league of individual causes of death (OPCS monitor, 1991). Table 23.1 indicates the contribution of different types of malignant disease to the total figure. Lung cancer constitutes the greatest overall number of cancer deaths, although amongst women carcinoma of the breast is more common. Cancer arising in the gastrointestinal tract constitutes 26.5% of all cancer deaths. Surgery has mainly a diagnostic and staging role in the management of the most common cancer, lung cancer. Surgeons most frequently con-

tribute to the therapeutic management of patients suffering from malignant disease of the breast and gastrointestinal tract, although similar principles apply to malignant disease managed by urologists (bladder, kidney, testis and prostate), head and neck surgeons, etc. The nature of modern cancer therapy demands considerable familiarity with the pathological basis of malignancy.

## PATHOLOGICAL BASIS OF THE ORIGINS AND SPREAD OF MALIGNANT DISEASE

A tumour results when an individual cell or group of cells escapes from the constraints which control normal cell replication. Controlled proliferation occurs during embryogenesis, hypertrophy, healing, regeneration, repair, and during the metabolic response to trauma and sepsis. Controlled cellular replication is mediated by small peptide growth factors which bind to their specific receptors on the cell surface. Growth factors may be autocrine (i.e. bind to receptors on the cell which produces them), paracrine (i.e. bind to receptors on a cell adjacent to the cell of origin), or classically endocrine (i.e. bind to receptors on a cell at some distance from the cell of origin, usually being transferred via the circulation). Once a growth factor binds to its cell surface receptor, intracellular signals are induced which, amongst other things, activate the nucleus and promote the cell to enter the cell cycle. Within the nucleus nucleoproteins ensure accurate DNA replication, DNA repair, and DNA transcription via messenger RNA (mRNA). Clearly the growth factors, their receptors, the enzymes which their binding activates and the nucleoproteins (e.g. DNA polymerase) which regulate DNA synthesis and repair

**Table 23.1** Causes of death

|                              | 1987    | 1988    | 1989    |
|------------------------------|---------|---------|---------|
| *All causes*                 | 556 994 | 571 408 | 576 872 |
| Cardiovascular disease       | 271 061 | 267 927 | 264 600 |
| (% of all causes)            | 47.8%   | 46.9%   | 45.9%   |
|                              |         |         |         |
| *All malignant*              |         |         |         |
| *neoplasms*                  | 140 768 | 142 540 | 143 439 |
| (% of all causes)            | 24.8%   | 24.95%  | 24.86%  |
|                              |         |         |         |
| *Numbers of deaths*          |         |         |         |
| *from individual tumour sites* |       |         |         |
|                              |         |         |         |
| Bronchus/lung                | 35 138  | 35 302  | 34 581  |
| Lip/oral cavity              | 1 689   | 1 687   | 1 716   |
| Oesophagus                   | 4 770   | 4 884   | 5 108   |
| Stomach                      | 9 509   | 9 425   | 9 062   |
| Small bowel                  | 204     | 242     | 220     |
| Colon                        | 11 378  | 11 494  | 11 626  |
| Rectum/anus                  | 5 675   | 5 755   | 5 756   |
| Pancreas                     | 6 065   | 6 009   | 6 116   |
| Primary liver                | 666     | 674     | 676     |
|                              |         |         |         |
| Genitourinary                | 22 188  | 22 527  | 24 145  |
| Carcinoma of                 |         |         |         |
| female breast                | 13 751  | 13 723  | 14 008  |
| Lymphoma                     | 9 489   | 9 718   | 9 913   |

are all coded for by codons within the human genome. They are therefore susceptible to modifications of their structure, either by mutations, deletions or amplifications of their corresponding genes or by errors of transcription of the code into the mature protein. Mutations occur either spontaneously or as result of the reaction of chemical carcinogens with DNA.

Tumours rarely grow simply because their cell cycle times or proportion of proliferating cells (growth fraction) are greater than those in normal tissues. Tumours grow because, unlike normal tissues where in general a cell divides only in order to replace one which has been lost, there is failure to respond to the constraints which regulate normal growth irrespective of cell loss. This is not to say that tumours do not also shed cells. It has been estimated that 50% of tumour cells are lost as a consequence of exfoliation, hypoxia, non-viability, metastasis and host defences. Tumour size therefore depends on three factors: the cell cycle time, the growth fraction and the numbers lost from the tumour surface. A tumour will become clinically palpable when it consists of $10^9$ or more cells but most tumours contain far more cells than this when they first present. Even the smallest radiologically detectable mammary carcinoma contains $10^7$–$10^8$ cells and patients usually die before a size of $10^{12}$ cells has been achieved. In rapidly proliferating tumours the cells de-differentiate and less and less resemble the parent cells. Failure to be inhibited by contact with neighbouring cells is an important characteristic of tumours but two further properties of this uncontrolled replication distinguish the malignant from the non-malignant tumour. These are the capacity to invade and destroy adjacent normal structures, and the ability to invade lymphatic and venous vessels and produce metastases.

## Oncogenes, growth factors and the multistep hypothesis of tumour progression

The concept has evolved that cancers proceed through multiple stages before reaching the point of invasive malignancy. This may involve the inheritance of a genetic change which provides susceptibility to the development of malignancy (e.g. the retinoblastoma (Rb) or familial polyposis (FAP) gene deletions on chromosomes 13 and 5 respectively), or exposure to environmental carcinogens which activate particular genes which, if dominant, will induce cellular proliferation. The resultant increase in cellular proliferation results in an increase in the frequency of mistakes in DNA synthesis which if unrepaired become permanent mutations. If a critical suppressor gene (e.g. the P53 gene which is coded for on chromosome 17p) is lost or mutated then the last molecular constraint over controlled cell growth disappears and further mutation leads to the development of cells with the capacity for invasion and metastasis. Thus the multistep hypothesis suggests that although a single activated gene or, perhaps more importantly, a lost suppressor gene may be necessary, it alone is insufficient to produce the complete malignant phenotype. Although the fine molecular details have not been fully elucidated, this is considered to be the basis of, for example, the well-known polyp–cancer sequence of carcinoma of the colon.

Many of these abnormalities involve genetic sequences known as oncogenes, which were originally identified as the genes within certain tumour-forming RNA viruses that were responsible for tumour formation, hence the expression v-*onc* (oncogene) to describe them when they are isolated from the virus in question. In fact it would appear that the viruses acquired the genes from the human genome during viral excision, and thus when identified in mammalian cells the sequences are given the prefix c-, as shown in Table 23.2. Cellular (c-) oncogenes or proto-oncogenes are *normal* genes which code for proteins (oncoproteins) that are implicated in *normal* cellular proliferation. They are expressed at certain stages in embryogenesis and during regeneration, healing, etc. Since oncoproteins are important components of the process of *regulated* cell division, their involvement in carcinogenesis is best understood by categorizing them as dominant oncogenes or recessive/suppressor oncogenes, but this needs to be combined with a knowledge of the site and function (if known) of their oncoproteins. Table 23.3 represents one such classification but it is important to reiterate that oncogenes and their corresponding oncoproteins *are normal components of cellular molecular physiology*. They become implicated in carcinogenesis when their encoded

**Table 23.2**  Oncoproteins and their functions

| Dominant oncogene products | | | | |
|---|---|---|---|---|
| Growth factors | Plasmalemmal | Cytoplasmic | Nuclear | |
| Ligands | Membrane receptors | Signal transducers | Transcription factors | Cell cycle factors |
| c-*sis* (platelet+derived growth factor, PDGF) | EGF-receptor c-*erb*B2 c-*kit* | GTP-binding c-Ha-*ras* c-Ki-*ras* c-N-*ras* c-*src* | c-*fos* c-*jun* c-*erb*A (thyroid hormone receptor) | c-*myc* c-*myb* |
| | PDGF-receptor c-*fms* | | | |

**Table 23.3**  Suppressor/recessive oncogene products

*Display a normal phenotype despite the inheritance of one abnormal parental gene but not if one is inherited from each parent, e.g.:*

1. *The Retinoblastoma (Rb) gene*
Only when the normal gene (13q14) undergoes spontaneous mutation in the eye and a homozygous genotype is present does retinoblastoma develop. Of couse retinoblastoma will develop if the child inherits the Rb gene from both parents

2. *The P53 oncogene*
Normally prevents malignant transformation unless mutated. Mutated P53 ptotein binds to normal (wild-type) P53 protein and inactivates it

3. *Wilms tumour gene*
The molecular genetics of this gene is similar to that of the Rb gene

proteins become over-expressed, truncated (mutated) or otherwise modified so that their function is constitutively expressed rather than declared in a regulated fashion as in the normal cell. Hence 60–70% of colorectal cancers possess a mutated Kirsten (*K*-) *ras* oncogene. Similarly the P53 oncoprotein, which is a normal suppressor of cell division and which prevents entry of the cell into S-phase, has been found to exist in mutated forms in at least 50% of tumours of the breast, colon, lung, bladder and hepatomas. The mutated forms can bind to and inactivate the 'wild-type' normal P53 and inactivate it, resulting in uncontrolled cellular replication.

The c-*erb*B2 oncogene product is over-expressed in 20% of breast cancers and correlates with increasing tumour grade but is independent of oestrogen receptor status, nodal involvement or any other risk factor for recurrence of breast cancer. It appears to have considerable prognostic significance independently of the aforementioned parameters even in those patients who are node negative.

It is this unregulated expression or neo-expression of deregulated genes that may also be responsible for the capacity of certain tumours to secrete proteins into the circulation which may be used to detect or monitor for the recurrence of certain tumours, e.g. carcinoembryonic antigen (CEA) for gastrointestinal, particularly colorectal, cancer or α-fetoprotein (AFP) for hepatomas.

## The concepts of early cancer, invasion and metastasis

A number of conditions are recognized which, although not being malignant per se, have the potential to become so and are categorized as premalignant. In the gastrointestinal tract these include leucoplakia of the oral mucosa, Barratt's columnar-lined oesophagus, certain types of severe gastric dysplasia, Peutz–Jehger syndrome and ulcerative colitis. However, in these conditions malignant cells may be present but they have not yet invaded the basement membrane. This defines carcinoma-in-situ which may be encountered in the breast (ductal carcinoma-in-situ), the cervix, the oral mucosa and a number of other sites. Depending on its site, carcinoma-in-situ may be treated by local resection, although in the breast removal of all breast tissue has been advocated because of the multicentricity of the condition. In the gastrointestinal tract it is necessary to distinguish carcinoma-in-situ from so-called 'early' lesions such as early gastric cancer and colorectal cancer of stage A in the Dukes' classification. 'Early cancer' of the digestive tract is therefore defined as frankly invasive cancer which has not yet breached the muscular layer of the intestine. Under these circumstances major resectional surgery is often curative and simple locally destructive approaches are inadequate.

The concept of early malignancy is also applied to malignant melanoma, where two main criteria are employed to express the invasiveness of the tumours. These are the thickness of the lesion (Breslow) and the histological level of invasion (Clarks level). Tumour thickness correlates well with overall prognosis, the so-called 'thin' melanomas (< 0.85 mm thick) rarely metastasizing following excision with a 1–2 cm clear margin. In contrast, the five-year survival rate of patients with melanomas thicker than 3.5 mm is only 38%.

Occasionally, primary malignancy in an organ is seen which is pathologically 'early' (e.g. has not yet invaded the muscularis mucosae of the gastrointestinal tract) but is associated with the presence of lymph node deposits. This is a scenario sometimes seen with gastric carcinoma or with a Dukes 'A' carcinoma which is accompanied by hepatic metastases, and these examples indicate the biological complexity of the process of metastasis. The mechanisms which underlie the development of metastasis have yet to be fully elucidated. Metastasis occurs via three distinct routes:

1. via the lymphatic drainage
2. via the venous drainage of the organ containing the tumour
3. via the body cavities, e.g trans-coelomic metastasis.

Rarely, metastasis may occur transluminally, as for example with the implantation of exfoliated viable colorectal cancer cells into distal healing sites such as haemorrhoidectomy wounds, anastomoses, etc.

These routes are surgically important. Because most common tumours spread via the lymphatics, and since lymphatic vessels and their associated lymph nodes commonly accompany the arterial supply to an organ, in many instances the surgery of malignant disease is based on the anatomy of the arterial supply to the organ containing the primary tumour. Similarly, the venous drainage of an organ is an important determinant of the haematogenous pattern of distribution of metastases from tumours arising from that organ.

The capacity of tumour cells to form a metastasis is a function of a complex sequence of events which involves direct invasion of a venous radical or lymphatic vessel by such processes as adhesion to the vascular endothelium and digestion of the basement membrane of the vessel in which the tumour cell has been arrested. These events relate to tumour cell receptors for the laminin of basement membrane and the release of enzymes such as collagenase which facilitate the invasion of tissue parenchyma. Also involved are host factors such as platelet/tumour cell aggregates, thrombosis, ischaemia and the further release of tumour cells into a growth factor-rich environment.

The organ distribution of metastases is determined by factors which are not necessarily related to the proportion of the cardiac output received by the organ. The 'soil' for metastatic implantation must be conducive to the growth of the metastatic 'seed'. However, anatomical considerations such as venous and lymphatic drainage cause metastatic disease to follow identifiable and predictable patterns, e.g. liver metastases from colorectal cancer, pulmonary metastases from renal cell cancer and malignant melanoma, lymphatic metastases from early gastric and breast cancers etc. Secondary metastatic sites such as the liver may in turn serve as a source of metastases such as from the liver to the lungs and from the lungs to the bones, adrenals, brain, etc.. The surgeon should appreciate these patterns of metastasis for individual tumours because: (1) modern management demands that patients be appropriately screened for recurrent disease which may be amenable to further excisional surgery (e.g. 'second-look' surgery following colorectal cancer excision, lymphadenectomy after excision of a limb melanoma etc.); (2) introduction of adjuvant therapies targeted at organs where recurrence is likely to occur or where surgery cannot completely guarantee the eradication of micrometastatic disease (e.g. radiotherapy to the breast and axilla following local excision and node sampling for carcinoma of the breast; (3) for monitoring those patients whose primary treatment modality may not be surgical but in whom subsequent recurrent disease may lead to the use of radical surgical excision as the next line of therapy (e.g. following radiotherapy to laryngeal carcinoma, bladder carcinoma, etc).

## Tumour staging and grading

Pathological tumour staging and grading have an impact on the choice of therapy, which increasingly is being individually tailored to the patient. Tumour grade mainly refers to the degree of differentiation of a particular tumour on histological examination using well-characterized criteria, such as the degree of nuclear polymorphism, capacity to resemble the parent histiotype, number of mitoses, etc.. Tumours are generally described as well, moderately or poorly differentiated, this being the best available separation obtainable by even the most experienced of pathologists. Unfortunately most tumours contain mixed elements of these grading systems and it is conventional to grade a tumour according to its worst area of differentiation. While poorly differentiated tumours tend to be more aggressive than well-differentiated lesions, the prognostic correlation with degree of differentiation is rather weak for most tumours.

Staging systems attempt to quantify the tumour mass in a manner which has clinical value for prognostic, therapeutic and comparative purposes. Most systems are based on an assessment of the size of the primary tumour (T), the presence of lymphatic metastases in lymph nodes (N) and the existence of distant metastases (M). For some tumours it is possible to make a clinical estimate of the stage of a tumour, as for example the clinical staging of carcinoma of the breast. However, for the purposes of comparing prognosis and the results of adjuvant therapy between different centres and therapeutic protocols, the TNM system based on pathological data is preferable. It provides prognostic guidelines and aids enormously in the decision for or against administering adjuvant therapy to an individual patient.

In general, nodal status plays a dominant role in determining prognosis but with certain tumours other factors may carry equal weight. For example, in the schema devised by the Japanese Society for the Study of Gastric Cancer, serosal involvement represents a major prognostic indicator with the albeit rare but interesting paradox of serosa-negative/node-positive tumours enjoying a better prognosis than those who are serosa positive but node negative, provided of course that radical lymphadenectomy is conducted during the course of the gastrectomy. In contrast, nodal status remains the strongest independent prognostic indicator in patients with operable carcinoma of the breast and this influences therapeutic strategies in the management of such patients.

Because lymphatics tend to accompany the main arterial supply to the organ in question, radical resectional surgery for malignant disease tends to be the surgery of blood vessels. For carcinoma of the stomach radical resection with lymphadenectomy can be achieved only by division of the left gastric artery at its origin, the right gastric artery at its origin, the splenic artery in the lesser sac and the right gastro epiploic artery at its origin, etc. These vessels are removed along with all their accompanying lymphoid tissue, including that along the hepatic artery and hilum of the liver, together with the pre- and paraaortic lymphatic tissue in the retroperitoneum. This inevitably necessitates removal of the body and tail of the pancreas. Of course such an extensive dissection is accompanied by greater morbidity and mortality than the somewhat less radical lymphatic resections more commonly undertaken for gastric carcinoma in the UK. This surgical risk is perhaps worthwhile if it is offset by a significant increase in disease-free interval and survival. Whereas this is true for gastric cancer in the Japanese it is as yet uncertain whether this is also the case in European patients, whose disease tends on the whole to be rather advanced at presentation. Nevertheless, the pathological staging of gastric cancer has led the Japanese Society for Gastric Cancer to devise a logical plan for the surgical treatment of gastric cancer.

Modern developments in cellular and molecular biology have also contributed to more accurate definition of prognosis for an individual patient. For example, in addition to the dominant influence of axillary lymph node status, it has now been determined that the expression of receptors for epidermal growth factor (EGF-r) and the c-*erb*B2 oncoprotein are also implicated as risk factors for metastatic breast cancer. The presence of nuclear oestrogen receptors is a good prognostic factor in such patients and is inversely related to the expression of EGF-r. The expression of EGF-r is second only to nodal status as an indicator of prognosis in breast cancer and further serves to discriminate a poor prognostic group in those who are node negative. It is likely that the identification of this latter marker will enter routine practice for the decision for administration or otherwise of adjuvant therapy for primary breast cancer. This is an important example of the incorporation of progress in molecular and cellular biology into the clinical arena which will undoubtedly be paralleled in the management of other tumour types. Other examples already exist, including, for example, the finding that the degree of amplification of the c-*myc* oncogene (N-*myc*) in childhood neuroblastoma correlates inversely with the disease-free interval following resection and also appears to render the tumour cells more resistant to chemotherapy.

It is obviously desirable that the patient be accurately staged before surgical intervention is applied. With certain tumours, e.g. carcinoma of the breast, this can be performed quite accurately. With many others, however, even with sophisticated imaging techniques such as ultrasound, computed tomography (CT) scans, magnetic resonance imaging (MRI) scans, positron emission tomography (PET) scans, various isotope scanning procedures and the more recent advent of scanning with radio-labelled monoclonal antibodies, the final decision as to the nature of the surgery to be undertaken and the necessity for surgical adjuvant therapy must await the operative findings and final pathological staging.

## POPULATION SCREENING FOR MALIGNANT DISEASE

The assumed relationship between detectability and cure rate shown in Figure 23.1 has resulted in the development of screening programmes for the more common malignant tumours. Routine endoscopic screening of the whole population has significantly improved the detection rate for early gastric cancer in Japan, where the disease is almost endemic. However, in countries such as the UK where the incidence is 11 000 new cases annually, a whole population endoscopic screening programme would not be cost effective (see Ch. 22).

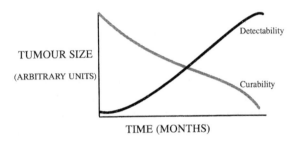

**Fig. 23.1**   Relationship between detectability and curability.

## The role of tumour markers in screening and follow-up after surgical excision

Genetic abnormalities are almost certainly responsible for the capacity of tumours to secrete certain proteins, which are not normally secreted in great quantities, into body fluids. Mostly these are normally detected in the plasma; and measurement of these 'tumour markers' is used predominantly for the monitoring of response to therapy or detection of recurrent disease following surgical excision of a primary or secondary tumour (see Ch. 26).

## SYMPTOMS, SIGNS AND DIAGNOSIS OF MALIGNANT DISEASE

Space does not permit a full description of all the symptoms to be expected with malignant disease of every organ. However, the symptoms and signs with which cancer commonly presents may be categorized as follows.

*1. As a palpable swelling.* This is most often painless until local structures are invaded.

Occasionally, as with inflammatory carcinoma of the breast, the swelling may be 'inflamed' but more usually it is not detected until ulceration and secondary infection supervene.

*2. With the symptoms of obstruction.* In tubular structures this is a most important and sinister group of symptoms. Examples are:

- dysphagia in carcinoma of the oesophagus
- the vomiting and succussion splash of gastric outflow obstruction due to gastric cancer
- obstructive jaudice
- small bowel colic
- large bowel colic
- spurious diarrhoea
- the bladder outflow symptoms associated with carcinoma of the prostate.

*3. With symptoms resulting from haemorrhage.* Anaemia, haemoptysis, haematuria, haematemesis, rectal bleeding, etc. Cutaneous lesions which itch and bleed should be viewed as highly suspicious.

*4. With symptoms due to local compression or invasion of local structures.* For example, caval compression, gastric or colonic outflow obstruction, nerve root pain, etc.

*5. With the symptoms and signs of metastatic spread.* Pleural effusion, ascites, hepatomegaly, isolated lymphadenopathy, anorexia and weight loss, pathological fractures, grand mal fits from cerebral metastases, etc.

*6. Asymptomatic incidental findings.* It should not be forgotten that cancer may be totally asymptomatic even when it is quite advanced, e.g. the silent pulmonary metastases discovered on a routine chest X-ray, asymptomatic axillary or groin metastses.

The investigation and final diagnosis of a patient with malignant disease will of course be determined by the site of the lesion and the symptoms which it produces, but again certain principles apply. First, it is rare that treatment of a particular tumour can be rationally prescribed without first obtaining a histological diagnosis. It is a tragedy for unnecessary major ablative surgery, irradiation or chemotherapy to be given to a patient who is suffering from a benign condition. *A histological diagnosis is, in the vast majority of instances, an absolute requirement for planning treatment.* Second, all investigations should aim not only to confirm the histological diagnosis but also to stage the tumour preoperatively as far as is possible. This is important not only to decide whether or not other treatments should also be administered preoperatively (e.g. neo-adjuvant therapy for carcinoma of the breast, radiotherapy for oesophageal cancer or rectal cancer), but also to avoid surgery where it is inappropriate. It is futile to undertake major resectional surgery for oesophageal cancer in the presence of extensive liver metastases. In contrast, the presence of a solitary liver metastasis or even more advanced disease should not necessarily deter the surgeon from resecting an obstructing primary colorectal carcinoma.

In general, the principles of investigation of a patient suffering from malignancy involves procedures which are as follows.

*1. Endoscopic.* The roles of oesophagogastroscopy, endoscopic retrograde cholangiopancreatographyl (ERCP), proctoscopy, sigmoidoscopy, colonoscopy and bronchoscopy are all widely appreciated. All abdominal surgeons involved in the management of patients with malignant disease should be able to perform a laparoscopy as part of the staging process. The 'open and close' laparotomy should rarely, if ever, be performed in this era of modern imaging technology.

*2. Radiological.* Most readers will be familiar with the principles of contrast radiology, particularly in relation to tubular structures such as the gastrointestinal and urological systems. Plain radiology still has a role in the evaluation of the patient with malignant disease, especially of the bones. Chest X-ray should never be omitted. Ultrasound remains the most sensitive preoperative modality for detecting tumours within the liver, with a sensitivity of around 75%. Ultrasound also affords an opportunity to obtain an ultrasound-guided biopsy of the lesion. Other information provided by ultrasound is that it can detect masses in the pancreas, kidneys, etc., and also detects the dilated biliary tree. Unfortunately ultrasound is not a terribly useful method for following the progress of a liver lesion which is being treated non-surgically, because it is very operator dependent and measurements of tumours can be quite difficult to make using ultrasound unless the same radiologist is available on every occasion. CAT scanning is much more useful in this regard, especially when combined with the administration of intravenous contrast, either as a 'CT portogram' or as a delayed CT scan after intravenous contrast injection.

It is now simply not enough to detect the presence of tumours within the liver. Their size, number and precise anatomical localization in relation to the anatomical segments of the liver must be determined. At the very worst this has a bearing on prognosis but may also enable surgical treatment for metastases to be adequately conducted. MRI does not appear to possess many advantages over contrast-enhanced CT scanning for the purposes of imaging the liver, and there is now little role for the adynamic sulphacolloid isotope scan of the liver for the detection of primary or secondary tumours.

Other radiological investigations include of course the use of other isotopes as, for example, bone scans using radioactive technetium, or the detection of cold non-functioning nodules within the thyroid using radioiodine. However, a modern development of isotope scanning is the conjugation of a radio-isotope to a monoclonal antibody which specifically identifies an epitope expressed on the surface of the tumour cell. Isotope-conjugated monoclonal antibodies to antigens related to the CEA molecule allow, in some cases, quite accurate determination of the localization of metastatic deposits from colorectal cancer. Monoclonal antibodies to antigens present on breast cancer, ovarian cancer and prostatic cancer have been developed and are being employed in a similar fashion.

**3. Pathology in the investigation of the patient with malignant disease.** The necessity of having an accurate histological diagnosis prior to initiating treatment in a patient with malignant disease cannot be over-emphasized. This may be obtained in a number of ways:

1. Via a fine needle — fine needle aspiration cytology (FNAC) can be performed on an outpatient basis and provides rapid diagnosis in the investigation of squamous tumours of the head and neck, tissue thyroid, breast, subcutaneous nodules, enlarged lymph nodes and within a variety of other scenarios including at CT scanning and endoscopy where the use of wider-bore needles than 19 to 21 gauge in relatively inaccessible sites might be hazardous. The false-positive rate for carcinoma of the breast is less than 1% but the false-negative rate is somewhat higher and is dependent on the skills of both the clinician performing the aspirate and the cytologist who reads it. However, further levels of refinement may be added with the use of monoclonal antibodies to particular antigens. Both the sensitivity and specificity of cytology for carcinoma of the breast are now so highly developed in most institutions that confidence in this particular mode of investigation enables the surgeon to proceed to definitive therapy without necessarily having histological proof via a needle biopsy or frozen section.

2. Needle biopsy — this should be distinguished from FNAC because it provides a core of tissue which is treated as a histological preparation and not a cytological one. It is used less frequently nowadays, having been largely replaced by FNAC. However, there are specific instances such as liver biopsy where it remains the procedure of choice and it is used when FNAC has failed to provide a definitive diagnosis.

3. Wedge biopsy is rarely used these days except perhaps at open operation on the liver. It is rarely indicated for skin lesions, where excisional biopsy is more appropriate.

4. Excision biopsy with a wide margin is the procedure most often performed for cutaneous lesions such as malignant melanoma.

Although the use of standard histological stains such as haematoxylin and eosin frequently provides definitive diagnostic information, difficulties occasionally arise in distinguishing the organ of origin of certain malignancies, particularly when they are poorly differentiated. Here again the use of a panel of monoclonal antibodies may facilitate diagnosis. For example, positive staining with an antibody to the common leucocyte antigen permits a diagnosis of lymphoma to be made when standard histological preparations may be unable to distinguish the lesion from anaplastic carcinoma. Clearly such a distinction is important because of the relatively successful treatment which can be applied to lymphoma compared with that available for anaplastic carcinoma. Use of the S-100 antibody may also categorize an undifferentiated lesion as malignant melanoma rather than a carcinoma, again with therapeutic implications.

Errors in histological or cytological diagnosis usually relate to sampling errors rather than errors of interpretation. The endoscopic biopsy forceps may have failed to take a bite from the tumour tissue and this may mistakenly be categorized as normal. Aspirates are occasionally unsuitable for cytodiagnosis because of insufficient material. Errors of interpretation occasionally occur, particularly where severe dysplasia occurs in a tissue known to have malignant potential. For example, many pathologists will differ on the classification of severe dysplasia in gastric biopsies. The presence of severe dysplasia in biopsies of a large polyp of the colon or rectum should always arouse clinical suspicion that this is in fact a carcinoma.

## PRINCIPLES OF SURGICAL TREATMENT OF MALIGNANT DISEASE

Sight must not be lost of the fact that the treatment of malignant disease is nowadays often based on a multimodality approach. The surgeon may play a central role in initiating treatment but also must coordinate the close teamwork between a group of clinicians which often includes radiotherapists and medical oncologists.

### Curative surgery for primary malignant disease

The modes of extension of malignant disease exert a dominant influence on the design of curative surgical procedures for cancer. Lymph nodes and their vessels lie along the major arterial supply to an organ and surgical excision involves not only the vascular isolation of the organ in question for the purpose of safety of its excision but also the removal, as far as is feasible, of any tumour-containing lymphoid organs. In addition, it must not be forgotten that tumours also spread directly to invade contiguous structures as well as into laterally placed tissues and longitudinally

along tubular organs. Thus in squamous carcinoma of the oesophagus involvement of the trachea or bronchus renders the tumour inoperable but because of its propensity to spread submucosally it is considered that total oesophagectomy is the procedure of choice for curative surgery for this condition. Oro-intestinal continuity is restored by full gastric mobilization and transthoracic routing of the gastric tube to form a neo-oesophagus which is anastomosed to the residual cervical oesophagus in the neck.

Similarly, although it was previously considered that a longitudinal margin of clearance of 5 cm was essential for curative surgery for carcinoma of the rectum, it is now recognized that clear lateral margins are of equal if not greater importance in avoiding local recurrence of rectal carcinoma. The recognition of the surgical significance of the lymphatic vessels present in the pelvic mesorectum has also contributed to the reduction of the incidence of local recurrence of rectal carcinoma. The slightly diminished importance of wide longitudinal margins of clearance of rectal carcinoma from 5 cm to 3 cm may also have permitted the more frequent performance of restorative (low anterior resection) rather than ablative (abdominoperineal excision) rectal excision, these low anastomoses also being facilitated by the use of intestinal stapling devices.

A further important principle in performing curative surgery for malignant disease is the avoidance of transecting lymphatic vessels en route to the regional lymph nodes. Thus whenever axillary dissection is performed during segmentectomy or mastectomy for breast cancer then this should be performed 'en bloc' with the main operative specimen to avoid local spillage of any metastatic tumour cells which may be in transit to the regional nodes, the aim being to minimize the risk of this causing a local recurrence. A similar principle is applied during the conduct of an R3 gastrectomy in which the body and tail of the pancreas, spleen and retroperitoneal lymph nodes are excised 'en bloc' together with the stomach.

### Curative surgery for secondary malignant disease

The development of local or locoregional recurrence of malignant disease should not necessarily be an occasion for surgical despair. Regional lymph node metastases following earlier excision of a malignant melanoma from the limb or trunk should be treated initially by a block dissection of the regional lymph nodes, provided that distant metastases are excluded by CT scanning. The five-year survival rates following this procedure are, as described earlier, dependent on the characteristics of the primary lesion but overall figures of 20–25% may be expected. A policy of 'second-look' surgery is also appropriate for recurrent colorectal malignant disease, which should be detected through regular monitoring with plasma CEA levels and liver ultrasound. Local recurrence of colorectal cancer is rarely amenable to curative resectional surgery but useful palliation can sometimes be achieved by further resection. In contrast, the detection of liver metastases from colorectal surgery should always lead to consideration for liver resection. Approximately 10% of all such patients will ultimately prove to have disease which is suitable for resection and if there are fewer than four metastases confined to fewer than two anatomical segments of the liver, then a 35% five-year survival rate may be accomplished following liver resection. Of course the presence of extrahepatic disease should be excluded as far as is possible before this is undertaken.

## Reconstructive surgery for malignant disease

The ablative nature of radical surgery for malignant disease means that there is often a need for reconstructive or restorative surgery. The basis of reconstructive surgery is a sound knowledge of the vascular supply to the tissues to be used to reconstruct the defect which has been created. For example, the use of the stomach to restore intestinal continuity following total oesophagectomy is based on the fact that provided the left gastric artery is divided at its origin from the coeliac axis, the stomach can be supplied totally by the right gastric and gastro-epiploic arteries. By dividing the short gastric arteries and mobilizing the duodenum the gastric fundus can be made to reach almost to the base of the skull and can be used to replace the pharynx and oesoph-agus even following full pharyngolaryngo-oesophagectomy.

Similarly the use of the rectus abdominis flap to reconstitute the breast following mastectomy is based on the anastomosis between the superior and inferior epigastric arteries. Another major myocutaneous flap commonly used for breast reconstruction is the latissimus dorsi flap which is based on the thoracodorsal vessels for its integrity. A number of other myocutaneous flaps such as the pectoralis flap are available for head and neck reconstruction, but several technological advances have been introduced which have greatly facilitated superficial reconstructive surgery. These are the use of subcutaneous tissue expanders to increase the amount of skin available to replace a defect and the advent of microvascular surgery to enable the transposition of large islands of tissue as free grafts.

## Palliative surgery for malignant disease

It is self-evident that surgery for malignant disease cannot always be curative because either the primary or the secondary disease cannot be totally eradicated by surgical means. However, there are many circumstances under which surgical procedures may be employed to alleviate symptoms. These may be variously categorized as follows:

1. For the alleviation of obstructive symptoms. Obstruction by tumours of the oesophagus, stomach, periampullary region, small bowel and colon can all be alleviated by appropriate bypass surgery if resectional surgery (even if palliative) is not feasible. However, for certain conditions less invasive intervention enables obstructive symptoms to be overcome. The endoscopic insertion of an Atkinson tube through an inoperable carcinoma of the oesophagus has largely replaced the perioperative insertion of a Mousseau–Barbin tube. However, modern technology has now intervened to permit the endoscopic use of a laser beam to burn a lumen through the tumour. Although this is never curative it at least facilitates swallowing but carries the disadvantage of having to be repeated at intervals. Similarly the insertion of stents through unresectable malignant strictures of the periampullary region, common bile duct and common, right and left hepatic ducts can be

procured via ERCP or the transhepatic route or a combination of the two. Unfortunately even with sophisticated scanning modalities it is often difficult to be certain that a stricture within the biliary tree is inoperable, and one should not lose sight of the fact that even with pancreatic cancer the five-year survival rate after resection is 5%, and with carcinoma of the ampulla 35% of patients will survive five years after a pancreatico-duodenectomy. The subject of bypass surgery versus stenting for obstructive jaundice is currently the subject of considerable controversy, partly because of the difficulty in deciding which lesions are inoperable preoperatively and partly because of the frequency with which stents tend to block, compared with the relatively complication-free, though invasive, surgical bypass procedures.

2. For the diminution of transfusion requirements. Ulcerated lesions of the stomach or colon may not necessarily be curable by surgical resection but their existence may result in chronic anaemia as a consequence of chronic occult haemorrhage. Even in those deemed incurable at operation, resection may alleviate the symptoms of anaemia suffered by these unfortunate patients.

3. For the relief of pain. Pain, other than that of intestinal colic, is seldom relieved by surgical resection of a locally invasive tumour. Occasionally neurectomy may be of help but this may also cause a degree of motor loss. For the deep infiltrating pain of conditions such as unresectable pancreatic cancer a coeliac axis block may be preferable to systemic analgesia.

## OTHER MODALITIES OF CLINICAL ONCOTHERAPY

It is unfortunate that for many tumours in which the surgeon plays a central management role, alternative treatments are seldom successful in providing a cure once surgery is no longer an appropriate therapeutic option. There are three types of non-surgical treatment for malignant disease. These are readily categorized into radiotherapy, chemotherapy and biological response modification.

## Radiotherapy

A detailed description of the way in which radiotherapy works is beyond the scope of this chapter. The principles of radiation therapy are well established but it is important to appreciate that there is no consistent difference between the radiosensitivity of normal and tumour tissue within a particular organ. The unit of absorbed radiation dose is the gray, 1 Gy being equivalent to 1 J of energy per kilogram. Cells in mitosis are those which are most susceptible to the lethal effects of irradiation but cells in the late S-phase when the nuclear material has been duplicated are more resistant. Nonetheless, such is the level of expertise with fractionated radiotherapy that not only is this modality used as palliative therapy for certain unresectable or metastatic lesions, but it is now also employed as adjunctive to surgery, as for example, following wide local excision of T1–T2 breast carcinoma or following excision of a rectal carcinoma. Unfortunately, a disappointingly large number of tumours remain relatively radioresistant, as for example, those arising in the adult kidney, adenocarcinomas of the stomach and malignant melanoma.

Irradiation depopulates a tumour of its malignant cells mainly via direct effects during mitosis, and thus the efficacy of fractionated irradiation is determined by the number of clonogenic cells which the tumour contains, its intrinsic radiosensitivity, and the mitotic rate. Since irradiation damage becomes manifest during mitosis it follows that the normal tissues and tumour cells with a high cellular turnover such as the bone marrow and enterocytes will show evidence of damage within a few hours of irradiation. Conversely it may be many weeks or months before the maximum effect of radiotherapy is apparent in more slowly proliferating tumours such as basal cell carcinoma of the skin. A more detailed description of the scope and clinical application of radiotherapy is referenced at the end of this chapter.

## Chemotherapy

As with radiotherapy, more sophisticated application of chemotherapeutic regimens, coupled in many instances with reduced systemic toxicity, has led chemotherapy from a palliative role to that of a surgical adjunct and, occasionally, sole curative therapy for some tumours. It may be used as an adjunct prior to surgery (so-called neo-adjuvant therapy), as in the treatment of locally advanced breast or oesophageal cancer, or post-operatively as in premenopausal women. Thus the scope of chemotherapy has broadened enormously in recent years.

Cytotoxic drugs interfere with cell division irrespective of whether the cell is normal or malignant. This means that the success of chemotherapy is dependent on the intrinsic resistance of the tumour cell to the drug and the dose-limiting toxicity of the drug against the normal tissues. In general, four main groups of anticancer drugs are categorized. These are as follow:

1.    Alkylating agents such as the nitrosoureas and epoxide groups (cyclophosphamide, melphalan, chlorambucil, etc.). These compounds contain an alkyl group (e.g. $CH_3$) which combines with other intracellular molecules such as nucleic acids, proteins (especially enzymes) and cell membranes. Damage to the enzymes which link DNA strands thus impairs mitosis during the S-phase of the cell cycle.

2.  Antimetabolites have a similar chemical structure to the compounds required for the elaboration of nucleic acids. They therefore disrupt the sequence of DNA by being incorporated instead of the normal nucleotide or irreversibly bind to the constituting enzyme and render it ineffective. This class of drugs includes methotrexate, 5-fluorouracil, cytosine arabinoside and 6-mercaptopurine.

3.  The *Vinca* alkaloids bind to intracellular tubulin and inhibit microtubule formation which constitutes the spindle during mitosis. Thus mitosis is arrested at metaphase. The components of this group are vincristine, vinblastine and vindesine.

4.  Antimitotic antibiotics are a large group of agents which includes adriamycin, epirubicin, actinomycin D, mitomycin C and bleomycin. The first two drugs act in a variety of ways, including intercalation between opposing DNA strands leading to disturbed DNA function. Actinomycin D and mitomycin C impair DNA and RNA synthesis and generate harmful toxic free oxygen radicals.

There also exists a further miscellaneous group of agents whose mechanisms of action are varied or unknown. Cisplatin and its less toxic derivative carboplatin react with the guanine in DNA and form cross-linkages along the DNA chain as well as between DNA strands. Other agents such as etoposide are tubular poisons derived from podophyllotoxin.

Clinically many of these agents are used in varying combinations which have been developed to maximize therapeutic efficacy without excessively augmenting toxicity. However, their effects on normal proliferating cells cause them to be especially toxic to bone marrow and intestinal cells.

**Biological response modifiers**

These are a miscellaneous group of compounds, many of which have been developed by recombinant DNA technology. Some, such as the interferons and tumour necrosis factor (TNF), act directly on tumour cells to produce cytostasis or cell death through as yet obscure mechanisms. Other act directly by augmenting endogenous host responses to the tumour, as for example interleukin-2, which activates cytotoxic T-lymphocytes in patients with malignant melanoma. A further group of agents, the colony-stimulating factors, are finding an important role in preventing the bone marrow suppression and septicaemic episodes commonly associated with high-dose chemotherapy. Whether this results in higher clinical response rates as a consequence of higher and more protracted chemotherapeutic dosages remains to be seen.

It seems not unreasonable to include endocrine manipulation under the heading of biological response modifiers. The concept that the trophic or stimulatory effects of a hormone can be abrogated by agents which block the activity of a receptor for that hormone is an important one in the management of patients with breast cancer where tamoxifen is employed to block the binding of oestrogen to its receptor. The discovery of receptors for autocrine hormones on tumour cells as described at the beginning of this chapter will undoubtedly lead to the construction of synthetic analogues of these autocrine growth factors so that their administration can be used to block the receptor binding sites for therapeutic purposes in the future.

As with surgery, the cost : benefit ratio of these various treatments must be considered carefully before they are administered to a particular patient. It is quite unreasonable to impair the quality of life of a patient in the terminal stages of his or her disease by administering a toxic therapy or the physical assault of surgery unless this is going to prolong life considerably, or relieve symptoms. This is one of the most difficult judgements which the oncologist has to make and the trainee must learn how to enter into a careful, informed and sympathetic discussion with the patient in order to reach a joint conclusion as to the desirability or otherwise of a therapeutic course of action.

## ACKNOWLEDGEMENT

I am grateful to Miss V France for her expert typographical assistance in the preparation of this chapter.

## FURTHER READING

Duncan W 1988 Ionising radiation and radiotherapy. In: Cuschieri A, Giles G R, Moosa A R (eds) Essential surgical practice (2nd edn). Wright, London pp 190–202

Guillou P J 1990 Biological response modifiers in the treatment of cancer. Clinical Oncology 2: 347–353

McArdle C 1990 Surgical Oncology. Butterworth, Oxford

Priestman T J 1989 Cancer chemotherapy: an introduction (3rd edn). Springer-Verlag, Berlin

# 24. The principles of radiotherapy

*R. A. Huddart    J. R. Yarnold*

## SOURCES OF IONIZING RADIATION

Radiotherapy is the therapeutic use of ionizing radiation for the treatment of malignant disorders. Natural sources of radiation include radioactive isotopes which decay with the production of β-particles (electrons) and γ-rays (a form of electromagnetic radiation). Originally radium was used but over the last 20 years it has been replaced by safer artificial isotopes such as cobalt-60, caesium-137, and iridium-192, which are generated in nuclear reactors. Isotopes are used mainly as sources implanted directly into tissues (e.g. iridium needles in the treatment of carcinoma of the tongue) or inserted into a cavity (e.g. caesium sources inserted into the uterus and vagina for the treatment of carcinoma of the cervix). Radioactive isotopes may also be given systemically (e.g. iodine-131 in the treatment of thyroid cancer).

External beam radiotherapy was revolutionized in the 1950s by the advent of megavoltage treatment machines; initially cobalt machines and later linear accelerators. The linear accelerator generates a stream of electrons which are accelerated to a high speed by microwave energy before hitting a tungsten target. This interaction results in the emission of high-energy X-rays. The high-energy X-ray beam produced by a linear accelerator has several properties which make it well suited for present day radiotherapy:

1. The greater penetration of the γ-rays means that a high proportion of the dose applied to the body surface reaches the tumour.

2. All X-ray beams have a fuzzy edge (called penumbra) due to the reflection and scattering of the beam by tissues. High-energy X-rays suffer relatively little sideways scatter as they pass through tissues, and this helps to keep the edge of the beam sharp.

3. The forward scattering effect is also indirectly responsible for the point of maximum dose being 1–2 cm below the skin surface. The skin therefore receives a low dose and is spared from radiation reactions. It was the high skin doses associated with low-energy X-ray machines that caused the uncomfortable skin reactions and limited treatments of deep-seated tumours.

In addition, cyclotrons can be used to produce ionizing beams of heavier particles such as

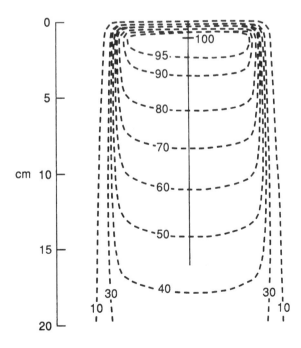

**Fig. 24.1** Dose distribution of a linear accelerator. Note the maximum dose is below the skin surface and 65% of the applied dose is present at 10 cm.

neutrons or protons. However, these machines are yet to find a place in routine clinical practice.

## ACTIONS OF IONIZING RADIATION

X-rays (from linear accelerators) and γ-rays (from isotopes) are both forms of electromagnetic radiation and are biologically indistinguishable. High-energy X-rays consist of packets of energy (photons) which interact with the molecules of body tissues to cause ionization and release electrons of high kinetic energy. These electrons cause secondary damage to adjacent molecules including DNA via an oxygen-dependent mechanism. The resultant DNA damage is mostly repaired by enzymes in a matter of hours but certain DNA lesions are irreparable. Non-repairable DNA damage causes a variety of chromosomal abnormalities which prevent normal mitosis from occurring. When the cell tries to divide it dies in the attempt. This DNA damage, however, does not stop most cells from performing their normal physiological functions effectively. Thus damage is expressed only if the cell attempts mitosis, and in fully differentiated cells incapable of further division (e.g. muscle cells) this damage may never be expressed. Hence:

1. Tissues may be severely damaged by irradiation but appear essentially normal. Damaged may be expressed only if they are stimulated to divide.

2. Response to radiotherapy by tumours may be delayed especially in tumours with slow rates of growth (e.g. pituitary tumours).

There are many data on the respective effects of radiotherapy on normal tissues and tumours. It appears that tumour cells are not intrinsically more sensitive than normal cells to single doses of radiotherapy though there may be differences in the ability of tumours and normal tissues to recover from the effects of cell damage. For example, normal tissues have a greater ability to respond to radiation-induced cell depletion by accelerated repopulation — an ability which seems to be less developed in tumours. To eradicate a tumour within the limits of tolerance of surrounding normal tissues, radiotherapy must exploit these and other subtle differences in DNA repair and regrowth of normal tissues.

In external beam treatments therapeutic advantage is generally achieved by dividing the total dose of radiotherapy into small parts over several weeks, a practice called *fractionation*. A full discussion of the effects of fractionation is not possible in this chapter but generally:

1. Reducing the dose per fraction allows certain critical normal tissues such as the nervous system, the lungs and other slowly proliferating tissues to repair damage more effectively than tumours.

2. Fractionation over a period of several days or weeks gives rapidly proliferating normal tissues such as skin and gut a chance to repopulate and hence recover from radiotherapy-induced damage faster than tumours.

3. Many tumours contain hypoxic areas. As radiotherapy's major effect is by an oxygen-dependent mechanism these areas are relatively resistant to radiotherapy. Each fraction of radiotherapy reduces the number of tumour cells and allows some hypoxic areas to become better oxygenated. Fractionation allows this process of reoxygenation which may take hours or days to occur and is thought to make tumours more radiocurable.

The above comments help to explain the empirical finding that radiotherapy is most effective when given daily over several weeks. A comparable effect to fractionation is seen with interstitial and intracavity treatments where a continuous low exposure over several days is biologically equivalent to multiple small fractions.

The ability to a cure a tumour probably depends on being able to eliminate every clonogenic tumour cell from the target volume. This is influenced by a variety of factors: size of tumour, radiosensitivity of tumour cells and tolerance of normal tissues.

### Size of tumour

In theory, successive doses of radiotherapy will eliminate equal fractions of the tumour cells. The larger the tumour the greater the number of cells present and hence a larger number of fractions will be necessary to have a high probability of eliminating the last clonogenic tumour cell. For example, the majority of 2 cm carcinomas can be controlled by 60 Gy whereas a 4 cm carcinoma needs 80 Gy for similar control rates. As discussed above, large tumours may also contain large hypoxic areas which are relatively radioresistant and reduce the chance of cure. Large tumours usually need a larger treatment volume than small tumours. This usually increases the volume of normal tissue irradiated; the greater the volume of normal tissue the higher the chance that a part of that tissue is damaged by the radiotherapy and hence the normal tissue complication rate rises. To reduce this complication rate a dose reduction is often necessary with a corresponding reduction in the chance of cure.

## Radiosensitivity of tumour cells

The commonest histological types of tumour have cells of similar radiosensitivities, e.g. squamous carcinoma cells, adenocarcinoma cells. Differences in tumour cure between these common histological types probably relate more to differences in tumour bulk, oxygenation and proliferation. There are exceptions, with the cells of some tumours being more radiosensitive, e.g. seminoma, lymphoma, and others being more radioresistant, e.g. melanoma, glioma, sarcomas. The reasons for these differences remains unclear, but there is evidence at least in vitro that a variety of mechanisms have a role, e.g. melanoma seems to be more resistant to radiotherapy due to an increased ability to repair DNA damage.

## Tolerance of normal tissues

The total dose which can be applied to a tumour is limited by the tolerance of the surrounding normal tissue. This varies greatly between tissues. If the tumour lies close to a sensitive organ, e.g. the spinal cord, then the total dose that can be safely delivered is much less than if the tumour lies within muscle or bone, for example. Hence the chance of cure may be reduced. The dose able to be applied will also depend on the volume needed to be irradiated. A good example of this is the lung. The tolerance dose for whole lung to be able to function after treatment is in the region of 20 Gy in ten fractions of 2 Gy. Therefore if the whole lung or large sections need to be treated (e.g. selected cases of Hodgkin's disease) this is the maximal fractionated tolerated dose. However, doses as high as 60 Gy can be given to portions of a lung such as lobe because small areas of permanent damage are acceptable and have little overall effect on lung function.

## RADIOTHERAPY PLANNING

The major principle of radiotherapy is to give the maximum possible dose to the smallest volume which will encompass all of the tumour. This volume, termed the *target volume*, consists of:

1. The macroscopic tumour volume determined from clinical findings, imaging (X-rays, computed tomography (CT) scans, radioisotope scans, etc.) and operative findings.
2. A biological margin (often 0.5–1 cm) which allows for microscopic tumour spread beyond the visible tumour. It may also include allowance for nodal spread.
3. A technical margin, usually 0.5 cm to allow for errors and variability in daily set-up (e.g. due to respiratory movements of the patient). Minimizing these errors and improving quality assurance is an area of active research. Techniques such as megavoltage imaging (in which an X-ray image of the patient is produced as the treatment beam passes through the tumour showing how well the area actually treated corresponds to the treatment plan) may enter clinical practice in the future.

Localizing the tumour in the patient accurately is essential to the success of radiotherapy. In most cases the tumour cannot be visualized directly and localization depends on physical examination, imaging and operative motes. The importance of accurate and detailed operative records cannot be over-emphasized. An operation is a unique opportunity to visualize the tumour directly and full advantage of this opportunity must be taken to describe the extent of disease and acquire as much additional information as possible about local pathology. Limited information invariably leads to larger target volumes, increased radiotherapy morbidity and reduced cure rates.

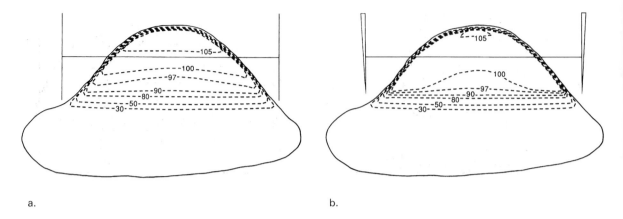

a.

b.

**Fig. 24.2**   Comparison of the dose distribution of different field arrangements. The parallel opposed field arrangement (**a**) adequately treats the target volume (the bladder) but gives a high rectal dose. A three-field arrangement (**b**) covers the target volume with a much reduced rectal dose and is therefore preferable.

Once the radiotherapist has determined the exact size, shape and location of the target volume the aim is to encompass the target volume with a radiation dose distributed as homogeneously as possible. A variation of under 10% is aimed for and achieved. Single fields are usually inadequate in this respect except for superficial tumours. Opposing two fields at 180° to each other treats intervening tissue homogeneously. This arrangement is very simple to plan and is suitable for  most low-dose palliative and a few radical treatments. Two opposed fields usually include more normal tissue in the high-dose volume than strictly necessary (Fig. 24.2). Therefore more complex multi-field arrangements are normal for curative treatments to confine the high dose volume to the target volume more closely. These are planned either by drawing the target volume on orthogonal anteroposterior and lateral X-ray films of the patient or more usually taking the cross-sectional target volume directly from CT scans of the patient in the treatment position.

Directing several beams of radiation accurately to intersect across the target volume does not necessarily guarantee an even dose distribution because the X-rays have to pass through different amounts of tissue on the way from the entry point on the skin to the target volume. In addition lung absorbs less energy than other tissues because of the air it contains. These potential sources of dose inhomogeneity throughout the target volume must be calculated and compensated for using a number of measures which alters beam shape and profile (such as different weighting on each X-ray beam and the introduction of wedge-shaped filters which absorb different amounts of energy across the beam) (Fig. 24.3). Production of homogeneous dose distributions has been greatly facilitated by the introduction of planning computers and CT planning which can visualize and allow for tissue inhomogeneities directly. This area continues to develop rapidly and in the future more sophisticated means of compensating for potential sources of uneven dose distribution will come into routine practice as well as more advanced beam-defining devices.

Once satisfactory dose distributions and treatment plans are produced and checked, treatment of the patient can begin. It is important that treatment is applied in a reproducible fashion. The patient must be positioned, lying in a recorded position, with appropriate supports to maintain stability. Lasers are frequently used now to help establish and monitor patient alignment. If extra accuracy is desirable (especially in the head and neck region) a light plastic shell may be used to immobilize the patient. The machine is then positioned according to skin markings and recorded settings, determined during planning, and treatment is commenced.

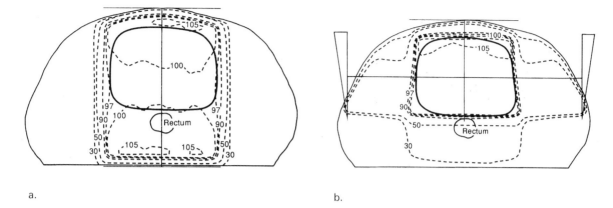

a.

b.

**Fig. 24.3** Treating the breast without compensation for breast curvature produces an inhomogeneous dose distribution (**a**). When this is compensated for by a wedge filter (**b**) the dose distribution is improved.

## RADIOTHERAPY : THE FUTURE

In recent years several new techniques have improved the therapeutic ratio in selected circumstances.

### Accelerated radiotherapy

This involves giving multiple daily treatments of the same size as used in conventional fractionation but given to shorten the overall treatment time from six weeks to less than three weeks. Recent research suggest that clonogenic tumour cells can proliferate significantly during a treatment course of six weeks and this could theoretically reduce the chance of tumour control. Reducing the overall treatment time could make an important difference, allowing less time for proliferation and leaving fewer tumour cells to kill. However, reducing treatment time also gives normal tissues less time to recover. Enhanced early skin and mucosal reactions may limit this approach.

### Hyperfractionation

This delivers two to three smaller fractions a day over the conventional treatment period (i.e. the number of treatment days remains the same but the number of fractions is increased). Reducing fraction size reduces late tissue damage with relatively less effect on tumour control. Theoretically,

this allows dose escalation to occur with an increased chance of cure.

### Chart

This stands for continuous hyperfractionated accelerated radiotherapy. This new regime aims to combine the advantages of accelerated and hyperfractionated radiotherapy by giving three treatments a day over a 12-day period with no gaps (including no breaks for weekends and bank holidays). Treatment can be completed before any acute reactions occur. Initial results are promising and are the subject of an ongoing multicentre trial in head and neck cancer.

### Neutrons and heavy ion therapy

Heavy ions, including neutrons, can be produced by cyclotrons which can now be used in the therapeutic situation. They damage DNA by a non-oxygen-dependent mechanism. Therefore hypoxic areas in tumours are not protected from the lethal effects of this form of ionizing radiation. Recent work, however, suggests that hypoxic areas are not as important as previously thought and it is also now recognized that neutron-induced damage is less well repaired by normal tissues. This means that the potential increase in local control achieved by more effective eradication of hypoxic cells is outweighed by a marked increase in late morbidity. At present neutrons have no role in common tumours though their role in selected tumours continues to be evaluated.

## Conformal therapy

Conventional therapy uses rectangular fields to encompass the target volume. As tumours are not cubes an unnecessary amount of normal tissue is included in the treated volume. This causes increased morbidity and limits the doses that can be given (e.g. for pelvic tumours the dose given is limited by the amount of small bowel included in the target volume). Conformal therapy uses new engineering and computer technology to generate irregularly shaped fields so that tumours can be encompassed by high dose volumes which correspond more precisely to the tumour's shape. The hope is that the same cure rate can be achieved with reduced morbidity, or that dose escalation can occur with increased cure rates for the same morbidity.

## ROLE OF RADIOTHERAPY

Radiotherapy may be used in the management of malignant disorders in the following ways:

1. as primary treatment
2. as adjuvant treatment prior to or following primary surgery (or chemotherapy)
3. for palliation of symptoms
4. as a systemic treatment, either in the form of external beam total body irradiation or systemic administration of a radioactive isotope.

## Radiotherapy as primary treatment

When radiotherapy is used as the primary treatment the aim is to effect cure with the minimum of side-effects. It is an alternative modality of local control to surgery. Radiotherapy, like surgery, is most effective at controlling small, well-localized and defined tumors but has the advantage of preserving normal function. For many cancers surgery and radiotherapy are equally effective modes of treatments and close liaison between surgeons and radiotherapists is essential if the appropriate modality of treatment is to be chosen for any given patient. This choice may vary between patients and depends on a variety of tumour (including site, stage and histology) and patient factors (including age and performance status). Choice of modality of treatment is not restricted just to either surgery alone or radiotherapy alone; a policy of initial radiotherapy followed by planned salvage surgery if this fails (as in many head and neck tumours) or initial combination therapy may best serve the patient.

Radiotherapy may be indicated as initial treatment by a variety of circumstances including:

1. Sites where surgery and radiotherapy are equally effective but radiotherapy gives better functional or cosmetic results (e.g. in bladder cancer where radical radiotherapy gives good results and avoids the necessity of cystectomy and ileal conduit, or laryngeal cancer where radiotherapy gives equal results to surgery but allows preservation of the voice).

2. Very radiosensitive tumours such as lymph node metastases from testicular cancers or early Hodgkin's disease.

3. Inoperable tumours. Occasionally radiotherapy can be used for attempted cure, e.g. brain stem gliomas or pelvic sarcomas.

4. At sites where operations carry a high morbidity/mortality and equivalent results are gained by radiotherapy (e.g. carcinoma of upper or mid-oesophagus).

5. In patients unfit for radical surgery when surgery is otherwise the treatment of choice (e.g. patients with bronchial cancer and chronic airways disease).

All cases, however, need to be carefully assessed to decide the appropriate treatment option. In some cases where radiotherapy would normally be indicated other factors may make surgery preferable in that patient. For instance, it may not be possible to apply a radical dose because of an adjacent sensitive structure (e.g. if small bowel is adherent to the bladder, giving a full radical dose may be impossible without a risk of severe morbidity. Cystectomy may therefore be indicated). Alternatively, bone or cartilage involvement by tumour may have occurred (especially in head and neck cancer). In such cases the risk of osteo-radionecrosis following radical radiotherapy is

**Table 24.1** Results of curative radiotherapy

| Site | Stage | Survival (5–year) | Comment |
|---|---|---|---|
| Skin | All | 90–95% | Equivalent to surgery. Choice depends on site |
| Head and neck | | | |
|   Tongue | TI | 91% | 50–60% for all stages |
|   Glottis | TI | 90% | |
|   Other sites | All | 30–80% | Local control rates with salvage surgery used for local relapse |
| Gastrointestinal tract | | | |
|   Oesophagus | All | 9% | Equivalent to surgery |
|   Anal canal | All | 66% | Better results than ano-perineal resection |
| Urology | | | |
|   Bladder | T2/3 | 34% | Salvage cystectomy for local relapse. Surgery only 28% 5–year Survival |
|   Prostate | T1/2 | 80% | Equivalent to surgery |
| | T3 | 60% | |
|   Penile | All | 75% | Over 90% cure for stage 1 tumours |
| Gynaecology | | | |
|   Cervix | 1B | 85–90% | Equivalent to surgery in randomized studies |
| | 2A/B | 61–85% | |
|   Endometrium | All | 60–65% | For patients unfit for surgery only |
|   Vagina | Stage 1 | 75% | |

**Table 24.2** Role of adjuvant radiotherapy

| Site | Stage | Criteria | No RT | RT | Comment |
|---|---|---|---|---|---|
| Breast | T1/2  N0 | LC | 63% | 88% | NSABP randomized trial of conservative |
| | T1/2  N+ | LC | 57% | 94% | surgery/radiotherapy |
| Central nervous system | | | | | |
|   Astrocytomas | Gd1 | S | 25% | 58% | |
|   Oligodendrogliomas | All | 10 yr S | 27% | 50% | |
|   Pituitary | All | 10 yr LC | 10% | 90% | RMH data |
|   Craniopharyngioma | Incomplete excision | S | 35% | 90% | 70% Survival for complete excision |
| Gastrointestinal tract | | | | | |
|   Pancreas | Operable tumour | 2 year S surv. | 15% | 42% | GITSG trial NO RT V RT with 5-FU |
|   Rectum | Dukes'C | LC | 65% | 90% | MRC 3rd trial survival advantage in some series |
|   Cholangiocarcinoma | Operable tumor | Median surv | 5mo. | 11mo. | Non-randomized data |
| Gynaecology | | | | | |
|   *Endometrium* | Stage 1 | LC | 88% | 99% | |
| | Stage 1 | S | 64% | 81% | |
| | Stage 2 | S | 20% | 56% | |
| *Parotid* | | | | | |
| Carcinomas | All | LC | 62% | 87% | |
| Pleomorphic adenomas | Incomplete excision | LC | 76% | 98% | |
| Bladder | T2/T3B | S | 28% | 45% | Non-randomized data |

LC, 5-year local control rate.
S, 5-year survival.

greatly increased, making surgery a preferred option.

## Adjuvant radiotherapy

For some tumours preoperative or postoperative radiotherapy may improve local control. Adjuvant radiotherapy achieves this by controlling microscopic spread beyond resection margins, tumour spilled at operation or lymph node metastases. The low tumour burden means that lower doses than normally used in radical treatments can be employed with a resultant reduced morbidity while obtaining a high rate of local control. If local control is an important determinant of survival then this may equate with an improvement in overall survival. Even if metastases limit survival, adjuvant radiotherapy often has a valuable role in improving locoregional control and quality of life. This may be especially important if symptoms of relapse cannot be easily controlled, e.g. rectal cancer.

Adjuvant treatment may be given to (a) the site of primary disease to reduce local recurrence or (b) sites of potential metastatic spread.

Postoperative radiotherapy has the advantages of the radiotherapist having details of surgical and pathological findings available in addition to clinical and radiological assessment. This allows for accurate staging and selection of those cases which would most benefit from radiotherapy.

However, the planning of postoperative radiotherapy can be more difficult as the radiotherapist can no longer directly image the tumour. Accurate operation notes greatly aid localization of treatment, as does marking the tumour bed with clips. If the need for postoperative radiotherapy is anticipated prior to operation it is often helpful for the radiotherapist to see the patient preoperatively (e.g. prior to wide local excision of a small breast cancer). Postoperative radiotherapy is of proven value in reducing local recurrence at many sites, some of which are listed below. At most sites postoperatively radiotherapy is of no proven benefit in prolonging survival after complete resection of the primary tumour.

In selected circumstances preoperative radiotherapy may be of value. Preoperative radiotherapy has the potential advantage of a downstaging effect which may allow an easier or less extensive operation to be performed (e.g. in rectal cancer or limb sarcomas). It may also reduce the risk of seeding at the time of operation and control microscopic disease at the edges of the tumour. Certain problems have limited the usefulness of this approach; foremost is the fear that radiotherapy increases the surgical morbidity. However, it is now thought that as long as the operation is performed within four weeks of radiotherapy this increase is minimal with doses of radiotherapy up to 40 Gy. A further problem is that the downstaging effect of the radiotherapy makes interpretation of the subsequent surgical specimen and pathological staging difficult. This also causes difficulties in comparing different series of patients, assessing prognosis and giving advice on further treatment . It is therefore a less established form of treatment but is used particularly in bladder cancer and sarcomas and, less often, in the treatment of rectal, oesophageal and endometrial cancers.

Radiotherapy to sites of lymph node spread has been used in the treatment of many cancers, especially when it was thought that blood-borne spread followed lymph node invasion. Increasingly studies suggest that lymph node metastasis may be a marker of synchronous blood-borne metastasis and at several sites prophylactic lymph node irradiation has been shown to be of little value in survival terms (e.g. bladder and prostatic cancer). Despite this, in a variety of cancers, lymph node irradiation is of value when initial spread is to lymph nodes and is an important determinant of survival, e.g. head and neck cancers, or relapse-free survival, as in seminoma.

Prophylactic lymph node irradiation is also justified in reducing the risk of macroscopic nodal disease when symptomatic relapse is difficult to salvage. An example of this is supraclavicular fossa irradiation in axillary lymph node-positive breast cancer. Node relapse at this site is difficult to salvage and has a high morbidity in terms of lymphoedema and brachial plexus neuropathy. The risk of such relapse is markedly reduced by applying adjuvant radiotherapy.

In a similar fashion, craniospinal irradiation improves prognosis when central nervous system (CNS) spread is common, e.g. medulloblastoma and ependymomas. Chemotherapy only poorly penetrates the CNS and for some otherwise chemosensitive tumours the CNS may act as a sanctuary site, e.g. acute lymphoblastic leukaemia (ALL), small cell lung cancer. If cerebrospinal fluid (CSF) metastases are common, cranial or craniospinal irradiation is a highly successful form of prophylaxis. For example, the incidence of CNS relapse was reduced from 67% to 4% in patients with ALL following the introduction of irradiation.

## Palliation

Of all modalities used to treat advanced cancer, radiotherapy is the most useful for the palliation of symptoms either from advanced primary or metastatic disease.

The criteria of success must be in terms of quality of life rather than survival. The aim is therefore to give sufficient treatment to relieve symptoms without short-term side-effects for as long as the patient is expected to survive. High-dose prolonged palliative courses are necessary in certain circumstances, especially if prognosis is relatively good and substantial growth delay is necessary, e.g. recurrent chest wall breast cancer or pelvic recurrences of rectal cancers. Nevertheless, the trend is towards short courses delivering a few large fractions of radiotherapy, thereby achieving maximum symptom relief with minimal interference in the patient's life. Frequently, a single large fraction of radiotherapy is all that is necessary to palliate symptoms.

Palliative radiotherapy may be used, justly, for symptomatic incurable primary cancer or locally recurrent disease. For example, most patients with lung cancer present with disease too advanced for any radical treatment. Such patients are frequently symptomatic with, for example, haemoptysis, dyspnoea, pain or cough. They are usually well controlled with one or two fractions of radiotherapy. At other sites, particularly in pelvic tumours, longer fractionated courses to higher doses are necessary to offer a good chance of sustained symptom relief. Secondly, palliative radiotherapy many be used for relief of symptoms due to metastases. The treatments of different types of metastasis are considered below.

### Bone metastasis

Symptomatic bone metastases affect approximately 20% of patients at some stage during their illness. Radiotherapy is a highly effective means of controlling local pain due to such bone involvement. Recent work has shown that a single 8 Gy fraction of radiotherapy will relieve pain partially or completely in 80% of patients four weeks after treatment. Lesions with substantial cortical bone erosion should, however, be considered for orthopaedic fixation followed by radiotherapy to prevent fracture. Patients with extensive bone metastases (as frequently seen in prostate cancer) obtain good palliation from wide-field hemibody irradiation given as a single treatment. The other half-body can be treated four to six weeks later and 67% of patients obtain good pain relief. An alternative approach is to use a radioactive isotope (strontium-89) which is taken up by bone metastases. It is given as a simple intravenous injection and may be repeated. Comparison with hemibody irradiation is awaited.

### Spinal cord compression

This is an emergency which can cause devastating motor, sensory and sphincter disturbances. Metastatic disease can cause cord compression by direct extension from vertebral disease, epidural deposits or rarely intramedullary disease. There has been no trial of radiotherapy versus surgery in the treatment of this disorder but it is generally considered that neurosurgical decompression gives the most rapid relief and should be considered for fit patients with short, single blocks. This should be followed by postoperative radiotherapy. Patients not fit for surgery (including patients with multiple levels of compression, anterior tumours and poor performance status) should receive urgent radiotherapy. Seventy per cent of patients will achieve good pain relief and 50% a useful response if treated before a major neurological deficit develops. Some patients will regain the ability to walk but only 10% of total paraplegics regain useful function.

### Brain metastases

This is a frequent complication of advanced cancer and is associated with a high morbidity. They are especially common in lung cancer, breast cancer (10% of all patients at some stage), melanoma, kidney and colon carcinomas. They are usually multiple and the prognosis is poor, with the median survival untreated being six weeks. A 50% symptomatic response rate to radiotherapy and dexamethasone is expected, the radiosensitive tumours such as small cell lung, breast and colon cancers responding better than average. A good response to dexamethasone and good performance status also predict for good outcome. Frail patients with poor performance status tend to gain little and treatment may not be indicated in such patients. Short courses of treatment seem to be as effective as longer courses and a current study organized by the Royal College of Radiologists is comparing 12 Gy in two fractions with a conventional course of 30 Gy in ten fractions.

Patients with a single metastasis have a better outlook, with a median survival of four to six months, and 30% of patients with breast cancer survive over one year. There is some evidence that surgical resection followed by whole brain irradiation is better than whole brain irradiation only (in selected patients fit for surgery). It is unclear whether whole brain irradiation with a local boost to the tumour would do equally well.

### Superior venal caval obstruction (SVCO)

SVCO is caused by enlarged right-sided mediastinal lymph nodes or tumours (especially lung cancers). It causes engorgement of veins to the neck, cyanosis, facial oedema and dyspnea. Seventy per cent of patients gain relief within 14 days following mediastinal radiotherapy.

Some other indications for palliative radiotherapy are retinal metastases, skin metastases and lymph node metastases.

### Radiotherapy for the treatment of systemic disease

Radiotherapy is generally used to treat local disease. There are, however, two areas where radiotherapy is used to treat systemic disease: total body irradiation and radioactive isotopes.

### Total body irradiation

A total body dose of >4 Gy will result in bone marrow failure. This has limited its usefulness for the treatment of malignant disease until the onset of bone marrow transplantation. Total body irradiation using a dose of 8–10 Gy as a single dose or a higher fractionated dose is a highly effective conditioning regimen for the treatment of leukaemias. It is also being examined in trials in the treatment of other radiosensitive tumours such as lymphomas.

### Radioactive isotopes

This technique uses radioactive isotopes which emit short-range $\beta$-particles and/or $\gamma$- rays. If the tumour concentrates the isotope compared to the surrounding tissues it will be preferentially irradiated. The best example is the use of iodine-131 in the treatment of follicular and papillary thyroid cancer. The malignant tissue takes up and concentrates iodine and hence residual tumour is irradiated to a high dose. Using this technique, lung and sometimes bone metatases can be eliminated. Other examples are the use of phosphorus-32 in polycythaemia rubra vera, strontium-89 in metastatic prostate cancer (see above) and meta-iodobenzylguanidine (MIBG) in neuroblastoma.

## COMPLICATIONS

Normal tissue side-effects are due to cellular damage inflicted at the time of irradiation. This damage is largely expressed at the time of mitosis, so the sensitivity to and the expression of this damage depends on the differing proliferative characteristics of each tissue.

In some tissues, such as the epidermal layers of the skin, the small intestine and bone marrow stem cells, turnover is rapid and damage is expressed early. Skin is the classical example of such a tissue. Stem cells in the basal layer of the skin divide; the daughter cells differentiate and move to the surface over a two-week period to replace shed cells. After irradiation, production of replacement cells is reduced or halted. The epidermis gradually thins and if sufficient damage is produced epidermal integrity is lost and desquamation occurs. Recovery will occur over a period of days or weeks after the end of treatment by surviving stem cells producing enough daughter cells to cover the deficient area.

It can be seen that:

1. The time to onset of side-effects is determined by the skin turnover time, i.e. two weeks for skin but five days for small intestine.

2. The severity and length of time to recovery depends on the amount of damage to the stem cells and hence radiation dose.

3. Provided there is a certain number of clonogenic cells surviving recovery is likely to be complete.

Although this mechanism is responsible for most acute reactions the clinical effect will vary from site to site. For example, in the upper gastrointestinal tract acute reactions cause inflammation and discomfort (mucositis and oesophagitis), while small or large bowel damage by similar mechanisms causes vomiting, diarrhoea or more rarely ulceration and bleeding.

Other acute reactions, however, may operate by different mechanisms and are less well understood, e.g. somnolence after cranial irradiation.

Stem cell damage as described above usually recovers completely but, if severe, long-lasting effects can occur. The most important example of this is gonadal damage. Oocytes are particularly radiosensitive and even moderate doses of a few grays of radiation precipitate premature menopause. Spermatogenesis is also sensitive to radiotherapy. Doses in the region of 3 Gy cause oligospermia or azoospermia which may last six months to a year, but higher doses (>6 Gy) cause permanent sterility.

In many tissues the parenchymal cells turn over very slowly (e.g. hepatocytes). As radiation damage is expressed at mitosis, lethal damage will not be expressed until cells divide weeks, months or even years later. In such tissues damage can be due to depletion of parenchymal or connective tissues, or to vascular damage.

## Depletion of parenchymal or connective tissues

Irradiation of the thyroid gland, for example, leads to gradual depletion of thyroid follicular cells and can cause hypothyroidism over a period of many years. Likewise, renal irradiation causes depletion of renal tubular cells and renal impairment over a period of years.

## Vascular damage

Damage to the vasculature is a common mechanism of damage, especially in tissues which never replicate, e.g. neurones or cardiac muscle, or which replicate only very slowly, e.g. fibroblasts. Radiation has a wide range of pathological effects on the vasculature due to damage to both endothelial cells and to connective tissue. This leads to impairment of the fine vasculature, often in a patchy fashion. The damage can result in poor wound healing, tissue atrophy, ulceration, strictures and formation of telangectasia.

The precise clinical effect depends on the organ involved. For example, in the bladder the telengectasia can cause haematuria, while fibrosis, ulceration and tissue atrophy can cause a constricted fibrotic bladder which causes frequency and nocturia. Similar changes in the gastrointestinal tract may cause bowel obstruction by stricturing of the viscus or by peritoneal adhesions.

At other sites vascular damage is manifest differently. In the CNS glial tissues are depleted as a direct effect of radiation and via vascular effects, causing secondary demyelination and neuronal loss. Damage to the cardiac vasculature may result in early ischaemic heart disease if the dose is high enough, with myocardial infarction being an increasingly recognized cause of late morbidity and mortality in a minority of patients 15 years after internal mammary irradiation for breast cancer.

High-dose radiotherapy can also damage lymphatic vessels, leading to reduced drainage and limb lymphoedema. The risk is increased if there has been previous or successive surgery. For example, radiotherapy to the axilla after complete axillary dissection for early-stage breast cancer carries a much higher risk of arm lymphoedema than either modality alone.

The incidence and severity of late damage tend to increase with time, but provided the treatment schedule has been carefully selected, planned and delivered, organs function normally for the remainder of the patient's life. Increasing the dose increases the risk of damage and this damage becomes clinically relevant at an earlier stage.

Late effects are usually irrecoverable and show a dose response. Low doses are less likely to cause damage, while progressively higher doses have a greater chance of causing complications. The radiation dose therefore has to be chosen carefully, taking into account normal tissue tolerance as well as predicted tumour cure dose. The actual dose chosen depends on a variety of factors. For each site an acceptable level of damage must first be decided and balanced against the chance of tumour control (see Fig. 24.4). Damage to the spinal cord has such disastrous consequences that no morbidity can be accepted. A lower dose than that used at many other sites has to be accepted, even at the expense of tumour cure probability. Damage to other soft tissues, e.g. muscle and fat, is undesirable but of lesser importance and a higher dose and higher risk are accepted. As mentioned previously, the volume treated is important; the larger the

volume the greater the risk of damage and the lower the tolerable dose (e.g. for the spinal cord a short length of cord can be treated to 50 Gy but long segments, i.e. over 10 cm will not tolerate over 40 Gy). Other factors affecting tolerance include age (children and the elderly being less tolerant), pre-existing vascular disease and previous surgery.

In addition to specific organ complications the problem of secondary malignancies is being increasingly recognized. This has been best studied in Hodgkins disease, where an increased incidence of acute leukaemias are seen three to ten years post irradiation, with a smaller increased risk of solid tumours following. The precise risk is difficult to quantify but data give an overall risk of leukaemia of approximately 1–2% at 15 years. The risk is greatest if radiotherapy is given in conjunction with or is followed by chemotherapy (especially chemotherapy with alkylating agents, e.g. cyclophosphamide, mustine) being 0.2% if no chemotherapy is used and 8.1% if the patient receives multiple courses. Similar increased incidence of leukaemia has been seen in other cohorts of patients, including those with ankylosing spondylitis who received spinal irradiation. The risk of solid malignancy is being increasingly recognized, estimates rising to 10% of patients surviving Hodgkin's disease 15–20 years following radiotherapy, though a disease-related phenomenon could also be responsible. The overall risk of secondary malignancy is, however, more than outweighed by the risks of dying from the primary disease in most cancer sufferers.

In conclusion, radiotherapy is set to remain the chief curative modality in patients with non-surgical cancer. As screening and other early detection methods diagnose an increasing percentage of individuals with truly localized disease its importance is likely to increase. This continued role in the curative treatment of cancer patients continues to stimulate research into the technical and biological bases of radiotherapy. In future years, further improvements in the efficacy and safety of radiotherapy should be expected to result from this research.

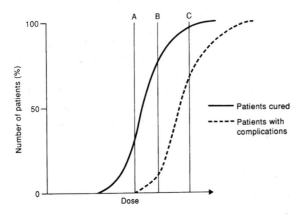

**Fig. 24.4** The relationship between cure and complications. A dose may be chosen with a very low risk of observable side-effects, but this may mean a very low chance of tumour cure as well (**A**). On the other hand, a high tumour cure rate may be associated with an unacceptable rate of complications (**C**)—forcing an intermediate dose to be chosen as optimal under a particular set of clinical circumstances (**B**).

# 25. Chemotherapy — principles, practice, complications and value

*C. A. E. Coulter*

Malignant tumours consist of cells that are able to invade throughout surrounding tissues and establish metastases. Localized tumours may be treated successfully by surgery or radiotherapy but metastases can only be cured by systemic treatment, which will normally be chemotherapy. The combination of chemotherapy with surgery and/or radiotherapy may also increase local tumour control. Chemotherapy given early when micrometastases are expected to be present is called adjuvant chemotherapy.

The word chemotherapy was first used by Paul Ehrlich. He used rodent models to develop antibiotics and this led George Clowes in the early 1900s to work on rodents which could carry transplanted tumours. The first modern chemotherapeutic agents were alkylating agents and their use followed the observation that seamen who were exposed to mustard gas had marrow and lymphoid hypoplasia. This led in the 1940s to the use of nitrogen mustard in humans with Hodgkin's disease and other lymphomas. The demonstration of successful regression of advanced cancer with these chemicals caused much excitement. Subsequent to this work at Yale, Sidney Farber's observations on the treatment of children with leukaemia and the successful treatment of children with Wilm's tumour led to a rapid increase in the number of cytotoxic drugs available and a rapid increase in the number of tumours in which they were used.

## BASIC PRINCIPLES

The aim of chemotherapy is to selectively destroy tumour cells while sparing normal tissues. Certain growth characteristics of tumour cells

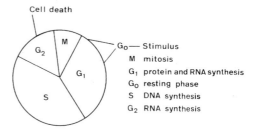

**Fig. 25.1** Growth characteristics of tumour cells.

allow relative selective tumour cell destruction and relative sparing of normal cells.

## KINETIC CLASSIFICATION OF ANTICANCER DRUGS

Non-phase-dependent drugs kill cells exponentially with increasing dose and are equally toxic for cells in cycle and in $G_0$.

Phase-dependent drugs kill cells at lower doses but reach a plateau kill if given at higher doses because they can only kill cells in a specific part of the cell cycle.

*Predominantly phase dependent*

- Etoposide
- Methotrexate
- Procarbazine
- Vinca alkaloids.

*Non-phase dependent*

- Alkylating agents
- Actinomycin D
- 5-fluorouracil
- Anthracyclines.

## GROWTH CHARACTERISTICS OF TUMOURS

The rate of proliferation during the lifetime of a tumour is not constant. In the early stages of tumour growth the growth fraction is high, but as the tumour enlarges the growth fraction is lower. The growth fraction peaks when the tumour is about 37% of its maximum size.

As the tumour enlarges the growth fraction falls and the growth rate slows. Chemotherapy will be less effective in larger tumours because the growth fraction is smaller and the number of cells killed by a therapeutic dose of chemotherapy will be smaller.

Skipper et al in 1964 formulated principles of tumour cell kill by drugs by using the Ll210 leukaemia in mice. He showed that the survival of the animal is inversely related to the tumour burden and that for most drugs there was a clear relationship between the dose of drug and the eradication of tumour cells. A given dose of drugs kills a constant fraction of cells, not a constant number. This means that cell destruction by drugs follows first-order kinetics and a treatment reducing a population from one million to ten cells should reduce a population of one hundred thousand to one cell. The implication of the fractional cell killing is that to eradicate a tumour population effectively it is necessary either to increase the dose of the drug or drugs within limits tolerated by the host, or to start treatment when the number of cells is small enough to allow tumour destruction at reasonably tolerated doses. The implication is not, as has sometimes been stated, that eradication of the last neoplastic cell is not possible with chemotherapy, but that the toxic effects on normal cells may be the limiting factor.

## DEVELOPMENT OF NEW CYTOTOXIC DRUGS

### Phase I

- Maximum tolerated dose
- Toxic effects
- Pharmacology.

### Phase II

- Evaluation of anticancer action.

If the drug has an objective response rate in a specific tumour type of 25% or more it may then proceed to phase III testing.

### Phase III

- Controlled clinical trials.

## PHARMACOLOGY OF CYTOTOXIC DRUGS

### Alkylating agents

These compounds probably produce their effects by linking an alkyl group (R-CH-) covalently to chemical moieties in protein and nucleic acids.

### Antimetabolites

Antimetabolites are agents that by virtue of their structural similarity with physiological intermediates are accepted as substrates for vital biochemical reactions and thus interfere with the required cell process.

### Antitumour antibiotics

These drugs produce their effect by binding to DNA and intercalating between the base pairs.

### The Vinca alkaloids and podophyllotoxins

These are mitotic spindle poisons that bind to tubulin, which is a protein of the cellular microtubules.

### Miscellaneous agent

Procarbazine: this drug is a weak monoamine oxidase inhibitor.

## USE OF DRUGS

### Alkylating agents

*Cyclophosphamide.* Breast cancer, small cell lung cancer, non-Hodgkin's lymphoma, leukaemia and sarcomas.

*Chlorambucil.* Low-grade non-Hodgkin's lymphoma, ovarian and breast cancer.

**Table 25.1**  Major cytotoxic agents

| Class | Route | Dose (guidelines only) | Acute toxicity Plasma WBC | Platelets | Nausea/vomiting | Other toxicity |
|---|---|---|---|---|---|---|
| *Alkylating agents* | | | | | | |
| Cyclophosphamide | i.v./p.o | 50 mg to 1.5 g | Marked | Mild | Moderate | Cystitis/alopecia |
| Chlorambucil | p.o. | 10 mg | Moderate | Moderate | Mild | Leukaemia |
| Melphalan | p.o. | 10 mg | Moderate | Moderate | Mild | Leukaemia |
| DTIC | i.v. | 500 mg | Mild | Mild | Marked | Flu-like syndrome, painful arm |
| Cisplatinum | i.v. | 150 mg | Moderate | Moderate | Severe | Neuropathy, ototoxicity Nephropathy |
| *Antimetabolites* | | | | | | |
| Methotrexate | i.v./p.o./i.t. | 50 mg to several grams (folinic acid given if dose greater than 50 mg m$^{-2}$) | Mild | Mild | Moderate | Renal and liver dysfunction Mucositis |
| 5 Fluorouracil | i.v. | 500 mg | Mild | Mild | Minimal | Diarrhoea Conjunctivitis Cerebellar syndrome Hand-foot syndrome |
| *Antitumour antibiotics* | | | | | | |
| Doxorubicin | i.v. | 40 mg | Marked | Marked | Marked | Alopecia Cardiomyopathy |
| *Antitumour antibiotics* | | | | | | |
| Mitozantrone | i.v. | 20 mg | Moderate | Moderate | Moderate | Mild alopecia |
| Bleomycin | i.v./i.m./i.p. | 30 mg | Minimal | Minimal | Minimal | Flu-like illnesses Discoloration and thickening of skin over joints Pulmonary fibrosis |
| Actinomycin D | i.v. | 1 mg | Marked | Marked | Minimal | Alopecia Mucositis |
| *Vinca alkaloids* | | | | | | |
| Vincristine | i.v. | 2 mg | Mild | Mild | Mild | Peripheral neuropathy |
| Vinblastine | i.v. | 10 mg | Marked | Marked | Mild | Mucositis |
| Vindesine | i.v. | 5 mg | Marked | Marked | Mild | Neuropathy |
| *Podophyllotoxins* | | | | | | |
| VP 16 (etoposide) | i.v./p.o. | 150 mg | Moderate | Moderate | Mild/moderate | Neuropathy |
| *Miscellaneous* | | | | | | |
| Procarbazine | p.o. | 150 mg | Moderate | Moderate | Mild | Incompatible with cheese and alcohol |

*DTIC.* Melanoma and soft tissue sarcoma.

*Cisplatin.* Testicular teratoma and seminoma, ovarian cancer, bladder cancer, small cell cancer of the lung, head and neck cancer.

## Antimetabolites

*Methotrexate.* Acute leukaemia, non-Hodgkin's lymphoma, breast cancer and sarcomas.
*5-Fluorouracil.* Breast and gastrointestinal cancer.

## Antiumour antibiotics

*Doxorubicin.* Breast cancer, lymphomas, small cell lung cancer, ovarian cancer and bladder cancer.

*Mitozantrone.* Leukaemia, lymphomas and breast cancer.

*Bleomycin.* Testicular tumours, head and neck cancers and lymphoma.

*Actinomycin D.* Teratomas, Wilm's tumour and paediatric sarcomas.

## Vinca alkaloids

*Vincristine.* Lymphomas, leukaemia, small cell lung cancer and breast cancer.

*Vinblastine.* Testicular tumours and lymphomas.

*Vindesine.* Melanoma.

## Podophyllotoxins

*VP16 (etoposide).* Testicular tumours, lymphomas, leukaemia, small cell lung cancer, Ewing's sarcoma.

## Miscellaneous

*Procarbazine.* Hodgkin's disease and brain tumours.

## PHARMACOLOGY

The susceptibility of a tumour cell to a drug depends on the sensitivity of the cell to the action of the drug, to the cycling of the tumour cell and to the concentration delivered to the tumour.

There is evidence of a dose–response relationship for some cytotoxic drugs and in breast cancer adriamycin has been shown to confer greater therapeutic benefit at high dose. Very high-dose chemotherapy, often with autologous bone marrow support, is an experimental technique in the treatment of lymphomas.

The dose given is usually defined on the basis of milligrams or grams per metre of the surface area.

The dose of an anticancer drug is limited by its toxic effect on normal tissues. The cells which normally are turning over rapidly are the usual sites of dose-limiting toxicity. The bone marrow and intestinal epithelium are therefore problem sites.

Dose schedules are also affected by the function of major organs such as the liver and kidneys.

## Liver

The liver is the principal site for metabolism and excretion of some drugs, and when the serum bilirubin is elevated doxorubicin, mitozantrone and the *Vinca* alkaloids should be used with caution and the dose of the drugs reduced.

## Kidneys

Drugs which are cleared by the kidney may cause increased toxicity if the patient has impaired renal function. Renal function must be checked carefully before each course of chemotherapy when certain drugs are given. The important drugs to note are cisplatin, cyclophosphamide, methotrexate, ifosfamide and procarbazine. When these drugs are given the patient should be well hydrated.

Carboplatin, which is similar in use to cisplatin, may be given with a low creatinine clearance.

## COMBINATION CHEMOTHERAPY

The potential circumvention of resistance to treatment has historically been the most important factor prompting studies of drug combinations. Human tumours present with a greatly reduced percentage of cells in the proliferating pool. Effective chemotherapy has in most cases to be repeated over long intervals and under these circumstances exposure of tumour cells to chemicals can lead to chemical resistance. Because of this combinations of drugs have been used to reduce resistance.

The major principles of combination chemotherapy are that all drugs included in the combination would be active against the tumour when used alone, that they should have different mechanisms of action and that they should have minimally overlapping toxicities.

## COMPLICATIONS

### Acute toxicity

*Local toxicity*

Doxorubicin and *Vinca* alkaloids cause tissue destruction when extravasated. This devastating toxicity can be avoided by ensuring that the needle is within the vein and that the vein is tested by a non-vesicant substance before the injection of the vesicant drug is started.

*Bone marrow toxicity*

For most drugs bone marrow toxicity is a dose-limiting factor. It is mandatory that a full blood count should be checked on the day of the treatment so that dose modifications or postponement of treatment can be considered.

Patients with granulocyte counts of $1.0 \times 10^9$ per litre should receive oral Septrin therapy. If patients have a fever of $38°C$ and have a granulocyte count of $0.5 \times 10^9$ per litre they should receive intravenous antibiotic therapy.

Bleeding does not usually occur until the platelet count falls to $20 \times 10^9$ but patients with low counts should be checked for signs of haemorrhage. Platelet support should be given if the count falls below $20 \times 10^9$ per litre.

### Gastrointestinal toxicity

Nausea and vomiting are caused by cisplatin, cyclophosphamide, doxorubicin and actinomycin C. This is probably due to a combination of stimuli from the chemoreceptor trigger zone, the gut and cerebral cortex.

Patients receiving less toxic combinations of chemotherapy treatment will respond to treatment with high-dose metoclopramide and dexamethasone. For patients receiving highly emetogenic drugs such as cisplatin treatment should be given prophylactically a 5-hydroxytryptamine antagonist. Ondansetron is currently available and is best given by continuous infusion for the most emetogenic drugs by a short infusion followed by oral therapy for somewhat less toxic compounds. An oral premedication with lorazepam 1–2 mg will help the patient to relax before treatment.

Methotrexate may cause mucositis and oral hygiene should be given particular attention. Vincristine may cause constipation and paralytic ileus. Treatment with laxatives is sometimes required. 5-Fluorouracil and cyclophosphamide may cause diarrhoea and prophylactic codeine may be given.

### Alopecia

Doxorubicin, cyclophosphamide, etoposide and vincristine cause alopecia. Hair loss due to doxorubicin may be much reduced by scalp cooling. All hair loss is temporary and patients can be reassured that there will be hair regrowth after treatment has been completed. Wigs are available and should be provided for patients before hair loss occurs. Hair loss will start at 18–21 days after the first injection of these drugs.

### Late toxicity

#### Carcinogenesis

Long-term treatment with alkylating agents such as chlorambucil and melphalan is associated with the development of acute leukaemia. The risk is directly related to the total dose of the drugs given. This is an important reason for reducing both the length of treatment and therefore the cumulative dose of these agents. The risk of developing a second solid tumour due to chemotherapy appears very low.

#### Gonadal damage

Alkylating agents are the drugs most commonly implicated in causing sterility. After combination chemotherapy for Hodgkin's disease the majority of men are azoospermic. This is thought to be due to the combination of chlorambucil and procarbazine. Sperm banking is available but unfortunately many patients are very ill with their lymphoma and have a poor sperm count at that time.

For women over 30 there is a very high risk of permanent amenorrhoea when they have received combination chemotherapy for Hodgkin's disease. Female patients need hormone replacement therapy whereas male patients do not.

Patients receiving chemotherapy must receive counselling about the risk of long-term infertility and the inadvisability of pregnancy during chemotherapy.

Men who receive treatment with cisplatin for germ cell tumours usually retain fertility as do women who have received chemotherapy for choriocarcinoma.

### VALUE

Chemotherapy can cure some of the patients with advanced cancers. Cure is possible in these tumours, which constitute about 12% of cancers.

*Advanced tumours which are potentially curable*

- Acute lymphoblastic leukaemia
- Germ cell tumours
- Choriocarcinoma
- Ewing's sarcoma
- ?Ovarian cancer
- Hodgkin's disease
- Wilm's tumour
- Diffuse large cell lymphoma
- ?Small cell lung cancer.

*Tumours which are potentially curable by local treatment and adjuvant chemotherapy*

- Breast cancer
- Osteogenic sarcoma.

*Tumours which have a response rate which leads to prolonged survival*

- Ovarian cancer
- Lymphoma
- Osteogenic sarcoma
- Breast cancer
- Acute myeloid leukaemia.

*Tumours which have an overall response rate of 50% but no definite survival benefit*

- Head and neck cancer
- Bladder cancer
- Cervical cancer.

*Tumours which are poorly responsive to chemotherapy*

- Pancreatic cancer
- Melanoma
- Soft tissue sarcoma
- Colorectal cancer
- Renal cancer
- Thyroid cancer
- Gastric cancer
- Non-small cell lung cancer.

FURTHER READING

Carmo-Pereira J, Costa F O, Henriques E et al 1987 A comparison of two doses of adriamycin in the primary chemotherapy of advanced breast cancer. British Journal of Cancer 56: 471–475

DeVita V T 1978 The evolution of therapeutic research in cancer. New England Journal of Medicine 907–910

Kaye S B, Cumming J, Kerr D 1985 How much does liver disease affect the pharmacokinetics of adriamycin? European Journal of Cancer 21: 893–895

Marshall E K 1964 Historical perspectives in chemotherapy. In: Goldin A, Hawking I F (eds) Advances in Chemotherapy, Vol 1. Academic Press, New York, pp 1–8

Skipper H E, Schabel F M, Wilcox W S 1964 Experimental evaluation of potential anticancer agents. Cancer Chemotherapy Reports 35: 1–11

# 26. Tumour Markers

*S. M. O'Reilly    G. J. S. Rustin*

Tumour markers are substances present in the body in a concentration which is related to the presence of a tumour. A tumour marker does not have to be tumour specific. It may be a substance secreted or shed into blood and other bodily fluids or expressed at the cell surface in larger quantities by malignant cells than by their non-malignant counterparts. Tumour markers can be detected either by measuring the concentration of the marker in body fluids (usually by immuno-assay) or by detecting the presence of the marker on the cell surface in paraffin sections or fresh biopsies (by immunohistochemistry).

Although the association between human cho-rionic gonadotrophin (HCG) and trophoblastic tumours was identified more than 60 years ago, measurement of tumour markers has, until recently, been confined to a small number of spe-cialized laboratories. However, with the con-tinuing development of monoclonal antibody technology, several new tumour markers have been isolated in the past five years, and commer-cial assays for tumour marker estimation are now widely available. This chapter examines critically those situations where estimation of circulating tumour marker levels may be of clinical value. The terms used to describe the usefulness of a tumour marker measurement are first defined, and the potential applications of tumour marker measurement are discussed. The role of tumour marker measurements in the management of pa-tients with specific tumour types is then outlined.

## DEFINITIONS

The terms most commonly used to describe the usefulness of a tumour marker are defined in

**Table 26.1** Tumour

|  | Present | Absent |
|---|---|---|
| Assay positive | TP | FP |
| Assay negative | FN | TN |

$$\text{Sensitivity} \quad = \quad \frac{TP}{TP + FN} \quad \times 100$$

$$\text{Specificity} \quad = \quad \frac{TN}{FP + TP} \quad \times 100$$

$$\text{Positive predictive value} \quad = \quad \frac{TP}{TP + FP} \quad \times 100$$

$$\text{Negative predictive value} \quad = \quad \frac{TN}{FN + TN} \quad \times 100$$

TP, true positive; FP, false positive;
FN, false negative; TN, true negative.

Table 26.1. Sensitivity is a measure of how commonly a tumour marker level is elevated in the presence of that particular tumour. Specificity measures the proportion of patients without tumour who have normal marker levels. The pre-dictive value of a positive result is the percentage of positive results (i.e. elevated marker levels) which are true positives. An ideal tumour marker would have 100% sensitivity, thus detecting all cases of a particular tumour, and 100% specificity, being elevated only in the presence of that tumour and not in any other situations.

## POTENTIAL USES OF TUMOUR MARKERS

The potential clinical uses of tumour marker estimation are summarized in Table 26.2. An ideal tumour marker would have sufficient

**Table 26.2**  Potential uses of tumour markers

Diagnosis and screening
Prognosis
Monitoring response to treatment
Early diagnosis of relapse
Tumour localization
Antibody-directed therapy

specificity and sensitivity to allow detection of a tumour in a large proportion of cases before it became clinically apparent and, in particular, before the development of metastatic spread. Such a tumour marker assay could thus be used for screening, either of the whole population or at least of selected high-risk groups. In addition, the detection of an elevated marker level would allow a diagnosis of tumour to be made without further investigations having to be performed. Unfortunately, such an ideal situation does not exist. The closest approximation, which will be described shortly, is measurement of HCG in patients with gestational trophoblastic disease.

In order to be of value in prognosis, the tumour marker level should correlate closely with tumour volume and/or aggressiveness. Ideally, estimation of the tumour marker level should provide prognostic information that is as good as, or better than, that provided by other available investigations. One of the best examples of an association between tumour marker levels and prognosis is the case of testicular germ cell tumours, where the degree of elevation of tumour markers before treatment is the best predictor of outcome.

The most common current use of tumour marker estimation is to monitor response of a tumour to treatment. Such measurements are essential in the management of patients with germ cell tumours and gestational trophoblastic disease, where treatment is undertaken with curative intent, and where the detection of the development of drug resistance can lead to a change to an alternative, effective therapy. Although information on response to treatment can also be deduced from serial tumour marker estimation in some of the more common solid tumours such as colorectal and ovarian tumours, a change in treatment is unlikely to lead to an

improved outcome. Nevertheless, early detection of resistance to treatment can lead to the cessation of ineffective, costly, potentially toxic treatment.

Another potential function of a tumour marker is to provide early evidence of tumour recurrence, before it becomes clinically apparent. Once again, this is of greatest use in those tumours where prompt detection of recurrence can lead to effective treatment. It is far from clear whether serial tumour marker estimations leading to the earlier diagnosis of recurrence of the commoner solid tumours such as colorectal, ovarian or breast cancers, where treatment on relapse is usually only palliative in nature, is actually of any benefit to the patient. Indeed, there are potential drawbacks to the early detection of asymptomatic, incurable recurrences, which may easily lead to anxiety for patients at a time when they would otherwise feel perfectly well.

Finally, although it will not be discussed in any further detail in this chapter, a number of clinical trials have attempted to exploit the existence of cell surface tumour markers to localize a tumour either for imaging purposes, using a radiolabelled antibody, or as a treatment modality, using antibodies to carry radioactivity or toxins selectively to the tumour.

## REVIEW OF THE USE OF TUMOUR MARKER ESTIMATION IN THE MANAGEMENT OF PARTICULAR TUMOURS

### Gestational trophoblastic tumours

HCG is a glycoprotein produced by trophoblast cells. The α-subunit is identical to that of follicle-stimulating hormone (FSH), luteinizing hormone (LH) and thyroid-stimulating hormone (TSH), but the C terminal end or the β-subunit is unique to HCG and provides the basis of the specific immunoassay. Although gestational trophoblastic tumours are uncommon, measurement of HCG in this condition is the closest to an ideal tumour marker assay currently available. The use of HCG measurement in the management of patients with gestational trophoblastic disease is therefore described in detail.

*Diagnosis and screening*

Elevated levels of HCG are found with as few as $10^5$ trophoblast cells, while the smallest number of cells detectable by clinical examination is over $10^9$ and even computed tomography (CT) scanning can only detect about $10^7$ cells. However, although HCG is a highly sensitive marker for gestational trophoblastic tumour (GTT) it is not specific. Elevated serum HCG levels are also found in normal pregnancy, in ectopic pregnancy, in patients with germ cell tumours and, occasionally, in patients with other non-germ cell tumours. Pelvic ultrasound examination therefore remains the best method for diagnosing hydatidiform mole.

The great sensitivity of HCG, however, allows it to be used to screen a high-risk population. The first national screening programme for any cancer was set up in 1972 by the Royal College of Obstetricians and Gynaecologists in the UK. Following a diagnosis of hydatidiform mole, all patients are centrally registered at Charing Cross Hospital, Sheffield or Dundee. Patients are then followed using serial HCG measurements to detect any evidence of recurrence for varying lengths of time, depending on the initial rate of fall to normal. Although most hydatidiform moles die out spontaneously after evacuation, approximately 8% of patients require chemotherapy. This screening allows these patients with persistent trophoblastic disease after evacuation of hydatidiform mole to be detected on the basis of plateauing or rising tumour markers before any clinical evidence of disease develops (Bagshawe et al 1986). Early detection reduces the risk of life-threatening side-effects such as uterine perforation or massive uterine haemorrhage, increasing the chance that the disease will be eradicated with less toxic therapy.

*Prognosis/monitoring response to treatment*

Since HCG levels in patients with GTT reflect the total body burden of viable tumour they constitute a significant prognostic factor, with high values contributing to high risk status. In patients with GTT, serial HCG estimation is used to monitor response to chemotherapy and to detect the development of drug resistance. The HCG value may initially increase after starting treatment. This initial surge in HCG has been attributed to either tumour lysis or to increased syncytial differentiation induced by therapy. The HCG level then falls at a rate which is a function of metabolic clearance and the rate of synthesis. Plateauing of HCG values or rising values during the course of chemotherapy indicate the development of drug resistance. The early detection of the development of drug resistance is particularly useful in GTT because, unlike many more common tumours, change to an effective second-line chemotherapy is still very likely to result in cure (Newlands 1991).

*Detection of recurrence*

Serial measurement of HCG will detect any recurrence of GTT with 100% sensitivity. This allows patients to be followed up by HCG monitoring, and obviates the need for frequent hospital visits. A rise in HCG is not, however, diagnostic of recurrent disease, and a new pregnancy must always be considered and ruled out by ultrasound examination. Patients who have had a hydatidiform mole have a slightly increased risk of choriocarcinoma after any subsequent pregnancy and should have further HCG estimations at four and twelve weeks post-partum.

## Germ cell tumours

Tumour marker measurement is essential for the correct management of patients with germ cell tumours of the testis or ovary. α-Fetoprotein (AFP) and HCG are elevated, either singly or in combination, in more than 80% of patients with disseminated non-seminomatous germ cell tumours (NSGCT) and in approximately 60% of patients with localized, stage I disease (Kohn & Ragavan 1981). Other markers which can also be measured in patients with germ cell tumours include lactate dehydrogenase (LDH), which rarely adds additional information for patients with NSGCT but can be a useful marker in patients with seminoma and dysgerminoma, and placental alkaline phosphatase (PLAP), which is elevated in about 50% of patients with seminomas.

## Diagnosis and staging

All patients who are suspected of having a germ cell tumour should have serum sent for tumour marker estimation before excision of the primary tumour. None of the markers mentioned above are sufficiently specific to be used alone to diagnose a germ cell tumour. However, patients whose clinical status could be compromised by a biopsy (e.g. a patient with severe dyspnea due to extensive lung metastases) should be considered to have an NSGCT if the distribution of the disease is compatible with such a tumour and there is significant elevation of either HCG or AFP. Measurement of HCG and AFP can also be a helpful adjunct to histological examination in the differential diagnosis of seminoma and NSGCT. It is important to distinguish these tumours as they differ in the optimal management for metastatic disease. Elevated HCG is associated with the presence of trophoblastic elements in an NSGCT. The presence of syncytial giant cells in a pure seminoma can be associated with a modest elevation of HCG, but any patients with a histologically pure seminoma but a substantially elevated HCG should be treated as if they had an NSGCT (Bosl et al 1981). AFP, a glycoprotein with a molecular weight of 63 000–70 000, is secreted by the yolk sac element of an NSGCT, and a patient with an elevated AFP should never be considered to have a pure seminoma regardless of the histological findings.

An additional reason for preoperative estimation of tumour markers in all patients with suspected germ cell tumours is the use of tumour marker measurement in initial staging and in the follow-up of patients with stage I disease. Complete resection of the primary tumour, in the absence of any metastatic disease, leads to a fall in tumour marker levels at a rate which is inversely proportional to their half-lives. Failure of tumour marker levels to fall to normal postoperatively indicates the presence of occult metastatic disease, even if all other staging investigations are normal. One further situation in which HCG estimation may be of diagnostic value is in the detection of brain metastases. A pretreatment cerebrospinal fluid HCG level that is more than one sixtieth the serum HCG level indicates the presence of brain metastases; the

normal ratio, however, does not exclude brain metastases (Bagshawe & Harland 1976).

## Prognosis

The prognostic value of tumour markers in germ cell tumours is well established. An initial HCG of >50 000 iu $l^{-1}$ and/or an AFP of >500 ku $l^{-1}$ were initially shown to be the most important indicators of failure to achieve complete response following chemotherapy (Germa-Luck et al 1980). Later studies have confirmed the prognostic significance of HCG and AFP values, with the largest studies using HCG levels of >1000 iu $l^{-1}$ or >5000 iu $l^{-1}$ as indicators of poor survival (MRC Working Party on Testicular Tumours 1985). LDH is raised in some patients with advanced NSGCT and has been found to be useful in predicting outcome in some patients (Bosl et al 1983), although it can rarely add additional information to that available from measurement of HCG and AFP. In seminoma, however, LDH can give information not provided by other means (Javadpour 1980). Although PLAP is frequently elevated in seminoma and is related to disease bulk, the high false-negative and false-positive results make it an unreliable marker for routine clinical use (Nielsen et al 1990).

## Monitoring response to treatment

In patients with elevated HCG or AFP, these markers are the most sensitive method for assessing response to treatment. Although, in general, successful chemotherapy is invariably accompanied by a fall in serial HCG and AFP levels, there are two situations in which this may not occur. Firstly, an initial rise in tumour marker levels may occur soon after starting the first course of chemotherapy. This is far more likely to be due to tumour lysis than drug resistance, and markers will usually begin to fall after a brief initial rise. The second situation in which a rise in marker levels may occur in the face of responding disease is a plateau or even a rise in AFP levels despite evidence of response from all other investigations (Coppack et al 1983). This is thought to be due to AFP production by the liver in response to toxicity and appears to be more common in those patients receiving hepatotoxic drugs such as methotrexate and ifosfamide. However, apart from this caveat regarding AFP levels, since the use of platinum-based chemotherapy there have been no recorded cases of patients having progressive malignant disease on scans or clinical examination during initial chemotherapy but response according to tumour markers. To date, half-life measurements of the fall of HCG or AFP during initial therapy have not been shown to be of unequivocal value.

*Early detection of recurrence*

The great sensitivity of HCG, and to a lesser extent of AFP, means that a rise in values is often the first indication of relapse. All patients with germ cell tumours should continue to have serial tumour marker estimation after completion of chemotherapy. Although most patients who enter complete remission will already be cured, early detection of relapse is of great importance since, unlike the situation with most other solid tumours, second-line treatment can still result in cure in a substantial proportion of cases.

The other situation in which serial marker estimation is invaluable in early detection of disease is in surveillance of patients with stage I disease following orchidectomy. In this situation, where there is no evidence of residual tumour on scans or marker measurement after orchidectomy, almost 75% of patients with NSGCT will never relapse (Freeman et al 1987). Close follow-up clinical examination, tumour markers, chest X-ray and at least one CT scan three months after orchidectomy will detect relapse early in the 25–30% of those in whom the disease is destined to recur and, with adequate treatment, virtually all patients will be cured. Such a policy avoids unnecessary therapy in the 70–75% of patients who are already cured, and there is no evidence that there is any adverse outcome in those stage I patients who relapse on surveillance compared with those treated with chemotherapy in the immediate postoperative period. However, in view of the potential for tumour markers to double rapidly, it is important that markers are measured frequently, with one recent study suggesting two-weekly markers for the first six months of surveillance (Seckl et al 1990).

**Gastrointestinal tumours**

There are a number of antibodies currently available which detect antigens expressed by gastrointestinal tumours. The most widely used are the antibodies which react with carcinoembryonic antigen (CEA), a 200 000 Da glycoprotein first described by Gold & Freedman in 1965. More recently described tumour markers include CA 19.9, an antigen derived from a human colon adenocarcinoma cell line with an epitope structurally identical to the sialysated Lewis[a] antigen and CA 50, which is similar but not identical to CA 19.9.

*Diagnosis and screening*

Serum CEA is elevated in fewer than 5% of patients with Dukes' grade A colorectal cancer, about 25% of Dukes' grade B, 44% of Dukes' grade C and about 65% of patients with distant metastases (Begent & Rustin 1989). It was initially thought that CEA was a specific tumour marker, but once sensitive radio-immunoassays became available CEA was found to be elevated not only in cancers of the gastrointestinal tract but in a variety of other conditions including severe benign liver disease, inflammatory lesions especially of the gastrointestinal tract, trauma, infarction, collagen disease, renal impairment and smoking. The low incidence of high serum CEA levels in early disease and its poor specificity explain its lack of value in screening normal populations for colorectal cancer. The low sensitivity precludes its being useful even for screening patients with ulcerative colitis or familial polyposis coli; although these patients are at high risk of developing colorectal cancer, both conditions may cause raised serum CEA in the absence of malignancy (Ziegenbein et al 1980, Dilowari et al 1975). No tumour markers currently available are sensitive enough to screen for oesophageal, gastric or pancreatic cancers. Although CA 19.9 is elevated in 75–90% of patients with pancreatic carcinomas, by the time the marker is elevated the tumour is already incurable by surgery in the vast majority of cases.

*Prognosis/monitoring treatment*

Although a raised preoperative CEA level has been shown to be associated with a poorer prognosis, this is in large part due to the fact that CEA level reflects tumour burden. The value of preoperative CEA as an independent prognostic factor is unclear. Serum CEA levels should fall to normal within four to six weeks of complete resection of a colorectal carcinoma, the mean half-life being about ten days. Levels usually rise with disease and fall with response to chemotherapy or radiotherapy. Failure of CEA to fall during radiotherapy usually indicates the presence of tumour outside the radiation field. Several studies have shown that survival is longer in patients who have a fall in serum CEA level during chemotherapy than in those in whom there is no change or an increased level (Allen-Mersh et al 1987).

*Detection of relapse*

In approximately two-thirds of patients with recurrent colorectal cancers, a rise in serial serum CEA values predicts recurrence four to six months before it becomes clinically apparent (Begent & Rustin 1989). Although early detection of recurrence might allow resection of recurrent disease, it is unclear whether resection of metastases detected in this way improves survival. A randomized, multicentre trial is currently in progress under the auspices of the Cancer Research Campaign trial centre at King's College Hospital, London, to address this question. Studies are also underway to assess whether the addition of serial CA 19.9 estimation to CEA measurement could improve the detection rate.

## Ovarian cancer

The site and pattern of spread of ovarian cancer make it very difficult to detect and monitor using conventional clinical and radiological techniques, so a circulating tumour marker is potentially very valuable. CA 125 is the most commonly used tumour marker for ovarian cancer. The CA 125 antigen was originally defined by its reactivity with a murine monoclonal antibody (OC 125 ) which was raised by immunization with a human cell line derived from a serous cystadenocarcinoma of the ovary. This antibody recognizes multiple antigenic determinants on a high-molecular-weight (>200 000 Da) glycoprotein. CA 125 is found in derivatives of coelomic epithelium including pleura, pericardium and peritoneum, but is not detected in normal ovarian tissue.

*Diagnosis*

CA 125 is elevated in over 90% of patients with advanced (stage III or IV) ovarian cancer, but in less than 50% of patients with stage I disease (Bast et al 1983). However, an elevated CA 125 is not diagnostic of ovarian cancer. Levels above 35 u ml$^{-1}$ are frequently seen during the first trimester of pregnancy, in patients with endometriosis or with cirrhosis, especially if ascites is present, and in 1% of healthy controls. In addition, over 40% of patients with advanced non-ovarian intra-abdominal malignancies have elevated CA 125 levels. Nonetheless, in a patient suspected of having ovarian cancer, the presence of an elevated CA 125 should prompt the surgeon either to refer the patient to a gynaecological oncologist or to perform the surgery through a more extensive midline incision to allow adequate debulking of tumour.

*Screening*

Despite the low sensitivity of CA 125 for potentially curable stage I tumours, large screening studies have been performed. One study at the Royal London Hospital measured serum CA 125 in >20 000 postmenopausal well women attending a screening clinic. Those women who had CA 125 levels > 30 u ml$^{-1}$ underwent pelvic ultrasound, and if that was positive a laparotomy was performed. In all there were 11 confirmed cases of epithelial ovarian cancer (true positives) and 11 cases in whom laparotomy did not reveal an ovarian tumour (false positives). Of note, however, is the fact that only 3 of the 11 patients with screen-detected ovarian cancers had stage I disease (Oram et al 1990). These findings led the UK Coordinating Committee on Cancer Research to recommend in 1989 that screening for ovarian cancer should not yet be offered to women outside a clinical trial.

*Assessing completeness of excision*

In order to decide optimum postoperative management, it is important to know whether one is dealing with a patient with completely excised, stage I disease, or whether the patient has residual tumour after surgery. A persistently elevated CA 125 after oophorectomy for suspected stage I disease is definite evidence of residual tumour. Such patients are candidates for chemotherapy rather than surveillance.

*Prognosis and response to treatment*

Very high CA 125 levels prior to surgery are associated with a worse prognosis, but knowledge of this is unlikely to lead to any alteration in management. Similarly, the fact that a patient with a CA 125 level > 250 u ml$^{-1}$ prior to starting chemotherapy has a poor prognosis is unlikely to prevent a trial of treatment (Parker et al 1988). However, information after one or two courses of chemotherapy that the patient had a poor prognosis or was not responding could influence the clinician to stop ineffective therapy. Several groups have shown that the CA 125 level after one, two or three courses of chemotherapy is the most important prognostic factor for survival. In addition, a long half-life and a greater than sevenfold fall in CA 125 level during the first month after chemotherapy have been shown to be adverse prognostic factors (Rustin et al 1989). Recently, an algorithm which defines response and progression based on serial CA 125 estimation during first-line chemotherapy has been described. Using this algorithm to define progression, the benefits which could have been obtained if the serial CA 125 results had been acted upon were calculated (Rustin et al 1992). These amounted to 11 ultrasound scans, 4 CT scans, 1 bone scan and 22 courses of carboplatin, costing a total of £7970 compared with the cost of CA 125 assays on all patients of £5467. Thus serial tumour marker estimation could be a cost-effective exercise, reducing the amount of ineffective, potentially toxic chemotherapy a patient receives and also the number of costly investigations necessary to assess response.

*Detection of relapse*

A serial rise of CA 125 levels of >25% has been shown in several studies to predict progression off-treatment with almost 100% specificity. However, although the use of CA 125 estimation to define progression may reduce the number of radiological investigations performed, as outlined above, there is no evidence at present that early reintroduction of chemotherapy or searching for a resectable site of relapse produces any survival benefit. Therefore, serial CA 125 measurements during follow-up off therapy cannot be recommended as a routine investigation. However, once there is any clinical suspicion of relapse, serial CA 125 levels at that point are likely to be the most effective investigation to confirm the presence of recurrent tumour.

**Prostate cancer**

Prostate specific antigen (PSA) is now widely accepted as the most useful tumour marker in patients with prostate cancer. PSA is a glycoprotein secreted exclusively by prostate epithelial cells, and is thus organ specific. Several studies have shown that PSA is elevated in a higher proportion of men with prostate cancer than prostatic acid phosphatase.

*Diagnosis and screening*

Elevated levels of PSA (>4 ng ml$^{-1}$) occur in about 65% of men with localized stage A prostatic cancer, but can also occur in 30–50% of men with benign prostatic hypertrophy, a condition common in men of similar age group to those who develop prostate cancer (Beastall et al 1991). Clearly, therefore, measurement of PSA alone is not sufficiently sensitive to be used in population screening for prostate cancer. The combination of PSA and rectal examination, followed by prostatic ultrasound in patients with abnormal findings, appears to be the best method of detecting early prostate cancer. Unfortunately, many screen-detected cancers will already have spread outside the prostate. In one recent study where healthy men with PSA > 4 ng ml$^{-1}$ underwent rectal examination and ultrasonography, only 59% of patients with PSA levels 4.0–9.9 ng ml$^{-1}$ and 13% with levels >10 ng ml$^{-1}$ with screen-detected cancers had localized tumours at surgical staging (Catalona et al 1991). Until the results of large-scale studies are available, it remains unclear whether screening can reduce the mortality from prostate cancer.

*Staging*

Although not of proven benefit in screening, PSA measurement may help to reduce the number of staging investigations in patients with prostate cancer. Patients with PSA levels of <20 ng ml$^{-1}$ can be assumed to have no bone metastases and do not necessarily need bone scans. However, as a PSA of >20 ng ml$^{-1}$ can occur in a patient with a bulky, poorly differentiated tumour without distant metastases, bone scanning is still necessary for patients with PSA of >20 ng ml$^{-1}$. PSA is inferior to transurethral ultrasound in the detection of capsular invasion, with 30% of patients overstaged and 25% understaged by PSA. Lymph node metastases are usually associated with elevated PSA, and a PSA value of 20 ng ml$^{-1}$ appears to have a positive and negative predictive value similar to CT scanning in the detection of nodal disease.

*Prognosis/monitoring response*

As the PSA level correlates with prostatic volume and tumour differentiation, it is not surprising that a high pretreatment PSA is associated with a poor prognosis. Serial changes in PSA level after initial treatment are potentially more useful in patient management, however, than a single PSA level at diagnosis. PSA levels fall rapidly to normal after complete removal of tumour by radical prostatectomy, although the rate of fall is slower after radiotherapy or endocrine therapy.

*Detection of recurrence*

There is evidence that a serial rise in PSA can precede other evidence of disease progression, although how useful such an observation is for a tumour for which there is no curative therapy on recurrence is unclear. PSA estimation can be of practical use, however, in the patient with a past history of prostate cancer who develops back pain, where the presence of a normal PSA level obviates the need for further investigation for metastatic disease.

## Hepatocellular carcinoma

*Diagnosis and screening*

Serum AFP is elevated at presentation in 50–80% of UK patients with hepatocellular carcinoma (HCC). Although HCC is one of the most common malignant tumours in the world today, the relatively low incidence in the UK does not justify general population screening, although such screening may be justified in areas such as China with high-incidence populations. In the UK, serial AFP estimation and ultrasound examination can be justified, however, for selective screening of high-risk populations (i.e. patients with cirrhosis, chronic hepatitis B or haemochromatosis) because patients who have successful resection of a solitary, screen-detected tumour have a higher chance of long-term survival.

Elevated AFP is not specific for the diagnosis of HCC and histological confirmation is essential. Patients with HCC may have a normal AFP, especially if the tumour arises in a non-cirrhotic liver. In addition, modest elevations of AFP occur in about 20% of patients with hepatitis, cirrhosis, biliary tract obstruction and alcoholic liver disease. Moreover, up to 10% of patients with hepatic metastases have elevated serum AFP. Despite these caveats, a massively elevated AFP in a patient with known cirrhosis is virtually diagnostic of HCC.

*Prognosis*

There is evidence that AFP provides prognostic information in patients with HCC. Patients with a low serum AFP have been reported to survive longer than patients with a high AFP. Although it was initially thought that this difference in prognosis was due to the association between high AFP and bulky tumours, the improved outlook associated with a low AFP is maintained after correction for tumour size. This longer survival associated with a low AFP may be related to the trend for patients with well-differentiated tumours to have a low AFP. Alternatively, the improved prognosis may be partly related to the observation that HCC with low AFP is more common in patients with non-cirrhotic livers.

## Breast cancer

A variety of tumour markers have been studied in patients with breast cancer, including CEA and tissue polypeptide antigen (TPA) and several polymorphic epithelial mucin markers (HMFG1, HMFG2, MSA, MCA, CAM–26, CAM–29, CA 15-3). The most widely investigated mucin marker in breast cancer is CA 15-3. The commercially available CA 15-3 kit utilized a sandwich technique which employs two monoclonal antibodies: the 115D8 antibody as the capture antibody and the DF3 antibody as the tracer antibody.

### Diagnosis and screening

Although elevated levels of CA 15-3 are found in 55–100% of patients with advanced breast cancer, serum CA 15-3 is raised in only 10–46% of patients with primary breast cancer and in about 10% of patients with early ($T_{1-2} N_0M_0$) operable disease. As 2–20% of patients with benign breast disease have elevated levels, it is clear that mucin assays such as CA 15-3 are lacking in both specificity and sensitivity as a screening tool. No other tumour marker or combination of markers contribute to the diagnosis of breast cancer (Nicolini et al 1991).

### Prognosis/monitoring response to treatment

Elevated preoperative levels of CA 15-3 have been shown to be associated with a poorer prognosis (Kallioniemi et al 1988). However, this may well be due to the association between CA 15-3 and tumour burden, and there is no convincing evidence to date that measurement of CA 15-3, or any other tumour marker, provides significant independent prognostic information. Although tumour marker levels can fall with reduction in tumour burden following systemic therapy, there is sufficient variation between patients to preclude the use of tumour marker estimation to define response.

### Early detection of relapse

The observation that over 60% of patients who develop recurrent breast cancer have raised levels of CA 15-3 suggests a potential value in early detection of recurrence. The use of a panel of tumour markers might further increase the pick-up of recurrent disease. However, it is questionable whether such early detection of relapse will alter survival and thus whether the patient will benefit.

## CONCLUSIONS

This chapter addresses the role of tumour marker estimation in the management of patients with the more common solid tumours. The rare gestational trophoblastic tumour has also been included as this is the situation in which a tumour marker is closest to the ideal. There are other rare situations in which tumour marker estimation may be of value, such as screening for neuroblastoma in children in a high-risk population or in the monitoring of tumour-associated hormones in gastrointestinal tract hormone-producing tumours such as carcinoid. In addition, measurement of immunoglobulins can be very useful as a marker for disease extent and response to treatment in patients with plasma cell tumours such as myeloma.

Although tumour marker estimation can be very helpful in the management of patients with certain, relatively uncommon tumours such as gestational trophoblastic tumours, germ cell tumours and hepatocellular carcinoma, the routine use of tumour marker estimation is of limited use in the management of patients with more common tumours. This is due to the fact that currently available markers are insufficiently sensitive and specific for routine use. It is to be hoped that the continuing expansion of monoclonal antibody research will result in more clinically useful markers being discovered.

## REFERENCES

Allen-Mersh T G, Kemeny N, Niedzwiechid et al 1987 Significance of a fall in serum CEA concentration in patients treated with cytotoxic chemotherapy for disseminated colorectal cancer. Gut 12: 1625–1629

Bagshawe K D, Harland S 1976 Immunodiagnosis and monitoring of gonadotrophin producing metastases in the central nervous system. Cancer 38: 112–118

Bagshawe K D, Dent J, Webb J 1986 Hydatidiform mole in England and Wales 1973–1983. Lancet ii: 673–677

Bast R C, Klug T L, St John E et al 1983 A radioimmunoassay using a monoclonal antibody to monitor the course of epithelial ovarian cancer. New England Journal of Medicine 308: 883–887

Beastall G H, Cook B, Rustin G J S, Jennings J 1990 A review of the role of established tumour markers. Annals of Clinical Biochemistry 28: 5–18

Begent R J, Rustin G J S 1989 Tumour markers : from carcinoembryonic antigen to products of hybridoma technology. Cancer Surveys 8: 107–121

Bosl G J, Lange P H, Nochomovitz L E 1981 Tumour markers in advanced non-seminomatous testicular cancer. Cancer 47:572–576

Bosl G J, Geller N L, Cirrincione C et al 1983 Multivariate analysis of prognostic variables in patients with metastatic testicular cancer. Cancer Research 43: 3403–3407

Catalona W J, Smith D S, Ratliff T L et al 1991 Measurement of prostate specific antigen in serum as a screening test for prostate cancer. New England Journal of Medicine 324: 1156–1161

Coppack S, Newlands E S, Dent J et al 1983 Problems of interpretation of serum concentrations of alphafoetoprotein (AFP) in patients receiving cytotoxic chemotherapy for malignant germ cell tumours. British Journal of Cancer 48: 335–340

Dilowari J B, Lennard Jones J E, Mackay A M 1975 Estimation of CEA in ulcerative colitis with special reference to malignant change. Gut 16: 225–260

Freedman L S, Parkinson M C, Jones W et al 1987 Histopathology in the prediction of relapse in patients with stage I testicular teratoma treated by orchidectomy alone: an MRC Collaborative Study. Lancet 8554: 294–297.

Germa-Luck J R, Begent R H J, Bagshawe K D 1980 Tumour marker levels and prognosis in malignant teratoma of the testis. British Journal of Cancer 42: 850

Gold P, Freedman D S 1965 Specific carcinoembryonic antigen of the human digestive system. Journal of Experimental Medicine 122: 468–481

Javadpour N 1980 Management of seminoma based on tumour markers. Urologic Clinics of North America 7: 773–781

Kallioniemi O P, Oksa H, Aaran R et al 1988 Serum CA 15-3 assay in the diagnosis and followup of breast cancer. British Journal of Cancer 58: 213–215

Kohn J, Ragavan D 1981 Tumour markers in malignant germ cell tumours. In: Peckham M (ed) The management of testicular tumours. Edward Arnold, London, pp 50–69

Medical Research Council Working Party on Testicular Tumours 1985 Prognostic factors in advanced, non-seminomatous germ cell testicular tumours: result of a multicentre study. Lancet i: 8.

Nielsen O S, Munro A J, Duncan W et al 1990 Is placental alkaline phosphatase (PLAP) a useful marker for seminoma? European Journal of Cancer 26 : 1049–1054

Newlands E S 1991 Gestational trophoblastic tumours. In: Blackledge G R P, Jordan J A, Shingleton M (eds) Textbook of gynaecological oncology. Saunders, London, pp 454–463

Nicolini A, Colombini C, Luciani L et al 1991 Evaluation of serum CA 15-3 determination with CEA and TPA in the postoperative followup of breast cancer patients. British Journal of Cancer 64: 154–158

Oram D H, Jacobs J, Brady L, Prys-davies A 1990 Early diagnosis of ovarian cancer. British Journal of Hospital Medicinel 44: 320–324

Parker D, Patel K, Alred E J et al 1988 CA 125 and survival in ovarian cancer: preliminary communication. Journal of the Royal Society of Medicine 81: 2

Rustin G J S, Gennings J N, Nelstrop A E et al 1989 Use of CA 125 to predict survival of patients with ovarian carcinoma. Journal of Clinical Oncology 7: 1667–1671

Rustin G J S, Nelstrop A, Stillwell M A 1992 Savings obtained by CA 125 measurements during therapy for ovarian cancer. European Journal of Cancer 28: 79–82

Seckl M J, Rustin G J S, Bagshawe K D 1990 Frequency of serum tumour marker monitoring in patients with non-seminomatous germ cell tumours. British Journal of Cancer 61: 916–918

Ziegenbein R, Jacobash K H, Pilgram G 1980 Determination of CEA in patients with colorectal carcinoma and polyps. Archiv fur Geschwulstforschung 50: 165–168

# 27. Clinical pharmacology

*M. Schachter*

## INTRODUCTION AND DEFINITIONS

A decade ago an eminent professor of clinical pharmacology could foresee a time when every district general hospital would have its own clinical pharmacologist. This has not happened and does not seem imminent. Indeed, many clinicians have reservations about the role of clinical pharmacology as a specialty, except perhaps within the pharmaceutical industry. In fact, clinical pharmacologists themselves have very divergent views on this issue. They have their own sub-specialties and cannot pretend to have comprehensive knowledge of all medicines. But clinical pharmacology does provide a framework of principles for evaluating the uses and dangers of new drugs, for comparing them with established agents, for detecting and even predicting both wanted and unwanted interactions, and for defining the ways in which drugs are handled in man. It is also involved in monitoring the effect of age, pregnancy and intercurrent disease on the use of drugs. This role is increasingly reinforced by the drug information services within hospital pharmacies, with access to extensive literature from many sources and to vast computer-linked databases. The readers of this chapter will be already be aware, with more or less enthusiasm, that surgeons are major prescribers of drugs of all kinds from analgesics to antibiotics. Some reminders of clinical pharmacological principles may therefore be helpful. It may be useful, first of all, to list some definitions, particularly relating to pharmacokinetics. These terms will be used frequently in other parts of the chapter. This will obviously not be an overview of all the drugs that might be used in surgical practice. Rather, it will consider the principles of drug usage in some of the circumstances outlined above.

### Half-life (or half-time)

This is almost always a measure of the rate of decline of drug plasma concentration, though occasionally it may have other meanings. The half-life (often written as $t_{1/2}$) is often easy to calculate, since the rate of decline of the drug concentration is usually exponential: if plotted as the logarithm of the concentration against time one therefore obtains a straight line (Fig. 27.1).

The knowledge of $t_{1/2}$ is clearly essential for the rational use of any drug (though prescribing practice does not always reflect this!). It allows the prescriber to calculate how rapidly a drug is eliminated from the body, both under normal and under pathological conditions. Equally important, it is an indication of the rate of accumulation of a drug during regular, fixed-interval dosing. For all practical purposes the $t_{1/2}$ is the only variable which determines the rate at which a drug accumulates under these circumstances, and also the time taken for plasma levels to reach a steady state (that is, where input and output of the drug are in approximate balance). This takes about five half-lives (Fig. 27.2). There is, of course, one special case of 'multiple' dosing of particular importance in surgical practice, namely intravenous infusion. In fact, this can be considered as the administration of an infinitely large number of separate doses separated by infinitesimally small time intervals. It still needs the same number of half-lives to reach steady state, but with a much smoother and less fluctuating increase in plasma levels. Finally another issue

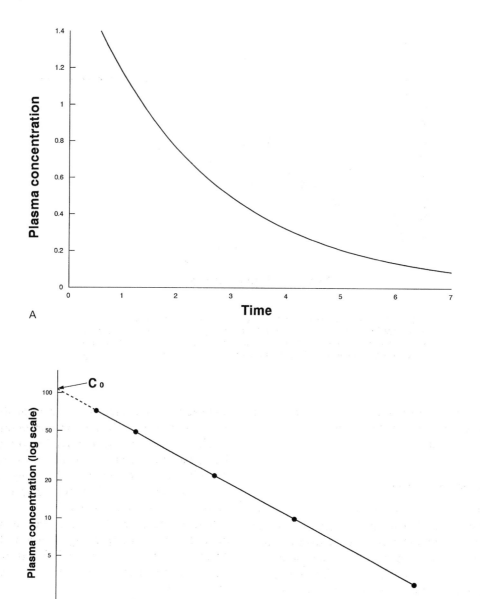

**Fig. 27.1**  Stylized representation of (**A**) decline in plasma drug concentration following single intravenous dose, and (**B**) logarithmic plot of the data. $C_0$ is the extrapolated drug concentration at time 0. Scales are arbitrary.

arises from the inflexible interaction of half-life and steady-state plasma drug concentrations. For drugs with long $t_{1/2}$ the time required to reach steady state may be unacceptably long. Therefore a loading dose may be given to achieve a thera- peutic level which can then be maintained as the steady-state concentration. Digoxin is much the best known example of this, with a $t_{1/2}$ of about 40 hours even in the presence of normal renal function. Of course, loading dose may also be

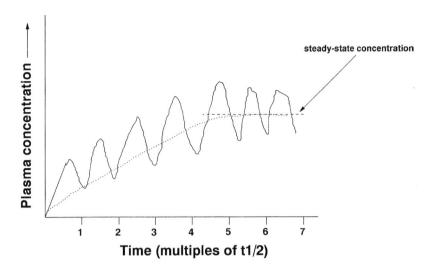

**Fig. 27.2** Stylized representation of the approach to steady-state plasma concentration of a drug after repeated oral dosing at approximate half-life intervals. The dotted line represents intravenous administration, by infusion. Note that the steady-state concentration is half-way between the peaks and troughs of drug level.

given for a drug with a short $t_{1/2}$ if a very rapid effect is essential (for instance, lignocaine with $t_{1/2}$ of about 1 hour).

### Volume of distribution

Many find this the most confusing term in pharmacokinetics. The volume of distribution (or more correctly apparent volume of distribution, abbreviated $V_d$), has units of litres per kilogram. This obviously leads, in some instances, to absurd figures totalling several thousand litres. This is not physically real, but does have practical relevance. The $V_d$ is calculated on the assumption that a drug distributes itself instantaneously throughout the body, with a concentration designated as $C_0$ (Fig. 27.1b). It is therefore most appropriate to think of $V_d$ as an indicator of the extent to which a drug is distributed in the tissues. Therefore:

$$V_d = Dose/C_0$$

Plasma and extracellular fluid may make only a modest contribution to the total volume. In this context plasma protein is not part of the tissues and, as a result, highly protein-bound drugs (such as warfarin and the sulphonylureas) have $V_d$ values approximating to plasma volume. On the other hand, very lipid-soluble drugs (tricyclics and neuroleptics, for instance) may have enormous volumes of distribution.

Knowledge of the $V_d$ of a particular drug may be useful in designing dosage regimes, though in practice it is not often used. $V_d$ is related to $t_{1/2}$ and clearance (see below) by a simple relationship:

$$Clearance = V_d \times 0.7/t_{1/2}$$

In other words, $t_{1/2}$ may be altered either by changes in clearance or in $V_d$. The clinical relevance of this will be discussed in other sections of this chapter. Knowledge of $V_d$ can also help in the evaluation of potential drug interactions: drugs with very large $V_d$s are, as already noted, likely to have low levels of plasma protein binding. They are therefore very unlikely to displace highly protein-bound drugs such as warfarin, while the converse is also true.

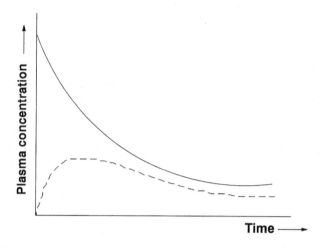

**Fig. 27.3** Stylized comparison of plasma concentrations after bolus intravenous administration (continuous line) and a single oral dose (dashed line) of a drug, illustrating how bioavailability can be derived from the comparison by area under dashed line/*total* area under continuous line.

### Clearance

This is a widely used term, though its exact meaning is not always appreciated. It is defined as that fraction of $V_d$ from which the drug is removed per unit time. It is usually expressed as millilitres per minute or millilitres per minute per kilogram. Total clearance is the sum of clearances by all routes of elimination, renal and non-renal. Much the most important of the non-renal routes is, of course, hepatic metabolism.

### Bioavailability

This term describes the proportion of the oral dose of a drug which reaches the systemic circulation, compared to intravenous dosing. It can easily be calculated from the areas under the time – concentration curves after intravenous and oral doses (Fig. 27.3). The main determinants of bioavailability are absorption and 'first-pass' metabolism. The latter usually refers to metabolism in the liver but sometimes significant metabolism can occur in the intestinal wall. Bioavailability may differ after chronic dosing, as compared to a single dose: metabolic enzymes may be induced or saturated during prolonged treatment. It must be appreciated that different brands and formulations of a particular drug may have widely differing bioavailability.

## DRUGS IN THE YOUNG AND OLD

### Neonates, infants and children

There is no lower age limit either for surgical intervention or drug therapy. It must therefore be appreciated that babies are not small adults. Every aspect of drug handling is drastically different in neonates and infants, as compared to adults. Firstly, the adult body has a lower water content than the neonate's (about 60% compared to 75%). Changes in fat content are less dramatic, but some may be surprised that fat represents 12–15% of body weight in the neonate and 18–20% in most adults (much more in some, of course). Renal function is initially much impaired in neonates, with glomerular filtration rate 5–10% that of the adult. However, adult values are reached in three to six months. Tubular function is also immature in the very young. Hepatic function presents a more complex picture. Some enzyme systems are grossly under-developed in neonates — chloramphenicol glucuronidation is a notorious example — but other processes are fully active: most sulphation for instance. In general, however, oxidative systems are not fully mature and this can be of clinical importance, as with theophylline.

The single most important alteration in gastro-intestinal function is the increase in gastric acidity with age. Higher pH leads to increased absorption of some drugs, such as amoxycillin and flucloxacillin. Gastric emptying is also impaired in the neonate. Finally, the blood–brain barrier is relatively permeable in the very young. This can have serious consequences both in disease — kernicterus — and after drug administration, as in the case of the antidiarrhoeal opiates diphenoxylate and loperamide. These can cause significant, even fatal, central nervous system (CNS) depression in infants. All of these considerations emphasize the importance of using the minimum number of drugs at the lowest possible doses: no different from any other patient, in fact! The principal difficulty lies in the calculation of the appropriate dose. Several approaches are possible, and none is universally applicable. Adjusting dose to surface area is considered the most appropriate method for neonates, but may not be accurate enough in premature babies. In these weight may be a more reliable guide, and this is sometimes also used in older children. Another system matches the age to a fixed percentage of the adult dose: for example, 12.5% at 1 month, 25% at 1 year, 50% at 7 years, 75% at 12 years. This is safe with relatively non-toxic drugs with a high therapeutic index, but is too approximate for more hazardous agents.

### Drugs and the elderly

The clinical pharmacology of the elderly has become a subspecialty in its own right. This is very welcome, and hardly surprising. The number of patients over the age of 65 is rising rapidly in all developed countries, as is the number of those over 80 or even 90. In parallel, the number of available drugs is also increasing, though at a rate constrained by the escalating costs of drug development and the growing anxiety of most governments at the budgetary implications of prescribed drugs. This section will summarize some of the most important considerations in prescribing for the elderly.

It is safe to assume that old patients will show increased sensitivity to the therapeutic and adverse effects of most drugs. Much of this can be explained by pharmacokinetic changes which are relatively easy to quantify. However, there are also examples where there seem to be alterations in pharmacodynamic responsiveness. These are usually very poorly understood but may be of considerable clinical relevance. For instance, it is well known that many CNS depressants, such as benzodiazepines, have an enhanced effect in the elderly: there is more prolonged sedation, often accompanied by confusion, disorientation or even hallucinations. For many benzodiazepines, including lorazepam and nitrazepam, conventional pharmacokinetic parameters differ little in the elderly and in young adults. The exaggerated response is often attributed to 'hypoxia', but the evidence for this is rarely convincing. This is in fact part of a broader area of ignorance: we know little about the determinants of individual response to psychoactive drugs, at any age. Similarly, warfarin often produces a disproportionate fall in clotting factor synthesis in the old, in the absence of impaired drug clearance or of significant interactions with other drugs. Another poorly understood phenomenon is the increased likelihood of diuretic-induced hypokalaemia. In some other instances there is a better understanding of the mechanisms of change. In the elderly there is a generalized reduction in adrenoceptor, particularly cardiovascular $\beta_1$-adrenoceptor, density. Consequently, the therapeutic efficacy of both β-agonists and β-antagonists (in angina and hypertension) is likely to be impaired. It should be noted that response to $\beta_2$-agonists in asthma seems to be undiminished. The relative lack of efficacy of β-blockers in the elderly hypertensive has been well characterized in large trials of hypotensive drugs in the elderly. A final example is the increased frequency and severity of drug-induced hypotension in aged patients, possibly due to reduced baroreceptor reflexes.

Much more is known about the altered pharmacokinetics characteristic of the elderly.

Drug absorption is not greatly affected, in the absence of specific gastrointestinal disease. Body composition is significantly different, with reduced muscle mass and total body weight, and a relative reduction in body water. There is therefore a compensatory increase in the percentage of body fat, though this may be drastically reversed in the very old. Plasma albumin concentration is often reduced, but this is rarely of practical importance. Changes in $V_d$ are complex and not always easy to predict. As examples, $V_d$ is higher for some benzodiazepines, including diazepam and chlordiazepoxide, and for gentamicin. By contrast, it is lower for digoxin and ethanol.

Renal function declines with age. This is true both of glomerular filtration rate and of tubular function, though the former is usually of greater clinical relevance: this will be considered in greater detail in another section of the chapter. Many important drugs are affected, including digoxin, the aminoglycoside antibiotics, tetracycline and lithium. Of these, the tetracyclines (except doxycycline and minocycline) should be avoided if there is significant renal impairment. Plasma levels of the other drugs can be monitored. Some other drugs — methyldopa and methotrexate are examples — are cleared by both renal and non-renal routes, and therapeutic monitoring is not usually available. If these drugs cannot be avoided doses can be reduced on an empirical basis, based on plasma creatinine levels or, preferably, on creatinine clearance. Changes in hepatic metabolism are more complex and more difficult to summarize. They are less often of therapeutic importance. There is usually a reduction in hepatic blood flow, reflecting diminished cardiac output, and this leads to reduced clearance of some highly metabolized drugs, such as propranolol and lignocaine (though there is some dispute about the latter). On the other hand, the clearance of other extensively metabolized drugs, including warfarin and ethanol, hardly changes with ageing. It should also be noted that the inducibility of hepatic microsomal enzymes tends to decline with age, possibly an actual advantage in avoiding some drug interactions.

From the clinician's point of view these are not necessarily the most challenging problems in prescribing for the aged. The real difficulties can be summarized as follows:

1. The elderly often have multiple illnesses, and tend to be prescribed numerous drugs — often far too many. This inevitably leads to additive side-effects and great potential for drug interactions.

2. There is a high incidence of non-compliance amongst the elderly, for a variety of reasons, notably failure to understand the prescriber's instructions and unwillingness (sometimes justified!) to take medication.

3. As an extension of the first two points, patients may be taking non-prescribed medication, often of unknown composition.

These points are, of course, relevant for any patient, of any age.

## DRUGS IN PREGNANCY

Unfortunately, prescribing is often unavoidable in pregnancy. Although there are considerable alterations in drug handling — increased plasma volume and glomerular filtration rate, decreased plasma albumin — this rarely necessitates alterations in drug usage. The overriding anxiety is the possibility of toxic effects on the fetus. Some of the most important teratogens and other drugs with potentially adverse actions are listed in Table 27.1.

## DRUG USAGE IN DISEASE

### Drugs in renal disease

It has already been pointed out that renal impairment almost inevitably accompanies ageing. Although this is significant it is rarely very severe. However, in many cases much more abnormal renal function has to be taken into account when using drugs. The consequences of diminished renal function are more complex than is often appreciated. Naturally, renal elimination of many drugs and their metabolites is impaired, but there are also changes in drug distribution. The plasma protein binding of many drugs, particularly acidic drugs such as phenytoin, warfarin and salicylates, is reduced. The reduction is proportionate to the severity of the renal failure, and may have several

**Table 27.1**  Drugs to be avoided in pregnancy

(a)  *In early pregnancy — potentially teratogenic*
Cytotoxic drugs
Sex steroids
Retinoids
Warfarin
Anticonvulsants*
Tetracyclines

(b)  *In later pregnancy — fetal and perinatal effects*
Sex steroids
Warfarin
Tetracyclines
Sulphonamides
Chloramphenicol
Alcohol
Tobacco
Non-steroidal anti-inflammatory drugs
Sulphonylureas

(c)  *Use with particular caution*
All CNS depressants
Lithium
Antithyroid drugs
Corticosteroids

* Some controversy, but probably all teratogenic. Sodium valproate may be most hazardous. However, danger of drugs must be weighed against danger of uncontrolled seizures.

causes. Firstly, there may be low plasma albumin due to proteinuria. Secondly, many endogenous acidic metabolites accumulate during renal failure, and these can compete for binding sites with the acidic drugs. Lastly, and most speculatively, the structure of the plasma proteins may be abnormal. The importance of these changes should not be overemphasized, as they often have been. Nonetheless, for drugs that are affected it will mean a higher free fraction in plasma: since this is the pharmacologically active component of the drug it will effectively lower the therapeutic range of the drug. It must be remembered, though, that the increased free fraction of the drug will also increase the clearance.

Many drugs will require dosage adjustment in the presence of renal failure: a few, discussed below, should be avoided altogether. In cases where a drug is used in reduced dosage the target steady-state blood level (if there is one) is the same as in healthy individuals. This can be achieved in two ways: by reducing the unit dose or by increasing the dosage interval. Both approaches are used in practice. Digoxin is produced in a low-dose formulation — 0.0625 mg

against the standard dose of 0.25 mg — specifically for use in the elderly or in other patients with renal impairment. Occasionally the standard dose unit is used at two- or three-day intervals, but this is generally done in hospital. Prolonged dosage intervals tend to have a negative effect on patient compliance. By contrast the aminoglycosides tend to be administered at prolonged intervals, but at standard unit doses. These drugs are classical examples of the usefulness of therapeutic plasma drug level monitoring to minimize toxicity in circumstances where drug clearance is abnormal. In fact, nomograms have been constructed which allow reasonable estimates of desirable dosages even if drug assays are not available. The nomograms are based on creatinine clearance or, if this is not known, on plasma creatinine. However, measurement of plasma levels is always preferable. For most other drugs this degree of monitoring is not available and dosage adjustment must be empirical. Important examples of such drugs are:

- atenolol, sotalol
- cephalosporins (most)
- methyldopa
- lithium — always monitor
- cimetidine, ranitidine (less significant).

Table 27.2 lists drug that should be avoided in renal failure, with the reasons for avoidance.

### Drugs in liver disease

Given the central role of the liver in drug handling, and so many other metabolic processes, it is to be expected that liver disease would have a dramatic impact on drug usage. This is the case, but in fact most of the problems arise from abnormal responses to drugs rather than to pharmacokinetic anomalies. These can be very complex, for several reasons. Firstly, severe liver disease is often accompanied by some degree of renal failure. Secondly, as in renal disease but often to a greater extent, plasma albumin levels may be depressed because of diminished synthesis. Thirdly, cirrhosis is often associated with an increase in total liver blood flow, but with a variable degree of shunting of blood within the liver. This can lead to increased flow to metabolically

**Table 27.2**  Drugs that should be avoided in severe renal failure (glomerular filtration rate $<10$ ml min$^{-1}$)

| | |
|---|---|
| Aspirin | Platelet dysfunction, gastrointestinal symptoms |
| Tetracyclines | Deterioration of renal function |
| (except doxycycline, minocycline) | |
| Nalidixic acid | Systemic lupus erythematosus-like syndrome due to metabolites |
| Nitrofurantoin | Peripheral neuropathy |
| Methotrexate | Nephrotoxic |
| Amiloride | Hyperkalaemia, acidosis |
| Thiazides | Ineffective, hyperuricaemia |
| Spironolactone | Hyperkalaemia, acidosis |
| Probenecid | Ineffective, possible uric acid stones |
| Chlorpropamide | Hypoglycaemia |
| Gallamine | Prolonged apnea |
| Pancuronium | Prolonged apnea |
| Penicillamine | Nephrotic syndrome |
| Aurothiomalate sodium | Nephrotoxic |

inactive areas. It will be seen that the ultimate outcome can be very difficult to predict, but can lead to increased bioavailability and possible toxicity of several important drugs such as metoprolol, propranolol, labetalol and chlormethiazole. More predictably, the clearance of many extensively metabolized drugs is reduced. These include theophylline, phenytoin, verapamil, chloramphenicol and most benzodiazepines.

The mention of these anxiolytics and anticonvulsants leads to consideration of drugs to avoid in severe liver disease. These are among the more important:

1. All CNS depressants, including benzodiazepines and opiate analgesics. These may precipitate or aggravate hepatic encephalopathy.
2. Diuretics, which may cause hyponatraemia and hypokalaemia and hence increase the likelihood of encephalopathy. However, the aldosterone antagonist spironolactone is widely used in cirrhosis-associated ascites.
3. Warfarin and other oral anticoagulants, since there is decreased synthesis of clotting factors.
4. Potentially hepatotoxic drugs, such as rifampicin and tetracyclines.

### Drugs in heart failure

Severe heart failure can have far-reaching effects on drug disposition. Reduced cardiac blood flow will lead to diminished perfusion of gut, liver and kidneys. The absorption of some drugs (for example, hydrochlorothiazide and frusemide) is therefore impaired. Hypoperfusion of the liver will diminish clearance of some extensively metabolized drugs: lignocaine may be particularly important in this context, with potentially serious toxicity. Altered renal blood flow will naturally result in reduced glomerular filtration rate and therefore reduced clearance of drugs such as digoxin. Abnormal distribution of blood flow within the kidney may cause increased reabsorption of some drugs, and thus further diminish clearance.

### DRUG INTERACTIONS

The number of possible drug interactions is astronomical, and lists of even the most important can occupy sizeable volumes. The intention of this section is to consider possible ways in which drugs can interact with one another. Usually, but not always, these interactions are unwanted. They can be considered under three major headings: pharmaceutical, pharmacodynamic and pharmacokinetic.

### *Pharmaceutical interactions*

These interactions occur outside the body, usually involving intravenous drugs which are incompatible with one another on the basis of chemical and physical reactions. Well-known examples include calcium salts and sodium bicarbonate, dopamine and sodium bicarbonate and amiodarone and sodium chloride. The British

National Formulary includes a very comprehensive list of permitted and incompatible intravenous mixtures and additives.

## Pharmacodynamic interactions

Two main types of interaction are possible under this heading. Drugs may have an additive or even synergistic effect, or they may antagonize each other's actions. The best-known example of the first type is the action of CNS depressants, which characteristically potentiate one another, generally acting through different mechanisms. Alcohol is very frequently one of the drugs involved, while others may be antidepressants, benzodiazepines, opioids or antihistamines. This interaction is potentially very serious and even fatal. A less well-known example, potentially of importance in anaesthetics, is the enhancement of the effect of non-depolarizing muscle relaxants by aminoglycoside antibiotics. As a final example, β-blockers and some calcium antagonists (notably verapamil and diltiazem) both produce bradycardia and can aggravate atrioventricular block. In combination they can produce severe bradycardia which may be associated with hypotension and heart failure. The latter might be further worsened by the negative inotropic action of both types of drug. Of these examples there is action at a common receptor only in the case of neuromuscular blockade.

## Pharmacokinetic interactions

This can encompass many different varieties of drug interactions, most of which will be listed here.

1. Drugs may interfere with each other's absorption. Well-known examples involve the tetracyclines, which chelate metal ions such as iron, aluminium and calcium. Iron supplements and antacids may therefore prevent absorption of tetracyclines, and the latter block the absorption of iron. Another example is the binding of warfarin by cholestyramine, inhibiting the former's absorption. Anticholinergics, including tricyclic antidepressants, and opiates, slow gastric emptying and therefore the rate of absorption of many drugs such as paracetamol, levodopa and diazepam.

2. The displacement of drugs from binding sites on plasma albumin is notorious, but its importance has been much overemphasized. Many supposed examples actually involve changes in drug metabolism which will be discussed below. Some authentic examples include, as ever, warfarin, together with tolbutamide and salicylates. Any drug that is involved must be over 95% protein bound.

3. By contrast, there are many well-documented examples of alterations in drug metabolizing systems. Enzyme inducers include most of the common anticonvulsants (phenytoin, carbamazepine, primidone and phenobarbitone), rifampicin and the antifungal griseofulvin. The list of target drugs is much longer and includes these drugs themselves as well as oral anticoagulants, oral contraceptives, corticosteroids and opiates. There are many other examples. In most instances drug effects are significantly reduced.

A well-known, if specialized, case of metabolic inhibition concerns monoamine oxidase inhibitors, which prevent the breakdown of amines such as levodopa, tyramine and dopamine, potentially causing a hypertensive crisis. On the other hand, tricylic antidepressants and pethidine can cause hypotension in combination with monoamine oxidase inhibitors. Another special interaction is the prevention of alcohol breakdown by disulfiram, metronidazole and some cephalosporins. Other drugs affect more general drug oxidizing enzymes: for instance, cimetidine, ketoconazole and isoniazid. The affected drugs include phenytoin, warfarin, theophylline and most benzodiazepines. As expected, this can produce drug accumulation, prolonged action and toxicity.

4. Finally, interactions can occur at the level of drug excretion. Urinary pH can alter the rate of drug clearance: alkaline urine enhances the elimination of salicylates, while acidification increases the excretion of amphetamines. There are some important examples of tubular interactions; probenecid inhibits the excretion of acidic drugs such as penicillin, salicylates and indomethacin. On the other hand, salicylates reduce the elimination of methotrexate, increasing the latter's toxicity. Finally, there is a very

important and potentially lethal interaction between lithium and thiazide diuretics. The diuretics promote the excretion of sodium ions at the expense of lithium, rapidly leading to toxic plasma levels of the ion.

## PHARMACOGENETICS

The genetic basis of variations in the handling of drugs, and in responses to them, is an area of growing interest. Apart from the well-investigated examples, some of which are described below, it is clear that there are many instances of more subtle but perhaps more important variations. For example, people of Chinese and Japanese origin appear to be more susceptible to the effect of β-blockers. This has far-reaching implications for drug usage, and for drug testing. Japanese licensing authorities in fact insist that clinical trials should be performed locally (though some suspect commercial motives may also play a part). This kind of variability is still incompletely understood. Most of the well-known pharmaco-genetic variations are based on alterations at a single gene. One of the earliest examples, and of particular relevance to surgeons and anaes-thetists, is suxamethonium apnea. The duration of action of the muscle relaxant suxamethonium is abnormally prolonged, because the enzyme that hydrolyses the drug (pseudocholinesterase) is abnormal or even totally inactive. Many abnor-mal alleles of the gene have now been identified. Mild forms of the syndrome are relatively com-mon and affect up to 4% of the population. The severe forms are fortunately extremely rare, with prevalence of one in 100 000 or less. Another well-defined genetic variation concerns the metabolism, by acetylation, of hydralazine, pro-cainamide and isoniazid. The minority of 'slow' acetylators, about a third or less of the population in the UK, have a greater likelihood of develop-ing a systemic lupus erythematosus-like syn-drome. A more recently described genetic dimorphism (that is to say, the presence of two genetically distinct populations) involves the oxidative metabolism of certain drugs in the liver. The prototype was the antihypertensive drug debrisoquine. More clinically relevant examples include propranolol, metoprolol, phenytoin,

nortryptiline and the now withdrawn hypo-glycaemic drug phenformin. Poor metabolizers were more likely to develop lactic acidosis while taking phenformin. However, a given dose of these drugs may also have greater efficacy in poor metabolisers.

A much more important genetic abnormality is the sex-linked deficiency of the red cell enzyme glucose 6-phosphate dehydrogenase. This plays a vital role in the protection of the erythrocyte from oxidants, including many drugs. There are at least two major variants of this syndrome, with up to a hundred rarer forms. These syndromes have a very wide geographical distribution among Africans, Chinese and several ethnic groups of the Mediterrenean basin: each of these groups has one or more abnormal variants of the enzyme. The more severe, Mediterranean, forms of this syndrome have a mild chronic anaemia with severe haemolysis on drug challenge. The African variant may not cause chronic anaemia. The drugs to be avoided include aspirin, sulphonamides, chloramphenicol, nitrofurantoin and, notoriously, the Fava bean — Pythagoras seemed to be aware of this danger! It is also inter-esting that antimalarial drugs, including quinine, chloroquine and primaquine, can also precipitate haemolysis: it is thought that the enzyme deficiency confers some protection to the red cell against malarial parasites.

Finally, a much rarer group of conditions must be mentioned, not all of them genetically deter-mined. These are the porphyrias, of which the best known is the autosomal dominant acute intermittent porphyria. Variegate porphyria is similar in manifestations and inheritance pattern, while a somehat milder form may accompany acquired liver disease such as cirrhosis. The bio-chemical abnormalities are extremely complex and the pathogenesis of the neuropsychiatric syn-dromes is very poorly understood. In general, it is necessary to avoid drugs which stimulate por-phyrin synthesis. This turns out to be an exten-sive list. Among the most important are the enzyme inducers already described, but also the short-acting barbiturates, chlordiazepoxide, chlorpropamide and tolbutamide, methyldopa, chloroquine, chloramphenicol, the contraceptive pill, and other oestrogens. It is *essential* to consider all potentially active drugs in patients with definite or suspected porphyria.

## CONCLUSION ˎ

It is hoped that this chapter may provide a brief guide to some practical aspects of clinical pharmacology and therapeutics. There are obviously many omissions. One area which must be mentioned, however, is that of adverse drug reactions. The monitoring system in this country relies entirely on voluntary reporting to the Committee on Safety of Medicines, using the 'yellow cards'. It is therefore very susceptible to doctors' apathy, or to the feeling that a particular adverse reaction is too well known to need further reporting. Often this is quite true — ampicillin and rashes, for instance — but it must be emphasized that *all* suspected adverse reactions must be reported for new drugs, marked with a black triangle in the *British National Formulary*. Even well-known reactions should be reported if they are serious or potentially life threatening.

No references have been cited in this chapter. The size of the literature is almost incalculably large, and it is usually safe to assume that clinicians do not look up primary references outside their own specialty: that is daunting enough. Instead, there is a short list of more or less comprehensive books which deal with all the above topics, and more, in far greater detail. By the very nature of books all are out of date to some extent and become more so almost daily. Fortunately, there are many sources of information which are regularly updated. The *British National Formulary* is an obvious example, as is the *Drug and Therapeutics Bulletin*. There are also many privately published magazines (e.g. *MIMS Magazine, Prescriber*) which provide valuable information on newly introduced drugs and put them in the context of existing agents. Some semi-official publications also provide data of this kind (for instance, from the Merseyside Resources Centre). As mentioned earlier, hospital and regional drug information centres can answer many questions relating to drug usage. Finally, it is occasionally worth talking to a clinical pharmacologist.

## FURTHER READING

Denham M J, George C E (eds) 1990 Drugs in old age: new perspectives (British Medical Bulletin Vol: 46 no. 1). Churchill Livingstone, Edinburgh

Dukes M N G 1988 Meyler's side effects of drugs, 11th edn. Elsevier, Amsterdam

Gillies H C, Rogers H J, Spector R G, Trounce J R 1986 A textbook of clinical pharmacology, 2nd. edn. Hodder and Stoughton, London

Gilman A G, Rall T W, Nies A S, Taylor P 1990 Goodman and Gilman's the pharmacological basis of therapeutics, 8th edn. Pergamon Press, New York

Grahame-Smith D G, Aronson J K 1992 Oxford textbook of clinical pharmacology and drug therapy. Oxford University press, Oxford

Rogers H, Spector R 1989 Aids to clinical pharmacology, 2nd edn. Churchill Livingstone, Edinburgh

Speight T M 1987 Avery's drug treatment, 3rd edn. ADIS Press/Churchill Livingstone, Auckland/ Edinburgh

Stockley I H 1991 Drug interactions, 2nd edn. Blackwell Scientific Publications, Oxford

Wingard L B, Brody T M, Larner J, Schwartz A 1991 Human pharmacology: molecular to clinical. Wolfe, London

# 28. Intensive care

*Jennifer Jones*

## FACILITIES

The Department of Health recommends that 1–2% of the acute beds in a hospital should be allocated to intensive care. The intensive care unit (ICU) demands space, equipment and, most importantly, staff.

### Space

The bed area should comprise only half the total space, so as to leave enough room for storage, staff, relatives' accommodation and a laboratory. An open-plan bed area is economical of staff, but there must be some cubicles or single rooms in which a patient can be isolated. Because the equipment at the bedside is bulky, the Intensive Care Society (1984) advises that there should be 20 m² space around each bed.

### Equipment

For the prevention of cross-infection and for the comfort of its staff, the ICU should be air-conditioned. Piped air, oxygen, suction, a monitor and a ventilator should be supplied to each bed (Intensive Care Society 1984).

### Staff

#### Nursing

The best bedside monitor is a competent nurse, and every ICU worthy of the name should have one at each bedside all the time that the bed is occupied. There should, in addition, be a senior nurse in charge of the unit. Shortages of suitably qualified nurses, and of the money with which to pay them, limit the availability of intensive care.

#### Medical

There must be a doctor always on duty within the ICU and free from commitments elsewhere. He or she does not have to be an anaesthetist, but must be able to intubate patients. A consultant should be immediately available. Although 75% of ICUs in the UK are run by anaesthetists, successful intensive care requires the cooperation of specialists of many disciplines (Intensive Care Service in the UK 1990).

#### Other

Technicians will be required to maintain the bedside and laboratory equipment. A large ICU may have its own physiotherapist. A ward clerk can save nurses from all but nursing duties.

### Scoring systems in intensive care

Scoring systems, such as APACHE, provide some quantification of the severity of a patient's illness, although their reliability as predictors of the outcome in an individual case is not established. Although time consuming, they should be invaluable for audit purposes (Intensive Care Audit 1990).

## INDICATIONS FOR ADMISSION

It should be clear from the above that intensive care is expensive, and should be offered only to patients who really need it, and who may be expected to benefit from it. Such patients fall, in descending order of priority, into three categories:

1. Those who need mechanical support of a

vital function. In practice, the mechanical support most frequently employed is a ventilator. It may also be a balloon pump, a machine for haemofiltration or haemodialysis, or even an extracorporeal oxygenator. None of these can safely be used anywhere but in an intensive care unit.

2. Those who need close monitoring. Patients who need intensive monitoring always require the continuous attention of a specially trained nurse, and often need frequent medical interventions in the shape of blood transfusions or inotropic drugs.

3. Those who need 'heavy' nursing. Under this heading fall patients (nearly always surgical) who need scrupulous care of skin, wounds and drains, and whose fluid balance and nutrition call for careful attention. Such patients need a great deal of nursing time, but a less sophisticated level of nursing skill than patients in the first two categories.

It is not reasonable to refuse admission to the ICU to a patient simply on the grounds that he or she is old. Old people can be very resilient, and have been shown to respond to intensive care just as well as younger ones with similar disorders. Equally, it is not good practice to make the ICU a final common pathway to the mortuary. For example, if a patient has respiratory failure due to diffuse metastatic infiltration of his lungs, he should not, as a rule, be supported with artificial respiration in the hope that chemotherapy will grant him a few more months of life.

## OXYGEN DELIVERY AND OXYGEN CONSUMPTION

The amount of oxygen available to the tissues is given by the equation:

oxygen delivery ($DO_2$) = cardiac output (CO) × arterial oxygen content ($C_aO_2$)

Normal values: 1000 ml min$^{-1}$ = 5000 ml min$^{-1}$ × 20 ml d$l^{-1}$ (Nunn & Freeman 1964).

Also: $C_aO_2$ = Hb concentration × ml oxygen carried g$^{-1}$ Hb

Normal values: 20 ml d$l^{-1}$ = 15 g d$l^{-1}$ × 1.34 ml g$^{-1}$ Hb at full saturation.

An adequate supply of oxygen to the tissues thus depends on:

- cardiac output (CO)
- Hb concentration
- % saturation of Hb ($SaO_2$).

The volume of oxygen consumed by the tissues at rest is given by:

oxygen consumption ($VO_2$) = CO × [$C_aO_2$ - mixed venous oxygen content ($C_vO_2$)]

Normal values: 250 ml min$^{-1}$ = 5000 ml min$^{-1}$ (20 ml d$l^{-1}$ - 15 ml d$l^{-1}$).

In normal circumstances, therefore, oxygen delivery exceeds consumption by a comfortable margin. In very sick patients, however, oxygen delivery may fall because of:

- a low cardiac output
- anaemia
- respiratory disorders causing the $SaO_2$ to fall.

Unfortunately, if they have sepsis, such patients may also have a higher than normal oxygen consumption, If oxygen delivery is inadequate to supply the tissues' needs, the consequences will be:

- lactic acidosis
- a low $C_vO_2$
- organ failure.

It is, therefore, crucial in intensive care to monitor and support the cardiovascular and respiratory systems in order to maintain a satisfactory tissue oxygen supply; and to monitor and support the function of the vital organs which demand adequate perfusion with oxygenated blood.

### Shock

Shock can be defined as inadequate tissue perfusion due to acute circulatory failure. It may be classified as hypovolaemic, cardiogenic, anaphylactic or septic (see Table 28.1). Oxygen delivery to the tissues is always reduced, sometimes critically.

*Hypovolaemic shock* is due to a reduction in the circulating volume, after haemorrhage, plasma loss (as in burns) or loss of water and electrolytes (e.g. intestinal obstruction; diabetic ketoacidosis; Addisonian crisis). The venous return to the heart is reduced, and the cardiac output and

**Table 28.1**

|  | HR | BP | CO | Extremities | CVP |
|---|---|---|---|---|---|
| Hypovolaemic | ↓ | ↓ | ↓ | Cold | ↓ |
| Cardiogenic Cold | ↑ | ↓ | ↓ | Cold | ↑ |
| Anaphylactic | ↑ | ↓ | ↓ | Rash sometimes warm at first | ↓ |
| Septic | ↑ | ↓ | ↑ at first Then ↓ | Warm at first Cold later | ↓ |

blood pressure fall. Tachycardia and peripheral vasoconstriction, reflexly mediated by the baroceptors, partially compensate for the hypotension.

In *cardiogenic shock*, the primary defect is a fall in cardiac output. Causes include myocardial infarction and cardiac tamponade. In the elderly, impaired myocardial perfusion secondary to hypovolaemia may cause acute cardiac failure. Hypotension, tachycardia and vasoconstriction are again seen, but the cardiac filling pressure (central venous pressure, CVP) will be raised because the heart is unable to eject all the blood that is returned to it.

The clinical features of *anaphylactic shock* are those of acute histamine release, often secondary to the administration of drugs to which the patient is sensitive, of plasma substitutes or of contrast medium. Profound vasodilatation causes hypotension with a fall in venous return and cardiac output. Urticarial rashes, bronchospasm and spasm of the gut also occur. There is an increase in capillary permeability, which may add an element of hypovolaemia.

*Septic shock* is due to overwhelming infection. The clinical features, which may be caused by the release of a variety of vasoactive substances such as bacterial endotoxin, are at first vasodilatation, opening of arteriovenous shunts and increased capillary permeability. The extremities are initially warm, and the cardiac output high. Later, loss of fluid from the circulation brings about the signs of hypovolaemia. Impaired organ function due to inadequate perfusion and oxygen delivery may occur in all forms of shock, but multiple organ failure, with the development of coagulopathy and the adult respiratory distress syndrome (ARDS), is a particular feature of continued sepsis.

The treatment of all forms of shock is, in part, supportive, and careful monitoring of the patient (see next section) is essential if support is to be appropriate. Support must be promptly given if organ failure is not to supervene. However, support is not all-important. Prompt treatment of the *cause* of shock may be crucial to the patient's survival. There is no point in relying simply on massive blood transfusion, attentively monitored, in a patient whose hypovolaemia is due to a ruptured ectopic pregnancy or to a leaking aortic aneurysm. Similarly, supportive treatment will not cure a patient with septic shock due to a ruptured bowel or to an empyema. Early surgery, after initial resuscitation, is the best treatment for patients of this sort.

## CARDIAC SUPPORT

### Monitoring the cardiovascular system

The measurement of cardiac output is an invasive procedure and, fortunately, is not essential in every patient in the ICU. Estimates of the adequacy of cardiac output can be made by monitoring other variables which are easier to measure. These include:

- the electrocardiogram (ECG)
- the blood pressure (BP)
- the core–peripheral temperature gradient
- the central venous pressure (CVP).

In addition, estimates of the adequacy of tissue perfusion can be made from simple clinical observations. A patient who is alert and passing urine must be supplying his brain and kidneys with enough oxygenated blood for them to function.

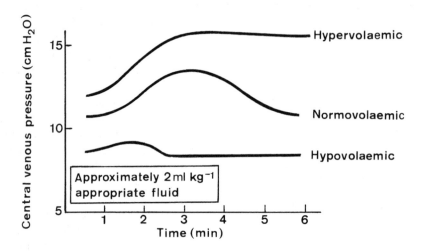

**Fig. 28.1**    Effect of rapid infusion of intravenous fluid on central venous pressure (Sykes 1963).

*ECG*

Since: CO = heart rate × stroke volume

continuous monitoring of the ECG provides reliable information of one determinant of the CO. The ECG will also demonstrate any arrhythmias; depression or elevation of the ST segments may be a warning of inadequate myocardial oxygenation.

*BP*

The BP may be measured intermittently using a cuff or displayed continuously on a monitor after arterial (usually radial) cannulation. Since:

$$BP = \frac{CO}{\text{systemic vascular resistance (SVR)}}$$

the BP is often a reliable guide to the adequacy of the cardiac output. However, in the presence of vasoconstriction, which may be secondary to inadequate filling of the circulation or to primary cardiac failure, a normal BP can be associated with a low CO. Further information on the state of the circulation can be obtained from the peripheral temperature.

*Peripheral temperature*

The core (rectal or oesophageal)–peripheral temperature gradient has been shown to be a reliable guide to the cardiac output (Joly & Weil 1969). Clearly, a patient with warm, pink feet cannot be vasoconstricted.

*CVP*

Clinical estimation of the jugular venous pressure is made by observing the level of the external jugular veins above the angle of Louis in a patient propped up to 45°. Cannulation of a central vein (usually the subclavian or internal jugular) enables the CVP to be measured, either intermittently using a water manometer or continuously using a transducer. Zero is taken from the level at which the right atrium is presumed to be (the mid-axillary line if the patient is lying flat). Because the zero level is somewhat arbitrary, and, in any event, alters when the patient moves to a different position, single measurements of the CVP are not very helpful. However, a low CVP (normal range 5–10 mmHg) which rises only transiently on the rapid administration of 200 ml intravenous fluid is strongly suggestive of an empty circulation. A persistently elevated CVP with a normal venous waveform (i.e. the high value is not due to a blocked cannula) in the presence of peripheral vasoconstriction suggests myocardial failure. (Sykes 1963. Fig. 28.1).

Central venous pressure measurement is an invasive procedure. The complications are:

1. pneumothorax
2. accidental arterial puncture causing haematoma or haemothorax
3. misplacement (check the position of the catheter with a chest X-ray)
4. air embolism if the catheter is opened to the atmosphere with the patient sitting up
5. infection—especially if the catheter is handled frequently or left in for too long.

If we monitor all the variables above, then, we shall in many patients be able to infer:

1. whether the cardiac output is adequate or not.
2. whether a low cardiac out put is due to:
   a. insufficient filling of the circulation
   b. impaired myocardial function.

We shall, further, be guided as to whether matters may be improved by infusing intravenous fluids, or using drugs to improve cardiac performance.

We shall, finally, be able to follow the results of whatever therapy we institute. In only a few patients will it be necessary to monitor any further variables.

*Pulmonary artery catheterization*

The CVP is a reliable indicator of cardiac filling (or preload) if both right and left ventricles are functioning similarly. Although the right and left ventricles function similarly in most patients, there are circumstances in which the performance of one may be impaired while the other continues to work normally.

The left ventricle is usually the one afflicted by ischaemic heart disease, with or without myocardial infarction. Left ventricular ischaemia, especially in the elderly, may follow hypovolaemic or septic shock. Some cardiac valvular lesions and cardiomyopathies affect solely or predominantly the left ventricle. Right ventricular performance may be impaired in the presence of normal left ventricular function in pulmonary hypertension of any cause. In all these circumstances, it is desirable to measure the left atrial pressure as

well as the right. It is also useful, in some patients with hypoxaemia and diffuse pulmonary shadowing, to monitor the left atrial pressure to ascertain whether the underlying cause is left ventricular failure or primary pulmonary disease, such as ARDS.

The least invasive way to measure left atrial pressure is to float a balloon-tipped catheter (often known as a Swan–Ganz catheter) into the pulmonary artery through an introducer placed in a central vein. The catheter is advanced until, with the balloon inflated, it 'wedges' in a branch of the pulmonary artery. The pressure at this point, the pulmonary capillary wedge pressure (PCWP), corresponds in most circumstances to the left atrial pressure. Deflation of the balloon reveals a pulmonary artery pressure tracing.

Pulmonary artery catheterization carries the risks of central venous catheterization, as listed above, and, in addition, those of:

1. dysrhythmia during passage
2. knotting and misplacement
3. trauma to cardiac valves
4. pulmonary infarction if the balloon is kept inflated all the time
5. pulmonary artery rupture
6. problems with the balloon:
   a. rupture
   b. leakage
   c. embolism
7. thrombosis and embolism of the catheter.

The septic complications of pulmonary artery catheterization include bacterial endocarditis, and it is recommended that, to minimize this risk, the catheter should be withdrawn after 72 hours.

*Measurement of the cardiac output*

Once a pulmonary artery catheter is correctly placed, it is possible to measure the cardiac output. If the catheter incorporates a thermistor, the method of thermal dilution may be employed. This is the method most commonly employed in ICUs. (Other methods employ the Fick principle or indicator dilution.)

Cardiac output computers are often programmed

**Table 28.2**   Properties of some sympathomimetic amines

|  | α-Receptors (agonists → vasoconstriction rise in B P) | β-Receptors (agonists → tachycardia, improved contractility, vasodilatation) | Other receptors |
|---|---|---|---|
| Adrenaline | α-agonist at high doses | β-effects predominate at low doses | |
| Noradrenaline | α-agonist | Some β₁ effects | |
| Isoprenaline | | β-Agonist | |
| Salbutamol | | β₂-Agonist | |
| Dopamine | Resembles noradrenaline at high doses | | Agonist at dopaminergic receptors → enhanced renal perfusion at low doses |
| Dobutamine | Closely resembles dopamine; believed by some to cause less tachycardia and to be a more effective inotrope | | |

to calculate additional physiological variables. For example, if the CO and BP are measured, the SVR can be calculated. Such more sophisticated information is extremely useful in patients with complicated disorders. For instance, the circulatory derangements in patients with trauma and sepsis may combine hypovolaemia with cardiac dysfunction; these patients may also have respiratory problems which further reduce oxygen delivery. The more information we have about cardiac performance, the better we shall be able to choose drugs which may improve it.

## Improving cardiac performance

*General measures*

1. Ensure that an optimal degree of cardiac filling has been achieved.

2. Correct any coexisting abnormalities such as hypoxaemia (see respiratory support), acidosis (lactic acidosis occurs if oxygen delivery is impaired), hyper-or hypokalaemia and hypocalcaemia.

3. Correct any dysrhythmias. (Apart from specific antidysrhythmic drugs, atropine raises the cardiac output in sinus brachycardia.)

*Drugs which increase cardiac output*

**Sympathomimetic drugs.** These agents act on α or β-adrenergic receptors or both (see Table 28.2 ). Dopamine in low doses improves renal perfusion through a direct effect on dopaminergic receptors (see section on Renal support). All of

these agents can increase CO at the cost of increased myocardial oxygen consumption. The α-agonists cause vasoconstriction, which may be of benefit in septic shock when SVR may be very low, but which increases cardiac work.

*Vasodilators.* (Examples: nitroglycerine, sodium nitroprusside.) These drugs bring about a fall in SVR, and reduce the work and oxygen consumption of the heart. Some of them act predominantly on the capacitance vessels and reduce CVP (or preload), which may improve the performance of the failing heart. Because the use of vasodilators is associated with a fall in BP, patients receiving these drugs must be closely monitored.

*Phosphodiesterase inhibitors.* (Examples: Enoximone, Milrinone.) Drugs in this recently introduced category increase CO and reduce SVR. Unlike β-adrenergic agonists, they do not cause tachycardia or a rise in myocardial oxygen consumption. They would appear to be most useful in cardiac dysfunction associated with peripheral vasoconstriction.

## RESPIRATORY SUPPORT

### Arterial oxygen saturation (SaO₂)

To recapitulate, Equations 28.1 and 28.2 (see above) have shown that oxygen delivery to the tissues depends on:

- cardiac output (discussed in cardiac support)
- haemoglobin concentration
- $SaO_2$.

$SaO_2$ is related to arterial oxygen tension ($PaO_2$),

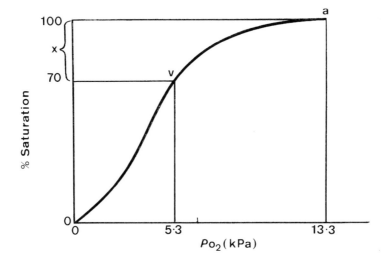

**Fig. 28.2**    The oxygen dissociation curve: a = arterial point; v = venous point; x = arteriovenous oxygen content difference.

as shown by the oxygen dissociation curve (Fig. 28.2).

Note that:

1. The normal $PaO_2$ in a healthy young person at sea level is 100 mmHg (13.3 kPa), and corresponds to an $SaO_2$ of almost 100%.

2. The $pO_2$ of mixed venous blood ($pVO_2$) is 40 mmHg (5.3 kPa), which is associated with an $SaO_2$ of 70%.

3. The normal $PaO_2$ falls with advancing age. The normal $PaO_2$ for an 80-year-old is 60 mmHg.

4. At a $PaO_2$ of 60 mmHg, Hb is 90% saturated.

*Measurement of arterial oxygen saturation*

$SaO_2$ may be continually and non-invasively monitored using a pulse oximeter. A sensing probe is attached to a finger or earlobe and the pulse rate and $SaO_2$ are digitally displayed. The device is generally reliable, although it may fail in the presence of intensive peripheral vasoconstriction, and can give inaccurate figures for $SaO_2$ if the patient has methaemoglobinaemia or jaundice. The pulse oximeter is an excellent simple guide to the adequacy of tissue oxygenation. If a patient has a peripheral pulse which can be sensed and an $SaO_2$ of 90% or more, he must be perfusing at least his finger or earlobe with oxygenated blood.

*Arterial blood gas analysis*

Most machines measure the pH, $pO_2$ and $pCO_2$ of a sample of blood directly, and will derive values for variables such as bicarbonate and base excess. It is essential to obtain a sample of arterial blood if $PaO_2$ is to be estimated, but an 'arterialized' capillary specimen from the back of the hand will give a reasonable idea of the arterial pH and $PaCO_2$. Normal values are shown in Table 28.3.

Blood gas analysis thus yields information on:

1. whether or not the patient is hypoxaemic
2. whether he is underventilating ($PaO_2$ elevated) or overventilating ($PaCO_2$ low) his alveoli
3. whether he is acidotic or alkalotic, and

**Table 28.3**    Blood gas analysis: normal values

| | |
|---|---|
| pH | 7.35–7.45 |
| $PaO_2$ | 75–100 mmHg, 10–13.3 kPa (see text) |
| $PaCO_2$ | 36–44 mmHg, 4.8–6.0 kPa |
| $SaO_2$ | 95–100% |
| Base deficit | ± 2.5 |
| $HCO_3^-$ | 22–26 mM $l^{-1}$ |

whether the acid–base disturbance is respiratory or metabolic.

### End-tidal carbon dioxide analysis

At the beginning of expiration, gas from the respiratory dead space leaves the airways first, with alveolar gas emerging at the end. Continuous monitoring of the expired carbon dioxide concentration (using infrared absorption) will therefore display a peak concentration of carbon dioxide at the end of each expiration. Since alveolar and arterial carbon dioxide tensions are closely matched, measurement of end-tidal carbon dioxide tension provides a guide to $PaCO_2$. Like pulse oximetry, end-tidal carbon dioxide analysis is a continuous and (in a patient connected to a breathing system) non-invasive method of assessment of respiratory function. An end-tidal carbon dioxide analyser is also a good warning of disconnection from a ventilator.

## Hypoxaemia (low $PaO_2$)

### General causes

1. Low inspired oxygen tension:
   a. high altitude
   b. negligent anaesthesia
2. Hypoventilation — see ventilatory failure (Table 28.3)
3. 'Shunting' of venous blood into the arterial system:
   a. pulmonary disease causing venous admixture (see hypoxaemic failure, Table 28.4)
   b. low cardiac output
   c. congenital cyanotic heart disease with right-to-left shunts.

In most patients, hypoxaemia has a respiratory cause.

### Hypoxaemia in the postoperative period

Immediately after surgery, a patient is liable to underventilate because of pain, or because of the residual effects of drugs used in anaesthesia (especially opiates and muscle relaxants). For reasons not fully understood, general anaesthesia causes a degree of venous admixture (ventilation/perfusion mismatch). If the patient's temperature has

**Table 28.4**  Causes of respiratory failure

Ventilatory failure ($PaCO_2 \uparrow$; $PaO_2 \downarrow$)
   Deranged mechanics
      Obstructive airways disease
      Chest wall lesions
         Kyphocoliosis
         Chest trauma—flail chest
   Deranged control
      Depression of the respiratory centre
         Drugs
         Trauma
         Increased intracranial pressure
      Spinal cord lesions
         Trauma above C3.4
         Motor neurone disease; poliomyelitis
   Peripheral neuropathy
   Neuromuscular lesions
      Myasthenia gravis
      Botulism
      Relaxants
Hypoxaemic failure ($PaO_2 \downarrow$; $PaCO_2 \downarrow$ or normal)
   Collapse
   Consolidation
   Contusion
   Oedema
      LVF
      ARDS
   Pulmonary emboli

been allowed to fall during the operation, he will start shivering as he wakes up and will consume an excess of oxygen.

If satisfactory pain relief is not achieved the patient will not breathe or cough properly, nor will he cooperate with physiotherapy. Retained respiratory secretions, pulmonary collapse and infection may follow. Obviously, the patient's prospects are worse if surgery has been major or if he has pre-existing chest disease, usually due to smoking. It has been explained elsewhere that poisoning the patient with large doses of opiates in the hope of providing pain relief will, in its turn, produce respiratory depression. More sophisticated analgesic techniques have complications of their own.

It may be helpful to admit a patient who is at high risk of chest complications to the ICU for a night or two after his operation. The ICU staff can provide the close supervision that a patient with, say, an epidural infusion requires. They can also monitor his $SaO_2$ and $PaO_2$, and maintain his oxygenation with controlled oxygen therapy. Chest physiotherapy always seems to be better performed in the ICU, possibly because the nursing staff here have a good understanding of it. It must be more economical to keep a patient for a short, elective period in the ICU than to admit him as an emergency with respiratory failure due to pneumonia a few days later and to ventilate him artificially for (perhaps) weeks.

## Artificial ventilation (intermittent positive pressure respiration—IPPR)

*Indications*

1. Respiratory failure, which may be ventilatory or hypoxaemic
2. cerebral oedema
3. prophylaxis.

***Respiratory failure***. A detailed list of the causes of both types of respiratory failure is given in Table 28.4.

*Ventilatory failure* is the consequence of inadequate movement of gas in and out of the lungs. Failure to excrete carbon dioxide causes the $PaCo_2$ to rise (hypercarbia), and the $PaO_2$ falls proportionately. The physical signs of hypercarbia are tachycardia, hypertension and vasodilatation in the cutaneous and cerebral circulations. The resultant rise in intracranial pressure may cause headache, confusion and papilloedema. Ventilatory failure is usually due to deranged respiratory mechanics or to disordered respiratory control (see Table 28.4). Excessive carbon dioxide production due to intravenous feeding has also been incriminated (Ashkenazi et al 1982).

*Hypoxaemic failure* occurs when large quantities of venous blood pass through the pulmonary circulation without participating in gas exchange, i.e. when non-ventilated or underventilated alveoli remain perfused. Ventilation/perfusion mismatch of a minor degree is normal; severe derangements occur if large numbers of alveoli are collapsed, or are filled with blood, pus or fluid instead of gas (see Table 28.3). The $PaCO_2$ does not rise in hypoxaemic failure; overventilation of the remaining functional alveoli keeps it at a normal level. If the $PaO_2$ falls below 60 mmHg, hypoxaemia reflexly stimulates the respiratory centre, and the $PaCO_2$ will fall below 40 mmHg. The physical signs of hypoxaemia are cyanosis and confusion.

***Cerebral oedema***. If the intracranial pressure is raised, hyperventilation can bring about a temporary fall in cerebral blood flow and in intracranial pressure. Artificial ventilation is also indicated in patients with cerebral oedema to prevent hypoxaemia or hypercarbia, both of which may cause the intracranial pressure to rise even further.

***Prophylaxis***. In a number of patients, respiratory failure may fairly confidently be predicted, and elective ventilation will prevent the development of dangerous hypoxaemia and/or hypercarbia. It has already been mentioned that some postoperative patients may benefit from a period of respiratory monitoring in the ICU. In others, usually those in whom the cardiac output, haemoglobin concentration and $SaO_2$ may all be erratic, artificial ventilation may be continued after surgery until the patient's condition has stabilized. Cardiac and major vascular surgery almost invariably demand a period of elective postoperative artificial ventilation.

### *Benefits of artificial ventilation*

In all the circumstances mentioned above, artificial ventilation will ensure:

1. the elimination of carbon dioxide
2. improved oxygenation by:
   a. reducing respiratory work and oxygen consumption by the respiratory muscles
   b. enabling very high inspired concentrations of oxygen to be administered
   c. recruiting collapsed or oedematous alveoli (especially if positive end-expiratory pressure is employed) in hypoxaemic respiratory failure.

### *Management of artificial ventilation*

1. Establish an artificial airway with
   ● endotrachial tube, oral or nasal
   ● tracheostomy.

This must subsequently be properly cared for. The inspired gases must be humidified to prevent drying of respiratory secretions, and great care must be taken not to introduce infection.

2. Suppress the patient's drive to spontaneous respiration.

a. Unless the patient is comatose or weak, it will probably be necessary to use drugs for the purpose, initially at least:

*Opiates* — provide analgesia as well as depression of the respiratory centre, and are the first choice for most surgical patients

*Benzodiazepines* — reduce anxiety and cause amnesia

*Muscle relaxants* — are inhumane in the conscious patient, and particularly hazardous if the patient is accidentally detached from the ventilator. Their place is extremely limited.

b. Once artificial ventilation is established, a moderate degree of hypocarbia or the choice of a mode of artificial ventilation which permits some spontaneous respiratory effects (e.g. synchronized intermittent mandatory ventilation (SIMV) may keep the patient 'settled' on the ventilator with minimal sedation.

3. Monitor the patient and the machine.

### Hazards of artificial ventilation

1. Complications of the artificial airway:
   - trauma from the endotracheal or tracheostomy tube
   - obstruction due to inspissated secretions
   - misplacement
2. Accidental disconnection of the patient from the ventilator
3. Barotrauma from positive pressure to the respiratory tract:
   - pneumothorax
   - surgical emphysema
4. Circulatory embarrassment — positive intrathoracic pressure may impede venous return to the heart
5. Acute gastric dilatation
6. Sodium and water retention
7. Introduction of microorganisms into the respiratory tract.

### Weaning from artificial ventilation

It may not be possible to wean a patient from his ventilator until he has recovered from the condition which brought him to it. This is a very simple point, but is constantly forgotten or ignored. For example, a patient with hypoxaemic respiratory failure due to a chest infection should be apyrexial, with clear sputum, resolution of the physical signs in the chest, a falling white cell count and some radiological improvement. It is not enough to demonstrate that the blood gases conform more closely to the ideal since IPPR was instituted. The longer the patient has been artificially ventilated, the more protracted the weaning process will be. Malnutrition, especially if associated with hypophosphataemia (Aubier et al 1985) can make weaning difficult.

A patient may be weaned by separating him from his ventilator for short periods of spontaneous respiration, which are gradually extended. Alternatively, the gradual and progressive reduction of support using a technique such as SIMV may be tried.

*Extubation* can be considered when the patient has demonstrated:

1. his capacity to breathe spontaneously for an indefinite period
2. his ability to cough effectively.

The longer the time of weaning has been, the longer the tube will have to be left in place after weaning is over.

## RENAL SUPPORT

Renal failure is a frequent occurrence in ICUs. An episode of hypotension, of any cause, may result in renal hypoperfusion and failure. Patients with sepsis may develop multiple organ failure, coagulopathy and ARDS, and in this group renal failure is often a terminal event. Generally, however, acute renal failure (acute tubular necrosis) is reversible, and the patient will recover if he is supported through his illness.

A patient who develops acute tubular necrosis will come to no immediate harm if his renal failure is diagnosed and promptly treated. Acute renal failure usually presents as oliguria, and it is crucial not to confuse it with oliguria due to some other cause. In a surgical patient in the ICU, the other causes of oliguria are:

1. obstruction to the flow of urine, most commonly due to a partially blocked catheter (NB — there are only two causes of anuria: renal cortical necrosis, which is irreversible,

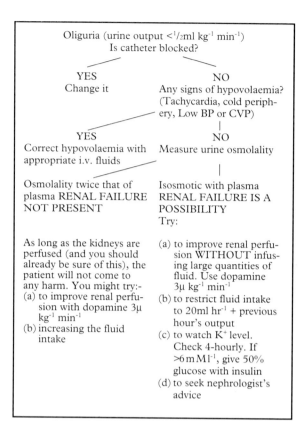

Oliguria (urine output <¹/₂ml kg⁻¹ min⁻¹)
Is catheter blocked?

YES
Change it

NO
Any signs of hypovolaemia?
(Tachycardia, cold periphery, Low BP or CVP)

YES
Correct hypovolaemia with appropriate i.v. fluids

NO
Measure urine osmolality

Osmolality twice that of plasma RENAL FAILURE NOT PRESENT

Isosmotic with plasma RENAL FAILURE IS A POSSIBILITY
Try:

As long as the kidneys are perfused (and you should already be sure of this), the patient will not come to any harm. You might try:-
(a) to improve renal perfusion with dopamine 3μ kg⁻¹ min⁻¹
(b) increasing the fluid intake

(a) to improve renal perfusion WITHOUT infusing large quantities of fluid. Use dopamine 3μ kg⁻¹ min⁻¹
(b) to restrict fluid intake to 20ml hr⁻¹ + previous hour's output
(c) to watch K⁺ level. Check 4-hourly. If >6 m Ml⁻¹, give 50% glucose with insulin
(d) to seek nephrologist's advice

**Fig. 28.3** First-aid management of oliguria in the surgical patient.

and a completely blocked catheter, which can be changed at once)
2. sodium and water retention occurring
   a. as part of the 'stress response' to surgery
   b. in response to an episode of renal hypoperfusion, past or present
   c. in response to an inadequate fluid intake.

Figure 28.3 outlines the immediate management of a surgical patient with oliguria. Having once excluded obstruction and hypovolaemia, the urine osmolality should be measured. An osmolality close to that of plasma (280–320 mosmol l⁻¹) is suggestive of renal failure, and the patient should, until the skilled advice of a specialist in renal medicine has been obtained, be treated as if the diagnosis were certain. There is little to do except:

1. infuse dopamine at 3 μg kg⁻¹ min⁻¹ to improve renal perfusion
2. restrict the basic fluid intake to 20 ml h⁻¹ plus the previous hour's output
3. watch the serum potassium, checking the level 4-hourly. If it is above 6 mm l⁻¹ it may be controlled, for some hours at least, with 50% glucose (50 ml boluses or 20 ml h⁻¹) with soluble insulin (1 unit for each 2–4 g glucose)
4. check blood gas measurements 4–6 hourly, to see if metabolic acidosis develops
5. measure and keep all the urine which is passed for 24 hours. Send 24-hourly aliquots for electrolyte and creatinine estimations. The serum creatinine level must be measured daily.

The other causes of oliguria are associated with a concentrated urine of high osmolality. As long as adequate renal perfusion is ensured, the patient will not develop renal failure. Attempts may be made to increase the urine volume by giving more fluid. They will not necessarily be successful in the presence of the stress response, but a good flow of urine is comforting to the doctor.

It is absolutely essential *not* to treat the patient who is passing isosmotic urine — i.e. a patient who may have renal failure — with repeated 'fluid challenges' amounting to several litres over a few hours. Remember the words of a wise nephrologist: 'No patient with renal failure ever died of dehydration, but, every day, one dies of pulmonary oedema'.

Of course, it is also essential to obtain expert advice as soon as possible. It is usual to persist with conservative treatment unless:

1. It is difficult to control the serum potassium
2. The serum creatinine is rising steeply
3. Fluid restriction is undesirable because of the need to feed the patient intravenously.

Active treatment, haemofiltration, or haemodialysis, is indicated in the above circumstances. Peritoneal dialysis is an alternative if the patient has not had recent abdominal surgery.

## ALIMENTARY SUPPORT

### The importance of feeding

It has been pointed elsewhere in this book

(Ch. 18) that patients who are starved break down their own tissues to meet their energy requirements. The catabolic response to surgery, trauma and sepsis promotes the breakdown of protein as well as of fat, so that many patients in the ICU are liable to sustain substantial nitrogen losses. Loss of muscle bulk in patients on ventilators may make weaning more difficult (Larca & Greenbaum 1982).

Enteral feeding is preferable to intravenous because it is:

1. cheaper
2. less fraught with complications
3. protective against stress ulceration of the stomach (Pingleton & Hadzima 1983).

Unfortunately, many surgical patients in the ICU are unable to absorb enteral feeds, and intravenous feeding must be resorted to. In some ICU patients, nutritional requirements are so large that only intravenous feeding can meet them. Enteral and parenteral feeding are discussed in Chapter 00. It has already been mentioned that intravenous feeding, especially if glucose is the main source of calories, increases carbon dioxide production, which can be a respiratory embarrassment.

### Prevention of stress ulceration

Very sick patients are liable to acute peptic ulceration, with consequent gastrointestinal haemorrhage. Routine prophylaxis is recommended, but it is uncertain which method is the best. The choices are as follows:

1. Enteral feeding, when it is feasible, is simple, safe and reliable.
2. Elevation of the gastric pH using one of the following:

a. Antacids, which may be instilled through a nasogastric tube, are effective, although large doses are required to raise the gastric pH above 4. Antacids containing magnesium may cause hypermagnesaemia in patients with renal failure.

b. $H_2$-receptor blockers (cimetidine or ranitidine) can be administered parenterally. These drugs are, however, expensive and have side-effects which include interference with the metabolism of other drugs, notably benzodiazepines, thrombocytopenia and arrhythmias.

The neutralization of gastric acidity, unfortunately, permits the colonization of the stomach by Gram-negative microorganisms, which may go on to infect the lungs.

3. Sucralfate, which has to be enterally administered, appears to have a protective effect on the gastric mucosa with very little effect on the pH of gastric juice. It has yet to be shown conclusively that its use in the prophylaxis of stress ulcers is associated with a lower incidence of hospital-acquired (nosocomial) pneumonia than is the use of $H_2$-receptor blockers. It is certainly cheaper.

### Selective decontamination of the digestive tract

Because the Gram-negative organisms which normally colonize the digestive tract have such deadly effects if they migrate, attempts have been made to decontaminate the bowel itself by the prophylactic administration of non-absorbable antibiotics. Routine selective decontamination has been claimed to reduce the incidence of infection in patients with trauma (Stroutenbeek et al 1984). The universal pursuit of the practice would certainly add to the cost of intensive care and might promote the emergence of resistant bacterial strains.

FURTHER READING

Hinds C J 1987 Intensive care: a concise textbook. Baillière Tindall, London


REFERENCES

Ashkenazi J, Weissman C, Rosenbaum S H et al 1982 Nutrition and the respiratory system. Critical Care Medicine 10: 163–172
Aubier M, Murciano D, Legogguic Y et al 1985 Effect of hypophosphataemia on diaphragmatic contractility in patients with acute respiratory failure. New England Journal of Medicine 313: 420–424
Intensive Care Audit 1990 Intensive Care Society, London
Intensive Care Service in the UK 1990 Intensive Care Society, London
Intensive Care Society 1984 Standards for intensive care unit. Biomedica, London
Joly H R, Weil M H 1969 Temperature of the great toe as an indication of the severity of shock. Circulation 39: 131
Larca L, Greenbaum D M 1982 Effectiveness of intensive nutritional regimes in patients who fail to wean from mechanical ventilations. Critical Care Medicine 10: 297–300

Nunn J F etc., Freeman J 1964 Problems of oxygenation and oxygen transport during haemorrhage. Anaesthesia 19: 206

Pingleton S K, Hadzima S K 1983 Enteral alimentation and gastro-intestinal bleeding in mechanically ventilated patients. Critical Care Medicine 11: 13–16

Stroutenbeck C P, van Saene H K F, Miranda D R et al 1984 The effect of selective decontamination of the digestive tract on colonisation and infection rate in multiple trauma patients. Critical Care Medicine 10: 185–192

Sykes M K 1963 Venous pressure as a clinical indication of adequacy of transfusion. Annals of the Royal College of Surgeons  33: 185–197

# 29. Dialysis

*J. E. Scoble   J. F. Moorhead*

## INDICATIONS

Dialysis therapy replaces the excretory functions of failed kidneys in patients with acute or chronic renal failure. As with all illnesses prevention is vital, encompassing optimal fluid, drug and infection management in acute renal failure and treatment of exacerbating factors, especially hypertension, in chronic renal failure.

It is important to realize that with most renal replacement therapies function equivalent to only 10% of normal renal function is provided. 'Dialysis therapy' uses two principles to imitate the kidney and provide effective renal therapy.

## PRINICPLES

### Diffusion

The first principle is diffusion of a solute from a region of high concentration to a region of low concentration as shown in Figure 29.1. In renal failure waste products such as urea or creatinine are present in high concentrations in the blood. Dialysis fluid, either peritoneal or haemo, contains neither, and provided the membrane between the two is permeable to these solutes, net movement will occur from the blood to the dialysis fluid. In peritoneal dialysis the membrane is the peritoneum and in haemodialysis it is an artificial membrane. It is important to note that some substances such as calcium and bicarbonate are present in low concentrations in the blood but in high concentrations in the dialysis fluid. Provided the membrane is permeable to these, net movement will occur from the dialysis fluid to the blood.

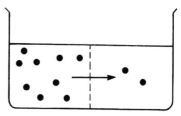

**DIFFUSION OF SOLUTE (MEMBRANE PERMEABLE TO SOLUTE)**

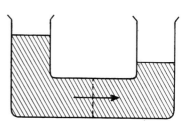

**ULTRAFILTRATION DUE TO HYDROSTATIC GRADIENT**

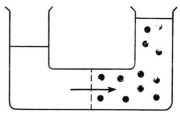

**ULTRAFILTRATION DUE TO OSMOTIC GRADIENT (MEMBRANE IMPERMEABLE TO SOLUTE)**

**Fig. 29.1** Diffusion of a solute from a region of high concentration to one of low concentration.

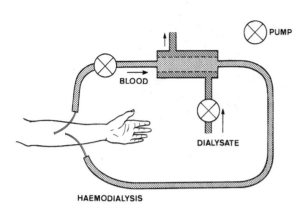

**Fig. 29.2** Ultrafiltration.

## Ultrafiltration

The second principle is ultrafiltration. This is where solvent moves through a membrane driven either by a hydrostatic or osmotic pressure difference as shown in Figure 29.2. The glomerulus in the kidney uses the hydrostatic pressure difference between the glomerular arteriole and the renal tubule to ultrafiltrate 180 litres per day under normal circumstances. In haemodialysis a pressure difference can be exerted between the blood and the dialysis fluid by using a blood pump. This results in net fluid movement. In fact under certain circumstances the dialysis fluid can be disconnected and pure ultrafiltration occurs from the blood to the perimembrane space in the artificial kidney. In peritoneal dialysis ultrafiltration occurs because of an increased osmotic pressure in the dialysis fluid, usually achieved by increasing the concentration of glucose in the dialysis fluid. As can be seen both haemodialysis and peritoneal dialysis as conventionally used rely on both diffusion and ultrafiltration.

## DEVELOPMENT OF METHODS

Although the principles of dialysis appear relatively simple the practical problems are very large. Kolf in Holland first introduced a haemodialysis machine and used it to dialyse a woman with acute renal failure. It is interesting to note that the patient was 69 years old and this underlines the point that since the beginning of dialysis the majority of patients have been in an older age group. The major problems with the early dialyses were the large extracorporeal volume of blood and access to the vasculature. The development by Schribner of a permanent arteriovenous external shunt which could be disconnected and attached to a machine transformed haemodialysis. The procedure could now be performed on a regular basis on patients with chronic renal failure rather than, as previously, once or twice on patients with acute renal failure. An arteriovenous shunt can be placed in the leg or arm, providing immediate vascular access for dialysis, but does involve the placement of foreign material in the body which may become infected. There is also the danger of accidental disconnection. Patients with shunts are limited in their ability to swim or bathe. The arteriovenous shunt still remains the best form of access for acute renal failure. The next step forward was the use of an arteriovenous fistula formed either in the fore or mid-arm. This usually involves the side-to-side anastomosis of an artery and vein. The vein then becomes large and arterialized over a period of four to six weeks. The vein can then be easily punctured by large-bore needles and large flows can be obtained. Once the needles are removed after dialysis there is no foreign material present and the patient can easily bathe or swim. The disadvantages are that steal syndromes can occur in the hand, aneurysms can form on the fistulae and, if the arteriovenous flow through a more proximal fistula is large, heart failure may be precipitated. The arteriovenous fistula is now the preferred form of vascular access in haemodialysis patients. There are, however, patients in whom it is impossible to form fistulae or in whom access is urgently required. In our unit this is achieved by a tunnelled subclavian catheter but there are many methods involving placement of a catheter into the internal jugular, subclavian or femoral veins. When suitable arteries and veins are not available or have already been used, some centres use a Gortex graft to link an artery and vein. The actual graft can be needled but if infection occurs it may prove impossible to eradicate.

Peritoneal dialysis has been used for the management of acute renal failure using a hard catheter inserted percutaneously midway between the umbilicus and pubic symphysis. This has the advantage of rapid placement in a unit not having access to haemodialysis. The disadvantages are that after 48 hours infection may occur and in many patients previous abdominal surgery makes placement of the catheter impossible. Although initially used on a weekly basis for chronic renal failure it came to be used only for acute renal failure until the late 1970s. Tenkhoff developed a soft catheter which needs to be placed surgically. This catheter has a number of cuffs on it which stimulate a local fibrous reaction. This seals the catheter track and stops both leakage and passage of infection around the catheter. The advantage of this system is that it can be used long term as chronic ambulatory peritoneal dialysis (CAPD). In this system the peritoneal fluid is changed four times a day. The advantages are that the patient is independent of any machine and is permanently undergoing dialysis, making fluid balance easier. The disadvantage is that it is relatively inefficient and peritonitis may occur, necessitating stopping this form of treatment.

## AVAILABLE DIALYSIS TREATMENTS

The dialysis treatments on offer seem confusing, with a large number of different names. The principles though are those already outlined. A glossary of what is available follows.

### Haemodialysis

This is a system whereby blood is pumped through an artificial kidney and dialysate is pumped around the fibres in a countercurrent direction as shown in Figure 29.2. The dialysate may contain either bicarbonate or acetate as a pH buffer. High-flux dialysers use a very permeable membrane but this requires specialized monitoring equipment because of potential large fluid fluxes. This method may enable shorter dialysis periods and may prevent dialysis amyloid by depletion of circulating $\beta_2$-microglobulin. Some units may still use intermittent haemodialysis in the management of acute renal failure but the management of fluid balance is more difficult using this method than the haemodiafiltration described below.

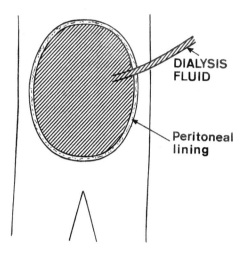

Fig. 29.3 Peritoneal dialysis.

### Peritoneal dialysis

This may be acute with a hard catheter or chronic with a Tenkhoff catheter as shown in Figure 29.3. Chronic ambulatory dialysis requires peritoneal dialysis solution to be changed four times a day with the fluid dwelling in the abdomen in between. Intermittent peritoneal dialysis is usually controlled by a machine and the patient is attached for a period of 6–8 hours and the cycle of fluid in, dwell, and out takes approximately 30 minutes.

### Haemofiltration

This is used mainly in the intensive care unit and depends on an ultrafiltrate being produced from blood driven through a filter usually by the arteriovenous pressure difference; it does not require the complicated air detectors required in a pumped system, as shown in Figure 29.4. These filters have a very low internal resistance to the passage of fluid from the blood through the membrane. If as well as this a dialysate solution is passed around the filter both dialysis and ultrafiltration can occur. With this method a clearance of approximately 20–30 ml min$^{-1}$ can be achieved. It is in essence a slow haemodialysis without requiring a haemodialysis machine.

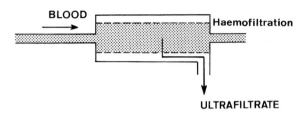

**Fig. 29.4**   Haemofiltration.

## PROBLEMS WITH DIALYSIS

Compared with a well-functioning transplant dialysis, therapy of any sort is always a second-best treatment. Many patients, however, await transplantation or have rejected a number of transplants, who need long-term dialysis therapy. The aim of dialysis is to maximize the well-being of the patient on the therapy. The quality of life on dialysis has been dramatically improved by erythropoietin. This treats the severe anaemia seen in many patients on dialysis. This in turn improves their exercise tolerance. The anaemia, however, is one of a number of long-term complications of dialysis. The first recognized was renal bone disease. Use of phosphate binders,

1,25-dihydroxycholecalciferol (or an analogue) and parathyroidectomy has meant that severe bone disease is no longer seen. The second major complication is a specific form of amyloid caused by the non-excretion of β-microglobulin. This causes severe arthropathy and may affect other organs. It is thought that some of the modern high-flux artificial kidneys for haemodialysis may decrease this problem. The third major problem is cystic changes which occur in the kidneys of patients on long-term dialysis. This may lead to haemorrhage or malignancy. This condition has been termed acquired multicystic kidney disease to differentiate it from the inherited polycystic kidney disease which pre-dates dialysis.

## CONCLUSION

Dialysis therapy replaces sufficient renal function to avoid death but it does not in any way provide normal renal function. The aims of dialysis treatment are to maximize the well-being of the patient until recovery occurs in acute renal failure or transplantation in chronic renal failure.

FURTHER READING

Sweny P, Farrington J F 1989 The kidney and its diseases. Blackwell Scientific, Oxford

# 30. Chronic illness, rehabilitation and terminal care

*A. C. Kurowska    A. Tookman*

In patients with chronic and terminal illness effective symptom control forms the basis of management. For such patients the primary aim of treatment is not necessarily to prolong life but to make life as comfortable and meaningful as possible. A significant number of patients experience functional limitations because of their disease or its treatment. Many of these can be treated by rehabilitation techniques which enable them to develop to their maximum potential.

A *terminally ill* patient is one in whom an accurate diagnosis has been made and cure is impossible. Usually prognosis is of the order of months or less. Treatment is aimed at relief of symptoms. The majority of such patients have far advanced cancer, but patients with non-malignant disease also fall under this definition, e.g. the end-stage of diseases such as renal failure, chronic obstructive airways disease, multiple sclerosis, AIDS and motor neurone disease.

A *chronically ill* patient has a longer and less predictable prognosis. Many of these patients are likely to have non-malignant disease, e.g. inflammatory bowel disease, peripheral vascular disease and post-trauma. However, some malignant conditions have a protracted course, e.g. breast and prostatic cancer.

Patients with malignancy will form a large proportion of the caseload of patients with chronic and terminal illness who are seen by general surgeons.

## OBJECTIVES

Since patients with incurable illness present with complex problems, an approach which focuses on the whole patient, rather than simply on the disease, is needed. It should:

- Address the psychological, social, spiritual and financial needs of the patient as well as their physical symptoms.
- Provide effective symptom control.
- Offer control, independence and choice. This will enable the patient to participate in decisions about the management of his problems. For the terminally ill patient this would include negotiating the most appropriate place for the patient to die (home, hospice or hospital).
- Support 'the family' (i.e. all those who are important to the patient) as well as the patient.
- Provide bereavement counselling for the terminally ill patient's 'family'.

To achieve these aims an interdisciplinary team approach is essential. The team includes the patient and their 'family'.

The proportion of all deaths occurring in hospital has increased over the last 15 years. Figures show that 65% of cancer deaths occur in hospital. The recent development of palliative care support teams, based in the hospital and/or the community, has led to marked changes in this trend in certain areas. Effective use of these teams will enable patients to choose the most appropriate place to spend their terminal illness. For example, one team has reported that of patients under their care 50% of deaths occur in the patient's own home and 34% in a hospice.

Such teams exist to provide support and expert advice to the professionals and other carers involved in the patient's management. It is therefore important that the surgeon be familiar with the local teams both within the hospital and in the community.

## COMMUNICATION

Communication with patients who have advanced incurable illness is always difficult. Chronic and terminal illness can be seen as a failure and can generate feelings of inadequacy, fear and despair in the doctors. These fears lead to the use of certain tactics in order to keep patients at a safe emotional distance.

Such tactics include prematurely reassuring patients of one's ability to control physical symptoms when the real issue is their underlying emotional fears. For example, when a patient complains of pain a quick reassurance is given that it can be got rid of rather than exploring the significance of the pain to the patient. Another tactic is the use of selective attention to physical symptoms — a patient may complain of losing weight and constipation and say 'I am worried'; the doctor ignores the worry expressed and proceeds to discuss the constipation! Other tactics include changing the topic when emotional issues are raised, asking closed questions and even physical avoidance by walking past the end of the patient's bed.

As well as avoiding the use of distancing tactics, clear explanations of the physical and functional outcome of surgery should be given. A better understanding of the rationale for treatment helps patients handle side-effects better and enhances trust in the physician. Studies of psychological reactions to cancer have shown that patients who are given accurate facts about their diagnosis and treatment adapt better to radical surgery. The opportunity to prepare psychologically for the major physical changes associated with procedures such as radical mastectomy, colostomy and head and neck surgery facilitates postoperative adaptation.

When patients have radical surgery, especially when associated with cosmetic deformity, issues surrounding 'loss' need to be explored. Such issues include altered body image, sexuality, social role and anxieties related to death and dying. The professionals involved must be sensitive to the psychological needs of patients and educate these patients in order to ease their acceptance of their new image and readjust their goals. Often these issues are not discussed at all. The rehabilitation process should start as soon as the diagnosis is made. Nurse specialists (e.g. breast, stoma, incontinence advisors, etc.) can be very useful.

There are some fundamental principles of good communication:

- The patient's concerns should be dealt with before professional concerns.
- Each topic should be fully covered before proceeding to the next.
- All the problems should be elicited before giving advice or attempting any solution.
- Non-verbal cues are very important.
- It is helpful to clarify and summarize what the patient reports.

Remember it is not always a question of 'What should the patient know?' but rather 'what does the patient want to know?'

## COMMON EMOTIONAL REACTIONS TO LIFE-THREATENING ILLNESS

### Anxiety

This is a normal reaction to a serious illness. One of the commonest emotional reactions to a life-threatening illness is fear. It is important to find out precisely what the patient fears since many anxieties are based on fears that can be resolved (see below). Normal levels of anxiety should be acknowledged and accepted; however, the patient must be assessed for signs of clinical anxiety.

Such signs include a persistently anxious mood which is subjectively different from normal worrying; difficulty in distracting the patient from his worries; feelings of tension and restlessness, insomnia, autonomic hyperactivity (e.g. palpitations, sensation of choking, etc.) and panic attacks. Anxiolytics may be helpful in this group of patients.

### Denial

It is important to assess whether the denial is causing harm (e.g. refusal of necessary medication, psychological turmoil). In many patients it represents a successful coping strategy, in which case breaking down the denial may cause unnecessary distress.

## Anger

This can be displaced onto staff and/or onto the relatives. It is important not to react with anger but to try to accept and understand. It needs to be explained to the relatives that the patient is not really angry with them, but is displacing the anger he feels towards the disease onto them.

## Despair/depression

Despair is a normal reaction to a life-threatening illness which should be recognized and acknowledged. However, it is important to look for signs of clinical depression.

The classical somatic symptoms of depression, e.g. weight loss, anorexia and lethargy, carry less importance in the assessment of patients with terminal illness as they are often a manifestation of the cancer. Important clues are a persistently depressed mood which is subjectively different from normal sadness; difficulty in distracting the patient; a lowering of interest in and enjoyment of social activities; crying, irritability, poor sleep and feelings of guilt. Suicidal ideas may be present. These patients should be treated with antidepressants.

*Common fears in patients with life-threatening illness*

- Fear of unrelieved symptoms especially pain
- Fear of death and the process of dying
- Fear of dying alone
- Fear of incompleted tasks (e.g. will has not been made)
- Fear of loss and separation (family, job, income, etc.)
- Fear of loss of dignity (confusion, incontinence, loss of control)
- Fear of altered body image
- Fear of retribution in the afterlife.

## UNDERLYING PRINCIPLES OF SYMPTOM CONTROL

A positive but realistic attitude should be encouraged and assurance given that a considerable amount can be achieved. A problem-oriented individualized approach is the key to effective symptom control. For each symptom:

1. *Diagnose the cause and treat appropriately.* An accurate diagnosis is important for good symptom control. A careful history and examination can be more revealing than extensive investigations, which can be impractical and distressing. Investigations may be important but should only be carried out if they alter the management.

The treatment of a symptom varies considerably depending on the underlying pathology. For example, in a patient with cancer, vomiting may be due to:

- raised intracranial pressure
- drugs
- hepatomegaly
- intestinal obstruction, etc.

each of which requires specific management.

Since many symptoms are multifactorial in origin it is important to recognize the contributory factors and address each as far as possible. Other intercurrent illnesses are common in debilitated patients, hence it is vital to consider non-malignant as well as malignant causes.

If the diagnosis is tentative but it is not appropriate to investigate further, symptomatic relief must be given. Very often a therapeutic trial will indicate the cause. For example, a trial of steroids would be appropriate in a confused patient with suspected cerebral metastases who is too unwell to undergo a computed tomography (CT) scan.

2. *Explain symptom to patient.* Fear is an important contributory factor in the patient's interpretation of any symptom they may have and therefore offering an explanation to the patient is important. The fact that the doctor understands the symptom and can treat it is reassuring.

3. *Discuss the treatment options.* Patients should be given adequate and accurate information on treatment options in order to make informed choices. This enhances the patient's sense of control. Therapy need not be limited to drugs. Other measures may be appropriate such as radiotherapy, nerve blocks, physiotherapy, psychological therapies (counselling, hypnotherapy), etc.

4. *Set objectives that are realistic.* It is frustrating for both patients and staff alike if expectations are set that will never be achieved.

5. *Anticipate.* In patients with advanced illness

symptoms may change rapidly; if such changes can be anticipated much distress may be avoided. For example, deterioration in a patient's condition may make it impossible for them to continue with oral medication. Such deterioration should be anticipated and injectable preparations should be available. This particularly applies in the home care setting and can avert an unnecessary crisis.

6. *Ensure relatives remain informed and supported.* It is important to treat the 'whole family'.

**Table 30.1** Approximate incidence of common symptoms in patients with far advanced cancer

| *Physical* | |
|---|---|
| Weakness | 80% |
| Pain | 70% |
| Anorexia | 70% |
| Dyspnea | 50% |
| Cough | 50% |
| Constipation | 50% |
| Nausea and vomiting | 40% |
| *Psychological* | |
| Depression | 30% |
| Anxiety | 30% |

## PAIN

Pain is a common symptom in chronic and terminal illness and one that is particularly feared by cancer patients. Pain can be alleviated or modified in all patients. Proper pain assessment leads to effective management. The principles outlined here have been developed in the context of management of patients with advanced cancer, but are applicable to patients who have non-malignant pain secondary to chronic disease.

### Diagnose the cause of the pain

The majority of patients with far advanced disease have pain at more than one site. Each pain should be evaluated individually.

In order to establish the cause of any pain it is essential to take a careful history, particularly noting:

- the site of pain and any radiation
- the type and severity of pain
- when the pain started and any subsequent changes
- exacerbating and alleviating factors.

Physical examination often confirms the diagnosis. On occasion it may be appropriate to investigate the patient with X rays, isotope bone scans, CT scans, etc..

Pain may be due to a malignant or non-malignant cause. In one third of patients with advanced cancer who complain of pain the underlying pathology is non-malignant.

It is always important to assess how significant the pain is for the individual patient — how does it affect him and alter his lifestyle?

### Common causes of pain in cancer patients

*Bone pain*

This is due to metastatic disease or local infiltration by adjacent tumour. It is characteristically a deep gnawing pain made worse by movement. The bone is often tender on percussion.

*Visceral pain*

Due to tumour mass in the lung or internal organs of the abdomen and pelvis. The tumour causes pain by a variety of mechanisms:

1. *Soft tissue infiltration.* Deep-seated pain which is due to complex pathology. The tumour invades and/or stretches pain-sensitive structures (e.g. parietal and visceral pleura, peritoneum, nerve plexuses, and local bony structures).

2. *Stretching of a capsule.* The capsule of an organ is sensitive when stretched. The most common example of this is right hypochondrial pain due to stretching of the liver capsule. The pain can be very severe, and a sudden exacerbation of liver pain may be due to a bleed into a local deposit.

3. *Stretching of a hollow organ.* Distension of hollow viscera (small and large intestines, bladder, ureters, etc.) can cause severe spasmodic pain that may be colicky in nature.

*Nerve pain*

Nerves can be infiltrated or compressed. Nerve destruction pain may be burning, lancinating, and associated with abnormal sensations (e.g. hyperaesthesia). Nerve compression pain is more often a deep ache. Destruction of nerve plexuses, nerve roots or peripheral nerves may result in deafferentation pain (dermatomal pain associated with sensory changes in the painful area). Pain of central origin (brain or spinal cord) is often unilateral and manifests itself as spontaneous pain and hypersensitivity, including dysaesthesiae of a disagreeable kind. Nerve compression and nerve destruction may, of course, coexist.

### Myofascial pain

Musculoskeletal pains are common in chronically ill patients. They radiate in a non-dermatomal pattern. Typically there are localized hypersensitive areas of muscle known as trigger points, which are tender to pressure.

### Superficial pain

In weak, debilitated patients bedsores may be unavoidable and give rise to distressing pain.

### Realistic objectives

In nearly all patients pain can be significantly modified and in many patients total freedom from pain can be achieved. In a few patients pain can prove to be an intractable symptom, unresponsive to most treatments. It is these patients that provide the greatest challenge and in whom all avenues of achieving pain relief must be explored.

### Realistic goals

- Freedom from pain at night — should always be achievable
- Freedom from pain at rest — usually achievable
- Freedom from pain on mobility — may not be achievable.

### Treat appropriately

This clearly depends on the cause — not all pain requires analgesia; e.g. the pain of constipation is best treated with laxatives, not analgesics! However, when indicated analgesics must be prescribed correctly.

### Analgesic treatment of pain

The variety of analgesics available for use in the treatment of pain can be daunting. It is better to use a few drugs really well than many badly. The following 'three-step' regimen is effective in the majority of situations:

Step 1: *'Non-opiates for Mild pain'*
    Paracetamol
If pain not relieved with two paracetamol 6-hourly move on to

Step 2: *Weak opiates for Mild/moderate pain*
    Coproxamol    Dextropropoxyphene
                      (central action)
                      + paracetamol
                      (peripheral action)
If pain not relieved with 2 coproxamol 4-6 hourly move on to

Step 3: *Strong opiates for Moderate/severe pain*
    Diamorphine/morphine (tabs/solution) or MST (morphine slow-release tablets).

### Principles of prescribing opiates

Opiates should be given so that pain is suppressed and, if possible, not allowed to break through: pain due to advanced disease is unlikely to remit. Therefore *regular prescribing* is essential.

Analgesia should be given in an adequate dose and the dose titrated upwards until the pain is controlled. Therefore there is *no maximum dose* of diamorphine.

Diamorphine/morphine *should not be prescribed* p.r.n. for pain unless it is for pain that breaks through the regular analgesia.

### Strong opiates of choice

**Diamorphine or morphine (tablets or solution).** Quick-acting preparations. Prescribe 4-hourly (day and night). The short duration of action means there is rapid response to alterations of dose. They are therefore used when the patient first starts on opiates in order to estimate the overall opiate requirement of that individual.

**Morphine sulphate slow release (MST).** Long-acting preparation. Prescribe 12-hourly. When the patient's pain is stable on 4-hourly diamorphine/morphine they should be converted to the equivalent dose of MST in order to simplify their regime.

In certain circumstances it is possible to start patients on MST straight away (e.g. out-patients with moderate pain where urgent control of pain is not necessary).

These two strong opiates will be suitable for virtually all needs. There are other strong opiates but none have significant advantages over diamorphine/morphine and most have significant disadvantages.

*Choosing the dose*

The dose depends on previous analgesic requirements.

If not on any previous analgesic start with 5 mg diamorphine/morphine 4-hourly or 10 mg MST 12-hourly.

If on weak opiate (e.g. coproxamol) start with 5–10 mg diamorphine/morphine 4 hourly or 30 mg MST 12-hourly.

If on other strong opiate use Table 30.2 to convert to equivalent dose of diamorphine/morphine 4-hourly. Titrate the dose as indicated by the level of pain control achieved.

For all practical purposes conversion of diamorphine to MST can be done on a milligram for milligram basis, e.g. Diamorphine 10 mg 4-hourly = Diamorphine 60 mg in 24 hours = MST 30 mg 12-hourly.

**Table 30.2**  Approximate opiate equivalents

| Drug | | Approximate Diamorphine equivalent (mg) | Duration of action (h) |
|---|---|---|---|
| Dextropropoxyphene (Coproxamol) | 32.5 mg | 3 | 5–6 |
| Dihydrocodeine (DF118) | 30 mg | 3 | 3–5 |
| Pethidine | 50 mg | 6 | 2–3 |
| Diconal (Dipipanone 10 mg) + cyclizine 30 mg) | 1 tab | 5 | 3–5 |
| Methadone | 5 mg | 5 | 6–8 |
| Dextromoramide (Palfium) | 5 mg | 10 | 2–3 |
| Buprenorphine (Temgesic) | 200 µg | 10 | 6–8 |
| Phenazocine | 5 mg | 15 | 5–6 |

*In summary*

If a patient has significant pain then adequate, effective analgesics should be started early.

Valuable time can be wasted using an array of ineffective moderate analgesics. In particular this can mean that the terminally ill patient may spend a substantial portion of his remaining life with uncontrolled pain. Opiates are the most effective strong analgesics.

**Routes of administration**

If the patient is able to swallow use the oral route. However, at times it may be necessary to give opiates rectally or parenterally.

*Indications for rectal/parenteral opiates*

- In the last few hours/days of life when the patient is unable to swallow
- Dysphagia
- Nausea and vomiting
- Gut obstruction
- Unable to tolerate taste/number of tablets.

Small-volume injections are more acceptable. Diamorphine hydrochloride is highly soluble (1 g in 1.6ml) and is therefore the drug of choice for parenteral use. *Subcutaneous* injections are effective and this is the route of choice. Diamorphine undergoes first-pass metabolism in the liver and therefore the subcutaneous dose should be half the oral dose.

If the patient is going to require more than two or three injections a subcutaneous infusion pump should be considered. This is a small battery-driven device that will inject the contents of a syringe over a 24-hour period. It can be used in the home as well as in the in-patient setting.

Examples of doses that are equipotent:

- 20 mg oral diamorphine 4-hourly
- 10 mg subcutaneous diamorphine 4-hourly
- 60 mg subcutaneous diamorphine per 24 hours in syringe pump.

**Fears of prescribing opiates**

Fears about prescribing opiates are common and

without foundation. They may lead to patients having effective analgesia with held.

### Fear of addiction

It has been shown in many studies that psychological addiction does not occur. Patients reduce and/or stop their opiate if their pain is controlled by another method (e.g. nerve block, surgical fixation). Since chemical dependence occurs (as is the case with many drugs) morphine should be gradually reduced. It must never be stopped abruptly.

### Fear of tolerance

This occurs only to a minor degree and for practical purposes is not relevant. If the dose of opiate needs to be increased it is as a result of an increase in pain secondary to further advance of the tumour.

### Fear of respiratory depression

With careful attention to dosage this does not occur. In fact opiates are used in the palliative care setting to alleviate dyspnea by reducing ventilatory demand and hence the sensation of breathlessness.

### Fear of hastening death

Opiates do not hasten death when correctly prescribed but the exhaustion caused by unrelieved pain can be a major contributory factor.

## Predictable side-effects of morphine/diamorphine

● *Constipation occurs in >95% of patients.* Regular prophylactic laxative should always be prescribed.
● *Nausea and vomiting occur in approximately 30% of patients.* An antiemetic should be prescribed if nausea or vomiting occurs but it is not necessary to prescribe antiemetics prophylactically unless the patient is primed to vomit (e.g. gastrointesinal tumour, already nauseated). The antiemetic of choice for opiate-induced nausea is haloperidol. Nausea due to opiates is usually self-limiting so the antiemetic can be withdrawn after 10–14 days.
● *Drowsiness occurs in about 20% of patients.* This side-effect wears off after approximately five days on a stable dose.
● *Other side-effects include:* Dry mouth, which is very common and should be treated with simple local measures; confusion and hallucinations are extremely rare (<1% of patients) and other causes should be excluded; twitching can occur on high doses.

## Narcotic-resistant pain

Some pains are either partically sensitive or insensitive to opiates. These pains will need to be managed with an additional or alternative drug or some other technique.

*Bone pain.* Although partially sensitive to opiates this pain frequently requires the addition of a non-steroidal anti-inflammatory drug (Froben 50–100mg t.d.s.). Localized bone pain can often be treated with radiotherapy. Surgical fixation may be indicated if there is a pathological fracture. Prophylactic fixation should be considered (if >75% of the cortex is eroded spontaneous fracture is highly likely).

*Nerve pain.* This is very often opiate insensitive. Steroids are useful in nerve compression. Nerve infiltration/irritation may respond to drugs which alter neurotransmission, e.g. low-dose tricyclic antidepressants, anticonvulsants. Radiotherapy and nerve blocks may also be indicated.

*Liver capsule.* This pain is partially opiate sensitive. Steroids are very useful in this context as they may reduce the liver swelling and relieve capsular stretching.

*Colic.* If due to constipation treat with laxatives! If due to tumour obstruction antispasmodics may be required.

*Meningeal pain/raised intracranial pressure.* Steroids are the drug of choice. Radiotherapy should be considered.

*Lymphoedema.* Non-steroidal anti-inflammatories and steroids can be helpful. Physical treatment plays an important role (massage, compression hosiery and intermittent pneumatic compression).

*Muscle spasm.* Benzodiazepines or baclofen can be used.

*Infection.* It may be appropriate to treat infections in order to relieve pain.

*Joint/myofascial pain.* Non-steroidal anti-inflammatories should be used in conjunction with opiates. Local injections of steroid into joints and trigger points may be of value. Physiotherapy can also be helpful.

*Superficial pain.* Patients with bedsores need to be kept off the pressure areas with regular turning. An effective patient support system (e.g. sheepskin, low-loss airbed, etc.) is helpful.

*Remember pain may be aggravated by psychological factors.* If management is solely directed at physical factors, one may fail to control pain adequately in some patients. It is important to treat coexistent depression or anxiety, and if appropriate offer counselling, diversionary activities, etc..

*Complementary therapies,* although scientifically unproven, seem to benefit some groups of patients. If the patient perceives these therapies as adding to their overall well-being then one should support the patient, provided the treatment does not harm the patient or interfere with their conventional management.

### Injection techniques in cancer pain

Nerve blocks have a place in palliative care. They are highly effective when used in a selected group of patients (approximately 4% of patients with pain will benefit). Various 'injection techniques' can be used. Although some of these techniques need expertise and specialized equipment to perform, simple techniques can be performed at the bedside.

*Nerve blocks*

Nerve blocks can be considered when there is:

- unilateral pain
- localized pain
- pain due to involvement of one or two nerve roots
- abdominal pain arising from 'upper' gut
- rib pain.

The patient needs careful assessment as to the cause of the pain before a block is carried out. This assessment will determine the exact site at which the pain pathways should be interrupted.

Many procedures can be performed using local anaesthetics and steroids. These blocks can give good pain relief outlasting the effect of the anaesthetic and are safe procedures. The pain relief from a nerve block may be transient and repeated blocks may be necessary. Careful patient selection is vital. A nerve block should not be offered as a 'last resort' but only if there is a reasonable chance of success.

Major neurolytic procedures may carry the risk of serious side-effects. For example:

- Intraspinal neurolysis for nerve root pain can produce urinary and faecal incontinence.
- Coeliac plexus block for upper abdominal pain can cause postural hypotension.
- Cordotomy for unilateral pain is a major procedure, with side-effects that can be permanent.

Once again careful patient assessment is vital.

### WEAKNESS AND IMMOBILITY

Weakness is a common and distressing symptom in patients with advanced illness. When due to general debility it is very difficult to treat. Reversible causes such as cord compression and cerebral metastases must be excluded.

It is important to acknowledge the problem and explain to the patient that it is a result of the illness. This allows realistic goals to be set, which in itself can reduce the patient's distress. Even very sick patients need to feel a sense of control of their lives and often simple measures such as a wheelchair can help them achieve this.

Steroids improve weakness in a proportion of patients. The response, however, is often short lived and side-effects, such as proximal myopathy and poor wound healing, must be taken into consideration. Therefore patients must be carefully selected and the time at which steroids are introduced has to be carefully assessed.

A patient who is immobile and confined to bed will lose muscle strength. A normal person loses 10–15% of his muscle strength when completely rested for one week and it takes 60 days to restore that strength. It is therefore not surprising that muscle weakness quickly develops in the immobile cancer patient, especially in the common situation where protein catabolism is increased. If immobility continues contractures can develop, leading to impaired ability to self-care. Contractures are more likely when soft tissue damage is present and with improper positioning in bed. Therefore in immobile patients good nursing care and regular physiotherapy are essential.

When patients are debilitated and immobile, pressure sores can rapidly develop. This is aggravated by increased protein catabolism and negative nitrogen balance as well as other factors, e.g. diabetes, steroids. Damage can be minimized if pressure on the skin is intermittent. Early prophylaxis with scrupulous nursing attention and the use of effective patient support systems e.g. special mattresses, low-loss airbeds, will limit damage and help prevent distressing pain.

Autonomic dysfunction and impaired peripheral circulation are the cardiovascular consequences of immobility. There is an increased likelihood of deep venous thrombosis and pulmonary embolism.

Atelectasis as a result of reduced aeration of the posterior lungs predisposes patients to chest infection.

Urinary retention and urinary infection are more common in immobile patients.

Immobility, anorexia and weakness lead to reduced peristalsis and constipation.

Loss of proprioceptors in skin of feet will lead to an inability to balance which can take many weeks to recover.

## ANOREXIA

This symptom is common. It occurs in approximately 70% of patients with advanced cancer. It is important to decide whose problem it is — the patient or the carers'. The family need to understand that as death approaches it is normal to lose interest in food. At this stage the goal of eating is enjoyment, not optimal nutrition.

### Causes

- tumour bulk and associated biochemical abnormalities (hypercalcaemia, uraemia, etc.)
- oral problems (e.g. thrush, oral tumour)
- constipation
- drugs, radiotherapy
- depression or anxiety.

It must be remembered that fear of vomiting may lead to avoidance of food (as opposed to true anorexia). Psychological factors such as anxiety and depression can manifest as lack of appetite. Presentation of food is important—it should be in small portions and well presented.

If the above factors have been attended to and it is still felt to be a problem for the patient, steroids can be tried as an appetite stimulant.

## DYSPHAGIA

### Site of dysphagia

The site of dysphagia can be predicted from the symptom complex. Drooling, leaking of food and retention of food in the mouth indicate a buccal cause; nasal regurgitation, gagging, choking and coughing suggest pharyngeal pathology; a sensation of food sticking behind the sternum and pain between the shoulder blades imply oesophageal obstruction.

**Table 30.3**

| Problem | Implication | Example of cause |
|---|---|---|
| Solids then liquids | Obstruction | Tumour mass External compression |
| Solids and liquids simultaneously | Neuromuscular cause | Terminal dysfunction in very weak patients Perineural tumour infiltration with head and neck tumours which damage cranial nerves (V, IX, X) Bulbar palsy |
| Painful | Mucosal causes | *Candida* (NB: only 50% of patients with oesophageal *Candida* have clinically apparent oral *Candida*) Post-radiotherapy |

## Management

It is important to explain the cause to the patient so that any dietary adjustments are understood. Restriction to liquids or soft foods may be necessary.

Any associated pain should be treated. Mucaine is useful for the local pain of *Candida* or radiotherapy, but many patients require opiates for satisfactory pain relief. *Candida* should be actively treated with topical or systemic antifungals. If patients are unable to swallow even liquids, drugs should be given by an appropriate route. A subcutaneous infusion of drugs (analgesics, etc.) is both effective and well tolerated.

If it is appropriate to attempt to relieve the obstruction, then possibilities include radiotherapy, endo-oesophageal tubes, dilatation and laser therapy. Steroids by reducing oedema may palliate dysphagia for a significant period. They can be particularly useful in the management of dysphagia syndrome associated with head and neck tumour.

Endo-oesophageal tubes should be considered in patients who are relatively independent and active, but are not appropriate for the moribund. Gastrostomy is rarely indicated in patients with incurable malignant obstruction. It does not solve the problem of saliva aspiration. In patients with carcinoma of the stomach or oesophagus, by the time severe obstruction occurs the prognosis is very short. Gastrostomy itself and its postoperative complications have a significant morbidity and mortality and can even contribute to terminal discomfort.

Nasogastric tubes and gastrostomies may be appropriate for patients with a longer prognosis (e.g. those with neurological problems, certain malignancies of the head and neck and cerebral tumours).

A belief that adequate nutrition is essential and the pressure to act may lead to overtreatment of dysphagic patients.

In irreversible total obstruction or terminal neuromuscular dysfunction secretions must be reduced to a minimum using hyoscine.

Dehydration should be looked on as a natural process in the last few days of life. It helps relieve a number of symptoms and intravenous fluids tend to exacerbate discomfort by increasing bronchial secretions, gastrointestinal fluid (thereby increased likelihood of vomiting), urine flow (leading to need for catheter), etc.

## NAUSEA AND VOMITING

Nausea and/or vomiting occur in approximately 40% of patients with far-advanced cancer. This is a symptom par excellence where the cause must be found in order that rational treatment can be offered.

**Table 30.4**

| Common causes in advanced cancer | Symptomatic treatment |
|---|---|
| Drugs | If possible withdraw the drug |
| Metabolic (hypercalcaemia, uraemia, etc.) | Treat with centrally acting antiemetics (e.g. cyclizine/haloperidol) |
| Bowel obstruction | |
| Gastric stasis | Treat with prokinetic |
| Squashed stomach syndrome* | antiemetic and/or asilone |
| Gastric irritation (e.g. non-steroidal anti-inflammatories/ gastric ulceration) | H2 antagonist |
| Constipation | Laxatives |
| Raised intracranial pressure | Steroids |

*Squashed/small stomach syndrome is a constellation of alimentary symptoms seen in patients with large epigastric mass/gross hepatomegaly. It is manifested as early satiation, epigastric fullness, epigastric pain, flatulence, hiccoughs, nausea, vomiting and heartburn.

If an antiemetic is appropriate most nausea and vomiting in patients with advanced illness can be controlled using just three antiemetic drugs. Most antiemetics act at one of the three sites shown in Table 30.5.

**Table 30.5**

| Main site of action | Class of drug | Example |
|---|---|---|
| *Central* | | |
| Chemoreceptor trigger zone | Neuroleptic | Haloperidol |
| Vomiting centre | Antihistamine | Cyclizine |
| *Peripheral* | Prokinetic | Domperidone |

Sometimes more than one antiemetic will be necessary to control the symptoms. If this is the case it is common sense to combine drugs which act at different sites, i.e. a neuroleptic with an antihistamine. The antiemetic must be delivered by the appropriate route. There is little point giving a drug orally if the patient is vomiting! Rectal or parenteral routes should be chosen in these situations. A 24-hour subcutaneous infusion by means of a syringe driver is a simple and effective method of drug delivery. (Syringe drivers are discussed in more detail later.)

## BOWEL OBSTRUCTION

Gastrointestinal obstruction occurs in approximately 4% of patients with advanced cancer. It occurs more commonly in those with colonic primary (10%) and ovarian primary (25%).

Surgical management in patients with known malignancy is indicated if the patients general condition is good, they have low-bulk disease and an easily reversible cause seems likely. Previous laparotomy findings must be taken into consideration. Surgery remains the primary treatment because 10% of obstructions in such patients prove to be non-malignant, 10% represent a new primary and approximately 60% will not reobstruct.

With conservative treatment (drip and suck) 30% of obstructions resolve spontaneously. Therefore this management should be considered prior to proceeding to surgery.

Neither of these strategies should form part of the management of irreversible obstruction in patients with far-advanced cancer. The majority of such patients have obstruction at multiple sites. The aim is symptom control with drugs. Intravenous fluids and nasogastric tubes are rarely needed.

### Medical management of bowel obstruction

Obstruction may be proximal, in which case the predominant symptom is vomiting, or distal, when the predominant symptom is colicky pain. Nausea is often more distressing than vomiting. The aim is to eliminate nausea, reduce vomiting to a maximum of once or twice a day and treat associated pain.

Baines et al (1985) reported on this form of

**Table 30.6**

| Diet | No restrictions but small meals appropriate |
|---|---|
| Nausea and vomiting | Cyclizine 150 mg per day via syringe pump If no success combine with Haloperidol 5–10 mg per day via syringe pump |
| Reverse obstruction | If constipated attempt to clear with softeners Docusate 100–200 mg t.d.s. tabs/syrup (Consider dexamethasone 8 mg b.d. to reduce oedema) |
| Pain | Diamorphine in appropriate dose in pump according to previous analgesic requirement and level of pain. Halve the oral dose to get equivalent subcutaneous dose, i.e. subcutaneous : oral potency = 2 : 1 |
| Colic | If colic persists despite the above add hyoscine hydrobromide 1.2 mg per day to pump |

*Gastrokinetic antiemetics such as metoclopramide or domperidone are contraindicated — they will exacerbate vomiting.*

management in 38 patients with advanced malignant disease. They found that nausea and vomiting was well controlled in 90% of patients, colic in 100% and pain relief was total in 90% with only mild residual pain in 10%. The median survival was three months and 24% survived >6 months.

## CONSTIPATION

The need to treat constipation is usually a consequence of failing to use prophylactic laxatives (virtually all patients on opiates should have a regular laxative). A rectal examination is essential on any patient complaining of constipation to assess for impaction. Use a laxative that combines a softener and stimulant, e.g. Codanthramer.

## SYRINGE DRIVERS IN SYMPTOM CONTROL

Syringe drivers delivering subcutaneous infusions of analgesics, antiemetics, anticholinergics and tranquillizers are commonly used in patients who would require regular parenteral medication. The subcutaneous route is simple, safe, effective and

**Table 30.7**    Drugs suitable for use in the syringe driver*

| Analgesics | Diamorphine | Dose according to need |
|---|---|---|
| Antiemetics | Haloperidol | 5–10 mg per 24 hours |
| | Cyclizine | 150 mg per 24 hours |
| | Methotrimeprazine | 100–200 mg per 24 hours |
| For bronchial secretions | Hyoscine hydrobromide | 1.2–1.8 mg per 24 hours |
| Terminal agitation | Methotrimeprazine | 200 mg per 24 hours |

*These drugs can all be combined in the same syringe.

acceptable to most patients. Indications for the use of such syringe drivers have already been discussed above in the context of pain control.

## THE MANAGEMENT OF THE TERMINAL PHASE OF THE ILLNESS

When a patient who has advanced illness enters into the terminal phase (normally a day or so prior to death) *all* medication should be reviewed. All drugs should be stopped apart from those aimed at symptom control. Communication is vital and explanation should be given to the patient and their carers about anticipated changes in the patient's condition. Reassurance should be given that symptoms will remain controlled and the patient kept comfortable. Often it is appropriate to use a syringe driver to administer medications.

*Analgesia.* This should be continued even if a patient becomes unconscious. The patient may still perceive pain and in addition abrupt withdrawal of opiates can result in an unpleasant withdrawal reaction. If a patient is on regular opiates, they will need to be continued at an equivalent dose subcutaneously. If the patient will require more than a few injections a syringe driver should be started.

*Agitation.* This can be a problem and causes must be looked for and treated appropriately, e.g. retention of urine requires catheterization. However, it is not uncommon for patients to become agitated and confused shortly before death. If a tranquillizer is indicated, use subcutaneous methotrimeprazine 25–50mg 6-hourly. Methotrimeprazine (up to 200 mg per 24 hours) can be combined with diamorphine in a syringe driver.

*Bronchial secretion* This can be controlled using subcutaneous hyoscine hydrobromide 600 µg 4-hourly as required. It can also be added into the syringe driver together with the diamorphine and methotrimeprazine. If this symptom does not respond to repeated doses of hyoscine, try bumetanide 2 mg i.m.

*Crises* In some circumstances it may be appropriate to prescribe drugs for a crisis. For example, if it is likely that the patient may have a major bleed (haemoptysis, haematemesis, etc.) prescribe diamorphine and diazepam as a 'crisis pack' to be given in the event of such an emergency. Such crises can be of great distress to the patient and the family and need to be handled with speed and sensitivity.

The rules of symptom control should always be followed, even at this stage of the illness. Symptoms should be evaluated and appropriate treatment instituted. It is important to anticipate problems and to communicate well with all concerned. It has been shown that 'peaceful' death leads to far fewer bereavement problems in the family.

## BEREAVEMENT

Support offered to the family both during the patient's illness and at the time of the patient's death not only helps them to cope better but reduces the likelihood of future complications. Evidence suggests there is higher physical and psychiatric morbidity and possibly increased mortality in those recently bereaved.

People avoid grieving individuals because they feel helpless, awkward, embarrassed, they do not wish to feel sad themselves and they fear releasing strong emotions.

## Normal stages in the process of grief

### Denial

Death represents an enormous threat to the individual. Even if the death is anticipated the reaction of the bereaved person is often one of shock and disbelief. They feel numb and immobilized. The response of the individual depends very much on the circumstances of the death. Religious beliefs and cultural background will influence their reactions.

### Developing awareness

Gradually an awareness of the reality of the loss develops and various emotional reactions can emerge such as depression/sadness, anger, guilt, loneliness. In addition outbursts of grief, with episodes of anxiety and anguish associated with crying, restlessness and preoccupation with the dead person are common. A strong sense of the physical presence of the deceased, at times amounting to a visual awareness, should not be misinterpreted as abnormal. It is during this phase that the bereaved often present to their GP with physical and psychological symptoms. Stress, irrational behaviour, lethargy and physical illness which mimicks the symptoms of the deceased are common complaints.

### Resolution

Ultimately the individual gains a new sense of self-identity and adjusts to their new role in society. Gradually there develops a resolve that they will cope, and a feeling that it is now appropriate to develop new social contacts.

## Bereavement counselling

It is important to intepret normal reactions to loss. Many people who are undergoing a normal grief reaction interpret their symptoms as evidence of psychiatric illness. For example, they may feel the dead person is present or actually see the dead person. Reassurance can be given that such reactions are expected and will resolve with time.

The survivor will need to accept the reality of the loss in order to deal with its emotional impact. It is vital that they have time to talk about the dead person so that they can identify and express their feelings. Anger and guilt are common emotions. Anger may be directed at the deceased, other family members, professionals involved in the patient's care, God, etc. Such anger needs ventilating. Depression may result from self-directed anger (guilt), thus it is important to check for clinical depression and suicidal ideas. Feelings of anxiety and helplessness may make the survivor feel unable to cope. Exploring the resources the bereaved person utilized before the loss will enable them to see that they can indeed cope. When sadness occurs the bereaved person needs to be given permission to cry.

The recently bereaved person needs to adjust to their new role. Major life-changing decisions in the immediate bereavement period should be actively discouraged. As time passes a degree of emotional withdrawal from the deceased and the formation of new social contacts should be encouraged.

It is important to identify those who are likely to have a difficult bereavement since they are at risk of developing psychiatric illness in the bereavement period (e.g. psychosis, clinical depression, extreme anxiety states) Some individuals may resort to alcohol, drugs, denial, idealization, etc., as a way of coping with loss. They should be referred early to the appropriate agency (psychiatrist, bereavement counsellor, etc.).

## Important risk factors for abnormal bereavement reaction

Those at increased risk of difficult bereavement include those:

- with a close, dependent or ambivalent relationship
- undergoing concurrent stress at the time of bereavement
- with memories of a 'bad' death (e.g. uncontrolled symptoms)
- who have a perceived low level of support (the carer's perception is more important than the actual support in determining outcome)
- experiencing strong feelings of guilt/reproach
- unable to say goodbye, who feel there are

things left unsaid (e.g. sudden or traumatic deaths or absence at the time of death).

## FURTHER READING

Baines M, Oliver D J, Carter R L 1985 Medical management of intestinal obstruction in patients with advanced malignant disease: a clinical and pathological study. Lancet ii: 990–993

Directory of Hospice Services in the UK and the Republic of Ireland 1990 St Christopher's Hospice Information Service

Maguire P, Faulkner A 1988a Communication with cancer patients: 1. Handling bad news and difficult questions. British Medical Journal 297: 907–909

Maguire P, Faulkner A 1988b Communication with cancer patients: 2. Handling uncertainty, collusion and denial. British Medical Journal 297:972–974

Parkes C M 1972 Bereavement: studies of grief in adult life. Tavistock and Pelican, London, International Universities Press, New York

Regnard C, Davies A 1986 A guide to symptom relief in advanced cancer. Haigh & Hochland, Manchester

Stedeford A 1985 Facing death. Heinemann, London

Twycross R G, Lack S A 1983 Symptom relief in advanced cancer: pain control. Pitman, London

Twycross R G, Lack S A 1986 Control of alimentary symptoms in far advanced cancer. Churchill Livingstone, Edinburgh

Twycross R G, Lack S A 1990 Therapeutics in terminal cancer, 2nd edition. Churchill Livingstone, Edinburgh

# 31. Statistics

*H. Dudley*

What James Calnan has called an 'alert' surgeon must have some knowledge of statistics for the following reasons:

1. To understand what he himself means when he uses terms such as 'probable' or 'likely'
2. To assess figures quoted in articles or textbooks for their veracity and relevance
3. To understand new methods by which diagnoses are reached
4. To participate intelligently in clinical experiments, including trials.

It is not permissible in modern clinical practice to hand a mass of figures over to a statistician for him to produce descriptions and interpretations out of a hat (more usually a computer these days but the magical element tends to persist). It is not necessary for the surgeon to have detailed knowledge of a wide range of statistical tests but some quite simple principles are as much a part of clinical education as are learning to use a knife or dissecting forceps with skill.

## THE TWO COMPONENTS OF CLINICAL STATISTICS

*Description* pools a varying number of observations into what might be called a statistical shorthand. We look for some measure of the *central tendency* (e.g. an average) of a group or series of observations such as height or metabolic rate. In addition we can calculate a measure of the *dispersion* of the individual values around our central figure (e.g. standard deviation — see p. 368 — or the range). Descriptions of these kinds may allow us to make some simple inferences — say about the usual or average height in the British, weight in Americans or metabolic rate in Bantus depending where our measurements have come from. As we shall see, measures of dispersion also allow us to say how often an observed difference from the average might occur.

*Analysis* takes two forms. First, *comparison* is the principle behind most simple statistical testing when, for example, we compare two groups of patients undergoing colonic surgery, one of whom has had antibiotic M and the other antibiotic N in order to try to prevent wound infection. Strict rules govern such comparisons if valid inferences are to be drawn. Second, analysis can break down the variability between observations into its components — such as that which may be the result of measurement errors and that which is truly a consequence of different treatments or different conditions to which patients are exposed.

## STATISTICAL INFERENCE

To draw conclusions from numerical observations involves two things. First it is very uncommon that, in making a numerical assessment, we can study all those subjects (the word is used in a general sense be they patients, rats or laboratory measurements) which create the 'population' about which we want to make an inference. It is not easy to measure the height of every Briton, or the weight of every American. In consequence we must *sample* from what we believe to be the population about which we want to draw conclusions. Obviously any such sample must represent (i.e. have the same characteristics) as the population. Here we have a circular argument: unless we know about the population we cannot take a representative sample; we do not know about it — that is why we are studying it. So the only hope we have is take what we believe is a *random sample* — i.e. one in which an individual in the population has an equal chance of being selected and consequently in which there is no bias towards, say, sex, age or any other characteristic. The detailed techniques for this are largely beyond this introductory account but we will give some guidelines later (p. 364).

If, as is usually the case, we have to sample, then any inference we make about the population must be hedged around with a statement of uncertainty or probability of how what constitutes the sample reflects the population. If we could have studied the whole population we would be certain about inferences — they would be 100% valid or have a probability of 1 of describing or analysing the population. The smaller the sample the less the probability that it necessarily predicts the behaviour of the population because, in spite of intention of taking a random sample, we may have more women than men in a proportion that is not found in the population, more old than young and so on.

## PROBABILITY

Before we consider probability further in this context let us try to define it. It is a somewhat elusive concept even though we use the term all the time in everyday speech. We can first of all define *mathematical* or *prior* probability, which is a prediction based on what we know about a system. An example would be the toss of an unbiased coin: if we concede that it will never land on its edge, then it is plausible to say that in a long run of tosses it will come down on half the occasions heads and the other half tails. We can say that the probability is 0.5 for a head and 0.5 for a tail. However, even with our prior understanding of the system, we cannot tell from this statement whether the next toss will be a tail or a head and therefore when we talk about probability in practice we usually mean the quantifying of the occurrence of events over a long run of experiences. This is sometimes called *numerical* or *frequentist* probability and in our coin-tossing example implies that if we toss a coin a hundred-

times we would expect to get roughly fifty heads and fifty tails, though we might observe some slight imbalance unless we carried on our experiment to many thousand tosses. So when we say that the probability of an occurrence of a serum bilirubin concentration of 2.5mmol $1^{-1}$ is 0.02 we are indicating that in a long series of observations that value will turn up twice in a hundred samples taken from what we believe to be a healthy population.

Such a definition of probability also applies to the interpretation of statistical analysis. If we say that it is *probable* ($p < 0.05$) that two treatments differ, what we mean is that if we were to repeat the comparison between them a hundred times only five times in those repetitions would we fail to find a difference. We will discuss later how we can transfer such a statistical statement into a biological one (p. 374).

There are some simple rules about probability which we need to assume not only for statistical purposes but also when we consider diagnosis (see p. 376). Their logicomathematical basis need not concern us. They are:

1. The sum of independent probabilities must always equal 1. Thus if we are thinking about three horses in a race one may have a probability of 0.5 of winning, one of 0.3 and one of 0.2 (always assuming that all three do not fall at the first fence which in this calculation is given a probability of zero). Similarly for diseases. Given that there are three diagnostic possibilities only, then each will have a probability based on the evidence available but their sum cannot equal more or less than one.

2. The simultaneous occurrence of two or more independent events is the multiplicand of their separate probabilities. The probability of my having an acute torsion of the testis (say 0.005) and acute appendicitis (say 0.2) together as the cause of my right iliac fossa pain would be 0.005 × 0.2 or 0.001.

From the foregoing it is apparent that the major task of statistics is to quantify uncertainty in terms of probability values and that this is done against the framework of what will happen if we try things over and over again.

## HYPOTHESES AND THEIR EVALUATION

When we use statistical description or analysis we most usually have some expectation of what we are going to find — what sort of central tendency and dispersion or what degree, if any, of difference in a comparison. In regard to the latter, statisticians and surgical biologists have a problem of communication because of the different way they tend to set up their expectations or, to use the technical word, hypotheses. A biologist is usually interested in a comparison that is expected to yield a difference and he *designs his experiment* accordingly, though in fairly rare circumstances he will want to disprove a difference, say between the outcome of two operations. The statistician by contrast, conducts his analysis using the concept of the 'null hypothesis' — i.e. the starting point is the assumption that a difference does not exist. There is of course nothing incompatible about the two approaches but it does sometimes cause confusion in writings about statistical analysis.

In clinical work there is an advantage in distinguishing between a *specific* and a *non-specific* hypothesis as a challenge to the null hypothesis. To explain more precisely what is meant by this, we may take as our starting point the null hypothesis that there is no difference in terms of local recurrence in a patient with breast cancer and positive axillary lymph nodes between simple mastectomy and axillary sampling with selective treatment for those positive and simple mastectomy and routine axillary clearance. The alternative hypothesis could take the form that there is a difference but its magnitude is not defined — it is merely a biological fact that we should be interested in demonstrating and then exploring further. This is a non-specific alternative and merely states that the null hypothesis is false. A specific alternative hypothesis is that we would be interested only in a difference of a defined magnitude — say a 10–20% reduction by one method of treatment with respect to the other. The one approach aims at explanation in a biological sense; the other at the practical side of how we are going to proceed. Choosing between the two objectives may be important in defining the size of the samples we have to take as well as in the non-statistical sense of deciding what is really important for our patients and the health system in which we work. A decision on whether we are out to establish or refute a non-specific or a specific hypothesis is thus an important part of the design of a comparison.

## PROBING THE TRUTH OF HYPOTHESES — WHAT NUMBERS DO WE NEED?

Because we have to sample, there is always, as we have seen, an element of uncertainty about our inferences in relation to the population from which we believe the sample has been taken. What we must now explore is how prepared we are:

1. to accept that the null hypothesis is true (a real difference does not exist) when our results suggest that it is false and
2. to risk that the null hypothesis is false (some difference really does exist) but that our sampling and testing has failed to detect the fact.

We have already, in considering probability, implied the answer to the first. When we say our results can be interpreted that there are less than five chances in a hundred repetitions of the experiment which will give us an answer we would interpret differently (though of course this does not mean exactly the same numerical answer) we are effectively rejecting the null hypothesis. Statisticians call this the $\alpha$ probability or the probability of a type I error. The conventional level is 0.05 but the stringency is determined by context. For example, it would not be satisfactory for interpretation of comparative data from two channels of data in an aircraft's blind landing system to accept that there would be five chances in a hundred that they could safely disagree. Similarly if we are going to base our clinical behaviour in a life-threatening problem or one with considerable morbidity on the outcome of some statistical comparison then we might want to set our level of falsely rejecting conventional practice (the null hypothesis) at one chance in a hundred or even one in a thousand. To achieve this goal will in many circumstances require a larger sample so that it is important in designing the experiment to decide what $\alpha$ probability we feel is necessary.

Our second statement is what Feinstein has termed 'the other side of statistical significance' — failing to reject the null hypothesis when there is a difference really present. Such is a type II error and the chance that we might commit it is known as the $\beta$ probability. The bigger our samples, the more precisely do they tend to define the underlying population and its variability and the more sensitive should be comparisons to detect a difference between subsamples. We can set a $\beta$ probability based on the importance of the difference we think may be there and of the need to detect it.

Finally, defining a specific alternative hypothesis is the last thing needed to determine sample size. If we want to reject the null hypothesis in favour only of a big difference then we may not need very large numbers to find out that we cannot do so. However, if we are interested in a very small difference we may have to take large samples so as not to miss it.

## POWER

We can conclude the foregoing discussion, and particularly that related to type II errors, by referring to what is currently an 'in' word — power. The power of an *investigation*, by which we mean the overall study, is its ability to avoid failing to find a difference which exists in nature. The power of a statistical *test* is its ability, given the size of the difference expected and the size of the sample, to detect such a difference. Ideally for both we would like power to be 100% but usually we have to settle for less. Surgeons, when designing statistical comparisons, need to make an estimate of power in both senses. Ultimately to ensure statistical respectability they need also to obtain statistical advice. Though they must heed this, they must also recognize that it is not always enlightened by a clear understanding of the clinical problem, particularly in terms of the alternative hypothesis. In practice, the best way of not becoming too involved in statistical subtleties is to choose a problem for which a large difference is likely to be found on biological grounds, to make sure that it is possible to recruit a very large sample and to refine measurement so that it is as precise as possible. Then statistics will either not

be needed or will be simple to carry out and should provide an unequivocal answer.

Given that we have followed the pathway outlined above and defined the size of a difference we are interested in (i.e., the alternative hypothesis) and the level of $\alpha$ and $\beta$ that we will accept, then there are statistical techniques and tables which will give us the appropriate sample size. A 'guesstimate' of this kind is an essential preliminary to undertaking a comparison especially in that it may tell you that the sample size is much larger than it is possible to achieve either from the pool of patients available or with the time and resources at your disposal.

## A LITTLE MORE ABOUT SAMPLING

We have defined random sampling as taking a number of individuals from a population using some technique to ensure that each member of it has an equal chance of being chosen. We have also said that this is difficult if we do not know about the population. However, in clinical practice we often have to deal with an 'available' sample such as all Mr W's out-patients or Miss M's in-patients operated upon for a particular condition. Because of this we must be careful not to make inferences beyond these boundaries to draw the same conclusion about, say, Professor N's patients unless it can be shown that the last group is comparable in a large number of ways — such as age, sex and stage of disease. Even then, it is wise to be cautious both in inference and in pooling Professor N's patients with those already studied (see meta-analysis, p. 373).

In clinical work we are more often interested in making what might be called an *internal comparison*. We have two antibiotic regimens proposed for the prophylaxis of wound infection. Which is the better? For this purpose we take all the patients at our disposal and randomly allocate them to one or other agent (Fig. 31.1). We are then creating two random *subsamples* in which we expect all characteristics to occur with approximately equal frequency, so that we do not introduce extraneous factors which might alter the outcome in one way or another. Two such subsamples would be the simplest but in theory we could have any number. The process of random

## SAMPLING

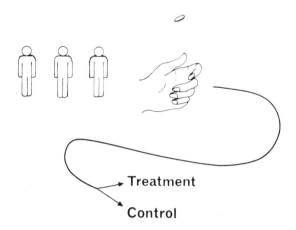

**Fig. 31.1**   Allocating to random treatment from an available queue of patients.

allocation into subsamples can be done using a table of random numbers (e.g. an odd number assigns to one subsample and an even to the other) a computer random number generator, envelopes drawn from a prepared pack or odd–even birth dates. Alternate allocation is *not* random.

### Checking the randomness of subsamples

We can obtain some (though not complete) reassurance that the chosen technique of randomization has worked  by carrying out an analysis of some biological features of the subsamples — for example, in the case of patients such matters as height, weight, age and sex. Unless our subsamples are enormous we would not expect them to be identical in these characteristics but we would think that they should be nearly so. Mathematically we can do this by the appropriate statistical comparison, which can give us a probability for how the observed numbers relate to chance. The details do not concern us here but it is worth noting that such a check is less often done than it should be. We must finally note that an internal comparison of the kind we have described means that we can only make *direct* inferences about the study subsamples. The same restraints apply to generalizing the information to all patients treat-

ed in the same way. We shall consider this matter in more detail below.

## SCALES OF MEASUREMENT AND THE CHOICE OF STATISTICAL DESCRIPTIONS AND COMPARISONS

Measurement is essential to our understanding of the physical–scientific world. We can, somewhat arbitrarily, distinguish three scales (Fig. 31.2): *Nominal* or *categorical*, such as male/female (Fig. 31.2A); *ordinal*, where we can state a difference but not its precise magnitude, such as taller/shorter, lighter/heavier (Fig. 31.2B); and *interval*, when we refer what we measure to an established scale such as a metre stick or a weighing machine usually with equal intervals specifying its points but, in its ideal form, continuous (Fig. 31.2C). It is obvious that our arbitrary scales shade into one another. Male may be male and female may be female but intermediate forms exist; black is black and white is white but we all recognize grey. Continuing the analogy, we recognize spectral colours in a rainbow but we can define light more precisely in terms of wavelength, though even here, as with all interval measures, how precisely we do so is determined by the instruments we have available. The scale against which a measurement is made has a considerable effect on both statistical description and analysis.

*Categorical scales* lead to descriptions which are usually expressed as proportions — the ratio of male to female or the percentages of a sample who are Caucasian or Caribbean. Proportions can lose a lot of their meaning if they are carried to absurdity, as for example when we say that for every female on the waiting list for hernia surgery there are 3.35 males. What is 0.35 of a male? For statistical comparison of proportions the tests used are usually based mathematically on the binomial theorem. The two commonest are the $x^2$ statistic (see Box 1, p. 366) and Fisher's exact test.

*Ordinal scales* tell us the position of individual values in the rank of all the measurements made — any value (except those at the two extremes) is greater than, less than or equal to some other. For descriptive purposes we can use the rank order to determine the central value, which is known as the *median*. In an odd-numbered series

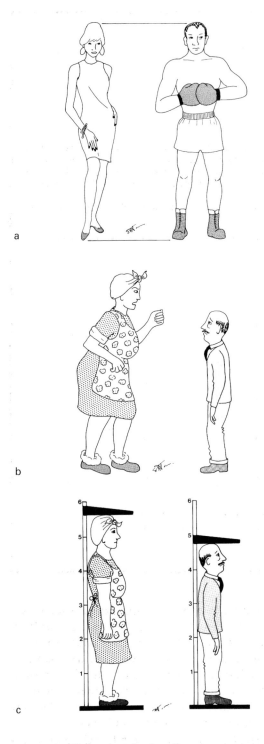

a

b

c

**Fig. 31.2** The concept of scales of measurement:
(a) Categorical — male and female; (b) Ordinal — I am
bigger than you; (c) Interval — I am 5ft. 9 inches; you are
4 ft. 10 inches.

---

**Box 1**

A $2 \times 2$ contingency table for two different methods of managing a condition reads as follows:

| Treatment | Outcome | | | | | | |
|---|---|---|---|---|---|---|---|
| | Death | | Survival | | | | |
| A | 41 | (a) | 216 | (b) | 257 | $(r_1)$ | |
| B | 64 | (c) | 244 | (d) | 244 | $(r_2)$ | |
| | 105 | $(s_1)$ | 396 | $(s_2)$ | 501 | $(N)$ | |

Where the letters in parentheses indicate the cells of the table.

The statistic we wish to calculate is a comparison of the observed values with those that would be expected if there was no difference between A and B. For example, the expected value for deaths under treatment A would be:

$$\frac{\text{total deaths } (105)}{\text{total patients } (501)} \times \text{total treated by A} \quad (257)$$

This is 54, so we have a difference between observed and expected of −13. To be able to manipulate this we square it (to get rid of any negative sign) and divide it by the expected value.
Our statistic is then:

$$\frac{(O-E)^2}{E}$$

or

$$\frac{(41-54)^2}{54} = 0.313$$

It is clear that the bigger the discrepancy between the observed and expected values, the bigger the statistic is going to be.

We make this calculation for each cell in the table and add them together. Statisticians have calculated the chance (probability) of values for this statistic $x^2$ occurring by chance and we can read these from a table. For example, $x^2$ for the table above is 7.37 (using a slightly more sophisticated method of calculation which includes a correction factor), for which $P < 0.05$. On statistical grounds, treatment A is preferable to treatment B.

**Box 2**

If we have two sets of data we can order them by rank using the convention: low value = lowest rank. We assign ranks to both sets in ascending order.

There are four possibilities shown below:

1.  All *x*s have a lower rank than all *y*s.
2.  All *y*s have a lower rank than all *x*s.
3.  The ranks of *x*s and *y*s alternate.
4.  There is a 'mix' of ranks between the *x*s and the *y*s.

It is intuitively obvious that for 1 and 2 the *x* and the *y* samples are not likely to have come from the same population, whereas in 3 there is no way of denying that they might have done. In 4 there is some probability that they might be either from the same or from different populations and this can be determined mathematically from a knowledge of the sample size and the rank sum for one sample (which automatically determines the rank sum for the other). The values are read off against probability tables.

(For more detail see Meddis 1983. For simplicity in this explanation paired values in the *x* and *y* samples have been ignored.)

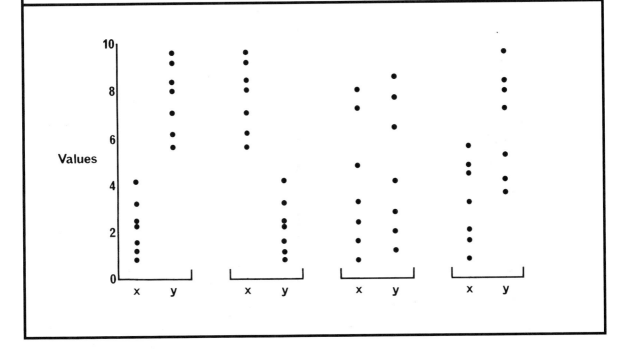

the median is truly the middle number; for an even numbered series it is defined as the average of the two central values. Dispersion of the values should strictly only be given by the range of the values from lowest to highest but we can refine that by looking at the range that encloses either a given proportion of the values observed (quartiles, for example). Comparative analysis of ordinal data must be done with a method which compares rank order (see Box 2). Such tests (also generically often referred to as *non-parametric*) have the additional advantage that they do not make any

assumptions about how the measurements are dispersed (*distributed* is the technical word) in some underlying population from which the samples have been drawn. Thus these tests are also often appropriate for comparisons of samples in which the measurements have been made on interval scales but we cannot assume the way they are distributed in the population.

*Interval scales* permit the relatively precise assignment of a number to a measurement and thus the use of arithmetic. The central value is the *average* or *mean* obtained by summing all the

## Box 3

Two normal curves are shown below. In the first is a set of values for the concentration of serum sodium in a large sample that we assume is biologically normal. The vertical lines are placed at one and two standard deviations from the mean (most frequent) value, which in this instance is 135 mmol 1⁻¹. Because of a mathematical relationship which need not concern us here, one standard deviation on either side of the mean encloses approximately 66% of the values and two standard deviations 95%. The two 'tails' shown as hatched areas thus each represent 2.5% of the population. The second figure shows this in graphical terms. Given a value of serum sodium concentration greater or less than the mean we can compare it with the curve and say that it lies either within one or two or more standard deviations from the mean: we can then translate that into a probability statement to say that it has a probability of 0.33, 0.25 or less of being representative of the normal population.

Statisticians generalize this argument by transforming the curve so that it has a mean of zero and as in the second figure is charted in terms of an *x*-axis expressed as standard deviations. It is then possible to calculate a *standardized deviate*, which is the ratio of the distance a value is from the mean to standard deviation (the measure of the dispersion of all values). When the curve is expressed in this way we can assign a probability to the values of the standardized deviate obtained. For example, a value of 145 mmol 1⁻¹ would have a standardized deviate of 1.194, the probability of occurrence of which would be $P > 0.05$.

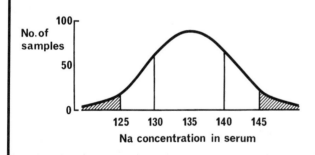

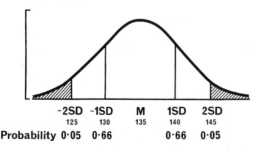

## Box 4

### SENSITIVITY AND SPECIFICITY

One hundred and eighty patients with suspected abdominal trauma undergo peritoneal lavage. A cut-off point of positive is selected at 50 000 red cells per cubic millilitre. All patients have an end-point confirmation by laparotomy, autopsy or a benign course without intervention. The results are:

No. of red cells in lavage

|  |  | >50 000 | <50 000 |
|---|---|---|---|
| Intervention | Yes | 75 | 25 |
|  | No | 18 | 62 |

False positive rate $= \dfrac{25}{100} = 25\%$

False negative rate $= \dfrac{18}{80} = 22.5\%$

Sensitivity $= 100 - 25 = 75\%$
Specificity $= 100 - 22.5 = 77.5\%$

Suppose we 'move the goal posts' and set the cut-off at 25 000 red cells per cubic millilitre:

No. of red cells in lavage

|  |  | >50 000 | <50 000 |
|---|---|---|---|
| Intervention | Yes | 90 | 10 |
|  | No | 70 | 10 |

False positive rate $= \dfrac{10}{100} = 10\%$

False negative rate $= \dfrac{70}{80} = 87.5\%$

Sensitivity $= 100 - 10 = 90\%$
Specificity $= 100 - 87.5 = 12.5\%$

By making this change we have increased the *sensitivity* of the test but have greatly reduced its *specificity*.

values and dividing by their number. Dispersion is summarized by squaring the deviations of the values from the mean, adding them together and again dividing by the number of observations (or more precisely in the case of a sample by one less than this). This gives an 'average' value for the squared deviations about the mean in both directions and is known technically as the variance. The square root of the variance is the *standard deviation* (SD). If the dispersion of values around the mean is symmetrical we can draw either an approximate (for a sample) or an ideal curve (for a population) which is the familiar bell-shaped one for which one standard deviation from the mean embraces about 66% and two standard deviations about 95% of the values (see Box 3). The mathematics of this curve are well understood by statisticians but not commonly (or necessarily) by surgeons. What we must note is that the word normal has not quite the same sense as it does in biology (see p. 375). A further descriptive measure of variation is the standard error of the mean (SEM), which is an estimate of the likely variation that would be found in the mean if the experiment was repeated many, many times. Its value is found by taking the square root of the standard deviation divided by the number of observations in the sample. It is *not* a good measure for description of the sample as a whole and when investigators show SEMs in diagrams it usually means that they are trying to minimize what is in fact a wide dispersion of their results. However, it has other important uses in relation to confidence intervals (see p. 375).

The analysis of data on an interval scale is often known as *parametric* and is based on the assumption that the observations are derived from a population in which the values are 'normally' distributed. We can redraw it as one of 'probability density'. The maximum frequency of values is at the mean and therefore the mean is the 'most probable' value. Moving away from the mean the values get less frequent so that by the time we reach two SDs the probability is down to five times in a hundred (0.05) that this value will be found (see Box 3 for further details).

We are less often interested in determining the probability of a single value wtih respect to a mean than we are in comparing two sets (samples) of values to see if they are probably or improbably drawn from the same population (this is a precise statistical statement but what we are really doing is seeing if they are different in some respect which would make it unlikely that if that population existed they would plausibly represent it). The principle is the same as that outlined in Box 3: a ratio is calculated which relates differences between the samples (differences of the means) to their dispersion (their standard errors). This ratio will be large if there is a large difference between the means and/or a small standard error and small if the reverse holds true. This is one form of the familiar '$t$' statistic that crops up in so much biological work.

Analysis of variance (ANOVA), which gives a partition of the variability within and between samples, is based on a similar argument but will not be gone into here.

*Note*. The statistical expert will point out that nothing has been said about either 'estimates' or 'degrees of freedom.' These are technical statistical terms which govern probability calculations. Degrees of freedom are equivalent to the number of independent comparisons that can be made between items in a sample, which in turn is usually one less than the number of observations. Any deeper consideration is beyond the immediate needs of the surgical biologist.

## OTHER FORMS OF STATISTICAL ANALYSIS

### Regression

It is sad that the general mathematics of statistics are beyond the comprehension of most of us, because it is possible to derive nearly all the common analytic techniques which are used in clinical work by starting with regression. To be able to do so would simplify the whole matter of trying to understand statistical reasoning because it would show that there is such a common and unified background. Anyone who is serious about more advanced statistical applications to clinical and biological work should attempt to grasp some of the theory of regression analysis, but most surgeons will probably be content with a nodding acquaintance.

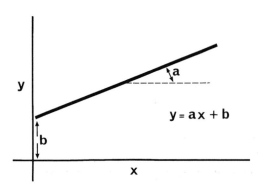

Fig. 31.3   Two dimensional Cartesian coordinates: *a* is the *slope* of the curve; *b* is the *intercept*.

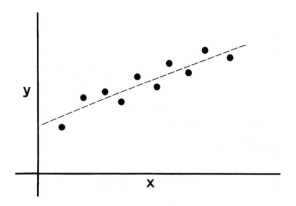

Fig. 31.4   A 'real life' curve with the values to one or other side of the perfect line.

Everyone is familiar with Cartesian coordinates (Fig. 31.3) and indeed they have already appeared in this account. A straight line drawn with reference to these can be described algebraically as a simple linear equation with three terms:

$$y = ax + b$$

which simply means that when $x = 0$ $y = b$ and as $x$ changes value so will $y$. In this sense the values of $x$ and $y$ are *co-related* and it is usual to say that $y$ is the *dependent* variable. Of course a lot of biological relationships are much more complicated than this but the linear model is the one most important for statistical work.

The relationship described by the equation is an ideal one — the sort we might hope to get, for example, when we calibrate a measuring instrument, when if it is a 'good' instrument we will get a series of values for $y$ which correspond to known values of $x$ so that a straight line can be drawn directly through them. However, in real life it is more usual to find — either because of the inaccuracies of the observations we make or because there are other 'disturbing' factors which affect the value of $y$ — a plot which looks more like Figure 31.4. There is still indubitably a relationship present — as $x$ gets bigger so does $y$, but it is now less precise.

We can do four things with the data in Figure 31.4:

1. we can 'fit' a straight line to it, which is done by finding the linear equation of a line that passes as close as possible to all the points. The mathematical way of doing this is to minimize the sums of the squares of deviations from the line and for this reason the method is known as 'least squares'. We will not give the details of the calculation — they can be found in any text on statistics and computer programs are available to do the work for you.

2. we can derive a statistic which gives some idea of how far from the line the individual values of $y$ are and thus how much of the value of $y$ can be ascribed to (or correlated with) the value of $x$. The usual statistic for this is the correlation coefficient ($r$) which, for mathematical reasons that do not concern us, ranges from $+1$ through 0 to $-1$. The correlation is 1 in Figure 31.3 and somewhat less than 1 in Figure 31.4; if there is no relationship of the values of $y$ to $x$ then the coefficient is 0; and if it is $-1$ then the relationship is again perfect but in this case as $x$ gets bigger, $y$ gets smaller.

Though the correlation coefficient has a distinguished statistical history it is not a very good measure and to the unsophisticated may be frankly misleading. It does not give a *direct* estimate of the amount of variability of $y$ that is related to change in $x$ though this can be obtained by squaring the coefficient. Thus a correlation coefficient of 0.5 means that a quarter of the variability of $y$ is associated with $x$. Further, it does not tell us anything about the *slope* of the regression line.

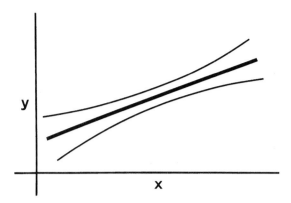

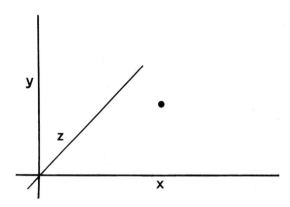

**Fig. 31.5** Confidence limits for the data shown in Fig. 31.4. Values within the confidence limits have a given probability (usually 95% or 0.95 is the level chosen) of being part of the population described by the curve.

**Fig. 31.6** Three dimensional Cartesian coordinates. A $y$ value for a given value of $x$ and $z$ will be found somewhere in the space enclosed by the coordinates.

Very precisely measured values of $x$ and $y$ may give us a coefficient which is highly significant (i.e. highly significantly different from 0) but in which there is only a very small change in $y$ for a given change in $x$, and the result is therefore not of much interest to us.

3. we can use a regression line to predict a value of $y$ from a value of $x$. How precisely this can be done depends on how tightly the observed values of $y$ relate to the regression line, which also means how close to 1 is the correlation coefficient. We can get a numerical idea of this by calculating a confidence interval — usually that which encloses 95% of the possible values of $y$ — shown as the curved lines in Figure 31.5. At the extremes of the range for measurements of $x$ these confidence lines get further away from the fitted line but the reason for this need not concern us — only that the prediction of $y$ from $x$ becomes less and less precise.

4. if we have two different sets of data which purport to relate $x$ and $y$ then we can draw two regression lines and see if either their slope and intercept are the same or different and calculate how likely this is the outcome of a real difference or could have arisen by chance. The difference can take two forms: differences in intercept and differences in slope. The techniques can be found in Gardner & Altman (1989).

So far this discussion has concentrated on the simplest case of two-dimensional Cartesian co-ordinates. However, we do not need to stop there. We can easily envisage a three-dimensional system where the value of $y$ is related to the value of two variables $x$ and $z$; the point shown in Figure 31.6 is in the three-dimensional 'space' defined by the $x$, $y$ and $z$ coordinates. Going beyond this into four or higher-dimensional spaces is not easy to visualize but is mathematically possible and is the basis for *multiple linear regression*, in which the dependence of $y$ on a defined number of variables is calculated. This gives the biologist (often an epidemiologist) the chance to work out how much, say, peripheral arterial disease (appropriately defined) is related to age, sex, smoking, serum cholesterol level and so on.

## CLINICAL TRIALS

### Prospective randomized controlled clinical trials (PRCCTs)

These are a special case of statistical comparison. There is an established treatment (this can be either an operation or a drug) and a new way of managing a clinical situation. How do we decide whether to adopt the new or persist with the old?

We set up an experiment so that by sampling as described on p. 364 we create two random sub-samples, one of which receives the standard treatment and the other the new one. We need the following to be considered carefully before such a study can be successful:

1. A precisely defined outcome measure — life or death, wound infection or no wound infection.

2. How big a difference (alternative hypothesis) are we interested in — i.e. how big a difference has there to be to alter our clinical behaviour?

3. In consequence of the size of the difference how many patients will we have to study in order to avoid type I and type II errors?

4. Can we find and randomize that number of patients for our study?

5. How 'blind' — by which is meant neither the patient, the investigator nor any assessor of outcome knows who has had what treatment — can we make the study? It is easy to blind both patient and investigator to a pill by having a dummy version to act as a placebo. It is more difficult to blind the surgeon to which operation he does or the patient to whether he has or has not had an operation.

Another important factor in surgical prospective randomized trials is what might be called 'technical efficiency'. Every surgeon knows that he or she is comfortable with a procedure which has been learnt well and done frequently; less so with a new but potentially better technique. Initially the new procedure may be associated with difficulties and complications or may simply be unsuccessful (as with some surgeons' initial attempts to do various refined types of vagotomy). If a comparison is begun during this phase then the new procedure is very likely to be shown to be less satisfactory than the old. In consequence comparative trials should not be set up until the 'learning curve' has been climbed. However, the difficulty is that if the start-up period makes both the patient and the surgeon feel that there are *perceived* advantages from the new, then mounting a randomized trial may prove impossible because either the patient is reluctant to be recruited or the surgeon is hesitant to request permission. Recent examples are simple mastectomy versus local excision for breast cancer and laparoscopic versus open cholecystectomy. In such circumstances we may have to admit that the full rigour of a PRCCT is impossible and try to make careful, continuous assessment of results to see if they conform to our expectations and ideals (see Audit, Ch. 32).

A final point about PRCCTs is that they become progressively more difficult to mount as results improve and the end-point for comparison — say wound infection, hernia recurrence or even death — gets less and less common. When wound infection rates are less than about 5% then it takes about a thousand patients to make a comparison between two techniques which might result in a further 3% reduction. This is often beyond available resources, or alternatively it is impossible to keep all the other factors that might influence the outcome stable over the period required. Multicentre studies can help there but they introduce their own problems.

PRCCTs, though they are a powerful tool, cannot be the only way that new knowledge comes to the surgical therapist.

## SURVIVAL ANALYSIS

Quite frequently in clinical practice we want to find out after something has been done to a patient what happens to him over the years — the influence of a treatment or a method of presentation, for example, on the outcome of patients with colorectal cancer. Ideally we would like to operate on a very large number of patients all at the same time and then follow them up to see how many die at every day over the next five or ten years. Usually this is impossible and patients have to accumulate over time. We also — in that we all die sometime — have to compare the deaths that occur in our group with those that would occur anyway from other causes. We may further be interested in subsampling, as already described, to compare two methods of management. All these give rise to statistical difficulties though they can all be allowed for. Detailed accounts of life table analysis and follow-up are beyond this simple introduction and advice should *always* be taken before embarking on such a study, though the rules given for controlled clinical trials

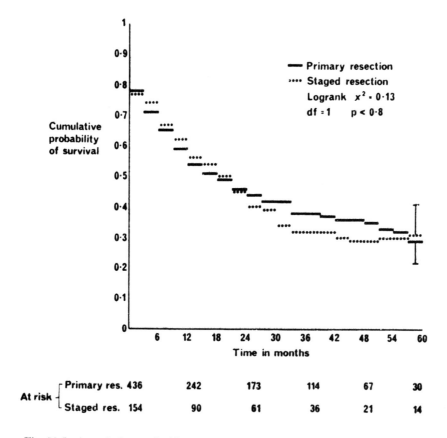

**Fig. 31.7**  A survival curve, in this case comparing primary versus staged resection for obstructing colon cancer. The curve has been constructed using what is known as the log-rank method. The horizontal bars at each probability level give the 95% confidence intervals. All these overlap.

do apply. An example of a life table analysis is shown Figure 31.7.

## META-ANALYSIS

In recent years techniques have been developed in statistics which permit the pooling of results from individual studies and their re-analysis by statistical means. As we pointed out on page 364 there must be good grounds for feeling that the studies are biologically comparable — for example, the operations done for varicose veins by one group are technically the same as those done by another — there being no statistical way one can compare chalk with cheese. Then, certain statistical rules must be observed and the new calculations must be done with methods which guard against over-interpretation. Finally it is doubly important to express results in terms of 'confidence', which we will discuss in more detail below. Though undoubtedly useful in trying to reach an overview or consensus on a new treatment, meta-analysis should be judged with considerable caution as a method which can give clear guidance to the clinician.

## ALTERNATIVES TO PRCCTS

The controlled trial as described on the previous pages has become something of a central dogma of clinical comparison. This is in some ways a good thing because its widespread adoption has got rid of a great deal of cant, opinion and rigid adherence to outmoded practices. Nevertheless, though in many respects it remains the ideal, it is not always feasible, for reasons we have already given. Are there any alternatives?

## Historical controls

The use of past experience to compare with what is currently being done is always criticized because the background may have changed from the past to the present: surgeons have become more skilled; the severity of the disease process under study may have changed; the population from which we draw samples has developed or lost some biological property such as immunity; and ancillary treatment — antibiotics, intensive care, nutrition — may more effectively support a new surgical procedure which is inherently no better or different from the old. All this is true, but even so it can be possible to draw some useful conclusions from comparison of the past with the present. Some rules which govern the use of historical controls are as follows:

1. Stability of the population — its nature and the outcome of treatment — from which the samples have been taken over several periods of previous study. The data for this are often lacking.

2. Caution in drawing conclusions from the outcome of a comparison. A formal statistical comparison is *not* usually justified on technical grounds, so that differences to which importance is ascribed must be large. There should be some collateral support from other studies or from scientific understanding of mechanisms for the inferences that are drawn.

3. Historically controlled studies which indicate a particular course of action should be confirmed by prospective analysis.

## Prospective studies

The last observation serves as an introduction to the *controlled prospective study*. This is a potential intermediate stage between a retrospective analysis and a PRCCT. It is no good starting out on the latter until a 'baseline' is established — i.e. we really know what is happening *now*. For example, it is vain to look for an improvement in survival in the surgical treatment of colon cancer

unless we know how good — or bad — the results are at the moment. Such studies in the real world can often direct us to critical points where improvements in surgical practice can be made with out recourse to elaborate controlled comparisons. They can also have a valuable 'halo' effect (sometimes known as the Hawthorn effect, after the town in which it was first demonstrated) in improving clinical practice, because it is well known that concentrating attention on a particular area nearly always improves results. In the often confused, multi-variable, circumstances of clinical practice, prospective studies with a recognition of their limitations still have an important place.

## Scenarios

There is a new proposal for diagnosis or management — for example, ultrasound or laparoscopy for the investigation of acute lower abdominal pain. In the scenario method, conventional management is taken to the point where the new technique would be used — after a full history and clinical examination and perhaps a white cell count in our example. A decision on how the clinician would proceed without the new technique being available is then requested (a 'scenario' for action). Then the new technique is deployed and the extra information which becomes available is used to modify that decision. The scenario and real outcomes are compared both with each other and with the final outcome. Clearly this approach has a considerable subjective element but it is an effective and economical way of first testing new ideas.

## STATISTICAL AND BIOLOGICAL INFERENCE

The foregoing account has been based almost entirely on the idea that we use statistics to analyse data so as to prove or disprove hypothesis at a predetermined level of probability. This in a way does not make very good sense in clinical practice because we are then faced with a second decision: given that we have established that repetitions of our experiment or trial will come out differently only five times in a hundred, what

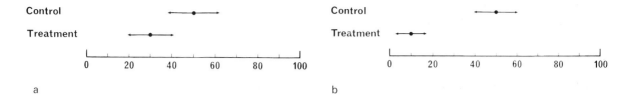

**Fig. 31.8**  Confidence intervals. Hypothetical values for a difference in mean between two methods of acid reduction. In (a) there is overlap of the 95% confidence intervals; in (b) there is not.

in fact do we do with our next patient? Do we or do we not give him the new treatment? The answer is that we usually do but sometimes we can have more confidence in making a dichotomized decision of this kind if we look at the confidence intervals which surround the difference which we have shown. We are not in fact using any new statistical information in doing this, just altering our attitude towards how we study the results.

Confidence intervals give us the values on either side of a mean or median within which we can find a given proportion of the results of the population about which we have drawn a conclusion (for their calculation see Gardner & Altman 1989). It is usual to calculate the 95% intervals. If we take a simple example of the effect of two acid-reducing agents on maximal acid output we might find the effects shown in Figure 31.8. In Figure 31.8A the mean of acid output with one agent is greater than the other and the difference is significant at the $p < 0.05$ level using a $t$ test. However, the 95% confidence levels overlap, so that we might find quite a number of subjects who got as good a result with either agent. If the confidence limits do not overlap, as in Figure 31.8B, then we would have greater confidence that the one agent was the better for us to use. In a sense, what confidence intervals tell us is the size of the mean difference and how widely the individual values are likely to be distributed around these means. Figure 31.7 shows how this method of display can be applied to a life table.

Similar calculations can be done on ordinal and categorical data, so when, for example, we are comparing outcomes in terms of life and death we can compare two survival curves and see if their 95% confidence intervals overlap or not.

## STATISTICAL AND BIOLOGICAL SIGNIFICANCE

Statistics is full of pitfalls about meaning. One of them involves the use of the word 'significance'. The previous pages have given its *statistical* meaning — it is the probability value assigned to the occurrence of events in a long run of 'trials' such as coin tossing or the outcomes of a repeatedly performed surgical operation or 'comparisons' such as the relative efficacy of two antibiotics. It tells us about *chance* or *likelihood* (though the latter word is sometimes used with a more specialized meaning we need not consider here). It does *not* tell us anything about the nature or magnitude of any difference we observe if we modify the conditions in a trial, and the same is true for a comparison. So when we say a difference is 'highly significant' or 'very highly significant' this just means that the outcome is less and less likely to have arisen by chance and not that it is bigger or more important. As we have seen (p. 370), the same is true for the correlation coefficient. Of course, a highly significant result may be important when our prime interest is not to do something which may turn out to be wrong — we have already given the example of a blind landing system (p. 363) — but this is not usually our objective in clinical practice. So in studying results we should be more interested in the size of the difference we observe and in the confidence which surrounds our measures — hence the current preference for expressing results in terms of the size of the difference and confidence intervals as we have described.

## DIAGNOSIS

Recently formal studies of how a diagnosis is reached have come to assume some importance. Much of the interest in the matter has been the result of pioneer work by surgeons and is especially relevant to their work. By diagnosis we mean either the definition of a pathological entity such as acute appendicitis, or the choice of a management option such as how to proceed in further investigation of acute lower abdominal pain — should it be by another investigation or by opening the abdomen? Clinical surgery and medicine have tended to concentrate on the former in spite of the recognition in some areas that the latter can be more important for the welfare of the patient. 'Better to look and see rather than wait and see' is an example of taking a management decision without having a clinicopathological diagnosis and, until recently, was rightly given priority over reaching a precise diagnosis in the management of the acute abdomen.

We can distinguish three interrelated methods by which diagnoses are made. *Pattern recognition* is probably the commonest way of both teaching diagnostic technique and of proceeding in clinical practice. It is the basis on which virtually all textbooks have been written since the Aphorisms of Hippocrates, which in effect are largely descriptions of patterns. If we have the 'running together' (the literal meaning of *syndrome*) of central abdominal pain, followed by pain, tenderness and guarding in the right iliac fossa, we say that this is the 'pattern' of acute appendicitis, just as a flat surface supported by four legs is the pattern of a table. The pattern does not need to be complete for us to make the inference that it is there: no central pain, as is not uncommon in the elderly if the appendix infarcts early in the course of the episode; no tenderness and guarding if the organ is in the pelvis. Similarly, if we see a drawing of a table with a leg missing, we would still be likely to infer that a table is what is meant to be depicted. However, the more items that are absent from the pattern the less confidence we

can put in our statement that this is appendicitis or that is a table. As we have seen in the section on statistics, confidence and probability are closely related and in recognition of an incomplete pattern we are saying: 'Given such and such items of history and clinical examination (perhaps supplemented by certain tests) appendicitis is *probably* present.'

Here we encouter the second method of diagnosis, which is almost certainly merely a numerical restatement of pattern recognition. It is based on a further term in the definition of probability. This is *conditional probability*. If there is a population of $N$ patients, $n$ of whom have appendicitis at any one time, then if we were to draw a patient from that population the probability that he or she has appendicitis is:

$$P_A = \frac{n}{N}$$

However, if instead of just drawing a patient at random we looked only at patients with acute abdominal pain, we should expect to find a different and somewhat higher probability, which is the *conditional probability* of the patient having acute appendicitis given that he or she also has acute abdominal pain. There are a variety of ways that this can be written but the usual one is:

$$P_{A|S}$$

where we have used S to indicate the symptom of acute abdominal pain.

Can we make use of this? The answer is yes, given that we have studied the population in the past for this symptom and its relation to the disease processes in which we are interested. A prior study of the population will tell us how often acute abdominal pain occurs in acute appendicitis and how often it is found in the same population without acute appendicitis being present or, what amounts to the same thing, when other disorders are present. Then we can write the equation:

$$P_A = \frac{P_A \times P_{S|A}}{P_S}$$

The more often acute abdominal pain without appendicitis is found in the population the smaller will be the probability of acute appendicitis, given acute abdominal pain in accordance with the probability axioms given on p. 362.

On its own this does not appear to add very much, but do not forget that we can add probabilities of this kind (p. 376); we can easily sum the probability of acute appendicitis, given acute abdominal pain, to the probability of appendicitis given pain in the right iliac fossa and also to the probability of acute appendicitis given tenderness in the right iliac fossa ... and so on. Therefore for an individual patient we can develop a probability value given any combination of symptoms and signs.

Calculations of this kind, which are known as Bayesian after the English divine who first tentatively described them, are mathematically trivial but arithmetically tedious, so that they are usually done on a computer. They have been extensively tested in such conditions as acute abdominal pain, back pain and dyspepsia. In the first they give an order of probabilities that is more precise than unaided clinical evaluation, particularly by the inexperienced. At the time of writing Bayesian techniques are most useful in:

1. Ensuring that data about the patient are properly gathered, because the computer forces the clinician to be precise.

2. Providing assistance to the clinician rather than taking over from him. They can also assist him to learn and so 'close the feedback loop' (see Audit, Ch. 32).

The third diagnostic technique that has achieved a good deal of prominence is *sequential reasoning*. Psychologists have established that we can only consider a small number of items at a time (unlike the computer using Bayesian methods) — not more than five or six. In such circumstances it is necessary to make a decision having considered these items and then to go on to consider more information or, what amounts to the same thing, take some course of action. For example, having put abdominal pain and tenderness and guarding in the right iliac fossa together to arrive at the conclusion that there is lower right quadrant peritoneal irritation we might then say: 'Is the patient male or female?' If the answer is male we might be prepared to explore the right iliac

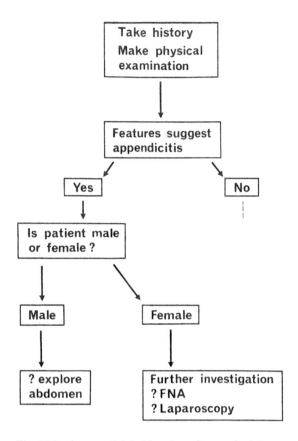

**Fig. 31.9** A sequential decision chart. See text for full explanation.

fossa; if female, and because of the more frequent occurrence of other causes, we might seek further evidence from an ultrasound examination or laparoscopy. This is an example of *binary decision making* (yes/no, go/no go) and can be built up into quite complex trees or algorithms (see Fig. 31.9). Algorithms are useful for sorting out how to make decisions in complicated circumstances and also for teaching purposes; they prove less satisfactory at the bedside. However, in the future they may form one basis for 'expert systems' in which knowledge is incorporated into a computer program to give an output which advises the clinician what he or she should, on the basis of the evidence, do next. A number of such systems have already been developed to deal with specific circumstances such as the prescription of antibiotics and more recently for the diagnosis of acute abdominal pain.

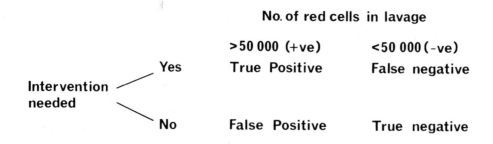

**Fig. 31.10**   Two by Two (four cell) table for the evaluation of a simple test. See text and Box 4 for full explanation.

It should be clear from the foregoing account that the three main methods by which we reach a diagnosis are interrelated. Pattern recognition can sometimes, when the pattern is incomplete, be based on probabilities of association. Bayes' theorem is a numerical way of creating a pattern of probabilities. Sequential reasoning takes a few items of a pattern, works on these and arrives at a binary decision (do this or do that) which though it appears exact is more often than not probabilistic (probably better to do this than to do that).

## ANALYSING DIAGNOSTIC TESTS

It is now common to analyse tests made to determine the presence or absence of a given condition (or more accurately for their ability to predict the presence or absence of a condition) in terms of their *sensitivity* and *specificity*. Many surgeons (including the writer) find this fairly confusing so we explain it here. For simplicity we shall first consider only a categorical variable (see p. 365), which is one when the outcome is yes/no or positive/negative. In practice we can set 'cut-off' points for most tests which are on interval scales (see p. 367) and we will briefly deal with that at the end.

Let us suppose that we want to work out the sensitivity of peritoneal lavage in the detection of intra-abdominal trauma. For the moment we will decide to call the lavage positive if there are more than 50 000 red cells per cubic millilitre of wash and negative if less than this figure. We also need a defined end-point with which to compare the test. It would be either the presence or absence

of an intra-abdominal lesion for which surgery was ultimately found to have been necessary (positive) or unnecessary (negative). With these definitions we can go on to study a number of patients with suspected abdominal trauma by peritoneal lavage and assign to one of the four cells of the table shown in Figure 31.10. If we find a positive peritoneal lavage but no lesion this is a 'false positive' for the test. If lavage is negative and there is a lesion this is a false negative. The false positive rate is given by

$$\frac{\text{no. of false positives}}{\text{no. with negative end-point}}$$

and the false negative rate is

$$\frac{\text{no. of false negatives}}{\text{no. with a positive end-point}}$$

If our test is to be of value in detecting abdominal trauma then we want it to have a low value for both false positives and false negatives — not to indicate abdominal trauma when it is absent and not to fail to do so when it is present. The lower the false positive rate the test has, the more *specific* it is said to be. The lower the false negative rate the more *sensitive*. In our example with a cut-off at 50 000 red cells per cubic millilitre we are not going to have many false positives, but we may well have some false negatives because of lightly bleeding, but nevertheless serious, lesions about which something should be done. If we were to change the cut-off to 25 000 then we would have more false positives but fewer false negatives (see Box 4 for further details).

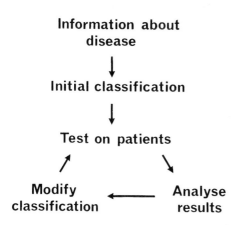

**Fig. 31.11** How disease is categorized.

## CATEGORIZING DISEASE

On p. 365 et seq. we considered the various forms of *scales*. For many years, clinicians and others have used either categorical or ordinal scales to classify diseases. Early attempts to stage breast cancer are an example of what amounts to a categorical scale — *the axilla is involved or it is not*. However, ordinal scales with 'more' meaning 'worse' or 'more advanced' soon superseded these, so that we reach, for example, Dukes' classification of colon cancer in which there were initially three stages based on histologically detectable tumour burden: confined to the mucosa (A); penetrating the bowel wall (B); and with lymph node metastases (C — sometimes subdivided further into I and II according to the extent of involvement).

The utility of such classifications relates to how they can predict the behaviour of the disease process and this is reflected in the way they are derived. There may be at the outset enough knowledge of the disease and its features that we can compare these with outcome; alternatively we may take what is initially an arbitrary but rational fact or set of facts which are then tested on a series of patients against some end-point — such as death. These processes form part of a circle (Fig. 31.11) so that an initially fairly rough classification is refined to improve its predictive value. Thus, though Dukes' staging works quite well to predict outcome, adding histological evidence of lymphatic permeation improves its predictive value, as does grading the tumour. The factors that go to make up the classification may not, however, be wholly independent — for example, undifferentiated tumours are more likely to have lymph node metastases. Some of the techniques of regression analysis (p. 369) can be used to find out if factors included in a staging of a disease are independent or not and this technique is now widely applied to establish what it is useful to measure as independent predictors.

As with other uses of measurement in clinical medicine, it is always conceivable that being able to base a classification or staging on an *interval* rather than a categorical or ordinal scale might increase its precision. One of the first successful attempts to do this was when the Birmingham Accident Hospital surgeons used their records to construct a table (more accurately a matrix) which related age and the extent of a burn to the probability of survival. This, at the time it was constructed, clearly told the clinician that, below and above certain ages, burns of a given percentage were non-survivable (had a probability of death of 1) and therefore that treatment should be directed to palliation only. More recently a similar approach has been used to develop *scores* for individual situations (trauma, sepsis, severe illness — e.g. the APACHE score). A number of items of data are pooled with or without being given some weighting factor to give them more or less relative importance and a total score produced by adding the values for the items together. What weight is given to an individual item is derived from a study of the predictive value of each alone or in combination. This is best undertaken by using regression analysis on a sample of patients with the condition under consideration and an outcome such as death or complications being the dependent variable. As more information becomes available and the size of the sample increases, these values can be modified and the score updated for its predictive capability.

Classifications and scores are very useful in giving us an overview of complex processes. It must be emphasized very firmly that they have some limitations. First, the score is only as good as the data that goes into it, and an ill-defined condition studied by analysing only a small or heterogeneous sample will yield values for the score which have wide confidence intervals. Second, the figures produced give outcomes which are applicable to groups of patients. Thus if, using the old Birmingham burns figures, a 45-year-old male with a 50% burn had a probability of surviving of 0.5 this meant only that if 100 patients of this kind were studied in the future 50 of them would die. It could not tell you *which* 50. Effort is usually directed to finding in numerical scores a 'cut-off' that will discriminate accurately between a favourable or unfavourable outcome, but the problem is the same as balancing the sensitivity and specificity of a test (p. 378).

The second point is that a grade or score predicts the mean of what has been achieved in management *so far*. It does not necessarily imply that a measurement which predicts a high mortality should lead us to abandon our efforts. New techniques and, for example, their application by an enthusiastic team can shift outcome so that a previously bad prognostic score is so no longer. The Birmingham burns probabilities have had to be updated several times as treatment at all stages of severe burns improves. It is for this reason that socio-economic decisions about individuals based on their classification or score should be made with great caution — if at all. The Quality Adjusted Life Year (QALY) is a recent example of assigning a value to the outcome of a procedure based on a scoring technique which can then be used to decide which patients should have priority for treatment. For example, hip replacements produce a large number of QALYs and are good value but oesophagectomies for cancer are the reverse. Again such techniques are of analytical value for groups but not necessarily the way to base decisions in practice.

Although these are legitimate criticisms of classifications and scores, there is no doubt that they are useful in terms of giving us yardsticks by which we can compare treatment and attempt to single out groups of patients who will or will not benefit from our use of particular techniques. In complex circumstances where outcome is determined by the interplay of many factors, they supply an important 'handle' for more precise study.

## SCREENING

Considerations of sensitivity and specificity for a diagnostic test relate directly to the subject of screening. It is widely assumed that if we can detect a disease process before it has led the patient to consult her doctor, then the disease is likely to be at a pathologically earlier stage in its evolution and its effects on the patient; it is, in effect, more susceptible to cure. Although this assumption is probably too simple, it is the basis for screening either to elicit symptoms which have not alerted the patient to the fact that she has something wrong (e.g., minor intermenstrual bleeding or a change in bowel habit) or to apply a test to a truly asymptomatic group (e.g. undertaking a cervical smear or looking for occult blood in the stool). Fundamental requirements for a screening programme are:

1. The condition for which the screening is being undertaken is treatable or, in the case of a possible genetic defect, can be pre-empted by some action such as a termination of pregnancy.

2. A 'target' population is identifiable which contains the great majority, if not necessarily all, of those at risk. It is not likely to be valuable to screen patients under 45 for occult blood in the stool and it is a waste of time (and can possibly be dangerous) undertaking mammography to look for breast cancer under the age of 40. In neither instance is the disease which is being sought completely absent from these age brackets but in both it is so rare as not to justify the work involved.

3. The resources are available to apply the screening technique. It is usual to distinguish between 'programmed' and 'opportunistic' screening. In the first, the target population which has been identified from prior epidemiological studies is approached and either invited or cajoled into taking part (cervical smears; stool occult blood; mammography). In the second, if patients present either for a routine examination/procedure or because they have a condition associated with screenable risk factors, the opportunity is taken to screen them (hypertension in patients undergoing hernia repair; hyperlipidaemia in patients with vascular disease).

4. Given that the condition can be identified

by screening, are the resources and techniques to manage it also available? It is not very useful to find a possible carcinoma of the breast at mammography and then not to have the facilities for targeted biopsy freely available.

5. Finally, there must be a test (or a battery of tests) which have a reasonably high sensitivity and specificity for the condition. Low sensitivity will mean too many false negatives, so negating the purpose of the screening programme. Low specificity (which as we have seen — p. 378 — can mean high sensitivity) will result in a large number of patients having to be alarmed by the possibility that they have the disease; considerable resources may need to be expended to show that most of them are in the 'false positive' zone.

Quite often screening programmes are started without due consideration for the above points. Nevertheless successful screening programmes for surgical disease are in progress — such as mammography for breast cancer and the search for positive occult blood in the stools to detect early colon cancer.

## ASSESSING PUBLISHED WORK

Only practice and living in a critical professional atmosphere will enable the surgeon to acquire and sustain the ability to assess published work. However, there are some ground rules which can help make it easier to tell the adequate from the bad. In theory, bad work should not get published because of the workings of 'peer review', by which papers submitted to journals are assessed by those who are supposed to know about their content and to possess rigorous standards of judgement about the scientific worth of a paper. However, this system can let a lot of papers through which when they are perused require a critical eye from the reader.

### Hypothesis

Although straightforward undirected observations still have a part to play in clinical science (what social scientists have called 'abstract empiricism'), most work that achieves publication is based on some sort of hypothesis. Some of the rules that govern generation of a scientific

hypothesis have already been discussed. In addition, the reader of a paper should ask the following questions:

1. Is there a hypothesis at all? If not, are the observations of interest without one?

2. Is the hypothesis well formulated? By this is meant, does it have a basis in science or in past experience or is it just a wild speculation?

3. Is the work and the analysis based on a prospective (a priori) as distinct from a retrospective (a posteriori) hypothesis? The exploitation of a hypothesis is likely to lead to more meaningful conclusions if it is set up before any studies are made simply because the collection of data or the conduct of an experiment will then be structured more adequately to test it. Thus the comparison of two methods of closure of the abdominal wall should, *before* the study begins, state the hypothesis (e.g. layered closure is better than mass), lay down criteria for the selection of patients, the difference which it is desired to detect and which is clinically important and the process of randomization. The hypothesis is then a priori and the study is prospective. The alternative that is frequently encountered in clinical practice is to have used (perhaps at random but usually not) different methods of closure in a surgical unit over a period of time and then come up with the hypothesis such as the one above and try to test it by looking back at outcome. Such an a posteriori hypothesis requires retrospective collection and analysis of information and usually lacks the same rigour as a prospective study simply because the data have not been collected with the hypothesis in mind. The same problems arise when data which have been collected to test one hypothesis are then reanalysed to test another one not originally part of the protocol or perhaps even thought of when the study began. Neither of these circumstances is fatal to the possibility of getting some useful information out of a study (and statisticians have techniques for dealing with subsidiary or a posteriori analysis) but both should be looked upon with caution, particularly in terms of the inferences drawn by the authors. Although audit is a useful method of quality control (see Ch. 32), it can suffer from the same problem in that a priori decisions are not neces-

sarily taken on the hypothesis of what special quality it is wished to control for.

## Design and conduct of the experiment

1. Has the sample been adequately constructed and taken and is it of sufficient size (see sampling, p. 364)? Do the authors give any calculations of power?

2. Have the observations/experiments that follow from the hypothesis been adequately made? In these days of high-technology measurement the investigative tools have to be taken largely on trust (though the referees who peer reviewed the paper should be able to assess these) but some assessment of the sensitivity of the measurements for the desired purpose is always welcome and often missing.

## Results

Are the differences claimed by the authors of biological as distinct from statistical significance (see p. 374)?

## Introduction and discussion

Do these adequately review the past information? This question begs to a certain extent that of whether the reader is already familiar with the other work done in the field but some clues can sometimes be gained from:

1. the number of personal comments such as 'it is the author's personal conviction', 'our experience is', 'we believe', all of which are evidence of special pleading
2. the reference list, which if it includes a large amount of self-quotation usually implies a selective and therefore biassed approach to the analysis of other publications.

The discussion should be firmly based on the work reported and correlated with similar work (if any) of others. It should state either explicitly or implicitly whether the expectations announced in the introduction — such as the confirmation or refutation of a hypothesis — were fulfilled. A long rambling discussion which includes an extended chain of inference such as 'we have shown *this* and if this means *that* and if at the same time we assume *something additional* then it is worth while *speculating* that *maybe* yet *another thing* follows' is unconvincing. Such tenuous chains of reasoning are not usually quite so blatant as this but they do tend to exist (often in an attempt to gain priority for new speculative ideas) and they call into doubt the scientific clarity of the authors (as well of course the critical faculties of peer reviewers and the editor of the journal in which it appears).

FURTHER READING

Explicable foundations of clinical statistics:
Campbell M J, Machin D 1990 Medical statistics: a commonsense approach. Wiley, Chichester
Gardner M J, Altman DG 1989 Statistics with confidence. British Medical Journal, London
Armitage P, Berry G 1987 Statistical methods in medical research, 2nd edn. Blackwell, Oxford (hard going but authoritative)
Feinstein A R 1977. Clinical biostatistics. Louis St Mosby, (full of useful insights though rather detailed)
Altmann D C 1991 Practical statistics for medical research. Chapman and Hall, London (more accessible than Berry and Armitage and excellent for the practising clinician)
Rank order methods:
Meddis R 1984 Statistics using ranks. Blackwell, Oxford (somewhat advanced but worth tackling of you are seriously interested)
A useful 'cookbook':
Swinscow D 1976 Statistics from square one. British Medical Journal, London
Research in general:
Mattie R T, Taylor K W, Calnan J S (eds) 1989 Principles of surgical research. Wright, London

# 32. Audit

*B. W. Ellis  J. Simpson*

## DEFINITIONS

*Clinical audit* is defined by the Department of Health (DoH) as: 'The systematic, critical analysis of the quality of medical care, including the procedures used for diagnosis and treatment, the use of resources, and the resulting outcome and quality of life for the patient', and states that 'an effective programme of medical audit will also help to provide reassurance to doctors, their patients, and managers that the best quality of service is being achieved, *having regard to the resources available*' (DoH 1989).

*Resource management* involves clinicians, managers and nurses in using financial and other management (including clinical) information to help achieve more efficient and effective use of resources. Thus clinical audit and resource management have much in common. The data required for both overlap considerably and the information derived in each is relevant to the other (Ellis et al 1990); the use of resources cannot be ignored but it is not the first priority of clinical audit.

Clinical audit is the responsibility of clinicians and must be led by them (Standing Committee on Postgraduate Medical Education 1989). The terms 'clinical audit' and 'medical audit' are often used interchangeably, but a consensus has developed whereby *medical audit* refers to the assessment by peer review of the medical care provided by the medical profession to the patient, and *clinical audit* refers to an assessment of the total care of the patient by nurses, professions allied to medicine such as physiotherapists as well as doctors (Standing Medical Advisory Committee 1990). These and other health professionals have an essential role in patient care and the quality of medical care cannot be determined by doctors alone.

## HISTORY AND BACKGROUND

While modern-day concepts of audit may be new to many, a critical appraisal of the care dispensed by clinicians is by no means new. There are many examples of audit activity in a number of guises over the last few centuries. Our forefathers in surgery very often had no option but to learn by trial and error. The openness of their writing, especially in their descriptions of surgical disasters, makes fascinating reading when we can look back with the benefit of hindsight and with our current state of knowledge:

The patient had complete retention. I was induced at length to try forcible catheterisation with a straight instrument — an operation which has been recommended by excellent surgeons, especially Dupytren. My attempt was unsuccessful; the instrument bent and did not penetrate the prostate gland. Retroperitoneal infiltration of urine followed and the patient died. I do not advise anyone to follow my example. In such a case puncture of the bladder by the rectum would have been the proper proceeding [sic]. (Bilroth 1881)

Nor were these expositions confined to the anecdotal. In the same book T. H. Bilroth, who was then Professor of Surgery in Vienna, noted: 'Of 118 operations on the breast alone, eight were fatal; the cause of death in all cases being erysipelas. Of 187 operations on the breast and axillary glands,. . . forty patients died from various causes; three deaths occurred from severe secondary haemorrhage, but many of the other cases, who were attacked with septicaemia, pyaemia or erysipelas had also haemorrhage from the axilla.' There then follows a critical appraisal of the various techniques of ligature of veins and the use of antiseptics and caustics.

The improvement in standards of care in surgery as a whole and in the practices of individual surgeons has, until recently, relied on the apprenticeship of the training years, the dissemination of new learning and good practice through the medium of the book, the journal and the lecture by the 'expert'. Those who were prepared to listen and read were able to change practice where appropriate. Even now many surgeons rely on the annual meetings of the various 'craft' associations for education in current surgical practice.

The roots of modern audit lie in the regular morbidity and mortality meetings held in many hospitals in the UK and the USA in the 1950s and 1960s. The value of these meetings as a means of learning was recognized and taken up by many departments while the scope of audit activity broadened.

In the early 1980s microcomputers made their first appearance on the audit scene and this made it possible to collect and analyse large amounts of information very swiftly. This then gave the clinician a powerful tool to assist in the interpretation of types of work done, throughput and complications. Audit systems are now very powerful and can rapidly highlight areas of high risk of complication, death, cost, etc. However, there is the danger that some surgeons believe ownership of an 'audit' system to be synonymous with the successful practice of audit. They must appreciate that such systems are merely tools with which we can get a grasp and some understanding of the activity for which we are responsible.

From April 1991 local medical audit committees are responsible for ensuring the development of medical audit *in which every doctor participates* (DoH 1989). Whereas before, audit was practised on a voluntary basis, and thus predominantly by enthusiasts, it has now become compulsory and the requirement for audit is written into the job descriptions of all new staff. Managers must also be given clear evidence that effective audit is being practised.

In the past there was no funding or allocation of time for audit activity. Now there are funds available; in 1991 £48 million was allocated by the DoH. The money was allocated to district health authorities by their regional health authorities.

## ATTITUDES TO AUDIT

### The clinician

Some will argue that medical audit is practised already; that ward rounds, clinical presentations, research and morbidity and mortality meetings fulfil this function. However, there are differences between these and medical audit. Medical audit must be seen as a systematic approach to the review of clinical care to highlight opportunities for improvement and to provide a mechanism for bringing them about. As such it endeavours to get away from the 'single interesting case' and look for patterns of care. There should also be a difference in emphasis in the type of case examined. Audit should initiate investigation into those areas of clinical care that are considered as high risk, high cost, or very common. Audit investigation is also suitable to resolve issues of contention or local interest. The rare and clinically interesting case should be left for the clinical conference.

There remains a view held by many clinicians that the time spent on audit could be much better spent on other activities, such as treating more patients. This is not a wholly spurious argument; few have attempted to audit the process of audit itself and the results have as yet failed to demonstrate overt value for money or effort expended (Lomas et al 1991). There is, nonetheless, general agreement that a regular review of his own practice by a clinician in the light of constructive criticism by his peers can lead to improved delivery of care for the patient. It is important that we do not lose sight of the concept that the principal beneficiary of the process should be the patient.

### The Manager

With the implementation of purchaser/provider contracts from April 1991 there is now a need to specify the quality of the service provided and to link quality of care with quantity and cost. More explicit quality standards and outcome measures will be specified in contracts between health authorities (the purchasers) and their hospital (the providers). Doctors and managers will be required to share medical audit information within agreed rules of confidentiality, and, generally, managers will want to show the value of their involvement in the audit process (Bowden & Walshe 1991).

## THE IMPLEMENTATION OF CHANGE

If audit is to be effective it must lead to change. Audit may be considered as a cycle, the first component of which is the observation of existing practice to establish what is actually happening. Then, standards of practice are set to define what ought to happen and a comparison made between observed practice with the standard. Finally change is implemented. Clinical practice is observed again to see whether what has been planned has been achieved. A decision can then be made as to whether practice needs to change further, or whether the standards were unrealistic or unobtainable. This process has become known as the 'cycle of audit' (Royal College of Physicians 1989) and the achievement of change has been termed 'closing the audit loop'.

The provision of information on clinical activity, without any evaluation or suggestions for improvement, has been judged to have almost no effect on clinical practice (Mitchell et al 1985), unless it is targeted at decision makers who had already agreed to review their practice (Mugford et al 1991). It was also judged to be most effective if presented close to the time of decision making (Mugford et al 1991). The most commonly used approach, and one of the most effective, involves the publication of guidelines, in the form of notes to junior staff, the display of posters or notices and the redesign of forms or charts. Changes in behaviour may occur. However, these are much less effective when developed by external 'experts'. Involvement in the development of guidelines seems to enhance compliance (Anderson et al 1988). Guidelines need to be regularly reviewed to establish 'ownership'. If they are not valued, they will not be used. Finally, it has been noted that the act of investigating clinical decisions has itself brought about improvements in clinical practice (Gabbay et al 1990).

## THE EDUCATIONAL COMPONENT

The educational benefits of clinical audit have been considered in depth by Batstone (1990). It is now seen as vital that doctors in training are taught the basic principles of audit. Equally, conclusions drawn from the audit process should be seen as an important feeder into education.

There can be little doubt that the critical review of current practice and comparisons against predefined standards encourages the acquisition and updating of knowledge. The audit process also enables the identification of key features of clinical practice which should help to make teaching more explicit. However, the evidence for the effectiveness of educational strategies on clinical practice is unclear (Mugford et al 1991).

Through audit, it is possible to identify particular areas where knowledge could be improved or is deficient, suggesting the need for research. Self-evaluation and peer review (common activities in audit) are important components of postgraduate education.

In order to fully realize the educational potential of audit it is essential that the lessons arising from previous audit meetings are reviewed, and the conclusions acted upon.

## STAFF FOR AUDIT

Most hospitals in the UK now have an audit officer and/or audit coordinator. It is their task to enable the implementation of audit and to assist where possible in the execution of the audit process.

While much still rests on the clinical staff to prepare for audit exercises, the audit staff should be able to provide support in:

- suggesting audit activities
- helping to prepare audit programmes
- helping to plan audit studies
- literature searching

- screening case records against clinically determined criteria
- computer assistance with databases/graphics and forms
- preparing audit reports.

## COMMITTEES FOR AUDIT

Shortly after the introduction of the White Paper (DoH 1989) health districts set up district medical audit committees to oversee the implementation of audit and report to management. Now that health districts are in effect the 'purchasers' and the hospitals (either as trusts or directly managed units) 'providers', most hospitals have their own audit committees reporting to their unit management. District committees still exist in some areas as the funding for audit is still allocated on a district basis (although this is likely to change).

An audit committee should draw members from a range of clinical backgrounds so that a wide perspective can be used in the planning of audit at a local level. The chairman needs to be well motivated and prepared to devote time on a regular basis to the task. There should be representation from the nursing profession, primary health care (general practice), education (usually the clinical tutor) and doctors in the training grades. In addition two or three other clinicians and the audit staff should sit on the local committee.

Hospital audit committees have the following functions. They must:

- coordinate and foster clinical audit for every doctor; attempt to minimize the perception that audit is a threat and highlight the benefits of the audit process to doctors and patients
- determine existing practice of audit and assist clinicians in the implementation of audit methods
- monitor the results and conclusions of the audit process and check the validity of data and reporting
- ensure that changes, where indicated by the outcome of audit, are implemented
- ensure that the outcome of audit is perceived as educational and that doctors are educated in the practice and process of audit

- train and direct audit officers
- ensure effective liaison with general practitioners and management
- maintain confidentiality
- estimate funding required for audit
- prepare annual report and forward programme.

## ROYAL COLLEGE OF SURGEONS OF ENGLAND GUIDELINES

In 1989 the college published *Guidelines to Clinical Audit in Surgical Practice.*

## TECHNIQUES IN AUDIT

Donabedian (1966) identified three main elements in the delivery of health care: structure, process and outcome.

*Structure.* This includes the quantity and type of resources available and is generally easy to measure. It is not a good indicator of the quality of care but should be taken into account in the assessment of process and outcome.

*Process.* This is what is done to the patient. A review of process can be done quickly and cheaply. It includes consideration of the way an operation was performed, what medications were prescribed, the adequacy of notes, and compliance with consensus policies. There is an underlying assumption that the activities under review have been previously shown to produce an acceptable medical outcome. This is the area of patient care that can be changed by education.

*Outcome.* This is the result of clinical intervention and may represent the success or failure of process. For example, outcome could be measured by studies of surgical fatality rates, incidence of complications, or patient satisfaction. It can be considered to be the most relevant indicator of patient care, but it is the most difficult to define and quantify. Mortality and length of stay in hospital are very easily measured outcome indicators but variations in these outcomes are rarely related to the quality of the service being delivered. It may be more important to consider whether patients perceive that their problems have been solved, their quality of life and, where appropriate, the duration of their survival.

It is essential when planning an audit exercise to consider which of the above elements of care are being examined and how the changes in each might bring about improved patient care.

A number of audit techniques have evolved and found a place in the regular assessment of clinical practice. These are as follows.

**Basic clinical audit.** This entails an analysis of throughput, a broad analysis of case type, complications and morbidity and mortality. It is suggested that review of such data is undertaken by each clinical firm at intervals of approximately three months. Where possible, figures derived from the data should be contrasted with previous periods of time, other clinical firms, other hospitals or information derived from global audit (see below). There is a danger that this exercise can become a boring repetition of figures. The essential ingredient is to distil out of the data any notable deviations from an accepted 'norm' and then to act upon such observation. Hence the need for a comparative 'yardstick'.

**Incident review.** This involves the discussion of strategies to be adopted under certain clinical scenarios. An incident may be taken to be anything from a patient suffering from a leaking aortic aneurysm to the use of a department for an investigation, e.g. emergency intravenous urography. It is expected that such discussions would lead to clear policies for future use, and may result in the production of local guidelines. This audit method is particularly suitable for multidisciplinary or interdisciplinary audit.

**Clinical record review.** A member of another firm of the same or similar specialty is invited to review a random selection of case notes. Where possible, criteria should be established for this review purpose. Clinical record audit has the advantage of simplicity and requires relatively little additional time or other resources. However, there is a potential disadvantage in that discus-sion might concentrate too much on the quality of record keeping and not enough on patient care — these two are distinct facets of the clinical process, although related. In practice, a balance between these two components of audit might be encouraged by having the audit meetings chaired by a third clinician who is neither 'auditing' nor 'being audited'.

**Criterion audit.** This is an approach that can be considered as a more advanced and structured form of incident audit. Retrospective analysis of clinical records is made and judged against a number of carefully chosen criteria. These criteria should encapsulate the key elements in management of a particular topic which should be capable of unambiguous interpretation from the medical record by a non-medical audit assistant. All cases falling within the scope of the topic in question are screened and those that fail to meet any of the criteria are brought forward for futher clinical review. The criteria may relate to administrative elements (e.g. waiting time), investigations ordered, treatments considered, outcome, follow-up strategies, etc. Criteria for adequate management of a particular condition can be easily derived from clinical guidelines, if these have been developed. Clinical time is necessary in the preliminary discussion but the majority of the work can be done by audit assistants. It is applicable to a variety of circumstances and allows the comparison of data between different hospitals (Shaw 1989).

**Adverse occurrence screening.** A clinical firm decides on a shortlist of events that are worthy of avoidance, e.g. wound infections, unplanned readmissions, delay or error in diagnosis. Details of occurrences are recorded and complex or serious occurrences are reviewed by clinicians. A database is built up which can then be interrogated to identify trends, perform comparative analyses, etc. Cases can be selected by considering all admissions or a sample of them. This technique can also be used for risk management (Bennett & Walshe 1990).

**Focused audit studies.** Outcome from any other area of audit may dictate the need for a more closely focused area of research. Such a study comes close to an academic research exercise.

***Global audit.*** In any one hospital the number of departments undertaking similar work is often very small. Even between two firms of general surgeons the case mix may be sufficiently different to negate the value of comparative audit. In other specialties there may not be anyone else in the hospital with whom to compare results. Global audit implies the collection of data and its comparison across units, districts and even through a whole region (Gruer et al 1986, Black 1991). The Royal College of Surgeons has already set up a confidential comparative audit service in which all surgeons are requested to supply information under a confidential number for comparison with their peers at regular meetings (Royal College of Surgeons 1991). Techniques in data presentation now allow such sensitive information to be widely disseminated and discussed while maintaining an individual clinician's confidentiality (Emberton et al 1991).

***Outcome audit.*** Outcome will depend on the whole of the process of health care delivery during a patient's episode in hospital and, as such, is a measure of the spectrum of the skills of the medical and nursing staff, the hospital administration and indeed, every person or department with whom the patient comes into contact. There will inevitably be a contrast between the perspectives on outcome between the patient, the GP and the clinician, and much work remains to be done to evolve satisfactory measures. Studies on outcome, especially in the surgical specialties, are likely to be seen as an important measure of the quality of care.

***National studies:*** These were first used over a decade ago to address the question of perinatal mortality in obstetric units. The report of the first confidential enquiry into perioperative deaths (CEPOD; Buck et al 1987) considered the factors involved in the deaths of patients who died within 30 days of surgery in three regional health authorities. Much was learnt from that exercise, especially the need for doctors in the training grades to be given adequate support and supervision. It was clear that disaster frequently arose when surgeons attempted procedures for which they possessed insufficient skill or training. Since the original report further studies have looked at deaths following surgery in children (Campling et al 1990).

## ETHICS AND CONFIDENTIALITY

Information used in audit about patients must protect the confidentiality of individual patients and also that of the professionals involved. The local audit committee must have clear guidelines on confidentiality. It is vital that there is a consistent policy on confidentiality particularly where audit activities cross boundaries between specialties or professional disciplines.

With regard to patient confidentiality, the same principles are involved as in the clinical conferences which form part of any academic programme. The matter becomes more complex if professionals other than doctors are involved in audit. It is important to secure an undertaking from all those involved not to talk about what was discussed in an audit meeting outside that meeting. Unless an explicit and convincing case can be made for inclusion of identifying details of a patient in verbal or written presentations, such details should be excluded.

The confidentiality of the professionals involved also requires protection. This is likely to prove difficult in some types of audit, for example where one consultant reviews the clinical records of another consultant's patient. Nevertheless, this type of audit can be successful provided that the necessary atmosphere of trust and collaboration is fostered. Some types of audit are more likely to precipitate interpersonal conflict than others. It is always necessary to obtain permission from all consultants involved before starting an audit exercise.

It is important to consider what should happen if audit reveals problems or deficiencies in a given individual's clinical practice. Such a situation is likely to occur infrequently, if at all, but this makes it the more important to anticipate such an eventuality and to make explicit provision for it (Ellis & Sensky 1991).

Ethical committee permission before interviewing patients is occasionally required, but this is usually a local requirement which needs to be checked. In general, audit projects need not involve ethical committees.

## COMPUTERS

The past decade has seen a staggering evolution in computing. In the mid-1970s computers were rarely seen outside large corporations and research centres. They were large and difficult for all but the expert to use. Paper tape and the punched card were the medium of storage for data and programs. Now, in the 1990s we have small, very portable 'notebook' machines whose power easily matches a computer of two decades ago that would have filled a room. Current desktop and deskside machines are now more powerful than almost *any* computer of the early 1970s.

The surgical trainee should have a good working knowledge of the basics of computing. He or she should be capable of installing application programs onto a personal computer and have a working knowledge of a word processor, the principles of a spreadsheet and database and be familiar with the use of a graphics program and the graphical user interface found in today's multitasking environments such as 'Windows' (Microsoft Ltd).

Computers offer many possible advantages to the surgical trainee, from the preparation of neatly presented data for meetings to the recording of useful references, the preparation of slides using graphics and the drafting of papers and theses. Perhaps the commonest use will be the updating of the personal curriculum vitae (CV).

Many postgraduate medical centres now offer the use of a microcomputer for the production of graphics and for word processing. Some centres have also installed CD-ROM drives to enable enquiry on those databases published in CD format. A 'data' compact disc, which looks identical to its audio counterpart, can hold well in excess of 500 mB of information. The best-known, and most useful, medical publication in this format is 'MEDLINE'. With regular update discs access to such a system will replace the need to search *Index Medicus;* furthermore computer-based searching is not only a great deal faster but it is also more comprehensive and permits searching in many different ways. For those trainees with access to a CD-ROM a 'download' facility allows the exportation of selected papers with or without abstracts into a database on a personal computer. Excellent programs are available for handling such information on a PC such as 'Reference Manager' (Reference Information Systems, Carslbad, California). Such software permits the rapid searching and manipulation of references and permits their exportation into word processors for use in papers, CVs, etc., in any desired journal format.

Computing skills are best acquired by practice on the computer itself. Books and manuals tend to get used only to solve problems. Thus the best application programs tend to be intuitive.

A number of programs are available as clinical information systems, which usually have outputs configured to help in the process of audit. For the college guidelines on the selection of these programs see Further Reading.

Despite some pioneering ventures into the realms of clinical decision-making systems and artificial intelligence there is still a great deal to be learnt about the clinical as opposed to the administrative capabilities of computing in medicine.

## HOSPITAL INFORMATION SYSTEMS

As personal computers have grown in power, so have the larger mini and mainframe computers. The role of large computers in hospitals in the UK is currently under review. The DoH has never been keen to prescribe solutions, and the result is that every hospital has the potential to find a different configuration of computer.

At one end of the spectrum are a small number of hospitals which have a completely integrated 'hospital information system' covering every function from the recording of clinical data, the scheduling of clinics, to the provision of financial and manpower reports, etc. Such systems are very costly and, at present, not well developed in the UK.

At the other end of this computing spectrum are those hospitals which have a mainframe type computer running a patient administration system (PAS), including the 'master index' (patients' demographic details) and records of admissions and diagnostic codes. This represents the minimum upon which a hospital manager can rely for information. PAS systems regularly pass aggregated information to a district information system (DIS); it is from the DIS that reports are usually generated.

In those hospitals with the latter configuration there are bound to be many departments which have implemented their own information systems. Surgeons may rely on proprietary clinical information systems, while the accident and emergency department is likely to have its own variant. Operating theatres and maternity departments frequently have departmental systems to help provide the reports necessary for management.

There may also be separate systems installed for manpower, finance, personnel, estates, etc.. All of these departmental systems may be required to pass information onto other departments, and, in the context of integrated computer systems, are known as 'feeder systems'.

Current trends seem to favour the introduction of so-called case-mix systems. These pull together information from the clinically orientated feeder systems (or provide their own input modules) and allow interrogation of the common pool of data for resource management, general management and audit. As yet these case-mix systems have yet to prove themselves in the realms of audit; the clinical information may not be derived with sufficient detail.

Only one thing is certain: that the surgical trainee will find himself involved in the collection of data for the common use of:

● the production of a discharge summary to the GP
● clinical information for audit
● information for resource management.

The better systems will provide the trainee with feedback and give him or her the ability to get useful information out of the system.

## REFERENCES

Anderson C M, Chambers S, Clamp M 1988 Can audit improve patient care? Effects of studying use of digoxin in general practice. British Medical Journal 297: 113–114

Batstone G F 1990 Educational aspects of medical audit. British Medical Journal 301: 326–328

Bennett J, Walshe K 1990 Occurrence screening as a method of audit. British Medical Journal 300: 1248–1251

Bilroth T H 1881 Clinical surgery: reports of surgical practice 1860–1876. The New Sydenham Society, London

Black N 1991 A regional computerised surgical audit project. Quality Assurance in Health Care 2: 263–270

Bowden D, Walshe K 1991 When medical audit starts to count. British Medical Journal 303: 101–103

Buck N, Devlin H B, Lunn J N 1987 Report of a confidential enquiry into perioperative deaths. Nuffield Provincial Hospitals Trust and Kings Fund, London

Campling E A, Devlin H B, Lunn J N 1990 Report of the national confidential enquiry into perioperative deaths. Department of Health 1989 Working for patients (paper no. 6). HMSO London

Donabedian A 1966 Evaluating the quality of medical care. Millbank Memorial Federation of Quality 3:2, 166–203

Ellis B W, Sensky T 1991 A clinician's guide to setting up audit. British Medical Journal 302: 704–707

Ellis B W, Rivett R C, Dudley H A F 1990 Extending the use of clinical audit data. British Medical Journal 301: 159–162

Emberton M, Rivett R C, Ellis B W 1991 Comparative audit: a new method of delivering audit: Bulletin of the Annals of the Royal College of Surgeons 73: 117–120

Gabbay J, McNicol M C, Spiby J, Davies S C, Layton A J 1990 What did audit achieve? Lessons from preliminary evaluation of a year's medical audit. British Medical Journal 301: 526–529

Gruer R, Gordon D S, Gunn A A, Ruckley C V 1986 Audit of surgical audit. Lancet i: 23–26

Lomas J, Elkin M, Anderson G A et al 1991 Opinion leaders versus audit and feedback to implement practice guidelines: delivery after previous Caesarian section. Journal of the American Medical Association 265: 2202–2207

Mitchell M W, Fowkes F G R 1990 Audit reviewed: does feedback on performance change clinical behaviour? Journal of the Royal College of Physicians 19: 251–254

Mugford M, Banfield P, O'Hanlon M 1991 Effects of feedback of information on clinical practice: a review. British Medical Journal 303: 398–402

Royal College of Physicians 1989 Medical audit. A first report—what, why and how? Royal College of Physicians, London

Royal College of Surgeons 1991 The Royal College of Surgeons Confidential Comparative Audit Service. Bulletin of the Annals of the Royal Coll Surgeons 73:96

Shaw C D 1989 Medical audit: a hospital hand book. King's Fund Centre, London

Shaw C D, Costain D W 1989 Guidelines for medical audit: seven principles. British Medical Journal 299: 498–499

Standing Committee on Postgraduate Medical Education 1989 Medical audit: the educational implications. SCOPME, London

Standing Medical Advisory Committee 1990 The quality of medical care. HMSO, London

## FURTHER READING

Guidelines for clinicians on medical records and notes 1990

Royal College of Surgeons of England, Clinical Audit and Quality Assurance Committee, London

Computers in medical audit: a guide for hospital consultants to personal computer based medical audit systems 1990 Royal Society of Medicine Services Ltd, London

Guidelines for surgical audit by computer 1991 Royal College of Surgeons of England, London

Walshe K, Bennet J 1991 Guidelines on medical audit and confidentiality. South East Thames Regional Health Authority, Bexhill on Sea

Confidentiality and medical audit: interim guidelines 1990 Scottish Home and Health Department, Edinburgh

# 33. Consent for surgical treatment

*L. Doyal*

For surgery to be successful, there must be a relationship of trust and confidence between surgeon and patient. Otherwise, patients will be reticent to present themselves for treatment or to divulge the detailed personal information required for recording accurate case histories and making successful diagnoses. Aside from the belief that their care will conform to a high clinical standard, the trust of patients also depends on their belief that their autonomy will be respected — that they will have the right to decide their own medical destiny, whatever anyone else may think. This general right can be subdivided into three principles — the right to informed consent, to the truth and to confidentiality. The latter two clearly follow from the first. Choices cannot be properly informed on the basis of deception and cannot be respected if what patients deem private is made public. Therefore, it is the principle of informed consent itself which is fundamental and on which both the morality and the legality of good surgery depends.

## THE MORAL IMPORTANCE OF INFORMED CONSENT

The moral unacceptability of anyone exercising unlimited power over others is at the heart of many of our liberal values. It is our capacity for rational choice that differentiates humans from other creatures. Respect for this capacity — especially our right to be the gatekeeper of our own bodies — is an indication of the seriousness, therefore, with which we respect the humanity and dignity of others.

## What is informed consent?

For patients to give their informed consent to surgery, they must receive enough accurate information about their illness, the proposed treatment and its prognosis, to be able to make a considered choice about whether or not it is in their own personal interest. For this to be a reality, the surgeon must complete four general tasks. First, the procedure itself must be described, including information about its practical implications and probable prognosis. Second, the probability of specific associated risks or complications should be revealed. Third, it should not be assumed that the patient already knows the risks of other aspects of surgical procedures, such as the complications that might result from a general anaesthetic, bed rest, intravenous fluids or a catheter. Finally, other surgical or medical alternatives to the proposed treatment — including non-treatment — should be outlined, along with their general advantages and disadvantages.

Ideally, the amount of such information should be that which mentally competent patients require to make their informed choice a realistic possibility. Surgeons should remember that the amount of information they are obligated to divulge may well change depending on what they should know about patients as individuals. For example, it may not be necessary for informed consent to occur for a manual labourer to be told of a very small operative risk of stiffness in one finger. This would obviously not be true of a concert pianist, underlining why the recording of the patient's employment in case notes and reference to it in the presentation of case histories is so important.

## Good consenting practice

As much as possible, the physical surroundings during the discussion should be conducive to easy, quiet discussion. Ideally, the place should be private and free of disturbances and interruptions by junior staff or medical students following in retinue on a busy Nightingale ward. The surgeon should not stand threateningly over a patient in bed and should avoid giving the appearance of being rushed by other duties.

The language with which the surgeon communicates should be as simple as possible, avoiding needless technicalities. When serious matters are being discussed, it is often helpful for a relative or friend to be present, both for support and to participate in ensuring — both at the time and later at home — that the patient really does understand. In the hospital ward, nurses with whom the patient is familiar can often fulfil this role very effectively. Appropriate leaflets or booklets can be of great help and innovative work is also being done with audio recording of interviews with transplant patients, for example, who are encouraged to take them home to discuss with others.

Having tried to provide clear information, it is then important to try to check that the patient has actually understood it. No doubt there will be time constraints on doing both. However it is clear that the surgeon is morally responsible for attempting both to an acceptable standard. There are a variety of ways in which this might be done — asking the patient to go back over what has been said in his own terms, for example, and, obviously, asking him at various times if he has any questions. The more confident surgeons generally become in this respect, the less time effective consenting will take.

Surgeons have often limited the amount of information given to patients on the grounds of the potential distress it would cause. This is unacceptable, if the long term aim is to keep the patient in ignorance. All competent individuals have a right to decide what is and is not in their best interest, even if what they decide is not endorsed by their professional advisors. It would be no more acceptable for a solicitor or accountant to delude their clients on the grounds that they did not want to distress them about the possibility of losing a court action or going bankrupt. Why should the moral obligations of the surgeon be any different?

## The consent form

In principle, the consent form which patients should sign before having surgery is their public and permanent affirmation that they have indeed agreed to it. All competent patients who are 16 or older should sign the form for all surgical procedures involving a general anaesthetic. A form should also be signed by the patient for procedures under local anaesthetic if there might be significant sequelae — for example, an excision of skin lesions. Clinicians obtaining the consent should also sign the form to indicate that to the best of their knowledge, the patient has both been given and understands the information necessary for him to make a considered judgement.

This being said, two things should be remembered about the consent form. First, it is not necessary for competent patients to sign it for all surgical interventions. Simple investigative procedures (e.g. sigmoidoscopy) which involve minimal risk of harm can be undertaken on the basis of a verbal explanation of what they physically entail. Consent can be assumed to be implied if the patient then accepts the procedure, even though he may not explicitly state that this is the case. Second, the consent form is not legal proof that consent has been given — something that should always be borne in mind when there is a temptation to cut corners as regards good consenting practice. At most, it is only one piece of evidence that some attempt was made to obtain informed consent, not that it was a morally or legally satisfactory attempt.

## THE LEGAL IMPORTANCE OF INFORMED CONSENT

Aside from its general moral and clinical importance, doctors also have a legal obligation to respect the patient's right to consent to treatment.

## Battery

In principle, it is a violation of the civil law pertaining to battery to touch another person without their consent. For example, two women won damages for battery because they were given hysterectomies to which they did not agree in the aftermath of operations for other problems. Also, in a case in Canada, a woman who made it clear that she wanted to be injected in one arm successfully sued when she received the injection in the other! The harm resulting from battery is not necessarily physical in nature since in law a battery can be committed without its occurrence. Rather harm should here be construed as the moral violation of the patient's right to exercise rational choice.

Of course, in many situations involving **minor** surgical procedures or tests, it will not be possible or advisable specifically to ask for the consent of patients every time they are touched. Were this the case, surgery would become practically impossible. But it does not follow that even here the patient's consent is legally irrelevant. Rather, as we have just seen, they can be said to have given their implied consent by virtue of the fact that they have presented themselves for treatment and have accepted what is offered. A woman once argued, for example, that a ship's surgeon had committed a battery because he vaccinated her without specifically asking if she wanted the injection. She lost on the grounds that her consent was implied since she was in a queue of people who were clearly waiting to be injected and she actually held out her arm when her turn came.

Clearly, there will be many situations which are much less clear cut. For example, is there a risk of battery if a patient claims that had they been given more information before surgery, they would have refused it? If the patient was generally informed in a way thought relevant to an informed choice and was not deliberately deceived, if they gave no indication of questioning their desire to proceed through asking for more information and if they signed the appropriate consent form then the answer is probably not. Of course, this presupposes that the surgeon has not deprived the patient of information about potential risks or discomfort that has been specifically requested or, returning to our example of an unwanted hysterectomy, has usurped a clinical choice commonly regarded as remaining with the patient.

## Negligence

Yet battery is not the only legal action surgeons risk for inadequately respecting their patients' right to informed consent. In an important case, Mrs Sidaway suffered paralysis resulting from spinal surgery to relieve pressure on a nerve root without being told of the small risk that this could occur. Here, it was judged that she had not been a victim of battery because, again, she had given her general consent to the surgery in question. However, her solicitors then claimed *negligence*, the action now recommended in such cases. The negligence concerns the professional duty of surgeons properly to advise patients not just about the proposed surgery but also about its potential hazards. In such situations, the patients argue that had they known the risks in question, they would not have proceeded with surgery.

It would again be wrong to assume that in these circumstances surgeons are protected from such accusations by a signed consent form for treatment. The patient might still successfully argue that even though he had signed the form, he was not given enough relevant information to make an informed decision before he signed and/or that he was not aware of the significance of the form. There is no escaping the surgeon's general duty to disclose information about potentially harmful side effects and to do so in a way that the patient can understand in principle. Thus, for example, in all cases other than those of acute emergencies, care must be taken to provide translations for non-English speaking patients.

How are we to establish whether or not compliance with this duty is sufficient — whether or not enough information has been disclosed about risks so that the rights of patients are seen to be respected? Legal judgements concerning negligent standards of adequate disclosure in the UK are still primarily set by the profession itself. Thus if recognised specialists all testify that they too would have communicated the same amount of information in the same circumstances then this will weigh strongly in favour of defendant surgeons who have not provided patients with more.

Recent legal developments have underlined this 'professional standard' in the determination of what constitutes negligent informed consent. In the Sidaway case, for example, a majority of appellate judges in the House of Lords agreed with this approach to determining negligence. However, most also warned of the dangers of completely equating the patient's right to information with standards set by the profession. Indeed, one argued in a minority decision that there will be some information about surgery, for example serious hazards, which any 'prudent patient' would wish to know before giving his consent to proceed. A similar standard of legal negligence as regards informed consent is widespread in North America and is increasingly being endorsed morally by the medical profession in the United Kingdom. Therefore, surgeons should respect the right of patients to a level of information about their treatment which is dictated by their need for self-determination. The fact that this need should be balanced against standards of professional practice does not entail that it is determined by them.

### The unconscious patient

Suppose that a surgeon on A&E is confronted with the victim of an automobile accident who requires an immediate operation. Here there is a clear duty to treat despite the fact that it is impossible to obtain the patient's consent. This is not because the surgeon becomes the proxy of the patient and makes a substituted judgement on his behalf, one which attempts to second guess what his own choice would have been. In such circumstances, there is no way of knowing for certain what the patient might choose. In the UK, no adult can act as a legal proxy for any other.

Therefore, the only thing that is relevant in justifying surgery without the consent of the competent patient is his dramatic need — its *necessity* for the preservation of life rather than convenience, and his inability to give consent. For example, the arrest of a life-threatening haemorrhage in an otherwise healthy patient would clearly be in order while the same could not be said of the repair of a hernia. Of course, if the patient is conscious and evidently capable of rational judgement then even in an emergency you must advise him of his condition and your proposed treatment. If it is physically possible, a patient should also sign a consent form as he would in normal circumstances. Verbal consent is adequate if the patient's condition prohibits it in writing. However, in these circumstances, it is advisable if possible for another health worker to act as a witness.

### Children

Ordinarily, consent for surgery on children must be obtained from a proxy, usually a parent, deemed competent to make informed choices which are in the child's best interests. This is not, however, to suggest that surgeons must always be guided solely by parental consent. If such decisions are believed to be inconsistent with the child's best interests then in life-threatening emergencies they can be overriden. Equally, if parents are proposing long term treatment (or non-treatment) options which are regarded as similarly inconsistent then the child can be made a ward of court — very quickly if necessary, and appropriate surgery administered.

Legally it is acceptable for surgeons to treat adolescents under the age of 16 without parental consent, just as it is for GPs to prescribe contraceptives, provided that care has been taken to insure that they are mature enough to understand the nature of their illness, their prognosis and their proposed treatment, including any important associated risks. This said, treatment without parental consent should be regarded as the exception and not the rule. Unless the adolescent has specifically refused permission, attempts should be made if possible to find and consult parents who are not already on site. Aside from serious emergencies, the point at which the acceptability of childhood consent morally and legally ceases and parental consent becomes compulsory is difficult to establish in practice.

Certainly, quite young children often have a

good grasp of their prospects and treatment, especially when they have already experienced distressing surgical therapy for an illness which they have had for some time. In such circumstances, before further surgery is embarked upon, attempts should be made to consult such children about their wishes. Where there is disagreement between parent and child about the best course of action, especially in instances of potentially terminal disease, both should be counselled about what appears clinically to be in the child's best interests. Such counselling will be particularly important in situations where there is disagreement between the surgeon and parent about the most appropriate way to proceed. Again, in the unusual event that a surgeon believes parental choice dramatically conflicts with the medical interests of the child, it is always open to approach the Court for a judgement.

**Mental handicap and psychiatric illness**

In the case of adults who are judged incompetent to choose for themselves, we have seen that no one may legally act as a proxy. However, decisions about incompetence are complex. For example, incompetence to consent to surgery does not follow from severe psychiatric illness. If a patient has been properly Sectioned under the 1983 Mental Health Act, he can be compulsorily treated for psychiatric illness without his consent. But this does not hold for other forms of surgical treatment. In such circumstances, attempts must therefore be made to obtain the patient's consent, even when communication is difficult and certainty of understanding not assured.

Where there is doubt (and with the exception of some specific interventions like psychosurgery) treatment can proceed, provided that the surgeon and the relevant psychiatric team agree that it is in the patient's best medical interest. But great care must be taken in establishing this fact. The reticence to allow surgery which may seem to some to be in the interest of the incompetent is witnessed by the refusal of some courts to permit the sterilisation of young women deemed incapable of giving their own consent to the procedure.

## TWO PRACTICAL PROBLEMS

The obligation to disclose information about both proposed treatment and its hazards is not something the surgeon has any choice about. However, putting this moral and legal principle into practice is not always easy for two reasons.

### 1. Limitations on the understanding of patients

It is sometimes unclear whether or not consent has really been obtained even if the surgeon has taken care to explain the proposed procedure and its potential hazards. The comprehension of competent patients can be compromised by their illness, their educational and social background and by other aspects of their personalities which make them overly anxious or unwilling to listen. Yet difficult as such instances of impaired autonomy can be, especially if some patients are facing acute and complex surgery, the fact remains that surgeons should be able to demonstrate the fact that they have disclosed adequate information for proper consent and that the patient has confirmed that they have understood it.

It would be absurd to suggest that patients have a right to something which on other grounds they cannot possess — a complete clinical understanding of their condition and treatment. But it does not follow that surgeons do not have the specific duties of disclosure already outlined.

Practically speaking, therefore, how should surgeons demonstrate to themselves (and if necessary a judge) that they have done their best in this regard? Most important of all, they need to work constantly to improve their ability to communicate. Both the GMC and BMA stress this point and its importance is underlined by the increasing importance placed on communication skills within medical education generally. Surgeons can do no more than their best in this respect. However, it follows from the moral importance of informed consent that they should always attempt to optimise their ability to do so.

Further, it is important to keep some written record in case notes of the main points about treatment which have been communicated prior to the signing of the consent form. If one sticks to the model of the prudent patient outlined above, information should certainly have been given on significant risks of mortality and other hazards to bodily functions relevant to normal social participation: swallowing, speaking, continence, mobility, pain, and sexual performance, for example. A brief indication in the notes that each of these variables has been mentioned should not be too onerous a task and if challenged, will provide surgeons with evidence of what the patient was informed. This approach can be reinforced by giving patients written information about their proposed treatment and possible side effects.

Even after they have followed good consenting practice, surgeons may conclude that patients still cannot be said properly to have given their consent to treatment. Here, life saving emergencies aside, there is no choice but to postpone therapy until better communication has been achieved. This may be inconvenient but it is necessary if the rights of patients are to be protected and if surgeons are to be able to demonstrate that they have taken their moral and legal duty to do so seriously. No reasonable person could expect more.

## 2. Limitations on patients' consent

There are things to which a patient cannot consent, or refuse since this is an expression of the same right — even if they wish. There is no professional duty to provide surgery which is requested by patients who have no need for it. But what if they clearly need surgery but don't want it? Here respect for the autonomy of patients may well conflict with the other moral obligation to protect their life and health. The situation where this conflict is often most acute is when, in considered and unambiguous terms, patients refuse surgery which will save their lives.

The moral and legal emphasis on respect for autonomy within medicine is so strong that even in these circumstances, treatment must not be forced without consent, again assuming that the patient is conscious and competent. This fact is sometimes obscured because patients who are terminally ill and do not wish further treatment are physically unable to resist it through discharging themselves if their wishes are not taken seriously. Where it becomes very clear, however,

is in the case of Jehovah's Witnesses who will only proceed with surgery on the understanding that if they haemorrhage, they will not be transfused. Legally, competent patients have every right to make such a demand. Having made it in a convincing way, a surgeon who proceeds to the contrary risks an action for battery. This said, surgeons do not have to operate under these terms if they believe them to be morally unacceptable. The patient can be referred elsewhere.

Another factor which complicates the right of patients to refuse treatment which can save their lives is the degree to which this legally and morally compromises surgeons who respect it. No patient can expect active steps to be taken to cause their life to end. However, the surgeon may decide, in consultation with the patient and relatives, that further surgical treatment is pointless given the irreversible and terminal character of a particular disease. Complying with the request to omit or to stop treatment, therefore, is neither actively killing nor aiding and abetting suicide. Unlike the potential suicide, the patient may well want desperately to live but not at any cost, as regards the quality and length of life which surgery might provide. Yet to go along with a request to be left alone in the face of dire surgical need is a very serious moral, and potentially, legal matter. Great care must be taken to ensure that the patient fully understands the implications of refusal of treatment and is competent to make an informed judgement. For in this situation, a mistake either about the patient's condition, or his wishes cannot be corrected.

## INFORMED CONSENT AND SURGICAL RESEARCH

The availability of surgical choices is dependent on the experimental research which makes them possible. Yet researchers must be careful. Without enthusiasm and conviction about the importance of their work, they will not have the commitment that successful research requires. Yet such commitment can lead to an underestimation of the risks or discomfort of experiments. Focusing for the moment on therapeutic research which might be to their benefit, patients have a right to informed consent for the same reasons described above. Further, allowing them to evaluate hazards for themselves is one of the best ways of regulating experimental zeal, a factor which has unquestionably led to moral abuses in the past. The clearest example is the notorious and needless experiments inflicted by some Nazi doctors and surgeons on Jewish prisoners.

The Nuremburg Code which was internationally adopted as a result declared that 'the voluntary consent of a patient is essential' in any medical research. The later Declaration of Helsinki is even more explicit. It states: 'In any research, each potential subject must be adequately informed of the aims, methods and anticipated benefits and potential hazards of the study and the discomfort it may entail'. And after this, their consent must be obtained.

The enforcement of the Helsinki Declaration in Britain is entrusted to research ethics committees. These exist for all hospitals and must approve all research proposals concerning work within them. In principle, research ethics committees are supposed to check that the protocol makes good scientific sense and poses no further risks than those of the best available treatment. Only then should patients be asked to consent to participate, employing information and a form of words on a consent form which have themselves been approved by the committee.

There is, however, one significant problem that does remain concerning research and informed consent. As a result of differing ability and willingness to understand and to question medical authority, we have seen that patients vary in their ability to understand the details of clinical information. Consequently, enthusiastic researchers are in a position, wittingly or not, to manipulate patients to do things that might not be proposed in ordinary treatment. Patients may be encouraged to agree to participate in the development of surgical procedures, for example, without realising how experimental they are. Here the general guidelines concerning informed consent should be followed with extra vigilance. Care must be taken to identify surgical procedures which might not be regarded as standard professional practice and to proceed only when the patient's written consent has been obtained in the knowledge that this is the case.

In non-therapeutic research with volunteers, it is equally important to avoid confusing agreement to participate with informed consent to do so. The researcher must try to ensure that the moral legitimacy of the consent of the volunteer is not obtained under financial, social or professional duress. The difficulty of doing so in some circumstances has led in the UK to medical research not ordinarily taking place among the prison population.

## INFORMED CONSENT AND CONFIDENTIALITY

As a corollary of their right to informed consent, patients also believe that they have the right to control access to information which they give to surgeons for the purposes of treatment. The GMC fully concurs through the importance it attaches to the principle of confidentiality — of respecting this right through obtaining the permission of patients before revealing clinical information about them to others. Few things can more quickly lead to a surgeon being professionally disciplined than a proven breach of confidence in unwarranted circumstances.

There are two types of arguments behind this concern. First, the right to be the moral gatekeeper of one's body extends to information divulged in clinical consultations. Second, if patients are frightened that their confidence might be breached, they may not be willing to provide the honest information on which successful diagnosis depends or even to turn up for treatment at all. This can pose a severe danger to them and possibly to the general public.

It is this latter potential conflict between the freedom of the individual and the interest of the public which creates circumstances where the surgeon either must or might divulge information otherwise regarded as private. The same professional codes which stress the importance of confidentiality, the GMC Blue Book, for example, also outline the exceptions to the rule which fall into two general categories.

### The public interest

Suppose that in a clinical consultation in A&E, a

surgeon discovers that a highly agitated patient is armed, has committed a robbery and has killed a bank clerk and a customer as a result. Here, it seems straightforward that the confidence should be broken and the police informed. The patient might strike again. Indeed, it is legally mandatory to breach confidentiality where patients are suspected of involvement in terrorism or where they are found to be suffering from a highly infectious and notifiable disease.

But how serious must this risk to the public actually be? For example, would a surgeon be just as willing to turn someone in who confessed in confidence that they had stolen a badly needed winter coat? The fact is that it is not always easy to balance the interests of the patient against those of the public. This can create difficult dilemmas for surgeons when the two seem in direct conflict and when, as is often the case, there is considerable professional discretion as to how morally to proceed. Debates about HIV and AIDS have recently underlined these issues.

Two things are clear. First, it does not follow from the claim by someone in authority that the public interest demands a breach of confidence that it actually does. For example, the police have no right to disclosure or to access to clinical records which may provide it. A judge may issue a warrant authorising such access or a subpoena demanding disclosure in court. However, even this does not make it inevitable. Some clinicians have felt so strongly about the immorality of breaking a patient's confidence that they have risked being charged with contempt of court for refusing to do so. Again, the law and morality should not be conflated, even though they often do overlap.

Second, patients have no right to harm others through the exercise of their right to confidentiality. There is an obvious link between this right and the right of individuals to control the use of their private property. Yet just as the legitimate exercise of this right stops at the point at which the safety of others is threatened, the same can be said about clinical information. Therefore, if a surgeon discovers that maintaining confidentiality will lead to the threat of serious harm to another specific individual – just the suspicion of a general threat is not sufficient – then a breach of

confidence may be warranted. For example, a psychiatrist in the United States was successfully sued for negligence for not informing a young woman that he had convincingly been told by a patient that he was going to kill her. He did.

### The interest of the individual patient

Breaches of confidence may not just be in the public interest. They may also be necessary in order to obtain information vital for successful treatment. Because of the physical or psychological effects of their illness, some patients are unable to communicate clearly about their medical history. Under such circumstances, relatives or friends may have to be consulted, especially in emergencies.

This said, attempts should still be made to obtain the patient's consent and to verify the identity of any others from whom information is sought. No more information about the patient's condition should be revealed than is necessary for the clinical purposes at hand. Knowledge about prognosis and treatment, for example, should remain confidential remembering how its unwarranted spread might drastically affect the patient's private and public life. Certainly, clinical information should never be communicated over the phone to those not involved in treatment, unless it is with the patient's prior consent.

The interests of patients are also served if the surgeons to whom they reveal clinical information share it with colleagues whose assistance they require. Patients are presumed to consent to such revelations by virtue of their general agreement to treatment. Given the complexity of its division of labour, surgery is an essentially cooperative exercise whose success depends on the free flow of relevant information. This said, only those professionals involved should have access to it, something which requires caution, especially on open wards.

## MORAL INDETERMINACY, INFORMED CONSENT AND OPEN COMMUNICATION

Thus far, we have examined the general principles governing informed consent which are endorsed by the profession of surgery and which are reinforced by statute and case law. Yet clear as these are, their correct interpretation may be much more obscure in practice. Such rules do not interpret themselves: individual surgeons interpret them faced with the complexities of specific cases.

In the majority of cases, there will be a consensus among the surgical team about the most appropriate interpretation. It will be reasonably clear, for example, how much information to attempt to communicate to a knowledgeable patient about the hazards of a particular treatment and whether or not they have understood enough of it to warrant proceeding. Yet in some situations, such agreement will not exist and interpretations will conflict. Here reference to the facts of the case themselves cannot solve the problem. Their openness to conflicting interpretation is what poses it.

Suppose, for example, that despite careful attempts to communicate the considerable risks of an urgently needed operative procedure to a patient, there is still disagreement among a surgical team about whether or not they have been understood. Here, and against the background of the necessity to come to a quick decision, there may be no 'right' interpretation as to how ethically to proceed. Another illustration might be conflicting beliefs about whether or not urgently to operate on a Jehovah's Witness who refuses a blood transfusion but seems partly to be doing so under pressure from her family or clergy.

What is crucial in such circumstances is that despite their disagreements, individual members of the surgical team accept that the final decision about how to proceed is reached after an open and rational discussion where everyone has the chance to present his arguments. As a result, clinicians will be much more willing to cooperate in the search for a common view, even when it involves a degree of what they may perceive as moral compromise. Open communication does not have to conflict with the recognition that it is the senior clinician who must take responsibility for the final choice. Surgeons in authority should always try to create space for such discussions, a practice which is increasingly common in the face of taxing moral dilemmas which have to be resolved in short periods of time — those, for example, concerning non-treatment.

## CONCLUSION

We have argued that patients have a moral and legal right to give their informed consent to surgical treatment and that the surgeon's duty of care extends to respecting this right, just as much as it does to providing a high standard of surgery per se. What such respect means in principle is clear — to allow competent patients to act as the gatekeepers of their own bodies and of clinical information about them, even if their decisions conflict with those of their clinicians. Unless there is a clinical diagnosis of incompetence, the expressed wishes of patients should only be overridden in serious surgical emergencies. If the patient is unconscious and incapable of choice, the necessity of the surgical intervention rather than its convenience must be the determining factor.

It has also been argued that in practice, gaining informed consent can be negatively affected by the education and/or receptiveness of the patient and the ability of the surgeon to communicate. As regards the latter, there is a range of opportunities for improvement which should be taken. Concerning patients, methods should be devised to ensure that they have understood as much as they are capable of and that really important information is always disclosed. Taking care to do so will reinforce the confidence of the patient and increase the quality of the clinical relationship for all of those concerned with the provision of good surgical care. Where there is disagreement about what this entails in practice, open discussion is essential. As much as possible, the importance of respecting the autonomy of patients should always extend to colleagues as well.

### Addendum

New case law has necessitated two additions to the existing text. First, as regards children, a court can now order treatment under the age of 18, irrespective of a patient's wishes. The case in question concerned a young woman of 16 suffering from anorexia who was regarded as competent to give her consent to treatment. However, she was not allowed to refuse it, once treatment was defined clinically to be in her best interests.

Second, competent patients may refuse life-saving treatment while conscious and then lapse into unconsciousness. However, their prior refusal must be respected only if it is judged to be an autonomous decision intended to apply in the circumstances that have arisen. For example, a young adult woman refused a blood transfusion on the grounds of her acceptance of the doctrine of the Jehovah's Witnesses. After she had become unconscious, the court overruled this refusal on the grounds that she had been unduly influenced by her mother and that her decision was based upon a false impression of her prognosis.

The upshot of both of these legal developments is that surgeons should do their best to ensure that any refusal to life saving care is made while adult patients are competent, are not under undue pressure from others and are as fully informed as possible about the consequences of their refusal. If a minor who is competent to consent to life saving treatment refuses it, the surgeon can ask the advice of a court and act accordingly.

## Acknowledgements

Many thanks to John Cochrane, Bob Cohen, Lesley Doyal, John Dickenson, Alastair McDonald, Rosanne Lord, Paul Lear, Norman Williams, Daniel Wilsher, Chris Wood and Richard Wood. Special thanks to Ian Kennedy.

SELECTED BIBLIOGRAPHY

Alderson P 1990 Choosing for children. Oxford University Press, Oxford
Appelbaum P, Lidz C, Meisel A 1987 Informed consent. Oxford University Press, New York
Beauchamp T, Childress J 1989 Principles of biomedical ethics. Oxford University Press, New York
Brazier M 1992 Medicine, patients and the law. Penguin, Harmondsworth
Faden R, Beauchamp T 1986 A history and theory of informed consent. Oxford University Press, New York
Faulder C 1985 Whose body is it? — the troubling issue of informed consent. Virago, London
Harris J 1985 The value of life. Routledge, London
Kennedy I 1988 Treat me right. Oxford University Press, Oxford
McLean S 1989 A patient's right to know: information disclosure, the doctor and the law. Dartmouth, Aldershot
Skegg P 1984 Law, ethics and medicine. Oxford University Press, Oxford

# 34. Clinical surgery in general examination

*A. O. Mansfield   R. M. Kirk*

The purpose of the FRCS examination is to determine whether candidates have the basic knowledge required for further training in surgery and are able to use this knowledge competently. All examinations are a compromise since the whole curriculum cannot be tested. We have concentrated on making the examination as comprehensive, as fair and as objective as possible. We recognize that objectivity is difficult — perhaps impossible to achieve in a clinical examination.

In order to cover the field as widely as possible the clinical part of the FRCS examination is split into sections, each intended to test different aspects and allow as many examiners as possible to assess each candidate to minimize bias. The examiner's responsibility is to cover as wide a range as possible, favouring essential topics. Different examiners emphasize different aspects. Similarly, two candidates may produce the same answer to a question but one imparts the answer clearly, confidently, with well-ordered priorities, and is awarded a higher mark. This is inevitable in a profession in which communication skills are so important.

In order to maintain standards as level as possible, new examiners are always partnered by a senior, experienced examiner. Many candidates believe that the Court has a 'rationing' system, allowing through a limited number on each day or during the whole examination. This is not true. The numbers passing on different days and throughout different examinations vary widely. The standard does not.

If you accept that the ability to utilize knowledge is at least as important as possessing it, you will realize that it is not enough merely to imbibe facts — you must arrange them so they are immediately accessible and practise using them. One of the overlooked benefits of the 'big bang' examinations over continuous assessment is that they give a stimulus to survey the whole field, identify deficiencies and correct them.

The clinical surgery in general section assesses competence in the basics of surgery. You are expected to possess, and to be able to use, the basic knowledge that will be required in any branch of surgery that you enter. Since all candidates do not have equal experience, you will be questioned within what is accepted as of general relevance, or in areas that you have experienced by reference to the surgical procedures which you have recorded in your log book.

## Written examination

Essay questions are devoted to topics of major importance, those that have undergone advances or are changing, and those in which recently instituted or newly evaluated management has been reported. The questions are selected so that reasonably knowledgeable candidates could write for three or four times the allotted period. Good answers display the ability to comprehend the question and the reason it was included, select essentials, arrange facts, discuss complex issues and communicate lucidly in writing.

Read every word of the question carefully, asking yourself, 'Why was this question asked?' Make notes but do not start writing the answer until you are sure how you will arrange it. As you start to write, remember that examiners can only mark what they can read.

You cannot write all you know so do not waste time with irrelevant or unimportant facts at the risk of omitting major points. Remember it is possible to fail even though everything you have written is correct. The reason you will have failed is because you have not answered the question that was asked or because you have failed to communicate priorities in management. Do not omit important points because you think they are obvious. It is safer to mention them.

Questions often start with the word 'discuss'. Identify all the aspects, including the contentious ones, that demand explanation or justification. You will not be expected to have great personal experience but you should be able to display the relevant arguments. You will be expected to have gained a greater depth of understanding since the MB or equivalent examination.

## Short notes questions

Here your knowledge in a wide range of subjects will be examined. The essentials can be set out briefly but careful planning will be required; merely writing correct but irrelevant information will not earn marks. Your ability to organize your knowledge is also being tested.

In the first examination the short notes questions were answered badly. It was apparent that candidates were not considering the questions fully and frequently omitted important aspects of the question while including facts that had not been asked for. Each question paper — essay and short answer — is marked independently by two examiners. This was introduced because the written paper now eliminates candidates who fail badly. In order to facilitate the photocopying you are asked to write with a black ball-point pen, which will be provided.

## Clinical examination

It is often difficult not to view examiners as adversaries, especially in face-to-face encounters. Remember they have a duty to the public and to the profession to maintain the standard of surgeons. They are not just influenced by your theoretical knowledge but they also take account of your communication skills with the patients and with themselves, your common sense and ability to make deductions and decisions even when the information is incomplete. This part of the examination is stressful but you should prepare yourself by seeing as many patients as possible and presenting your findings to a critical instructor.

## Long case

The intention of this part of the examination is to test your ability to gather clinical information in a limited period of time, interpret it, draw conclusions, make decisions and present your findings professionally. You will spend 20–25 minutes alone with the patient and you can make notes for your own use. After taking the history and examining the patient, spend a few moments deciding how you should present the facts of the case to the examiner.

The patient may tell you the diagnosis. This does not exonerate you from the need to assess it critically and consider differential diagnoses. Consider how to test the diagnosis and how to determine its severity. Examine other systems to find out whether they are involved. Think about possible treatments. Do not be dismayed if you cannot make a diagnosis. You often cannot make a diagnosis in the out-patient clinic but you should be able to indicate how you will proceed with investigations and management.

The discussion with the examiner lasts about 10 minutes. Unless requested by the examiner to do otherwise you should present the patient in the way you would during a ward round with your consultant. This entails introducing the basic facts about the patient and progressing purposefully towards your conclusions. Report incidentals briefly, without distracting attention from the main line of reasoning. Report only those negative findings that are relevant to the diagnostic problem. Expect to be interrupted by questions.

The presentation is followed by your conclusion. You should present your diagnosis and be prepared to justify it, together with the incidental and differential diagnoses. Continue with the investigations you would request in order to confirm your diagnosis and determine the extent of the disease, exclude others, and to assess the patient's general condition. Follow this with a discussion of treatment choices, indicating and justifying your selection.

Do not be upset if the examiner interrupts and guides you along another path, asks you to explain or expand a detail, asks you to justify a statement, or changes the subject of discussion entirely. The examiner needs to determine the depth and range of your knowledge.

You may be shown the patient's investigations such as X-rays and laboratory test results and asked to discuss them.

### Short cases

The objective is to assess your ability to observe and elicit a variety of physical signs and interpret them. It gives your examiners the opportunity to observe your approach to patients and the way you examine them. Time does not permit you to take a full history and examine the whole patient so you will be directed by the examiner to the affected area. In case of doubt ask the patient if the part you are to examine is painful or tender. Above all else treat the patient with kindness and consideration. Do not obsessively repeat the examination. Carry it out once, carefully, making sure that you obtain all the information you need. You may ask the patient to move if this will help you to make the diagnosis.

Even though this is a short case you should observe the patient in general because the age, sex and general condition of the patient will influence your choice of management. Surgical practice depends on accurate diagnosis, assessment of the severity of the disease and choosing the appropriate management for the particular patient. Your abilities to observe, and to deduce from those observations, are tested in the clinical part of the examination.

Decide what is the most likely diagnosis and consider where else you should look. What differential diagnoses are possible and how can you confirm the diagnosis? What advice and treatment, if any, should you offer the patient?

Be sufficiently confident in your clinical findings to state them boldly but word them in such a way as not to alarm the patient. Do not continue to examine the patient while reporting your findings.

### Oral examinations

Each of the two oral examinations is conducted by two examiners. The topics which may be included will be found in the guide to the examination and as this guide will be revised from time to time you must make sure that you read the most recent one. You will be questioned by each examiner in turn, and the examiner may cover a number of different topics.

### Principles of operative surgery

There are certain essentials, such as aseptic technique, surgical access, haemostasis and effects of foreign materials, that are common to all branches of surgery.

Secondly, there are certain life-saving procedures that must be learned by anyone practising in any branch of surgery and some of these might reasonably be asked in an undergraduate examination. These include the maintenace or provision of an adequate airway, cardiac massage, chest drainage and intravenous access. There are others that should lie within the scope of any surgeon, such as cranial burr holes, thoracotomy, abdominal surgery for peritonitis, intestinal obstruction or intra-abdominal bleeding. Similarly you must know the management of trauma and the principles of surgery for malignant disease.

The examiners will look at your log book and ask questions about the procedures listed in it. This tests your knowledge of particular operations in which you have participated. They will not normally ask details of operations that you have not seen except for those that they consider within the competence of most trainees and those that are life saving.

### Surgical topics

Topics here are wide ranging and frequently include the application of basic sciences in clinical surgery. A pathological 'pot' may be used to introduce a surgical topic. Resuscitation, diagnostic methods, intensive therapy and terminal care are a few of the many subjects to be found in the guide. Knowledge of medical ethics, methods of evaluation of surgical practice and critical reading of the surgical literature will all be tested here.

## MARKING AND ASSESSMENT

You are identified by number throughout the examination in order to reduce any bias to a minimum. If you have worked for one of the examiners you may be passed to an independent examiner. In all you will normally be examined by eight examiners. They record the questions asked and the responses given and each pair will agree a mark for that section but without any knowledge of the mark given in any other part of the examination.

The marks from the four sections are added together at the end of the day.

At this time the whole Court of Examiners meets to check and to discuss the marks under the chairmanship of the senior examiner of the day. Candidates fall into three groups. Those with a pass mark are not discussed further. Those who have failed badly are also not discussed further. However, all the candidates who have just failed are fully discussed by the whole Court. The questions asked and the responses received are individually reported by the examiners. The Chairman, who has made notes, sums up and the Court votes to pass or fail that candidate. A majority decision is made, with the Chairman having a casting vote when necessary.

This method allows the Court as a body to monitor the difficulty of questions and to make allowances if it considers that a candidate has been unfairly marked down. It also allows some compensation between subjects — a candidate who has been outstanding in one part may be voted through if the failure in another part is minimal. Examiners are usually reluctant to allow a candidate to pass who has performed badly in the clinical examination. If all the candidates achieved the pass standard they would all pass. There is no quota.

## THE FUTURE

It is well recognized that there are many qualities required of a surgeon that are not assessed in the FRCS examination. The Court is continuously reviewing the examination and taking advice with the intention of keeping the examination relevant and appropriate as a basic test of surgery in general. Consequently the format may change again when the examiners are convinced that worthwhile improvements can be made.

# 35. Annotated references

*R. M. Kirk*

## INTRODUCTION
*R. M. Kirk*

We have made it clear that this is not a standard textbook of surgery. There are many excellent ones available from which to choose. However, we accept that young surgeons seek guidance in reading, apart from these. It is valuable to read widely, both among original articles, reviews, and particular chapters in textbooks and monographs.

We have asked distinguished specialist surgeons, many of whom are present or past examiners for the FRCS, to offer suggestions for reading on clinical topics. In each case they have stated why they have made their recommendations. As far as possible the references are to easily accessible journals and books.

The list from which to choose is vast and we all differ in what we think is important. Look through them to identify written accounts of topics which interest you.

## PART 35.1
## UPPER GASTROINTESTINAL TRACT AND THE ACUTE ABDOMEN
*R. M. Kirk*

Akiyama H 1990 Surgery for cancer of the esophagus. Williams and Wilkins, Baltimore

The Japanese have made very great contributions to surgery of oesophageal cancer by carefully studying the operative findings and resected specimens. As a result they have placed on a firm basis the planning of treatment.

Professor Hiroshi Akiyama has been a leader in the field, producing remarkably low operative mortality and excellent five year survival figures. He has achieved this by scrupulous attention to detail. As he says in the preface to his book, '... major operations are a sum or combination of numerous small procedures, and therefore each individual component procedure must be carried out with maximum care'. This is a good philosophy for all surgeons to adhere to.

Cotton P B, Williams C B 1982 Practical gastrointestinal endoscopy, 2nd edition. Blackwell, Oxford

Every surgeon who wishes to operate on the gastrointestinal tract, or accept surgical emergencies, should be skilled in passing endoscopes and in interpreting the findings. In this classic book by two leading endoscopists, Professor Peter Cotton gives authoritative advice on upper gastrointestinal endoscopy.

Cuschieri A, Giles G R, Moosa A R (eds) 1988 Essential surgical practice, 2nd edition. Wright, London, pp 904–988, 1136–1192, 1232–1255

This textbook offers outstandingly succinct advice on the surgery of the upper gastrointestinal tract, small intestine and acute abdomen. Although young surgeons should keep up to date with the literature, it is necessary to have at hand easily accessible information on established practice.

DeMeester T R, Wang C I, Wernly J A et al 1980 Technique, indications and clinical use of 24 hour esophageal pH monitoring. Journal of Thoracic and Cardiovascular Surgery 79: 656–670
DeMeester T R, Attwood S E A, Smyrk T C et al 1990 Surgical therapy in Barrett's esophagus. Annals of Surgery 212: 528–542

Dr DeMeester has made valuable contributions to our knowledge of the physiology and pathology of the lower oesophagus. He and his team have carried out careful studies of the function, reflux and management of disorders in this area.

Jones P F 1990 Practicalities in the management of the acute abdomen. British Journal of Surgery 77: 365–367

Professor Peter Jones has made many contributions to our management of the acute abdomen, including his classical textbook on the subject: *Emergency Abdominal Surgery in Infancy, Childhood and Adult Life,* 2nd edition, 1987. In this article he considers the difficult problem of pain in the right iliac fossa.

Khoury G A: Squamous cell carcinoma of the oesophagus: 10 years on; Earlam R: An MRC prospective randomised trial of radiotherapy versus surgery for operable squamous cell carcinoma of the oesophagus; Cuschieri A: Invited introduction. Annals of the Royal College of Surgeons of England 1991, 73: 1–12

This mini-symposium debates a controversial problem in surgery. Each of the protagonists puts forward a viewpoint supported by arguments and a senior authority sums up. There are many areas in which differing views are held and which are resistant to efforts to resolve them.

Kirk R M, Stoddard C J 1986 Complications of surgery of the upper gastrointestinal tract. Baillière Tindall, London

We have attempted not only to display the complications of surgery in this region but also to give advice on avoiding and treating them. This involves avoiding rigid attitudes towards decision-making, care in every detail of management, and anticipation of impending trouble to avoid it if possible or to deal with it early if it has already occurred.

Monro A, McMillan I 1991 Adhesions and recurrent intestinal obstruction. Current Surgical Practice 3: 57–62

Abdominal adhesions are a great boon and a great cause of difficulty for surgeons. This article reviews the aetiology, presentation and management of complications caused by them.

Paterson-Brown S, Vipond M N 1990 Modern aids to clinical decision-making in the acute abdomen. British Journal of Surgery 77: 13–18

Management of the acute abdomen can be exceedingly difficult. It is too easy, though, to order investigations that have poor discimination,

thus wasting time, money and endangering the patient. Make sure that you can justify the investigations you order, and can rely upon them.

Thompson J C 1990 Hormonal control of gut function. American Journal of Surgery 161: 6–18

This topic may seem rather obscure as surgical reading. However, the gut is the largest endocrine organ in the body. Gut hormones play an important part in its function and its diseases, many of which impinge on surgical practice.

Tytgat G N J, Blankenstein M van 1990 Current topics in gastroenterology. George Thieme, Stuttgart

Review publications contain invited reports on important and changing areas. Although we should all like to read original research articles, there are far too many and we have to rely for balanced views on such as this. For example, on pages 530–544, Mills J G and Wood J R give a balanced review of recent developments in the treatment of peptic ulcer.

---

## PART 35.2
# HEPATOBILIARY SURGERY
*E. R. Howard    N. D. Heaton*

---

### Anatomy of the liver

Smadja C, Blumgart L H 1985. The biliary tract and the anatomy of biliary exposure. In: Blumgart L H (ed) Surgery of the liver and biliary tract. Churchill Livingstone, Edinburgh, pp 11-22

A thorough knowledge of the anatomy and blood supply of the liver and biliary tree is essential for any general surgeon performing hepatobiliary surgery. Bile duct injury will occur during cholecystectomy, for example, if variations in bile duct or vascular anatomy are not recognized. This article highlights the 'normal' biliary anatomy and the more common variations encountered. The segmental nature of the blood supply and biliary drainage of the liver is also described. The recognition of the segmental organization of the liver by Couinaud has been the key to improvements in the surgical management of liver trauma and the resection of tumours.

## Surgical liver disease in childhood

Howard E R 1985. Paediatric liver disease. In: Wright R, Millward-Sadler G H, Alberti K G M M, Karran S (eds) Liver and biliary disease, 2nd edn. London: Baillière Tindall/W O Saunders, London, pp 1219–1244

There are many congenital surgical conditions of the liver and biliary tract which usually present in childhood. Although they are rare they are of considerable interest to the general surgeon as they may be encountered occasionally at the time of a laparotomy in an older patient (e.g. chole-dochal cyst). The text also includes a description of tumours of the liver and biliary tract in children, which tend to be of the embryonic type (e.g. hepatoblastoma) and which differ considerably from adult tumours in their response to treatment. The management of portal hypertension in the younger age groups is also reviewed. In summary, this chapter is a comprehensive review of congenital, inflammatory and neoplastic hepatobiliary disease in childhood, and it includes an extensive review of the literature.

## Investigation of the gall bladder, cholecystectomy, and bile duct strictures

Johnson A G 1991 Biliary tract. In: O'Higgins N J, Chisholm G D, Williamson R C N (eds) Surgical management, 2nd edn. Butterworth–Heinemann, Oxford, pp 475–505

This review outlines the investigations used in biliary tract disease, and is particularly useful for the account of inflammatory conditions of the gall bladder, their treatment and the management of complications. Benign strictures and tumours of the bile ducts are included. The references at the end of each section contain a good selection of the key papers of the last ten years.

## Laparoscopic cholecystectomy

American Journal of Surgery 1991 161: March issue (multiple authors)

This edition of the *American Journal of Surgery* covers the initial American and European experience of laparoscopic surgery. The articles report the results of laparoscopic cholecystectomy and consider the developments that are occurring in this field. Other approaches to minimal access surgery are considered and the technical requirements, such as improved optical and imaging systems and changes in surgical instrumentation, are discussed. Laparoscopic surgery had previously been practised by a limited number of enthusiasts, but has now been taken up by a large number of surgeons. The place of laparoscopic surgery is as yet uncertain, but it seems certain to expand over the next few years, replacing many types of 'open' surgery as expertise and instrument design improve. This edition of the *American Journal of Surgery* reviews the present state of interventional laparoscopy; it is likely to continue to change rapidly in the future.

## Cholangiocarcinoma and carcinoma of the pancreas

Preece A, Cuschieri D, Rosin 1989 Cancer of the bile ducts and pancreas. Harcourt Brace Jonanovich, London

The prognosis of patients presenting with carcinoma of the head of the pancreas is poor, with fewer than 3% surviving five years. It has been described as a 'dismal disease', but the label could equally well be applied to cholangiocarcinoma, which is resectable in fewer than 10% of cases. Mean survival for the majority of patients is 6–12 months.

This book provides an excellent overview of a difficult subject. Clear guidelines are given for the investigation of the bile ducts and pancreas. Recent advances in the diagnosis and assessment of tumours, such as ultrasound scanning, cholangiography and angiography have failed to affect survival rates significantly although fewer patients are now subjected to an unnecessary laparotomy.

Surgical procedures including pancreaticoduodenectomy and resection of proximal biliary tumours are discussed and palliative endoscopic stenting reviewed. The importance of right and left hepatic duct drainage for adequate palliation is emphasized. Adjuvant therapy with cytotoxic drugs and/or radiotherapy is reviewed with the results of recent controlled trials. The diagnosis, management and surgery of rare endocrine tumours are also reviewed. The concluding chapter is a practical account of pain management including the technique of coeliac plexus block. This is a readable, critical account of the current management of biliary and pancreatic neoplasms.

## Benign and malignant liver tumours

### Benign liver tumours

Ishak K G, Rabin L 1975 Benign tumours of the liver.
Medical Clinics of North America 59: 995–1013

This paper, based on the study of a large number
of patients from the Armed Forces Institute of
Pathology, Washington, DC, provides a comprehensive account of benign tumours of the liver. It
differentiates between focal nodular hyperplasia
and adenoma, although the premalignant nature
of the latter is not stressed. The clinical and
pathological features of cavernous haemangiomas
and infantile haemangioendotheliomas, the commonest benign liver tumours, are discussed, and
their treatment briefly reviewed. Other rare miscellaneous tumours are also described in this
short but comprehensive chapter.

### Malignant liver tumours

Adson M A 1988 Primary hepatocellular cancers: western
experience. In: Blumgart L H (ed) Surgery of the liver and
biliary tract, Vol 90. Churchill Livingstone, Edinburgh pp
1153–1165

Hepatoma is the commonest cancer in man
worldwide. However, there are wide geographical
variations and the tumour is less common in the
West, reflecting aetiological factors such as viral
hepatitis, nutritional deficiencies or specific toxins. The difficulty in assessing resection rates in
the cirrhotic and non-cirrhotic liver is addressed.
The author presents his personal experience of
hepatic resection for hepatoma together with
other published series which suggest that survival
rates do justify the aggressive surgery needed to
excise these lesions. Improved management of
these tumours in cirrhotic patients by surgeons in
the Far East is also acknowledged. This includes
the recognition of small lesions, the use of limited
resections and the intensive perioperative management of cirrhotic patients.

### Liver tumours: colonic metastases

Hughes K S, Simon R, Soughovabodi S et al 1988 Resection
of the liver for colorectal carcinoma metastases: a
multi-institutional study of indications for resection.
Surgery 103: 278–288

Hepatic secondaries from the gut have been
regarded as untreatable in the past. Hepatic
resection for secondary disease has been associated with a high surgical mortality and extreme
morbidity. These views have been challenged in
recent years and several reports have now suggested a five-year survival of between 25% and
35% after resection of hepatic secondaries from
carcinoma of the colon and rectum. The paper of
Hughes et al analysed the results of surgery in
859 patients from 24 institutions, and with such
a large number of cases they were able to define
the benefits of surgical treatment and also the
contraindications. There was an overall actuarial
survival rate of 33%. The analysis revealed that
positive hepatic lymph nodes and the presence of
more than four lesions were associated with poor
prognosis. The stage of the primary tumour was
also important, with Dukes' C patients showing
poorer survival data than those with Dukes' B
lesions. The discussion includes a useful review
of the reports, which show almost no survival in
1650 patients with untreated hepatic metastases.
The large number of patients in this paper makes
it an important contribution to the literature on
hepatic metastases.

## Portal hypertension

Benhamou J-P, Lebrec D 1985 Portal hypertension. Clinics
in Gastroenterology 14: 1–288

Some of the interesting and clinically important
problems associated with portal hypertension are
covered by this issue. The aetiology and management of extrahepatic portal hypertension in children and adults are well summarized. The management of acute variceal bleeding is described
and medical and surgical approaches to the prevention of recurrent bleeding from oesophageal
varices reviewed, with a useful list of references.
The problems posed by ectopic varices in the
duodenum, small and large bowel, stomal and
intraperitoneal sites are comprehensively reviewed
and the management clearly defined.

American Journal of Surgery 1990 160: July issue (multiple
authors)

This edition of the *American Journal of Surgery*
was devoted to the current views of the management of portal hypertension. It is important in
that it presents differing personal views of the

current management of oesophageal varices and the complications of portal hypertension. The place of injection sclerotherapy in the treatment of acute variceal bleeding and in the prevention of recurrent haemorrhage is now of proven benefit. Doubt still remains about the benefit of prophylactic injection. The place of surgery now appears to be limited to those patients who fail to respond to injection sclerotherapy. Liver transplantation offers patients with advanced liver disease and bleeding oesophageal varices the best chance of long-term survival.

## Liver trauma

Feliciano D V, Pachter H L 1989 Hepatic trauma revisited. Current Problems in Surgery 26: 458–524
Feliciano D V, Jordan G L, Bitondo C G et al 1986 Management of 1000 consecutive cases of hepatic trauma (1979–1984). Annals of Surgery 204: 438–443

The management of liver trauma in recent years has tended to become more conservative, with a greater use of packs at the initial operation and a consequent reduction in the number of emergency hepatic resections. These two papers highlight the various approaches required for effective management and provide a remarkable record of a huge number of injuries. Decisions on treatment modalities, e.g. suture, hepatic resection or perihepatic packing, and the surgical results are clearly presented and the paper contains some interesting comments on the original work of J H Pringle (1908).

Moore E E 1984 Critical decisions in the management of hepatic trauma. American Journal of Surgery 148: 712–716

This paper gives a good classification of liver injuries and outlines the surgical management for each type — a short but useful guide.

## Liver Transplantation

Starzl T E, Demetris A J, Thiel D Van 1989 Liver transplantation (first of two parts). New England Journal of Medicine 321: 1014–1021
Starzl T E, Demetris A J, Thiel D Van 1989 Liver transplantation (second of two parts). New England Journal of Medicine 321: 1092–1099

This article, published in two parts, provides an up-to-date and authoritative summary by one of the pioneers of liver transplantation. Part one covers the topics of organ donation and indications for transplantation in non-neoplastic disease, putting risk factors such as age, previous operation and portomesenteric occlusion into context. Transplantation for inborn errors of metabolism that result from deficiencies of specific liver enzymes or from abnormal products of hepatic synthesis are also considered. The main indication for transplantation in these patients is deterioration of liver function, and correction of the underlying abnormality has been incidental. The disappointing results of transplantation for primary and secondary malignancy are briefly reviewed and the treatment of fulminant hepatic failure placed in context.

The operative details of the surgery are only briefly dealt with, but are in sufficient depth for the FRCS exam. The interesting problems associated with graft failure and monitoring of graft function are described.

Part two covers the problems of early and late graft dysfunction and the recognition and differentiation of immunological and non-immunological causes. Prevention and treatment of graft rejection, including the use of newer agents such as FK506, and late postoperative problems such as viral infection and recurrence of native disease are also covered. The article ends by mentioning the possibility of auxiliary transplantation in the management of acute liver failure.

## Liver infection

### Hydatid disease

Kune G A, Morris D L 1989 Hydatid disease. Schwarkz S I, Ellis H (eds) Maingot's abdominal operations, 9th edn. Appleton and Lange, Norwalk, C T, pp 1225–1240

Hydatid disease is a major worldwide health problem and surgery is still the only consistent and effective management for hepatic involvement. This chapter has been written by two of the recognized authorities on the subject. It is a very good summary of the pathology, relevant investigations, medical management and surgical techniques necessary for effective management. The bibliography includes references to the recent advances in drug therapy.

*Pyogenic liver abscess and amoebic abscess*

Barnes P F, Cock K M De, Reynolds T N, Ralls P W 1987 A comparison of amebic and pyogenic abscess of the liver. Medicine 66: 472–483

This paper reviews the clinical presentation and management of amoebic and pyogenic abscesses of the liver. Important features which help in the management of these patients are based on experience with a large group of patients. The value of ultrasound in the diagnosis of amoebic abscess is emphasized. Almost all amoebic abscesses respond to amoebicidal agents without the need for aspiration. In contrast, pyogenic abscesses should be aspirated to guide antibiotic therapy and a significant number will need to be drained surgically.

**Further reading**

Blumgart L M 1988 Surgery of the liver and biliary tract. Churchill Livingstone, Edinburgh

This textbook provides a comprehensive and authoritative review of the surgical management of hepatobiliary disorders.

PART 35.3

**COLORECTAL SURGERY**
*W. S. Shand*

Rob C G, Smith E R Alimentary tract and abdominal wall. 3. Rectum and anus. 1983 In: Todd I P, Fielding L P (eds) Operative Surgery, 4th edn. Butterworths, London

This extremely well-illustrated book gives a very good overview of the practical points of the various surgical procedures relating to colorectal surgery.

In the examination you will be expected to talk about operations which you have done yourself and at which you have assisted. When assisting the various steps of a procedure are not always obvious. Reference to this book with its superb and copious illustrations will fill gaps in your knowledge and also refresh your memory about procedures which you have undertaken yourself. It covers all the principal operations in colorectal and anal surgery. It covers the practical steps of anal procedures such as haemorrhoidectomy and

sphincterotomy particularly well.

You may find difficulty in getting hold of a copy from your hospital library, as all members of the surgical team from consultant down refer to it regularly.

Dudley H, Carter D C, Russell R C G 1986 Atlas of general surgery, 2nd edn. Butterworths, London

This book covers the principal procedures outlined in the above volume. Again it is the copious illustrations which are particularly helpful.

Fielding L P, Welch J P 1987 Intestinal obstruction. Churchill Livingstone, Edinburgh.

This book gives a very good overview of the subject of intestinal obstruction. The anatomy and pathophysiology of the subject are well covered. Chapter 8 on radiological evaluation is particularly good. Chapter 12 covers intraoperative techniques in large bowel obstruction in order to achieve safer resection with primary anastomosis.

Frontiers in colorectal disease. British Journal of Surgery 72. 1985 and supplement.

The following articles are of particular interest:

S 53–54 Morson B C.

This article covers the histological criteria for local excision of rectal tumours. It is written by a pathologist who is generally regarded as the leading authority on this subject.

S 59–66 Duncan W, Porter N H, Nicholls R J, Cummings B J (Three articles)

These articles cover the use of radiotherapy in rectal cancer, a frontier subject which is of particular importance.

S 97–103 Greenall M J, Quan SHQ, De Cosse J J.

This article covers epidermoid cancer of the anus. Considerable advance has been made in the treatment of malignancy of the anal canal and this article is a very good review of the subject.

This supplement covers much else besides the above subjects. Although it might be regarded as getting a little out of date it is in fact an extremely good review of the whole of colorectal surgery.

De Cosse J J, Todd IP (eds) 1988 Clinical surgery international. Vol 15, Anorectal surgery. Churchill Livingstone, Edinburgh

This volume covers a number of small subjects about which relatively little has been written. I would commend Chapter 2 on the subject of incontinence, Chapter 5 on fistula surgery, Chapter 8 on the difficult problem of sexually transmitted diseases and Chapter 15 on injuries to anus and rectum.

Lee E. C, Nolan D J (eds) 1987 Clinical surgery international Vol 14, Surgery of inflammatory bowel disorders. Churchill Livingstone, Edinburgh

In this volume ulcerative colitis and Crohn's disease are compared and contrasted. It refers to all the important contributors to the management of these diseases over the years. It gives a very good overview of a very difficult subject.

Marti M C, Givel J C 1990 Surgery of anorectal diseases. Springer-Verlag, Berlin

The chapter on malignant anal tumours by G. Pipard (pp. 162–186) is worth reading as a comprehensive review of the subject. This volume covers many other aspects of the surgery of the anus and rectum. In my opinion it would be better not to read the chapter on Haemorrhoid and fistula surgery.

Corman M L 1989 Colon and rectal surgery, 2nd edn. Lippincott, Philadelphia, pp 1051

This textbook covers the subject of colorectal surgery comprehensively. It is a single-author book which won the American Medical Writers Association prize. The text is clearly written and is complemented by excellent operative illustrations. The book has rightly been described as the American alternative to Goligher but is of course somewhat more contemporary.

Welch J P 1990 Bowel obstruction: differential diagnosis and clinical management. Saunders, Philadelphia, pp 711

As the title suggests, this is a thorough guide to the subject of bowel obstruction. The book starts with a description of the general principles of obstruction, including pathophysiology. Both mechanical causes and motility disorders are covered, both in adults and children. The last nine chapters apply specifically to large bowel obstruction. References are extensive for those who wish to obtain an in-depth knowledge of the subject.

Goligher J 1984 Surgery of the anus, rectum and colon, 5th edn. Ballière Tindall, London

This is the classical work on the subject, which was first published in 1961. It is extremely well written, extremely detailed, extremely well illustrated, but sadly now somewhat out of date. Well worth dipping into, however.

Hughes E, Cuthbertson A M, Killingback M K 1983 Colorectal surgery. Churchill Livingstone, Edinburgh

This is a shorter book than Goligher's by a group from Australia who are very well known for their contributions to colorectal surgery. Again this is well written and well illustrated but is now becoming a little out of date. It is worth dipping into, however, for a slightly different perspective.

Thomson J P S, Nicholls R J, Williams C B 1981 Colorectal disease: an introduction for surgeons and physicians. Heinemann Medical, London

This book is short and easy to read. It provides a very good introduction and easily assimilated overview of the subject. Again it is becoming out of date in some respects so don't spend too long with it.

## PART 35.4
## ENDOCRINE SURGERY
### M. H. Wheeler

Lennquist S 1987 The thyroid nodule: diagnosis and surgical treatment. Surgical Clinics of North America 67: 213–232

This account by one of the world's leading endocrine surgeons describes the management of the thyroid nodule — probably the commonest indication for thyroid surgery in the Western world. It is an important paper because it describes very clearly the correct assessment of the thyroid nodule, placing emphasis on the role of fine-needle aspiration and highlighting the limitations of traditional isotope-scanning techniques. This paper's most important contribution is to firmly state the rationale for advising total unilateral lobectomy and isthmusectomy as the treatment of choice for the thyroid nodule, rather than the time-honoured but inadequate operation of subtotal unilateral lobectomy. There are many excellent practical tips relating to the actual surgical technique.

Lennquist S 1986 Surgical strategy in thyroid carcinoma: a clinical review. Acta Chirurgica Scandinavica 152: 321–338

This important article, also from Professor Lennquist, should be studied in conjunction with his 1987 paper on the thyroid nodule (see previous reference). It is an excellent guide to the management of thyroid malignancy (excluding tumours of C-cell origin) and argues very clearly the case for an aggressive surgical strategy in the majority of tumours. The description of surgical technique could only have been written by an expert and is a first-class description of how to perform thyroidectomy safely without damage to vital structures, such as the parathyroid glands and recurrent laryngeal nerves. There are 130 references, many of which should be regarded as key papers on the subject of thyroid malignancy.

Harada T, Shimaoka K, Mimura T, Ito K 1987 Current Treatment of Graves' disease. Surgical Clinics of North America 67: 299–314

Hyperthyroidism due to Graves' disease can be treated by radioiodine, antithyroid drugs or surgery. Each method has its advantages and disadvantages and, not surprisingly, there is little agreement worldwide on the ideal strategy for the patient with Graves' disease. Dr Harada and his colleagues discuss the relative merits of these treatment modalities and describe how factors such as patient age, size of goitre, severity of disease, and pregnancy might affect this treatment selection. I think the article is particularly relevant as it advocates policies almost identical to those practised in most UK centres. In particular, caution is urged in the use of radioiodine and a plea made for surgery to be offered to more patients on the basis of the predictable outcome of such treatment.

Sizemore G W, van Heerden J A, Carney J A 1983 Medullary carcinoma of the thyroid gland and the multiple endocrine neoplasia type II syndrome. In: Kaplan E L (ed) Surgery of the thyroid and parathyroid glands. Churchill Livingstone, Edinburgh, pp 75–102

Although medullary carcinoma of the thyroid is relatively rare, accounting for only 8% of all thyroid malignancies, it has proved to be a disease of enormous interest to the endocrine surgeon, partly because of the existence of the tumour marker calcitonin and also because of the familial variety of the disease with associated MEN II syndromes. This chapter is a most comprehensive account of management of the disorder and

is based on the enormous clinical experience of the Mayo Clinic group.

Clark O H 1989 Surgical treatment of hyperparathyroidism (indications for surgical exploration and intra-operative strategy). In: van Heerden J A (ed) Common problems in endocrine surgery. Yearbook Medical Publishers, Chicago pp 164–172

This book chapter written by a surgeon extremely experienced in the field is concise, yet contains almost everything the potential endocrine surgeon needs to know about the management of primary hyperparathyroidism. Dr Clark not only describes the surgical approach to the typical case, but also identifies and discusses the problems which present when there are variations in parathyroid anatomy, particularly those resulting from supernumerary or ectopic glands. All surgeons and physicians who manage patients with hypercalcaemia should read this contribution carefully and repeatedly because of the many pearls of wisdom within it.

Grant J S, van Heerden J A, Charboneau J W, James E M, Reading C C 1986 Clinical management of persistent and/or recurrent Primary Hyperparathyroidism. World Journal of surgery 10: 555–565

Persistent or recurrent hypercalcaemia following surgery for primary hyperparathyroidism (HPT) remains one of the most challenging problems in endocrine surgery. This report from the Mayo Clinic is important because it describes results of treatment of a very large series of 157 patients undergoing re-exploration. The approach to selection of localization procedures is well addressed and the authors remind us of the fact that the disease site in persistent or recurrent HPT is usually in the neck, the pathological parathyroid gland often being located in a normal position. Dr Grant and his colleagues show that reoperative parathyroid surgery can be extremely successful (89%) and performed with fairly low morbidity and extremely low mortality. The value of this paper is enormously enhanced by the excellent invited commentary at the end.

Thompson N W 1983 Surgical consideration in the MEN I Syndrome. In: Johnston I D A, Thompson N W (eds) Endocrine surgery. Butterworths, London, pp 144–163

Management of the inherited disorder MEN I syndrome remains a difficult challenge in endocrine surgery. This article by Professor

Thompson is based on a large personal clinical experience and addresses the problems posed by the parathyroid, pancreatic and pituitary components of the syndrome in a clear and comprehensive manner. Although the author does not side-step the controversies, he has managed skilfully to cover the surgical considerations and produce a chapter which should be an invaluable guide to any surgeon treating patients with this syndrome.

Thompson N W, Cheung P S Y 1987 Diagnosis and treatment of functioning and non-functioning adreno-cortical neoplasms including incidentalomas. Surgical Clinics of North America 67: 423–436

Most adrenocortical tumours secrete cortisol and cause Cushing's syndrome. This article is to be commended for describing the investigation of the syndrome in a logical and step-wise manner, removing much of the confusion and difficulty which frequently surrounds the topic. Diagnostic imaging necessary for localizing adrenocortical neoplasms is well covered, as are the principles of surgical management. Since the advent of computed tomography scanning, the new disease of 'incidentaloma' has appeared and the principles of management of this entity are expertly discussed.

Granberg P O, Adamson U, Cohn K H, Hamberger B, Lins P E 1982 The management of patients with primary aldosteronism. World Journal of Surgery 6: 757–764

This very well-written article provides all the essential information necessary to recognize, investigate and diagnose primary aldorsteronism. The differentiation between adenoma and hyperplasia, so important because the latter condition does not require surgery, is clarified. The essential steps in the posterior approach to the involved adrenal gland are described. Operative results of the authors' personal experience are recorded and attention paid to remaining controversies in the management of this condition.

Welbourn R B, Manolas K J 1983 The role of adrenalectomy in the management of Cushing's syndrome. In: Johnston I D A, Thompson N W (eds) Endocrine surgery. Butterworths, London, pp 53–75

There are several different forms of therapy appropriate for the various types of Cushing's syndrome and Professor Welbourn carefully discusses the relative merits of these treatments used to reduce the secretion of cortisol to normal.

With the advent and development of pituitary microsurgery, the precise role of adrenalectomy became a matter of some debate and in this article the technique is put into proper prospective. The authors' analysis of indications for adrenal exploration in their own personal experience of 95 cases of patients with Cushing's syndrome helps to define further the role of adrenalectomy.

Norton J A, Jensen R T 1991 Unresolved surgical issues in the management of patients with Zollinger Ellison syndrome. World Journal of Surgery 15: 151–159

Management of Zollinger Ellison syndrome remains a complex and difficult issue, although advances in understanding of the disease, the availability of sophisticated localizing studies and powerful antisecretory drugs have made total gastrectomy almost an obsolete procedure. In this article Drs Norton and Jensen discuss a series of important questions and issues in a way which helps to define the precise role of surgery in the management of the syndrome.

Edis A J, McIlrath D C, van Heerden J A et al 1976 Insulinoma: current diagnosis and surgical management. Current Problems in Surgery 10: 1–45

Although this publication is now 15 years old it is still a key article on the subject of insulinoma. The historical description of Wilder's first case in 1927 and the section on clinical features illustrate and underline how difficult the diagnosis can be. With the passage of time there have been changes in emphasis in the use of localization techniques and one would nowadays no longer rely heavily on angiography as stated in this review. The approach to the surgical management of the condition is well described and illustrated, showing that careful inspection and palpation of the pancreas are crucial localizing techniques. The majority of these tumours can be treated by simple enucleation and the success rate in expert hands is very high.

Gorman B, Charboneau J W, James E M et al 1986 Benign pancreatic insulinoma: pre-operative and intra-operative sonographic localisation. American Journal of Roentgenology 147: 929–934

This article describes the localizing techniques which should now form an essential part of the armamentarium of the surgeon treating insulinoma. It is an important publication because it demonstrates how the highly sensitive technique of intraoperative high-frequency ultrasound may detect tumours which are not palpable at surgery. This accurate localization facilitates tumour excision and reduces the need for blind pancreatic resection.

Wheeler M H, Chare M J B, Austin T R, Lazarus J H 1982 The management of the patient with catecholamine excess. World Journal of Surgery, 6: 735–747

This review article covers historical aspects, clinical presentation, investigation and treatment of phaeochromocytoma. Emphasis is placed on the methods of preoperative preparation, techniques for safe anaesthesia and the essential steps of surgical exploration. Particular variations of phaeochromocytoma including acute phaeochromocytoma, malignant phaeochromocytoma and phaeochromocytoma in children and pregnancy are discussed.

## PART 35.5
# BREAST SURGERY
*T. G. Brennan*

Hughes L E, Mansell R 1988 Benign disorders and diseases of the breast: concepts and clinical management. Baillière Tindall, London

This is the only comprehensive book on benign disorders of the breast. It is easy to read and beautifully illustrated. It contains important new concepts on the nature of some of the more common benign diseases of the breast.

Fentiman I S 1990 Detection and treatment of early breast cancer. Martin Dunitz, London

This book is a comprehensive and up-to-date look at the detection and treatment of early breast cancer. It contains 15 chapters and some of the more important of these are:

Chapter  2  Presenting features of breast cancer
3  Making a diagnosis
4  Screening
5  Breast conservation
6  The role of mastectomy
7  Aduvant therapy

Cady B, Bland K I (eds) 1990 Breast cancer: Strategies for the 1990s II. Surgical clinics of North America 70 (5)

Fifteen different groups of authors contribute on different aspects in the management of breast malignancy. There is a very good account of reconstruction after mastectomy. The possible strategies in the management of stage III breast cancer are throughly discussed. Another chapter deals with the 'clinical problems in the follow-up of patients after conservative surgery and radiotherapy'. Also discussed is the substantial overlap in the X-ray appearances of benign and malignant lesions after radiotherapy.

Lancet No 8784 Vol 339 Jan 4 1992, pp 1–15, 27
Lancet No 8785 Vol 339 Jan 11 1992, pp 71–85, 94–97

These two very recent articles address in great detail the value of aduvant therapy in early breast cancer. They look at the more wide experience of all aspects of aduvant therapy, hormonal, cytotoxic, etc. These strongly emphasize and highlight the important role of aduvant therapy in early breast cancer.

DHSS Breast Cancer Screening: Report to the Health Minister of England, Wales, Scotland and Northern Ireland by a working group chaired by Sir Patrick Forrest

The report forms the basis of the breast cancer screening programme which is ongoing in Great Britain. It discusses the pros and cons and pitfalls of screening and looks at the results of screening programmes carried out elsewhere.

## PART 35.6
# VASCULAR SURGERY
*J. H. N. Wolfe*

Ingoldby, C J H, Wujanto R, Mitchell J E Impact of vascular surgery on community mortality from ruptured aortic aneurysms. British Journal of Surgery 73: 551–553

The approach to abdominal aortic aneurysms is slowly changing. This is an excellent community-based study based on Swansea (population 248 000). During a ten-year period 260 patients had ruptured aneurysms and only 101 (38%) reached hospital alive; 52 of these (50%) survived. The overall survival rate is thus 19.8% from a ruptured abdominal aortic aneurysm. This has led to a more extensive screening programme.

Scott R A P, Ashton H A, Kay D N 1991 Abdominal aortic aneurysm in 4237 screened patients: prevalence, development and management over 6 years. British Journal of Surgery 78: 1122–1125

This is the report of one of the most extensive screening programmes, in which 7200 men and women aged between 65 and 80 were contacted, 4237 of whom were screened. Of these patients 4.3% had an abdominal aortic aneurysm of greater than 3 cm in diameter. The patients did not have surgery unless the aneurysm became symptomatic, had expanded to a diameter of 6 cm, or increased by more than 1 cm in a year. Their follow-up over six years indicates that patients with aneurysms of less than 6 cm without symptoms may be followed with repeat ultrasonography scans.

Crawford E S, Crawford J L , Safi H J et al 1986 Thoraco-abdominal aortic aneurysms: pre-operative and intra-operative factors determining immediate and long term results of operation in 605 patients. Journal of Vascular Surgery 3: 389–404

With modern techniques it is also possible to treat more extensive aneurysms surgically.

This is the most extensive experience in the world literature. During a 15-year period 605 patients underwent repair of a thoraco-abdominal aneurysm, 80% of which were due to medial degenerative disease, and 17% were due to aortic dissection. The 30-day mortality rate was 8.9% and 60% of patients were alive at five years. Paraplegia remains a major problem.

Anton J E, Hertzer N R, Beven E G, O'Hara P J, Krajewski L P 1986 Surgical management of popliteal aneurysms: trends in presentation, treatment and results from 1952 to 1984. Journal of Vascular Surgery 3: 125–134

Popliteal aneurysms occur in 10% of patients with an abdominal aortic aneurysm and represent a risk to the limb.

The above reviewed 110 patients and found that the incidence of bilateral aneurysms rose from 30% to 61% over the study period and that 56% of these were asymptomatic. The ten-year cumulative patency rate was 56% and limb salvage rate 83% subsequent to graft replacement, but these results are significantly improved in patients who underwent vein bypass (limb salvage 98%, cumulative patency rate 94%) rather than a prosthetic graft. Recently two British papers have expressed contradictory views. One suggests the conventional approach that asymptomatic aneurysms should be treated early since the results are poor in those patients who have to be treated acutely:

Halliday A W, Taylor P R, Wolfe J H, Mansfield A O 1991 The management of popliteal aneurysm: the importance of early surgical repair. Annals of the Royal College of Surgeons of England 73: (4) 253–257

The other suggests that the results are just as good if a conservative approach to asymptomatic aneurysms is adopted:

Hands L, Collin J, Morris P J 1988 A warning from 12 years of popliteal aneurysm treatment. British Journal of Surgery 76:416
European Consensus on Critical Ischaemia 1989 Lancet i: 737–738

Critical leg ischaemia has, in the past, been poorly defined but this consensus defines this group of patients and is a brief guide from a useful document.

Leather R P, Shah D M, Chang B B, Caufman J L 1988 Resurrection of the in situ saphenous vein bypass: 1 000 cases later. Annals of Surgery 208: 435–442

Good results can now be achieved with femoro-crural arterial bypasses. The in situ technique has again become popular.

During a 12-year period the authors performed 1038 in situ saphenous vein bypasses to the popliteal or crural arteries, with a 30-day patency of 95% and a five-year patency of 76%. These results confirm that the prevention of amputation is one of the greatest recent contributions of vascular surgery to the ageing population. However, there is no clear evidence that the in situ technique confers any benefit over the reversed vein technique as shown in a randomised study:

Harris P L, Jones D, Howe T 1987 A prospective randomised clinical trial to compare reversed and in situ vein grafts for femoro-popliteal bypass. British Journal of Surgery 74: 252–255
Taylor P R, Wolfe J H N, Tyrrell M R, et al 1990 Graft stenosis: justification for 1 year surveillance. British Journal of Surgery 1125–1128

Graft surveillance and correction of graft stenoses is now well established as an important adjunct to femorodistal grafting:

In this study 412 femorodistal grafts were prospectively studied with treadmill Doppler assessment, duplex scanning and intravenous digital subtraction angiography. The overall incidence of stenoses was 16% and approximately half of these required correction. Mean follow-up was 22 months (range 9–48 months) but all the stenoses started to develop during the first year. It is likely that a few stenoses would develop after this but surveillanece is no longer cost effective.

Wiseman S, Kenchington G, Dain R et al 1989 Influence of smoking and plasma factors on patency of femoro-popliteal vein grafts. British Medical Journal 299: 643–646

Smoking has also been shown to have a deleterious effect on graft patency.

Of 154 patients studied prospectively for a year 44 had occluded their grafts during that time. Blood concentrations of carboxyhaemoglobin, thiocyanate and fibrinogen were significantly higher in patients with occluded grafts (serum cholesterol levels were higher in the patients with patent grafts). One quarter of all patients untruthfully claimed to have stopped smoking.

European Carotid Surgery Trialists' Collaborative Group 1991 MRC European carotid surgery trial: interim results for symptomatic patients with severe (70–90%) or with mild (0–29%) carotid stenosis. Lancet 337: 1235–1243
North American Symptomatic Carotid Endarterectomy Trial Collaborators 1991 Beneficial effect of carotid endarterectomy in symptomatic patients with high grade carotid stenosis. New England Journal of Medicine 325: 445–453

Twenty-five to thirty per cent of strokes are due to internal carotid artery disease but the place of carotid endarterectomy has remained controversial until two significant and similar reports. Both of these studies deal with symptomatic stenoses of the internal carotid artery.

The European Multicentre Study and the NASCET Study in the USA entered 2518 and 659 patients respectively. They have both shown (1) that in patients with stenoses of less than 30% surgery *does not* confer any advantage; (2) that in stenoses of greater than 70% surgery confers a significant advantage; (3) that in stenoses between 30% and 70% the randomized study should continue. Asymptomatic carotid bruits, however, do not justify invasive diagnostic procedures according to

Hayman A, Wilkinson W E, Hayden S et al 1980 Risk of stroke in asymptomatic persons with cervical artery bruits. New England Journal of Medicine 302: 838–841

A survey in a rural community revealed cervical bruits in 72 of 1620 patients aged 45 or older (4.4%). The presence of an asymptomatic bruit was associated with a higher risk of stroke in men but not women, but there was no correlation between the location of the bruit and the site of the subsequent stroke. Cervical bruits were, however, a risk factor for death from myocardial ischaemia.

Prevention of fatal post-operative pulmonary embolism by low dose heparin. Lancet ii: 45–51

Pulmonary embolism remains an important cause of postoperative mortality and there have been many studies in this area.

The International Multicentre Trial addressed this issue in 4121 patients over 40, half of whom were treated with 5000 units of heparin subcutaneously 8-hourly. There were 16 deaths with pulmonary embolism in the control group and 2 in those treated with heparin. Isotopic evidence of deep vein thrombosis was present in 24.6% of the control group and 7.7% of those treated with heparin. Like all studies, there were criticisms but surgical practice was nevertheless altered. The other major complication of deep vein thrombosis is venous ulceration and this was studied by

Callum M J, Harper D R, Dale J J, Ruckley C V 1987 Chronic ulcer of the leg: clinical history. British Medical Journal 294: 1389–1391

In this study 600 patients were studied and in those over 40 there were significantly more females. In females, but not males, there were significantly more left leg ulcers than right. The median duration of ulceration was nine months and 20% had remined unhealed for two years. Recurrence was common and 66% of patients had a greater than five-year history of recurrent ulceration.

Browse N L, Burnand K G 1982 The cause of venous viceration. Lancet ii: 243–244

The final cause of this ulceration has been hotly debated but a significant contribution has been made by this paper.

From biopsy specimens they were able to show an abnormal thick fibrin cuff surrounding the capillaries and postulated that this blocked permeability, with resulting breakdown of the tissues.

## PART 35.7
# NEUROSURGERY
## *R. S. Maurice-Williams*

Miller J D (ed) 1987 Northfield's surgery of the central
nervous system, 2nd edn. Blackwell Scientific
Publications, Oxford

This is the only British textbook of neurosurgery,
being a multi-author revision of Northfield's original textbook which was published in the early
1970s. It provides an attractive, well set out and
clearly written account of the whole field of
neurosurgery. It is of course too detailed for the
general surgical trainee but is a good starting
point for the neurosurgical trainee and a useful
source of reference for those in other specialties.

Jennett B, Teasdale G 1981 Management of head injuries.
Davis, Philadelphia

This provides a useful basic guide to head
injuries, their epidemiology, pathology and
management. It was written by the two profes-
sors of neurosurgery, Glasgow, who have revolutionized the management of head injuries in the
UK. Again, it is clearly written, well laid out and
a most useful source of reference.

Maurice-Williams R S 1987 Neurosurgery. In: Kirk R M,
Williamson R C N (eds) General surgical operations, 2nd
edn. Churchill Livingstone, Edinburgh, pp 590–604

This provides all the general surgical trainee
needs to know about neurosurgery from an operative point of view. It describes the basic procedures which a non-neurosurgeon might be called
upon to carry out from time to time and also provides an outline of what is involved in those other
parts of neurosurgery which the general trainee
does not need to know about other than an
outline.

Jennett B, Bond M 1975 Assessment of outcome after severe
brain damage: a practical scale. Lancet i: 480–484

The functional assessment of outcome after head
injury and after neurosurgical procedures has
always been problematical. Numerous scales and
scores of different complexity have been devised
but the only one which has gained anything like
general acceptance is the simplest one, the
Glasgow Outcome Scale. This paper outlines the
thinking behind the GOS and describes it in detail.

Teasdale G, Jennett B 1974 Assessment of coma and
impaired consciousness: a practical scale. Lancet ii: 81–83

Even more successful than the Glasgow Outcome
Scale has been the Glasgow Coma Scale, now
used in the management of head injuries
throughout the world. The GCS provides a simple and easily communicated measure of the
severity of obtundation after any form of cerebral
insult. This is the paper in which it was originally
described. It is a beautiful example of how some
of the most worthwhile advances in clinical practice are based on quite simple ideas.

Mendelow A D, Teasdale G, Jennett B et al 1983 Risks of
intracranial haematoma in head injured adults. British
Medical Journal 287: 1173–1176

This is a further paper based on a very simple
idea which has completely revolutionized the
management of head injuries. This is the first
paper which attempted to make any assessment
of the risk of a patient with a head injury harbouring an intracranial haematoma based on just
two parameters — whether or not a skull fracture
is present and whether or not the level of consciousness is clouded. The authors were able to
demonstrate that a patient with clouded consciousness who also has a skull fracture has a one
in four chance of developing a traumatic intracranial haematoma, thus pinpointing a group of
patients who are at a specially high risk after a
head injury.

## PART 35.8
# WAR SURGERY
## *I. R. Haywood*

War surgery is taken to cover all aspects of the
management of those physically injured in conventional war, war-type situations such as terrorist violence and by weapons normally only used
in war. Long-term reconstructive surgery or rehabilitation is not covered here.

Cooper G J, Ryan J M 1990 The interaction of penetrating
missiles with tissues: some common misapprehensions,
and the implications for wound management in peace and
war. British Journal of Surgery 77: 660–710.

This article reviews the present state of knowledge as described and places in perspective many of the recent controversial issues between war surgeons. It should be read in conjunction with Ryan et al (1991) below.

Dufour D, Kromen S, Owen-Smith M S et al 1988 Surgery for victims of war. International committee of the Red Cross, Geneva.

This is the Red Cross surgical pocket book providing didactic instruction for the surgeon faced with war injuries. Its basic surgical teaching is sound but its sections on analgesia and anaesthesia are weak. Remember that ICRC hospitals for which this is a doctrine are neither military hospitals on a battlefield where evacuation of patients is paramount, nor civilian peacetime hospitals in developed countries with modern facilities and technology.

Eisemann B, Swann K 1988 Military strategy in trauma. In: Maddox K L, Moore E E, Feliciano D V (eds) Trauma. Appleton and Lange, San Mateo

This chapter, in what is possibly the most comprehensive single-volume textbook on trauma management, is designed to educate the civilian surgeon why if mobilized for war he may have to change his conventional surgical habits — a point it makes better than any other published work.

Fackler M L, Bretau J P L, Courbill L J et al 1988 Open wound drainage versus wound excision on the modern battlefield. Letterman Army Institute of Research: report 256

Over the last few years the authors, in particular Fackler, have openly challenged many of the conventional hallowed tenets of war surgery. This paper contains the scientific evidence from their own research upon which many of their arguments are based.

Fackler M L 1988 Wound ballistics: a review of common misconceptions. Journal of the American Medical Association 259: 2730–2736

The author continues to elaborate on his theme which challenges the standard teaching based on the research in the previous reference and critically analyses the whole subject.

Haywood I R 1984 Triage. Journal of the British Association of Immediate Care 7: 31–35

Triage or the sorting of multiple casualties into priorities for evacuation and treatment has for

two centuries been part of military surgery. Over the last few years, probably as a result of an apparent spate of major disasters and accidents, the principles have become a recognized part of civilian trauma management. *It is now part of the syllabus for the new FRCS.* This is one of the few publications on the subject.

Haywood I R 1988 Terrorism: general aspects, aetiology and pathophysiology. In: Baskett P, Weller R (eds) Medicine for disasters. Wright, London, p 401

Injuries from bombs and bullets were traditionally the province of the war surgeon, but the advent of the terrorist has brought them to the catchment area of any surgeon anywhere. As well as describing the nature and treatment of injuries caused by these agents, these chapters contain advice on associated matters which the FRCS candidate should now know. These include organizational problems, the forensic and legal responsibilities of surgeons, and the psychological aspects which all who may have to look after these casualties should understand.

Haywood I R 1989 Missile injury. In: Ellis H, Lamont P M (eds) Problems in general surgery wound healing 6 (2): 330

This chapter summarizes the pathophysiology of wounds induced by missiles, be they bomb fragments or bullets, to form a rational basis upon which treatment may be based. Secondary contamination is given greater significance than in most articles on the subject.

Kirby N G, Blackburn G 1981 The field surgery pocket book. HMSO, London

This is the standard didactic instruction book on war surgery produced by the Surgical Directorate of the British Army Medical Services. Unlike those produced by other armies it was produced as a civilian textbook to make it easily available to surgeons anywhere. This edition is now, however, significantly out of date in many areas, but a new edition is scheduled for publication in 1993.

Owen-Smith M S 1981 High velocity missile wounds. Edward Arnold, London

Possibly the only textbook in the world confining itself to all aspects of these injuries which form a significant part of the problem facing the surgeon at war. Some of the theses proposed, however, are now considered by many to be controversial if not outdated, and of course the technology of weaponry has advanced.

Ryan J M, Cooper J G, Milner S M, Haywood I R 1991 Field surgery on a future conventional battlefield: strategy and wound management. Annals of the Royal College of Surgeons of England 73: 13–20

This article was written to update surgeons in war surgery. It outlines the basis of many present controversies and suggests practical compromises. Weapon manufacturers have produced a large range of new weapons over the last few years which have never been used in combat, and hence their wounding effects are largely conjectural. The article was submitted for publication just before the onset of the Persian Gulf crisis and ironically was published a few days before the start of the Gulf War, where the effects of some of these weapons were experienced for the first time. Initial analysis suggests that the theses on effects and treatment proposed were generally correct.

Scott R 1984 War wounds. In: Harding Rains A J, Ritchie H D (eds) Bailey and Love's short practice of surgery. Lewis, London

Every candidate for the FRCS will read some or all of this textbook. This chapter contains the essential principles that the candidate must know on the subject.

Trueta J 1943 The principles and practice of war surgery. Mosby, St Louis

Finally a paper for those with a historical bent. Trueta was one of Spain's greatest surgeons. He learnt war surgery from Americans towards the end of the First World War, and then found himself heavily involved in the Civil War in his own country. He perfected much of what he had been taught under difficult conditions, subsequently passing this on to allied surgeons at Oxford, where he was senior lecturer during the Second World War. He was the first war surgeon to use antibacterial chemotherapy (sulphonamides) and the operative techniques he developed and describes for contaminated wound management could not be bettered today. Also the early chapters are probably the best on the history of war surgery up to that time.

## PART 35.9
## PAEDIATRIC SURGERY
## *L. Kapila*

Gough M H 1989 Cryptorchidism. British Journal of Surgery 76: 109–112

This article clarifies the otherwise confused terminology of undescended testis and differentiates between a normal and abnormal testis. Changes in the incidence and management are well described.

Atwell J D 1988 Inguinal hernia and hydrocele. In: Spitz L, Nixon H H (eds) Rob and Smith's operative surgery. Paediatric surgery, 4th edn. Butterworths, London, pp 207–215

An inguinal hernia or hydrocele in a child requires a different surgical approach from that in an adult.

This chapter gives a step-by-step description of the operations, with diagrams illustrating each stage of the operation. The reason for surgery and complications are also dealt with.

Stevenson R J 1985 Gastrointestinal bleeding in children. Surgical Clinics of North America 65: 1455–1480

Gastrointestinal bleeding in children is a common symptom for emergency referral and the causes for bleeding vary from those seen in adults and do not carry the same implications.

This paper describes in detail the procedure of upper and lower endoscopy in children and the causes and management of patients with special reference to the age-related sources of bleeding.

Rowe M I, Lloyd D A 1988 Preoperative and postoperative management. In: Spitz L, Nixon H H (eds) Rob and Smith's operative surgery. Paediatric surgery, 4th edn. Butterworths, London, pp 4–10

For a surgeon in training it is essential to acquire knowledge about the physiological and metabolic variations that occur from birth to adolescence.

For any child undergoing surgery consideration must be given to the fluid and electrolyte balance in relation to the patient's age and maturity, as the physiological response to surgery is quite different from that seen in adults.

Kapila L 1987 Intussusception in children. Surgery 40: 945–947

Intussusception still gives rise to a higher incidence of morbidity and mortality than acute appendicitis in children. Recent advances in ultrasound scanning and non-operative hydrostatic or air insufflation reduction have reduced the mortality following non-operative treatment.

The indication and contra-indications for the correct mode of treatment are listed.

Spitz L 1988 Pyloromyotomy. In: Spitz L, Nixon H H (eds) Rob and Smith's operative surgery. Paediatric surgery. Butterworths, London, pp 267–272

Since 1912, when Ramstedt described the operation of extramucosal pyloromyotomy, surgery has totally replaced medical treatment for pyloric stenosis. Early diagnosis using ultrasonography and a better understanding of fluid and electrolyte balance have considerably reduced the morbidity and mortality.

The operative procedure has not changed since Ramstedt's original description, although general anaesthesia is preferable to local.

Jones P G, Woodward A A 1986 External genitalia. In: Jones P G, Woodward A A (eds) Clinical paediatric surgery, 3rd edn. Blackwell, Oxford, pp 329–337

Circumcision is the most frequent surgical operation performed. The majority are done for religious reasons. The precise surgical indications for the operation are given and the pros and cons discussed.

Dickson J A S 1989 Cysts of the thyroglossal tract. Surgery 68: 1618–1622

Fifty per cent of thyroglossal cysts present in childhood. A sound understanding of the embryology of this condition is essential for correct operative management and avoidance of recurrence. The article is well illustrated with clinical and histological photographs. The differential diagnosis is listed.

Neblett III W W, Pietsch M D, Holcomb Jr. G W 1988 Acute abdominal conditions in children and adolescents. Surgical Clinics of North America 68: 415–430

The cause of an acute abdomen in a child may be congenital or acquired, and can be arbitrarily divided into three groups according to the age of presentation: infant, childhood or adolescent, with some overlap. Appendicitis spans all three age groups and may present with a wide range of signs and symptoms. The postoperative complications encountered in children differ from those seen in adults.

Jones P G, Woodward A A 1986 Trauma in childhood. In: Jones P G, Woodward A A (eds) Clinical paediatric surgery, 3rd edn. Blackwell, Oxford, Ch 55, 467–478

Trauma is the most common cause of death in children after the neonatal period. The principles of resuscitation of a severely injured child are outlined. Non-accidental injury frequently presents to the surgical unit and aspects of presentation are discussed.

## PART 35.10
# PLASTIC SURGERY
## D. M. Davies

Mackin R M 1989 Pictorial record of both macro and micro skin tumours and their management. Martin Dunitz, London

This is a good colour-illustrated atlas of common skin tumours and gives a good account of their management.

Smith J W, Aston S J 1991 Grabb and Smith's plastic surgery, 4th edn. Little Brown, Boston

This is an excellent complete textbook of plastic surgery. The chapters on skin grafting and wound repair would be of benefit to the FRCS candidate, as would other chapters such as breast reconstruction.

McGregor I A 1989 Fundamental techniques of plastic surgery and their surgical applications, 8th edn. Churchill Livingstone, London

This book is a standard basic textbook in plastic surgery and the main emphasis is on practical aspects of wound care and suture. To be highly recommended to any surgeon at any stage in his career.

Muir I F K, Barclay T L, Settle J 1987 Burns and their treatment, 3rd edn. Butterworth, London

This is a standard British textbook on the care of the burned patient and the chapters on wound pathology and resuscitation are important for any casualty officer/young surgeon, who will occasionally see these injuries.

Lister G 1984 The hand, 2nd edn. Churchill Livingstone, London.

This is an illustrated atlas on examining the hand. It is one of the great classic textbooks and the chapters on nerve injury and trauma should be read by any FRCS candidate.

Shaw W (ed) 1986 Clinics in plastic surgery: lower extremity trauma and reconstrucion. Saunders, Philadelphia, pp 619–620

This is an excellent volume on the management of lower limb trauma. In particular the chapter by the Late Marco Godina: Early Microsurgical reconstruction of the complex trauma of the extremities, pages 619–620, reinforces the principle of early skin cover for compound lower extremity injuries.

---

## PART 35.11
## ORTHOPAEDIC SURGERY
*N. J. Goddard*

---

Aids to the examination of the peripheral nervous system 1976 Medical Research Council, Memorandum No. 45, HMSO, London

This little booklet was first published in 1941, has been revised comprehensively since then and still remains an indispensable text. Its 62 pages are crammed full of the type of information which is paramount for sound clinical practice. There is a wealth of advice on examination technique as well as the expected data on individual peripheral nerves, muscle innervation, root values, dermatomes and myotomes. Moreover it slips easily into a white coat pocket and makes for ideal browsing material in between cases.

Bauer G C H et al 1990 Hip fracture in the elderly: a mini symposium. Current Orthopaedics 4: 147–183

To those who have held junior posts in an orthopaedic department this series of articles will probably be unnecessary. For others, however, it provides a wonderful overview of the problems posed by hip fractures in the elderly (currently running at 43/100 000 population). The social impact of this rising epidemic is discussed and

the section on epidemiology by Professor Grimley-Evans is a nugget. There are tips on requesting and interpreting the appropriate radiological investigations — not only X-rays. The classifications and differences between extra-and intracapsular fractures are clearly explained, so making differences between their management more comprehensible. Finally the section on complications makes salutary reading for all.

Conventry MB et al 1990 Osteo-arthritis of the knee: a mini symposium. Current Orthopaedics 4: 77–106

Over the past decade there has been a great deal of change in the management of osteoarthritis of the knee which has yet to find its way into the text books. Many of the 'traditional' methods of treatment have been superseded and there has been a massive increase in total knee replacement (TKR). Indeed TKR is one of the fastest-growing fields in orthopaedics today. This symposium covers all aspects of treatment of osteoarthritis of the knee, concentrating on the assessment, the role of osteotomy and especially the indications for joint replacement and management of the failed joint replacement. It is completely up to date and extremely relevant to current orthopaedic practice.

The hand: examination and diagnosis 1983 American Academy of Orthopaedic Surgeons, Churchill Livingstone, London

This book is included to satisfy my own interest in hands. It is a short, pocket-sized manual outlining the examination and assessment of the hand as well as including details of the fractures, deformities, congenital anomalies, tumours and infection. Its especial value lies in that many hand and upper limb cases make ideal short cases at examinations.

Grundy D, Russell J, Swain A 1986 ABC of spinal cord injury. British Medical Journal, London

This would possibly appear to be an unusual selection for the orthopaedic section, being one of a series of booklets reprinted from the original articles from the British Medical Journal. Its value lies in that it provides an extremely clear and concise account of the treatment of spinal cord injury from the site of the accident, through the early management, complications and finally rehabilitation into the community. The subject matter itself affects most fields of surgery but especially orthopaedics, neurosurgery, urology, and occasionally plastics. In addition many of those aspects of management frequently overlooked by surgeons are especially valuable to us all, i.e. nursing, physiotherapy, occupational therapy and the social needs of the patients and their family. This is a subject that has been known to appear in past papers but the booklet is worth more than just the exam. It is one of those rare nuggets that should be purchased by all and kept on the shelf handy for immediate access for the next spinal cord injury admitted to your department.

Johnson K D, Cadambi A, Seibert G B 1985 Incidence of adult respiratory distress syndrome in patients with multiple musculo-skeletal injuries: effect of early operative stabilization of fractures. Journal of Trauma 25: 375–384

This paper is truly one of those that can be said to have changed orthopaedic practice. It fundamentally altered our approach from 'This patient is too sick to go to theatre' to 'This patient is too sick *not* to go to theatre.' It was based around 132 patients presenting with multiple injuries with an injury severity score of greater than 18. They conclusively showed a threefold increase in adult respiratory distress syndrome and mortality rates in those patients where there was a delay in operative stabilization of the long bone fractures beyond 24 hours. Early operative treatment in these patients also resulted in a reduction in time spent in the intensive therapy unit by a factor of two and a 20% reduction of total hospital stay. The conclusions are irrefutable and the consequences far reaching. It is essential reading.

Kirkaldy-Wallis W H et al 1988 Bone and joint infection: a mini symposium. Current Orthopaedics 2: 63–89

The Hunterian Museum at the Royal College of Surgeons has many examples of the late results of bone and joint infection. Lack of knowledge in this field therefore puts the candidate at risk lest one of these specimens (Prefix E) appear on the appointed day. This mini symposium provides a valuable update on the presentation, radiological evaluation, pathology and treatment of bone and joint infection. To derive maximum benefit it should be read in conjunction with a visit to the Hunterian Museum to study the pathological

specimens. Don't forget to look at the preparations of chronic osteomyelitis, however.

McRae R 1981 Practical fracture treatment. Churchill Livingstone, Edinburgh

The preface of this book says it all in that it 'assumes little prior knowledge of the subject'. As such it seems an ideal and invaluable book for the candidate facing examination in a subject in which he or she may have little or no experience. It is a gem, full of line drawings (by the author himself) and pertinent X-rays laid out in a comic-strip style. The first section is confined to the general principles of treatment and forms a solid foundation on which to build. The remainder of the book deals with particular fractures region by region. On the whole a safe, middle-of-the-road treatment rationale is proposed without being didactic or too contentious. Alternative methods of treatment are discussed whenever possible. On balance this is a book that has seen many an aspiring orthopaedic SHO or registrar through their early clinical experience and will doubtless help many more in the future.

Rang M 1966 Anthology of orthopaedics. Churchill Livingstone, Edinburgh

I have included this book out of sheer indulgence, being one of those people more interested in the footnotes in Bailey & Love than the text. I have always had a fascination in knowing the man behind the eponym and this book fulfils my requirements. It makes light reading and provides a welcome break from cramming in the hard facts which are perceived necessary to pass the exam. Moreover it makes for a more enjoyable viva and impresses the examiners no end if you actually *know* who Esmarch was and that Langenbeck described the bandage first!

Skinner D, Driscoll P, Earlam R 1991 ABC of major trauma. British Medical Journal, London

The Advanced Trauma Life Support course is now a regular feature in the UK and many (ideally all) surgical trainees will have attended a Provider course. The *ABC of Major Trauma* is based around the syllabus of the ATLS course and is essentially a condensation and more readable version of the course manual. No candidate can afford to go into the exam without a thorough knowledge of the modern management of major trauma as presented in this book (many examiners are also ATLS instructors). Each chapter is short, comprehensive, and deals with individual clinical problems in a clear and occasionally didactic fashion. Photographs and diagrams are used to best advantage and for those of short concentration span (or the night before the exam) the salient points are summarized in boxes throughout the text.

Souhami R L, Craft A W 1988 Progress in management of malignant bone tumours. Journal of Bone and Joint Surgery 70 (B): 345–347
Grimer R J, Sneath R S 1990 Diagnosing malignant bone tumours. Journal of Bone and Joint Surgery 72 (B): 754–756

These two papers should be considered together since they deal with the same seemingly esoteric subject. The subject, however, is extremely relevant and attitudes have changed considerably since the days of Stanford Cade. Whenever possible the current trend is for limb conservation surgery combined with chemotherapy and radiotherapy. Modern treatment protocols, carefully planned by all involved parties, have greatly increased both limb and importantly, life expectancy in many primary bone tumours. Fifty per cent five-year survival rates are now the norm for osteosarcoma and Ewing's tumours. The two papers summarize current thinking on bone tumour management and in especially emphasizing the need for early diagnosis and referral to specialist centres for treatment. Remember that many specimens of primary bone tumours exist in the Hunterian Museum and make excellent viva material.

---

## PART 35.12
## CARDIOTHORACIC SURGERY
*T. Treasure*

---

### BOOKS

Moghissis K 1986 Essentials of thoracic and cardiac surgery. Heinemann, London

This is a small textbook of under 500 pages which has more than enough information about all aspects of thoracic surgery for the FRCS candidate, including enough operative detail for trainees in the generality of surgery. Its strength is its thoracic teaching. The small cardiac section was contributed by a physician.

Sturridge M, Treasure T 1985 Belcher's thoracic surgical management, 5th edn. Baillière Tindall, London

This small paperback, 200 pages in total, was written to describe the day-to-day practicalities of management on cardiothoracic wards. It describes bronchoscopy, under water seal drainage and many other procedures and investigations in what is intended to be a logical and readable way. Some aspects are specialized and perhaps dated, for example bronchograms are rarely performed and certainly not by the surgical SHO, but many of the basics of thoracic surgical management remain unchanged.

### CHAPTERS

Zorab JSM (ed) 1988 Surgery for anaesthetists. Blackwell, Oxford

Chapter 19    Cardiothoracic surgery: general considerations
Chapter 20    Acquired heart disease
Chapter 22    The lungs, pleura and mediastinum

It may seem odd to recommend surgeons in training to read a book written for anaesthetists, but it is about surgery, not anaesthesia. The principles of cardiopulmonary bypass and the essentials of cardiac operations are described, with line diagrams at the level of detail which a junior surgeon might reasonably be expected to know in an examination.

Treasure T, Griffin S 1990 Post operative thromboembolic disease: a tantalizing enigma. In: Hadfield J, Hobsley M, Treasure T (eds) Current surgical practice, Vol 5. Edward Arnold, London, Ch 4

All surgeons should know about this problem, its prophylaxis, diagnosis and management at each stage of its presentation. This is one chapter of a 300-page book full of articles by specialists, offering current teaching, for those in general training.

### CORONARY ARTERY SURGERY: A CHAPTER, A LANDMARK PAPER AND A REVIEW

Hadfield J, Hobsley M (eds) 1987 Surgery for coronary artery disease. In: Current surgical practice, Vol 4, Ch 8. Edward Arnold, London

This is one of the commonest and most thoroughly documented major operations and yet surgical trainees have only vague ideas about indications and results.

Floyd Loop and ten others 1986 Influence of the internal mammary artery graft on 10-year survival and other cardiac events. New England Journal of Medicine 314: 1–6

The landmark paper on the use of the internal mammary (or internal thoracic) artery from the Cleveland `Clinic.

Treasure T 1990 Coronary surgery : an up date. British Journal of Hospital Medicine 43: 459–463

A recent topical review on indications and results, with some comments on health economics and resource implications for this expensive operaion.

## TEACHING ARTICLES

The 'add-on' monthly Journal *Surgery* (Medicine Group) publishes articles specifically aimed at the trainee in the generality of surgery. These are contemporary, authoritative and designed to be read, rather than left on a shelf as a definitive and enduring statement, as is sometimes the case with textbooks. They were written and edited with the surgical trainee in mind and their purpose is to provide quite enough but not over-specialized information.

Cheslyn-Curtis S, Treasure T 1989 Pleural effusion in malignant disease. Surgery (June) 69

A common problem in breast carcinoma, for example.

Lock C, Smith J 1989 Thoracic trauma. Surgery (June) 69: 1645–1649

Trauma is an inescapable responsibility for all surgeons in training and continues to be a concern for all general, A&E, and orthopaedic surgeons.

Hamilton D I 1989 Congenital heart defects. Surgery (September) 72: 1724–1731

This is all that most surgeons ever need to know — the simple and the potentially complex, illustrated and explained.

Murphy J T, Treasure T 1989 Aortic dissection. Surgery (November) 74: 1765–1770

A very surgical condition that can present in several ways to different departments of a hospital and provides a challenge in management.

Griffin D, Treasure T 1989 Coronary artery surgery. Surgery (November) 74: 1771–1776

Colourful illustrations may make this an easier read than textbook chapters.

Treasure T, Murphy J 1989 Pneumothorax. Surgery (December) 75: 1780–1786

A deceptively easy condition with serious pitfalls.

Treasure T 1990 Surgical correction of valvular heart disease. Surgery (January) 76: 1809–1815

Valve repair and replacement are amongst the most technically satisfying of all operations. Souttar wrote in 1925 that diseases of the valves of the heart would be amenable to a 'mechanical' solution although physicians of his day could not tolerate what they saw as surgical hubris.

Treasure T, Bosworth P 1990 Cardiopulmonary bypass. Surgery (March) 78: 1860–1863

The essential plumbing of the bypass circuit and its complications.

McGoldrick J T, Purut C M 1990 Surgery for the complications of myocardial infarction. Surgery (April) 79: 1876–1881

Amongst the more exacting forms of cardiac surgery.

---

PART 35.13
## UROLOGY
*C. A. C. Charlton*

---

## BRITISH JOURNAL OF UROLOGY: REVIEW ARTICLES

Glesson M J, Griffith D G 1990 Urinary diversion. British Journal of Urology 66: 113–122
Jones D J, Russell G L, Kellett M J et al 1990 The changing practice of percutaneous stone surgery: review of 1000 cases 1981–1988. British Journal of Urology 66: 1–5
McLoughlin J, Williams G 1990 Alternatives to prostatectomy. British Journal of Urology 65: 313–316
Mundy A R 1988 Detruser instability. British Journal of Urology 62: 393–397
Mundy A R 1991 Artificial sphincters. British Journal of Urology 67: 225–229
Russell P J, Brown J L, Grimond S M et al 1990 Molecular biology of urological tumours. British Journal of Urology 66: 121–130
Sherar R J 1991 Prostatic specific antigen. British Journal of Urology 67: 1–5
Thomas E F M 1990 Fetal uropathy. British Journal of

Urology 66: 225–231
Waxman J 1990 Chemotherapy for metastatic bladder cancer: is there new hope? British Journal of Urology 65: 1–5

## UROLOGICAL REFERENCES

Mundy A R 1988 Detrusor instability. British Journal of Urology 62: 393–397

Unstable bladder was first defined in 1971 by means of urodynamics. Detrusor instability is due either to (a) neurological disease, (b) bladder outflow obstruction in the male or (c) is idiopathic.

Blockade of the sacral nerve roots abolishes the involuntary detrusor contractions, hence implicating the local reflex arcs. If the contractions are due to neurological disease, this is termed detrusor hyper-reflexia, as opposed to those with no evidence of neurological disease, when it is termed detrusor instability.

Treatment with anticholinergic drugs has mixed results. (Psychotherapy) support with bladder training is of short-term benefit only. Thereafter phenol (5%) injections in the older female (over 55 years) and clam cystoplasty are alternatives. The operation makes both the involuntary and voluntary detrusor contractions ineffective and voiding problems will result.

Waxman J 1990 Chemotherapy for metastatic bladder cancer. Is there new hope? British Journal of Urology 65: 1–5

The average age of patients with metastatic bladder cancer is 70 years, with a very poor outlook (worse prognosis than lung cancer or acute leukaemia) and a mean duration of survival if untreated of three months. This paper reviews the mode of action of cytotoxic agents and results if given singly and in combination. The main use is probably in using drugs in early-stage disease (i.e. G3 TI, in which survival is 20% at five years) since in this group patients die of metastatic disease despite 'cure' of their local bladder disease. Regard these early 'aggressive' types as a systemic malignancy that requires systemic therapy.

McLoughlin J, Williams G 1990 Alternatives to prostatectomy. British Journal of Urology 65: 313–316

Benign prostatic hyperplasia is found in 70% of men in their 70s. The mortality rate from a transurethral resection (TUR) is as low as 0.2% and is the optimal treatment for patients with prostatic outflow obstruction. Something like 70% of patients obtain symptomatic relief following a TUR. Patients who are symptomatic, but without evidence of detrusor decompensation or embarrassment of their upper urinary tract, should be considered for a conservative approach to management, which may also result in symptomatic relief.

The alternatives to prostatectomy are hormonal manipulation, hyperthermia and prostatic dilatation using balloons and none of these is proven to have long-term benefits to date. Alpha blockade still requires long-term follow-up studies assess patient compliance and the effects of treatment. Similar information is required for hyperthermia in patients with retention. There does seem to be a place for prostatic stents, but once again long-term follow-up later is required.

Gleeson M J, Griffith D G 1990 Urinary diversion. British Journal of Urology 66: 113–122

Permanent forms of urinary diversion are primarily applicable to patients with bladder cancer and some benign vesical conditions. They take two forms:

1. Wet — incontinent abdominal stomas needing collection devices. The generally accepted type is the ileal conduit, although long-term follow-up studies show an 80% complication rate, e.g. loss of renal function, pyelonephritis, stones, stoma problems. Large bowel predisposes to malignancy.
2. Dry — continent abdominal stomas needing intermittent self-catheterization. In addition to having anti-reflux ureteric components, a non-leaking abdominal wall fistula has been developed. There are many ingenious variants, using small and large bowel for reservoirs, and the development of nipples to solve these problems; yet a totally satisfactory form has not yet been created.

Other forms of diversion include ureterosigmoidostomy and rectal bladders (with and without colostomy). Bladder substitution, whereby reservoirs made of ileum with or without caecum or sigmoid colon are sewn to the membranous urethra, tends to be limited to males, unless a prosthetic sphincter is used to achieve continence in the female.

Thomas E F M 1990 Fetal uropathy. British Journal of Urology 66: 225–231

Prenatal ultrasound diagnosis requires careful evaluation since as many as four-fifths of neonates with prenatally diagnosed uropathies have neither signs nor symptoms at birth.

Fetal urine production starts at eight weeks gestation, and this forms the amniotic liquor, reaching a maximum volume of 1 litre at 38 weeks. A normal full-term fetus produces 1 litre of urine per 24 hours, but after birth this drops to a quarter of that value, hence the common finding of upper tract dilatation reverting to normal within the first year of postnatal life. In the second trimester, i.e. at 17–19 weeks, normal kidneys can always be identified and severely dilated systems can be identified at 12–14 weeks. Lethal effects of renal dysplasia and pulmonary hypoplasia are irreversible by the time they can be detected by ultrasound.

Hence prenatal ultrasound serves two roles: (1) severely affected fetuses which may therefore be appropriately terminated; (2) degrees of dilatation to investigate postnatally. Intrauterine operations are only justified in severe cases of bilateral uropathy.

Shearer R J 1991 Prostatic specific antigen. British Journal of Urology 67: 1–5

The antigen is a glycoprotein (molecular weight 33 000 Da) found in the cytoplasm of prostatic epithelial (in the ducts) cells. Prostatic specific antigen (PSA) estimation is time consuming, labour intensive and expensive. It is also used in immunohistochemical techniques such that it will identify the origin of the tumours and secondary deposits and in bone marrow. PSA is detectable in the serum of women. Levels above normal (4 ng ml$^{-1}$) are seen following instrumentation, rectal examination and needle biopsy. One-third of males with uncomplicated benign prostatic hyperplasia have levels above 10 ng ml$^{-1}$. The only diagnostic criteria for carcinoma of the prostate is biopsy.

The positive accuracy of PSA levels greater than 20 ng ml$^{-1}$ for bone metastases is 63%, i.e. one-third of patients with these levels do not have metastases. Furthermore the negative accuracy is 92%, and so patients with this level (20 ng l$^{-1}$) or less are most unlikely to have metastases.

The measurement of PSA is occasionally used if there is a long waiting list for TURs, so as to help decide which are malignant and deserve priority admission. Recognising that at least 10% of patients on the waiting list will have unrecognised carcinoma, and that over one-third of patients with uncomplicated benign prostatic hyperplasia have PSA levels above 10 ng/ml, the positive accuracy using this PSA level is 35%, i.e. only one-third of patients on the waiting list with this level will have carcinoma.

Fowler C H 1991 Flexible cystoscopy and laser surgery. In: Hendry W F (ed) Recent advances in urology/andrology 5. Churchill Livingstone, London, pp 71–84

A flexible cystoscope is an expensive steerable urethral catheter provided with fibre-optic viewing and illumination bundles. A major advantage is that, unlike conventional rigid cystoscopy, it can be performed with the patient lying in a comfortable supine position. For the majority of patients, topical urethral anaesthesia with 15 ml of 1% lignocaine gel is enough. The main use of the flexible cystoscope is a means of screening the lower urinary tract in those patients who probably *do not* have a lesion which requires more than biopsy, and in whom an examination under anaesthesia is not needed. A major drawback of the use of this instrument was its inability to deal with bladder tumours other than by using a laser beam. For this purpose the neodymium: YAG beam with a wavelength in the infrared range (1064 nm) is used, which raises the tissue temperature to 60°C to a depth of approximately 1cm. The laser beam can be directed down a flexible quartz fibre for use through the operating channel of an endoscope. The limitation of the tumour size is 1cm. The role of a laser as an alternative to surgical diathermy in the treatment of bladder cancer remains in dispute. The main clinical danger from Nd: YAG laser treatment of bladder tumours is late perforation caused by inadvertent heating of adjacent loops of bowel.

Christmas T J 1991 Interstitial cystitis: immunological aspects and progress in treatment. In: Hendry W F (ed) Recent advances in urology/andrology 5. Churchill Livingstone, London, pp 103–117

In interstitial cystitis there is no evidence of infection, and the classical Hunner's ulcer is present in only 29% of cases. It is found predominantly in middle-aged females, often in association with Hashimoto's thyroiditis, and it has been shown to have an autoimmune basis. Although circulating antibodies capable of binding to the bladder are found in interstitial cystitis, their true specificity and significance are not understood. In this disease the bladder wall contains a chronic inflammatory cell infiltrate, which appears to be more active within the urothelium and lamina propria. The disease is initially best treated by cysto-distension at the time of diagnosis, but this is unlikely to cure the condition. Intravesical dimethyl sulphoxide may relieve the symptoms, but if this fails, systemic therapy with corticosteroids with or without azathioprine may be effective. If the above treatment modalities fail to ameliorate symptoms, surgical intervention is indicated. If the patient is suffering predominantly from severe bladder pain with a normal-sized bladder, then an extravesical supratrigonal denervation is undertaken. If, however, the bladder is shrunken, then a subtotal cystectomy with substitution enterocystoplasty is preferred.

Gingell J C Gilbert H W 1991 Erectile impotence: diagnosis and management. In: Hendry W F (ed) Recent advances in urology/andrology. Churchill Livingstone, London, pp 203–216

The diagnosis is made by taking a careful history, enquiring into drugs taken and establishing whether there has been any previous trauma. The causes may be due to arterial, neurogenic or endocrine problems, or to congenital and acquired abnormalities of the penis. The disease can usually be classified from a practical treatment point of view into those patients who do and do not respond to intracorporeal injection of a vasoactive agent, e.g. papaverine. This drug will produce an erection in patients with psychogenic or neurogenic erectile failure but not in those with severe vascular impairment. The papaverine is injected into the corpora cavernosa, and to avoid a prolonged erection the initial dose of papaverine should be low, starting with 15 mg, which will be enough in the neuropathic or obvious psychogenic patient. In those in whom the problem is likely to be vasculogenic, start with 30 mg, rising to 60 mg. The development of a rigid erection implies normal penile haemodynamics. If, however, this drug is not effective, prostaglandin $E_1$ may be used. If the response to these two drugs is minimal or fails, then from a practical point of view there are two possible management strategies. The first is to establish whether there is a venous leakage occurring. Controversy surrounds the mechanism by which blood is retained within the penis, but whether or not this occurs can be measured by pharmacocavernosometry. If in fact a leakage of blood is shown, then various veins have been ligated but it has to be admitted that the success rate does not extend beyond 50% at the end of one year.

The alternative is either to use a penile prosthesis, which is inserted into the corpora cavernosa, or an external suction constriction device. The prosthesis is particularly useful in patients who may have associated Peryronie's disease, while a problem with external suction devices is the initial capital outlay.

Berthelsen J G, Giwercman A, Muller J, Skakkebaek N E 1991 Carcinoma in situ of the testis: screening and treatment. In: Hendry W F (ed) Recent advances in urology/andrology 5. Churchill Livingstone, London, pp 217–228

Carcinoma in situ (CIS) of the testis is a precursor of both seminomatous and non-germ cell testicular cancer. The pre-invasive state may last for more than ten years, however, approximately half of the cases develop invasive growth within five years, and most if not all will sooner or later develop into overt tumour. To diagnose this condition, open biopsy is indicated in those who are at increased risk. These include those patients who have had a carcinoma of the testicle, since in 5% the contra lateral testis will have CIS, as will 1% of men who are infertile. Those with undescended testes have a 2% chance of developing CIS in either testicle, and patients with intersex problems with a karyotype which includes a Y chromosome have a high risk of developing a cancer of the testis. Needle biopsy is of no value in this condition and an open biopsy in the postpubertal male is justified. In addition, the seminal specimen can be examined for monoclonal antibodies to the CIS cells. The value of ultrasound for identifying this condition is not yet established.

The treatment should be orchidectomy if the other testicle is normal. If the CIS is in a solitary testicle or both testicles, then local radiation seems the appropriate treatment.

---

# PART 35.14
## THE METABOLIC RESPONSE TO SURGERY
*M. Jourdan*

---

Cutherbertson D P 1935–6 British Journal of Surgery 23: 505–520 Further observations on the disturbance of metabolism caused by injury, with particular reference to the dietary requirements of fracture cases.

This paper records observations and dietary experiments on patients suffering fractures. The catabolic disturbance following injury is confirmed, namely in increased basal consumption of oxygen, increased pulse rate and temperature, and an increased urinary excretion of nitrogen, sulphur, phosphorus and to a lesser extent potassium. All of these latter point to a breakdown of body protein, and the skeletal muscle seemed the major contributor in this respect, since creatine was also excreted in increased quantities. Cuthbertson also found that diets rich in high-quality protein (e.g. meat extract) and calories diminished, but did not abolish this metabolic response to trauma, with a period of negative nitrogen balance, part of which therefore seemed obligatory.

Cuthbertson coined the terms ebb and flow for the phases of the response to trauma. The *ebb phase* is defined as the period of diminished vitality or shock following injury associated with poor peripheral perfusion, diminished metabolism and nitrogen retention associated with a poor urinary output. This phase was either followed by death if the injury was sufficiently severe, or by the *flow phase*, in which there was increased metabolism, increased body temperature, increased blood glu-cose concentration and increased pulse rate and respiration, presumed to be associated with an increase in protein turnover and healing. These phases are clearly much dependent upon the severity and duration of the injury as well as the nature of the treatment instituted.

Moore F D, Ball M R 1952 The metabolic response to surgery. Thomas, Springfield

This mammoth volume condensing the work undertaken in Francis Moore's department at the Massachusetts General Hospital in Boston summarizes all that was known up to the early 1950s and still forms the core of what we know today. Since then there has been much investigation into the *mechanisms* of the metabolic response to injury, but the actual changes were fully recorded at this time. It is worth looking at simply to see the magnitude of the studies that were undertaken and the ramifications surrounding the metabolic response to trauma and surgery. It is very much a reference book of the period.

Moore F D 1953 Bodily changes in surgical convalescence I. The normal sequence: observations and interpretations. Annals of Surgery 137: 289–315

This paper records a lecture given by Moore at Pittsburgh in October 1952, and summarizes his own work along with a philosophical consideration of the significance of the metabolic response to trauma. All the phases of response are again outlined, pointing out that teleologically the changes represent a process of physiological 'homeostasis' tending to return the body to its 'normal' composition. He details four phases of convalescence from surgery, namely:

1. The adrenergic–corticoid phase
2. The corticoid withdrawal phase
3. The spontaneous anabolic phase
4. The fat-gain phase.

Dudley H A F, Robson J S, Smith M, Stewart C P 1959 The permissive role of adrenal cortical hormones after injury in man. Metabolism 8: 895–903
Cooper C E, Nelson D H 1962 ACTH levels in plasma in pre-operative and surgically stressed patients. Journal of Clinical Investigation 41: 1599–1605

These two papers address the question as to the role of the adrenocortical hormones in the metabolic response to surgery. Both ACTH and cortical hormone levels in the plasma increased following surgery, returning towards normal 24–48 hours after the operation. The known effects of adrenocorticoid hormones on protein, fat and carbohydrate metabolism are consistent with their playing a role in the metabolic response to surgery, although this appears to be permissive. In patients being given a fixed level of steroid replacement following surgical removal of the adrenal glands, the metabolic response to surgery still occurs despite no elevation in the plasma steroid levels.

Daniel P M, Pratt O E, Spargo E 1977 The metabolic homoeostatic role of muscle and its function as a store of protein. Lancet ii: 446–448

In this 'occasional survey' paper the evidence is reviewed for the concept that the skeletal muscle, which weighs 21 times as much as the liver, forms a major store for protein, and acts as 'a great metabolic regulatory organ which helps to maintain acceptable levels of amino acids and glucose in the circulation'. The importance of the gluconeogenic amino acids alanine and glutamine, released from skeletal muscle in starvation, is stressed and the authors conclude that in their opinion 'the storage, metabolic and homoeostatic activities of skeletal muscle are almost as vital as are its primary functions of maintaining posture and providing the power for movement'.

Wilmore D W, Aulick L H, Becker R A 1983 Hormones and the control of metabolism. In: Fischer J (ed) Surgical nutrition. Little Brown, Boston, pp 65–95

These two chapters, in a very excellent book looking at all aspects of surgical nutrition, comprehensively summarize the actual nature of the metabolic response to surgery and trauma. The respiratory response, with an increased oxygen consumption, the change in respiratory fuels, including the mobilization of fat and the process of gluconeogenesis and the breakdown of skeletal muscle to yield amino acids, are all considered.

Dudrick S J, Wilmore D W, Vars H M, Rhoads J E 1968 Long term total parenteral nutrition with growth, development and positive nitrogen balance. Surgery 64: 134–142

This reference is worth studying since it is the first to demonstrate that it is possible, in certain circumstances, to maintain an overall anabolic effect with growth and the build-up of protein by the provison of all the basic nutritional building blocks intravenously. Emphasis in recent years has swung away from intravenous feeding back to the more logical use of the intestinal tract whenever possible, even if this has to be achieved by a jejunostomy. Not only is enteral feeding safer, metabolically more effective and cheaper than intravenous feeding, but it helps to maintain the blood perfusion of the gut, thus preventing a breakdown in the mucosal integrity which might otherwise lead to bacteraemia and endotoxaemia in the portal venous circulation. There is much evidence now to suggest that these factors leaking from the gut into the portal circulation might be responsible for sepsis, which may prejudice recovery from major trauma by damaging other organs such as the liver, kidneys and lungs, leading to multiple organ failure.

Tsuji H, Shirasaka, C, Asoh T, Uchida I 1987 Effects of epidural administration of local anaesthetics or morphine on post-operative nitrogen loss and catabolic hormones. British Journal of Surgery 74: 421–425

Patients undergoing elective gastrectomy were studied, and the urinary excretion of nitrogen and catecholamines, along with plasma concentrations of cortisol and glucagon were measured. Three groups of patients were studied, each containing 20 or 30 patients. One group was subjected to general anaesthetic and given postoperative opiates, one group epidural analgesia with local anaesthetics, and one group epidural analgesia with epidural morphine postoperatively. The two epidural groups showed a reduction in nitrogen loss postoperatively, and reduced excretion of catecholamines and cortisol as well as lower plasma levels of glucagon, cortisol and catecholamines. The results suggest that although the metabolic response to surgery was not abolished, epidural blockade markedly reduced it, presumably by reducing the sympathetic activity produced by pain stimuli and sympathetic nervous afferent stimulation, reducing the noradrenaline secretion in particular, and thus reducing the stimulus to glucagon and cortisol secretion. This paper represents another attempt to dissect the mechanisms of the metabolic response to surgery, but does confirm the importance of afferent stimulation from the site of the trauma.

Three recent papers have looked in more detail

at the humoral and cellular mechanisms which might play a part in the metabolic response to injury:

C. Weissman, Armour Forse R, Milic-Emili J et al 1986 The metabolic and ventilatory response to the infusion to stress hormones. Annals of Surgery 203: 408–412

Michie H R, Manogue K R, Spriggs D R et al 1988 Detection of circulating tumour necrosis factor after administration of endotoxin in humans. New England Journal of Medicine 318: 1481–1486

Hamish R, Michie et al 1988 Interleukin-2 initiates metabolic responses associated with critical illness in humans. Annals of Surgery 208: 493–503

Wilkinson A W 1973 Body fluids and electrolytes in surgery, 4th edn. Churchill Livingstone, Edinburgh

Apart from the protein and energy changes which occur in the body in response to trauma and surgery there is a major effect on electrolytes and water balance. In particular, there is retention of sodium, increased loss of potassium and retention of water, and this topic is well summarized in Chapter 8 of this volume, written by a surgeon who was Nuffield Professor of Paediatric Surgery at the Institute of Child Health and had a major interest in this problem. Although it has been subsequently established that the magnitude of these changes can be influenced by fluid replacement and drug therapy, the underlying facts of the metabolic change were well established at this point in time. Another point that emerges from this reference, which at one stage attracted much interest, was the effect of body temperature on the metabolic response to injury. As might be expected, if the body temperature is allowed to fall as a result of heat loss during surgical procedures, the postoperative metabolic response with heat production is likely to increase, resulting in some futher breakdown of muscle protein. Preventing this drop in temperature by maintaining the body fluid volume and infusing fluids at body temperature was shown to decrease the size of the metabolic response to trauma.

# Index